Blood Flow in Arteries

Donald A. McDonald

M.A., D.M.(Oxon.), D.Sc.(Lond.)
Professor of Physiology and Biophysics
at the University of Alabama, Birmingham, USA

'The dance along the artery
The circulation of the lymph
Are figured in the drift of stars'

> T. S. Eliot, *Burnt Norton*
>
> (From *Collected Poems 1909–1962*,
> Faber & Faber Ltd)

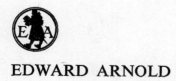

EDWARD ARNOLD

LQMK

First published 1960
by Edward Arnold (Publishers) Ltd.
25 Hill Street, London W1X 8LL

Second Edition 1974

ISBN: 0 7131 4213 8

TO

John Ronald Womersley
June 20, 1907–March 7, 1958

Samuel Armstrong Talbot
April 19, 1903–February 20, 1967

Kenneth James Franklin
November 25, 1897–May 8, 1966

Printed in Great Britain by
The Camelot Press Ltd, Southampton

Foreword

Donald Arthur McDonald died on May 24, 1973, in Birmingham, Alabama. At the time of his death he had not yet finished correcting and amending the galley proofs of this second edition. The remainder of this task, and the final editing of page proofs, were undertaken by his daughter Miss Alison McDonald, his former student and collaborator Dr. Wilmer W. Nichols, and myself. We share with many others a continued affection and admiration for a scientist whose work speaks for itself.

William R. Milnor, M.D.

Baltimore, Maryland
October 1973

The author's wife and family are grateful to the publishers for giving them this opportunity of expressing their great indebtedness to William R. Milnor and Wilmer W. Nichols without whose generosity with their time and expertise this second edition of *Blood Flow in Arteries* would not have reached the final stages of publication.

v

Preface

The present book is the direct offspring of the monograph *Blood Flow in Arteries* which was published in 1960 as one of a series sponsored by the Physiological Society of Great Britain and Ireland. In technical terms, it may be regarded as a second edition of that work and it does indeed hope to serve the same purposes as the original monograph. Thus, it remains as the work of a single author, a physiologist, and it is designed primarily for a readership of physiologists and physicians in cardiovascular medicine. Conversely, it also aspires to provide readers from the physical sciences with a survey of the achievements and problems of the biological field.

As stated in the Acknowledgments to the original work, my own entry into this field started when I was fortunate enough to meet that talented mathematician, the late John Womersley, just at a time when I found myself quite unable to interpret the relationship between the pulsatile flow curves and arterial pressure waves that I had been recording in the dog femoral artery. Our collaboration, however, appeared to be quite infertile for a period of well over a year when suddenly it blossomed and yielded a rich harvest until it was cut short by his untimely death. In retrospect, it was clear that the first period had, in fact, been a necessary time of incubation during which he was learning the elementary biological aspects of the problem and I was learning enough mathematics and physics to formulate the problem in a manner that a mathematician could interpret. Far too many attempts at collaboration between men reared in different disciplines of science have failed because they did not realize that such an exploratory period to learn their colleagues' scientific language is necessary.

It might properly be said that what is presented here is an introductory text in haemodynamics and indeed that had been suggested as a title for this new book. However, as I had set forth in a recent review (McDonald, 1968*b*) my doubts as to the philological legitimacy of the word haemodynamics it appeared to give the work a dubious christening. In that review, I defined haemodynamics as being in fact 'cardiovascular biophysics' and with that definition I am quite happy to describe this book; as a title it is only inaccurate in that limitations of space have not permitted the inclusion of a survey of the large volume of work on the physical analysis of the heart's function as a

vii

pump. *Blood Flow in Arteries* may appear to be rather neglectful of the studies of vascular pressure that take up a large part of it but as a title it emphasizes an *obiter dictum* of my first, and in many ways, my only teacher in physiology, the late Professor Kenneth Franklin. He declared that 'the fundamental problems in the circulation derive from that fact that the supply of adequate amounts of blood to the organs of the body is the main purpose of the circulation and the pressures that are necessary to achieve it are of secondary importance; but the measurement of flow is difficult while that of pressure is easy so that our knowledge of flow is usually derivatory' (with his usual modesty Kenneth Franklin attributed the saying to Karl Ludwig (1816–1895), but I have never been able to trace it).

Perhaps we both might have been better advised to go back another century or so to the original progenitor of most of our present lines of work to Stephen Hales who opened his great work *Haemastaticks* in 1733 as follows:

'As an animal Body consists not only a wonderful texture of solid Parts, but also a large proportion of Fluids, which are continually circulating and flowing, thro' an inimitable Embroidery of Blood-Vessels, and other inconceivably minute Canals: and as the healthy State of an Animal principally consists, in the maintaining of a due *Equilibrium* between those Solids and Fluids; it has ever since the important Discovery of the Circulation of the Blood, been looked upon as a Matter well worth the enquiring into, to find the Force and Velocity with which these Fluids are impelled; as a likely means to give a considerable Insight into the Animal Œconomy.'

And with that ancient blessing, as it were, we will define this work as 'an enquiry into the Force and Velocity with which these Fluids are impelled' with the ultimate aim that some of it at least will give us 'a considerable Insight into the Animal Œconomy' which, being interpreted, may be taken as an understanding of the disorders of the circulation which beset our human species.

The arrangement of the book follows approximately that of its forerunner. The properties of steady flow are considered in Ch. 2 and a short account of the large amount of work on the viscous properties of blood in Ch. 3. The extrapolation of this work to non-steady flow conditions such as turbulence in the circulation comprises Ch. 4. The hydrodynamic equations applicable to pulsatile flow and the simplifications of them that have been used then follows in Chs. 5 and 6. Before considering the experimental work of the later part of the book the techniques used are examined in the next three chapters on the use of Fourier analysis, manometers and flowmeters. To clarify the theoretical analysis of pulse wave propagation, the available data on the elastic properties of the wall are surveyed, with an introduction to the theory of elasticity in Ch. 10. Wave-propagation without reflection is discussed in Ch. 11 and the effects of reflection and the evidence for it are surveyed in Ch. 12. This extends to the more detailed experimental work on arterial impedance, wave velocity and damping in the following two chapters. The applications of all this work to the important clinical need to monitor the cardiac output on a continuous beat-by-beat basis form the topic of the last chapter.

To prevent the book from becoming unwieldy in view of the increase of experimental work in all these fields since 1960 the old chapter on pulsatile flow patterns has been omitted. The widespread use of good flowmeters which is perhaps the most striking change that has occurred in this period, would seem to have made this unnecessary in a purely descriptive way. The section on the generation of cardiovascular sound in the old book has been reduced to a very short reference to some important contributions to this special topic.

The *acknowledgments* of all the help, collaboration and stimulating discussions I have had over the years from my friends which I would like to list would be too enormous to expect any reader to tolerate. My debt to the midwives of my early interests and work in this field I tried to express in *Blood Flow in Arteries*. After coming to the United States in 1963 at the very kind invitation of Ernst Attinger, I spent nearly three valuable years in Philadelphia with him.

I had always kept in close contact with Dr. Sam Talbot of Johns Hopkins University ever since we had first met in 1956. In 1966 he invited me to join a Department of Biomedical Engineering which he was going to start at the University of Alabama Medical Center but, sadly, soon after he moved he incurred the illness which led to his premature death.

Thus, I came to join the active cardiovascular team at the University of Alabama in Birmingham, where we have close ties between the basic medical sciences and the clinical departments; in my particular case with the Department of Medicine and its chairman, Dr. T. J. Reeves, and especially the Division of Cardiology under Dr. Lloyd Hefner, and the Department of Surgery and its chairman, Dr. John Kirklin. The collaboration with Dr. Kirklin's vigorous cardiac surgery team began early when Dr. Nicholas Kouchoukos spent a whole year researching with me in developing methods of monitoring output and Lou Sheppard, as head of the computer services for Dr. Kirklin, has proved a close friend and mentor in this specialized field. And, above all, I have derived tremendous pleasure and help from my graduate students. Dr. Wilmer Nichols, as the first one, was undoubtedly the most invaluable, as from the beginning of 1967 he put in yeoman service in building up the laboratory equipment and training his successors in the experimental arts. Then followed Marshall Boone, who now also bears the title of Ph.D. and the work of Dr. Michel Gerin, who came from Louvain with an International Fellowship from the National Institutes of Health to study haemodynamics. Dr. Roger Lloyd came to me from our training programme in Biomedical Engineering to do his thesis work, James Webster from the

Tuskegee Institute, with which we have close ties, and Eladio Ruiz-de-Molina, originally from Cuba, but now an American citizen, from our bioengineering programme.

Ideas have also flowed from my invaluable collection of friends in America who have in some cases actually suffered me to make them offer opinions on parts of the book, such as Bill Milnor at Johns Hopkins and Dali Patel at N.I.H., from my close ties with Max Anliker at Stanford and with Urs Gessner at Baltimore, from my guidance in matters ultrasonic with Fred Stegall at Seattle and from my stimulating contacts with Dr. Daniel Kalmanson in Paris. The old English team also remains functional with visits from Derek Bergel, now at Oxford, and, above all, with Professor Michael Taylor, now in Sydney, who is a Visiting Professor in the Physiology Department here. On his last visit, he went through the whole of the book and offered much helpful advice and criticism, thus providing the final link with the original *Blood Flow in Arteries* for which he was also the spiritual midwife.

Acknowledgments *en masse* are all offered to all my friends (and their journal publishers) who have allowed me to use their work and figures. The generous financial aid from the National Institutes of Health research grants, initially in a personal grant, HE-10889, to be followed by the large Program Project Grant in 1967, HE-11310, in which I have been funded as the section on 'Cardiovascular Biophysics'.

Finally, I offer the most grateful thanks to my family; to my daughter, Alison, who, as my secretary, has borne the burden of typing several drafts of illegible text and verified references and also kept me straight in the paths of English style; to my son, Robin, who, as the artist in the family, has helped a lot in his vacations from college with the illustrations and in a meticulous check of the final draft. And, above all, to my dear wife, Renée, who over what must have seemed an interminable time, has borne the burden of the moods and strains of tending a struggling, fractious author.

D. A. McD.

Acknowledgments

(reprinted from the First Edition)

The goddess of Chance is rarely thanked on occasions such as this. I am sure that this is not so much due to the ingratitude of scientists as to the fact that she plays some part in starting almost any research. In my case her interventions have been so helpful and so perfectly timed that I feel I must pay her homage. For, although this book appears under my name alone, it could never have been written—for there would have been little of any value to write about—without the immense help I have had from my principal collaborators, John Womersley and Michael Taylor.

My interest in the present subject arose from the chance observation of streamline flow in the basilar artery of the rabbit (Fig. 4.2). This was in the course of a severely 'practical' research, with Dr. (now Mr.) J. M. Potter, into some problems arising from cerebral radioangiography. This led to the use of high-speed cinematography as the only method we could think of to measure the flow velocity in the basilar artery. I then thought it would be interesting to exploit the technique in a study of pulsatile flow in other systemic arteries— sliding, as it were, into circulatory physiology down the vertebral arteries.

In 1949, and again in 1951, I had the honour to work with Professor W. R. Hess in Zürich (on neurophysiological problems) and although his own great contributions to circulatory physics were made many years ago he gave me most stimulating help in this field, for which, and for his continuing encouragement, I am most grateful.

The collection of records of pulsatile flow velocity in arteries was interesting but proved unsatisfying because their interpretation was difficult in the absence of a quantitative method of analyis. Progress was only achieved when I had the great good fortune to arouse the interest and enthusiasm of that distinguished mathematician, the late J. R. Womersley, in these problems.

Womersley's career has been so well described by Sir Charles Darwin in his obituary notice (*Nature*, 3 May, 1958) that I need say little of it, except that he had a wide experience in many fields of applied mathematics and so was thoroughly familiar with the experimental approach so necessary in this type of work. Quite apart from the most valuable analyses he did, and the stimulation of his personality as a friend, the three years over which we collaborated were a most valuable experience in the problems of working with someone trained in a different scientific discipline. Long periods of discussion during the first eighteen months of our collaboration (during which Womersley only had his leisure hours to devote to it) were necessary before I could formulate the physiological problems in a way that would make physical sense. Equally it was a long time before he knew enough about the physiology of the circulation to tackle it in a realistic way. Once the main objectives were clearly seen, advance was very rapid, especially as he was able to spend a whole year in this department (June, 1954–55) supported by a personal grant from the Medical Research Council. I feel that unless colleagues from the physical sciences are prepared to spend a comparable amount of time in learning some physiology, then the value of such collaboration will always be limited. This field is littered with abstract analyses of the circulation by talented mathematicians which are of slight use because they have little contact with physiological reality. If only brief consultations are available, then my own experience indicates that we, as physiologists, must first get the problem into a mathematical form and use, as it were, our colleague as a translator, skilled in a language we cannot handle with any fluency. For no mathematical treatment is ever better than the primary assumptions on which it is based.

Womersley went to the USA in 1955 but good luck was still with me for, six months earlier, Dr. Michael Taylor had one day arrived on the doorstep (unannounced from Adelaide), asking if he could work at Bart's for a year during the tenure of a C. J. Martin Research Fellowship. He was thus able to spend a few months in collaboration with John Womersley before the latter's departure. While he remained in England my problems of collaborating with expert mathematicians were over. Taylor, with a training in medicine and physiological research, has also a passion for mathematics such that he is technically the equal of many professionals in this field. If I do not here sufficiently express my admiration and gratitude for his contribution to this work it is only because, while we are exhorted to speak only good of the dead, it is deemed fulsome (or at least un-English) to speak too well of the living—especially one's close friends. Let it suffice to say that the organization of the ideas on wave reflection and arterial input impedance (the chapters in the latter part of this book) are almost entirely due to discussions with him. In addition the whole text has been subjected to his critical scrutiny—but I should also apologize to him for not always acceding to his demands for more rigour (in the mathematical sense); any inaccuracies that physicists may find will almost certainly be due to my omissions, for the sake of simplicity, of this kind.

To Professor K. J. Franklin, FRS, I owe a debt of gratitude for over twenty years of teaching and encouragement. I am also very grateful to John Potter, Peter Helps and John Hale who in the past ten years have severally been most helpful colleagues, and to Derek Bergel who is here at present.

Thanks are also freely offered to Miss Mary Morse for typing so painstakingly the many versions of the text, and to Mr. D. C. Moore for lettering and photographing the figures.

All the high-speed cinematography was done by Mr. John Hadland and his expert team, and financed by a grant over several years from the Medical Research Council (who also purchased essential apparatus); the most superficial perusal will show how fundamental this support was for this investigation. Photographic apparatus was also generously provided by the Central Research Fund of the University of London, and the counter-chronometer by the Research Fund of this Medical College.

An important part in the clarification of my ideas (however relative that term may appear) was due to the innumerable discussions I had with my American friends during a visit to the States in the later part of 1956. This tour was due to a most generous travelling Fellowship from the Rockefeller Foundation and to them, and especially to Dr. Pomerat, I offer very grateful thanks. To mention all the physiologists, and physicians, who helped me at that time, whether by providing additional data, or merely by vigorous dispute, would be impossibly long. I must, however, thank Dr. Sam Talbot, of Johns Hopkins, for reading the whole of the first draft of this book so carefully in October–November 1956, and for the advice he gave me. It was particularly stimulating in the USA to find that this work aroused interest in Departments of Medicine quite as often as in Departments of Biophysics, or of Physiology, in spite of the theoretical or 'pure' nature of the research.

I am also very grateful for most helpful suggestions about the final draft from Dr. D. S. Parsons, Dr. L. E. Bayliss and Professor H. Barcroft.

I am also grateful to the Editors of the *Journal of Physiology* and of *Physics in Medicine and Biology* for permission to use blocks from their publications.

Finally, may I thank all those who have allowed me to use their data either in the text, or as figures (with permission often belatedly sought). In the case of figures their names are given in the relevant legends—where there is no attribution figures are from original graphs of my own.

February, 1960

Contents

1
Introduction

An interval of thirteen years between the completion of the first version of a book and its successor must always be a little difficult to bridge but here we seem almost to have moved into a different world. The opening sentence of the original monograph was the forthright statement that 'the most obvious feature of' blood flow in arteries 'is that it is pulsatile'. And in the late 50s the field of haemodynamics, in this sense, was but a small child; its biography in the first *Blood Flow in Arteries* thus had some of the freshness and innocence of childhood. Much of the material discussed was essentially a speculation on its experimental future. Its growth, in the intervening decade, has been, in terms of experimental, theoretical and analogue model work, positively Gargantuan —and hence, in terms of this metaphor, would need a (scientific) Rabelais to describe it.

I have no pretensions of being such a man. The material is, therefore, selective in terms of my best judgment and makes no attempt to be encyclopaedic, as was implied by the earlier reference to its introductory character. The child, however, is father to the man and because we were interpreting circulatory phenomena in terms of well-established physical laws the fundamental structure remained sound and indeed I am happy to say that most of the speculative parts have been justified by the experimental evidence that has accumulated since—because they were, as we understood them then, based on those physical laws.

So much has been written since 1960 that it might almost seem to be a superfluity to produce another book. This field of biophysics is, essentially, an exercise in bridge-building between the separated territories of physiology, mathematics, physics and engineering. The book literature of the 60s is thus thick with published symposia which inevitably lack a coherent aim, being made up of specialized reviews, and in addition are difficult to track down unless one's library facilities have an enormously wide range. This period may well be coming to an end with the appearance of the authoritative work edited by D. H. Bergel, but this will be in two large volumes and have some of the features of a symposium in that it is many-authored. To write a book on one's own in such a field would almost seem to be arrogant in claiming a mastery of all these fields as a polymath, or to have the appearance of foolhardiness. I do not feel apologetic, however, for I am old-fashioned to the extent that I believe that science should cover all knowledge and a scientist should have some familiarity with all of it; furthermore, I hope that the omissions that I will inevitably make will be compensated sufficiently by the coherence that comes from but a single pen. Finally, I would make the plea that the material that is required of a beginner or student to master should not be beyond the ability of one professor to produce! In any case, I am humbled by the large and wholly authoritative book from the single pen of my friend and colleague, Willem Klip, in *The Theoretical Foundations of Medical Physics* (1969), which far surpasses in erudition and comprehensiveness this present book. It is very detailed and aims at establishing mathematical rigour for the areas of mathematics that are most especially used in haemodynamics and other fields of medicine. Another most valuable book (for those that read German) is that by Wetterer and Kenner (1968). This concentrates on the problems of wave transmission and goes into the Windkessel theory and its relation to later work in much more detail than I am able to. In addition, there have been a considerable number of reviews of the whole or specific parts of the field. There is an excellent review on wave transmission in visco-elastic tubes by Hardung (1962). The symposium edited by Attinger (1964) was something of a landmark and the ASME symposium of 1966 entitled *Biomechanics* has some excellent review articles in it, notably the one by Skalak and Stathis (1966) on wave transmission. A more recent review by Noordergraaf (1970) on Haemodynamics (in a volume edited by Schwann, 1970) is also recommended. The important field of instrumentation is covered in *Methods in Medical Research*, vol. 11 (1966), and a more recent symposium devoted to flowmeters (Cappelen, 1970).

A review with a wide survey that is especially recommended is that by Bergel and Schultz (1971). An elementary book with strong practical emphasis on flow problems by Weale (1967) can be recommended. In addition, *Annual Reviews in Physiology* have fairly frequent reviews of haemodynamics. Copley is organizing congresses in Haemorheology of which the first was published in 1968 (e.g. McDonald, 1968b; Taylor, 1973). Finally, the annual meetings of the Annual Conference on Engineering in Medicine and Biology (ACEMB) and those of the Biomedical Engineering Society (since 1971) survey the field annually.

THE DEVELOPMENT OF HAEMODYNAMICS AS A SCIENCE

In the Preface, I observed that because the word haemodynamics has gained such a wide footing we must needs accept it, although it was clearly used in a looser sense than its derivation as the hydrodynamics of blood. Therefore, McDonald (1968b) proposed that it be defined as the physical study of flowing blood and of all the solid structures (such as arteries) through which it flows. The use of the word physical implies the study of these tissues as inanimate materials; this provides some tenuous separation of haemodynamics from physiology in which the living function is the specific aim of study.

The use of the term physics immediately emphasizes the importance of measurement which had been persuasively linked with science by Lord Kelvin in his oft-quoted (and more often mis-quoted) passage:

'. . . when you can measure what you are speaking about, and express it in numbers, you know something about it; but when you cannot measure it, when you cannot express it in numbers, your knowledge is of a meagre and unsatisfactory kind; it may be the beginning of knowledge, but you have scarcely, in your thoughts, advanced to the stage of *Science* whatever the matter may be.'

While expressing profound thought on the nature of science it is not, of itself, a complete definition and the quotation has, alas, been misused by men who, so often, are apt to seize on one idea to the exclusion of all others. This is best illustrated by the crabbed, misquoted form in which I first met it, which ran, 'Unless you can measure it and write it down in numbers it is *not* science.' The thought behind this formulation led to the concept of the 'exact' sciences such as physics and chemistry as distinct from the descriptive (and by implication 'inexact') science of biology which still persisted in my youth, and led to the class-conscious feeling that the latter was inferior. The persistence of this idea lies at the back of much of the difficulties biologists meet when attempting to collaborate with brash young physicists and engineers. In fact, a good case can be made for the fact that biology, in its ultimate problems, is more complex than the sciences of the inanimate world, an insight which Einstein's great mind perhaps grasped when he responded to a suggestion (in the 1920s) that he might investigate some biological problems, whereat he is reported to have recoiled and said, 'No, never, they are too difficult for me' (Clark, 1971).

Measurement and quantitation is then one of the hallmarks of science; generalizing, we may say that it is the simplest way of recording phenomena with complete objectivity. That this alone does not constitute Science is clear when we consider the other steps that comprise the scientific method. To this wider overview we shall return later, but for the present we may use the neatly compressed sequence that Johns (1968) uses: (i) The acquisition of measured data, (ii) data analysis, (iii) formulation of an hypothesis, (iv) experimental testing of the hypothesis leading back to the acquisition possibly of new data which confirm or overthrow the hypothesis, and so on, in an ever-widening circle. In essence, this necessitates that the fruits of man's speculation on the nature of things should always be referred back to the judgment of the nature of observed facts. And it is by this criterion that we distinguish the modern world of science from the teachings of the ancient world.

HISTORICAL LANDMARKS* IN THE DEVELOPMENT OF HAEMODYNAMICS

The sudden swing from medieval 'natural philosophy' into modern science is most vividly characterized in the person of Galileo Galilei (1564–1642). From 1598 to 1610 he was Professor of Mathematics at Padua. During this period, William Harvey (1578–1657) was studying medicine there, and although he never mentions Galileo in his book *De Motu Cordis* (1628) it is difficult to believe that he was not influenced by the new teaching in his approach to the problem of the circulation of the blood. We think of him as the Father of Cardiovascular Physiology, for in his analysis he resorts to experiments, even though they are simple observational exercises, to aid his argument. The bulk of the book is, in fact, couched in the form of the old Galenical teaching, a world he had been brought up in and from which he was only with difficulty freeing himself. Nevertheless, his demonstration that the valves in the veins would only allow the flow of blood towards the heart is a great intellectual advance over the views of his teacher at Padua (whose classical work *De venarum ostiolis* is a magnificent first anatomical description of these structures); it was his appeal to a quantitative argument in relation to the cardiac output which entitles him clearly as the first of the moderns. The classical Galenical teaching was that the blood was constantly being created in the liver and absorbed by the tissues to which it was conveyed with an oscillatory motion mainly by the veins. At the end of a long series of observations, in a wide range of species, relating the contractions of the ventricles and the flow of blood into, and consequent dilatation of, the arteries, he finally and rather diffidently offers a quantitative argument. For example, if the ventricle ejects, let us say, half an ounce of blood with each systole, and in half an hour it makes over a thousand beats, then the ventricle will have pumped out 'over five hundred ounces and this is far more blood than can be found in the whole body'. He then repeats it for small hypothetical stroke volumes, but this takes him into calculations in drachms and is not forceful enough to pursue in these obsolete units of weight. Had Harvey had the real figures the argument could have been overwhelming, for the resting cardiac output is very close to one total blood volume per minute in nearly all mammals for which we have reliable figures.

* Sources for the historical notes that have been used are E. T. Bell's *Men of Mathematics* (1965) which provides a fascinating overview of the science together with vignettes of the personalities involved. Also, Williams' *Biographical Dictionary of Scientists* (1969) is both interesting and valuable. Actual biographies of individuals have only been used for Harvey (Franklin, 1961) and Clark-Kennedy's detailed life of Stephen Hales, which was long out of print and has now appeared again (1965). Franklin's translation of Harvey's classic work is recommended as the best one available and was prepared for the tercentenary of the celebrations of his death (1957)—for scholars, it is accompanied by a reprint of the original Latin text. Facsimile editions of *Stephen Hales: Statical Essays* are now available (1964).

Although Harvey's description of the circulation of the blood (in 1628) so clearly, to us, opens up wide fields of understanding it was far from being immediately accepted. For example, Thomas Willis (1621–75) in his famous treatise on the anatomy of the brain, and, more particularly, its system of anastomizing arteries which bears his name in the Circle of Willis (De Cerebri Anatome, published 1664) still openly rejects Harvey's ideas and clings to the teachings of Galen (129–99) which had persisted with little question since the second century A.D. We may be more tolerant of this intellectual stubbornness when we realize that there was no descriptive evidence about the connections between the arteries and veins in the tissues which Harvey had to postulate. The capillaries were not observed and described until the publication, in 1660–61, of the studies of the frog lung under the microscope of Malpighi (1628–94). Nevertheless, Richard Lower (1631–91), although he had been a pupil of Thomas Willis, fully believed in Harvey's views and developed his concepts on the cardiac output in his *Tractatus de Corde* (published 1669).

This sketches lightly the state of circulatory physiology when Stephen Hales (1677–1761) first went to Cambridge in 1696. This was the year that Isaac Newton left the University to become Warden of the Mint but it is ten years after he had presented his great work, *Principia Mathematica*, to the Royal Society for publication. As is noted in Ch. 2, it is in one of the propositions appended to this book that the concept of viscosity of a fluid is first defined, so that, to this day, we still speak of Newtonian viscosity.* Hales did devote some of his time to physics, more particularly astronomy, but his importance to science is not to any theoretical advances but as a great biological experimenter. Nevertheless, his handling of concepts such as force and velocity of flow (which we can see in his Preface) is in the modern Newtonian sense. Although it is his great series of investigations of circulatory function that particularly concern us here and which were published as the volume *Haemastaticks* (1733), these were, in fact, the second volume of *Statical Essays,* and the first, subtitled *Vegetable Staticks* (1727), is concerned with a thorough investigation of the forces necessary to get the sap to the top of very tall trees; his conclusions on this are amazingly complete and have formed the basis of all work to this day. In addition, he devotes a lot of attention to the force problems associated with respiration in vertebrates. Why the circulatory experimental findings were not given priority in publication is not clear, but in his biography of Hales, Clark-Kennedy (1929, 1965) demonstrates quite clearly that they were started in his later years at Cambridge (1703–9) although they were mainly done in the years 1709 onwards, when he had just

* Newton, in the years 1669–1696, occupied the Lucasian Chair of Mathematics; it seems particularly apt in this context to note that the present occupant of that Chair, Dr. M. J. Lighthill, who is especially distinguished in the field of Fluid Dynamics, also made several investigations into problems of blood flow while he was at Imperial College, London, and collaborating with the Physiological Flow Unit there under Dr. C. G. Caro (Lighthill, 1969; Wolstenholme and Knight, 1969).

left Cambridge to take up his duties as Curate at Teddington, Middlesex (although he did study medicine for a while in his early years at Cambridge he graduated in the School of Theology).

To most physiologists, Stephen Hales is only remembered as the man who measured the arterial blood pressure in the horse; the famous passage beginning: 'In December I caused a mare to be tied down on her back . . .; Having laid open the left crural Artery about three Inches from her Belly, I inserted into it a brass Pipe whose Bore was one sixth of an Inch in Diameter; and to that, by means of another brass Pipe which was fitly adapted to it, I fixed a glass Tube, of nearly the same Diameter, which was nine Feet in Length; then untying the Ligature on the Artery, the Blood rose in the Tube eight Feet and three Inches perpendicular above the left Ventricle of the Heart . . .' is indeed the opening description of Experiment I* in *Haemastaticks* and was republished by Fulton (1966).

The pressures in both large arteries and veins were measured together with their pulsations and careful observations made of the changes due to muscular straining but in particular the progressive changes due to successive measured bleeding. He noted that the animal can compensate initially for quite a considerable haemorrhage but that there was a rapid collapse until death once a critical level was reached.

Hales also made the first real advance in computing the cardiac output since the tentative speculations of Harvey and Lower. Realizing that the venous pressure determined the diastolic volume of the heart he made wax casts of the ventricles at the normal distending pressure in diastole and then measured the volume of the cast. Although we know that the ventricle does not empty at each systole, nevertheless his estimates were surprisingly reasonable (e.g. in one of the two human hearts he studied his estimate of the cardiac output was 4·4 l/min—within the normal range). With his experimental measurements, he was able to refute the quite impossible estimations of the forces in ventricular muscle which Borelli, the highly influential founder of the school of iatrophysics, had made late in the seventeenth century.

Hales also deduced from the change in pulsatile flow in the arteries to the

---

* The use of an unanaesthetized horse has always seemed heroic and Dr. Otto Edholm has told me that when he first went to occupy the Chair of Physiology at the Royal Veterinary School in London, he attempted to repeat the experiments described as exactly as possible. But although Stephen Hales gives explicit details of how he used a field gate to tie the animals to, Dr. Edholm points out that he omits to say how many helpers he had. Edholm concluded from his own partially successful efforts that either Hales had a very large body of helpers or unusually placid horses; modern horses, it would appear, strongly resent the idea of being tied to a gate!

Actually, it is clear from the whole book that he used more dogs than any other species but he also used sheep and deer. In my own less ambitious way, I have always used an anaesthetized dog to demonstrate Hales' direct way of measuring arterial and venous blood pressure; there is a vividness in looking at a tall column of blood and saying 'the blood pressure is now four feet eight inches' that appeals to a student more than converting the trace on a cathode-ray oscilloscope into mm Hg.

steady flow in veins that this 'smoothing' action is largely due to the distensible properties of the arteries comprising an 'elastic reservoir' during ventricular systole. (In the first German translation, in 1784, of *Haemastaticks*, this phrase is rendered as '*Windkessel*'. Thus originated the term which figures so largely in the haemodynamics of the first half of the present century due to the large body of work by Otto Frank and his pupils.) Finally, by perfusing the vessels of the intestine at a fixed head of pressure, Hales was the man who introduced the concept of the peripheral resistance and realized the main site of this resistance was in the minute vessels in the tissues. His experimental design was beautifully simple. First, he made a longitudinal cut through the wall of the intestine on the outer side, away from the entry of the supplying arteries; he carefully timed the slow emptying of his liquid reservoir through the cut surface of the gut. He then cut through the small arteries just at the centre of the intestinal wall and observed that the emptying rate was greatly increased. He immediately deduced that the main resistance was sited in the minute vessels in the wall. To extend this concept he then showed that various agents, e.g. water at different temperatures, and, in particular, brandy, could change the rate of flow, presumably by altering the size of these small vessels. It was not until about 1870 when Claude Bernard did his classic experiments on the vessels of the rabbit ear that the concepts of vasoconstriction and vaso-dilatation were much advanced. Truly, Stephen Hales deserves the title 'The Father of Haemodynamics'.

Although Hales' books went into several editions, his own experimental work did not apparently influence any followers. The eighteenth century was notable, in our present context, for the great development of the theoretical mathematical treatment of fluid dynamics. The great name in this field is that of Leonhard Euler (1707–83) who is described as the most prolific mathematician that ever lived. In our field of interest, he is important as the author of Euler's equations of fluid motion. He enormously developed the power of the Newtonian calculus but he did not develop the Newtonian concept of viscosity, presumably because of the difficulty of introducing it into the universal laws of motion. Euler was a close friend of the Bernoulli family and particularly of Daniel Bernoulli (1700–82) who also devoted his life to mathematics. His great contribution was the treatise *Hydrodynamica*, from which we still use Bernoulli's Law (Ch. 2, p. 35). (It is said, however, by Bell (1965) that the only really rigorous derivation of this law was by Euler.) The treatment of fluids in the work of both Daniel Bernoulli and Euler was of 'ideal' liquids (i.e. without viscosity), and little attention was paid to practical problems. This is particularly curious in the case of Daniel Bernoulli who graduated initially in medicine and held the Chair of Anatomy at Basel for many years. Cournand (1964) in his introductory essay to the Stephen Hales facsimile reprint says that between 1733 and 1738 he 'enumerated the principles of the correct calculation of the work of the heart and compared the laws of fluid flow in tubes and in living vessels'. I have, however, found no other reference to this work, nor to the treatise in which (Cournand says) his pupil, Passavent (De Vi Cordis, 1748) used the data from *Haemastaticks* to calculate the work of the heart. I can only assume that these were minor excursions into this field for I have found no other reference to them. The tremendous impetus that Euler gave to the analytic treatment of the problems of liquid motion was so great that, to this day, a large part of theoretical hydrodynamics is concerned solely with ideal, non-viscous, liquids; some of the practical results of this are discussed by Birkhoff (1960) which are further discussed below (p. 15).

The work which actually led to the equations of pressure and flow was scattered rather haphazardly by a few experimentalists culminating in the classic and meticulous work of Jean Louis M. Poiseuille (1797–1869) which established the relationship of the flow of a viscous liquid and the pressure-gradient in a tube. (Good brief reviews of his life and work are by Joly (1968) and Herrick (1942).) This is reviewed briefly in Ch. 2 where it is also noted that the mathematical derivation of this flow problem was not made until nearly twenty years later. In the meantime, Stokes had extended the equations of motion of Euler in 1845 and added on another set of terms to allow for viscosity to form what are now called the Navier–Stokes equations (Ch. 5, p. 101). Nevertheless, the approach here was still highly theoretical for the derivation that Hagenbach made of the Poiseuille problem makes no use of the Navier–Stokes equations whatsoever.

WORK ON ARTERIAL ELASTICITY AND WAVE-VELOCITY

Poiseuille was fundamentally a physician with a training in physics and a man with a similar background but covering an even greater range was Thomas Young (1773–1829). The most famous of Young's researches in biophysics was concerned with human vision and particularly in the perception of colour. The theory that colour vision is based on the perception of three primary colours, red, green, and violet, is commemorated today in the fact that it is called the Young–Helmholtz theory. In fact, his work on the nature of light went much deeper and his work on interference gratings led to the acceptance of the wave nature of light. One short biography (Williams, 1969) names this as his main claim to fame; Newton in his great work on Optics had treated it as particulate in nature. It was not until the work of Einstein and the great period of nuclear physics in the early part of this century that a compromise was made in the acceptance of a dual nature for light. However, the other great body of work that Young did was into the nature of elasticity and, in particular, the relation between the elastic properties of arteries and the velocity of propagation of the arterial pulse (Young, 1808, 1809). His work on the nature of elasticity led to the concept of the elastic modulus to which his name is still attached. In determining the wave-velocity he derived the formula (given as eqn. 10.54) which Bramwell and Hill (1922) attributed to A. V. Hill and which other writers (e.g. Bergel and Schultz, 1971) attribute to Otto Frank.* It is finally of great interest to note that this polymath also had forays outside the sciences for he was the first man to do any considerable deciphering of Egyptian hieroglyphics after the discovery of the Rosetta stone.

(The reference to Egypt creates a link with Fourier (1768–1830) who was one of the band of 'savants' that Napoleon first took with him to Egypt, and who were stranded there for several years when Bonaparte had to beat a quick retreat to France after his defeat by Nelson at the Battle of the Nile. Thus, a lot of the analytical work that led to the Fourier series for the analysis of periodic functions was presumably carried out in Egypt. This was first published in his monograph on heat (*Théorie analytique de la Chaleur*, 1822). Fourier never contributed anything to haemodynamics but his name occurs so frequently in this book that it could hardly be omitted in a historical survey, however brief.)

The next work of interest in the field of wave-transmission was the result of a collaboration between two of the brothers Weber in the monograph of W. E. and E. H. Weber entitled *Wellenlehre* (1825) which established many of the fundamental properties of propagated and reflected waves. Here the bridge between physics and medicine was because the younger brother Wilhelm Eduard (1804–91) was a physicist while his brother Ernst Heinrich (1795–1878) was a Professor of Anatomy. E. H. Weber continued a lot of work on his own (see Weber, E. H., 1851 which reviews most of it). (There was a third brother, Eduard Friedrich (1806–71) who was also an anatomist and who collaborated with W. E. Weber in a famous monograph on the mechanisms of walking.)

This work of the Webers on wave propagation was soon followed by the experimental work of Moens in Leiden, published in his short monograph of 1878. The mathematical work of Korteweg and Résal on his data gave us the equation written here as eqn. 10.56 and which remains the most useful relationship, simple as it is and stringent in its basic assumptions (assuming a thin perfectly elastic wall and a non-viscous liquid).

This brings us to the threshold of our present era in haemodynamics. In terms of the fundamental parameters of 'the Force and Velocity by which these Fluids are impelled' that Hales had urged us to study there had been no real advance in pressure measurement beyond the measures of mean pressure that Hales had made. It had been made more convenient by Poiseuille's intro-

---

* This does not imply plagiarism because the mathematical nomenclature of Young's time is unfamiliar to us in these days; in fact, a careful perusal of Young's paper, mainly the 1808 one, will show that much of his reasoning had much in common with the foundations of Otto Frank's Windkessel theory of a century later. I am grateful to my friend, Robert Jones, for pointing this out to me.

duction of the U-tube mercury manometer with the addition, by Ludwig, of the float and pointer which inscribed on a smoked-paper kymograph. The development of manometers which could measure pulsatile pressure had to await Otto Frank's (1865–1944) great work of 1903, with all the theoretical developments that were to follow.

With regards to flow, it has become traditional within the last twenty-five years to accept the statement that pulsatile flows could not be measured in arteries. By some curious chance English workers seem completely to have overlooked the work of E. H. Marey (1830–1904) who, in a popular textbook of 1881, has a very full chapter on the velocity of blood in arteries. The technique he used was that of a double Pitot tube (see Ch. 9) which is based on Bernoulli's principle. The earliest paper he quotes is by Chauveau *et al.* (1860) in which an early form of the bristle flowmeter was used (see Ch. 9) and was rather large, for Chauveau only seems to have used it on horses. The Marey tracings look surprisingly like those that we accept as normal today— for example, they clearly show the back flow phase in the carotid and femoral arteries; had this work not been lost sight of, a lot of heated controversy over the form of the femoral flow wave could have been avoided in the 1950s.

The early twentieth century was completely dominated by Otto Frank and his pupils. Frank had been highly trained in physics and mathematics and does not seem to have turned to physiology until he was in his thirties. His first major papers were on the force-length behaviour of cardiac muscle. From this sprang the need to produce a manometer that could measure pulsatile pressures accurately (Frank, 1903, and later papers). This was based on a very sound physical analysis of the requirements of such a manometer and this remains valid to this day. Frank's approach to the analysis of the circulation was to conceive of the whole system as analogous to a model in which the heart pumped into a central elastic reservoir (the Windkessel) from which the blood drained to the tissues through essentially non-elastic conduits. The Windkessel was defined as the 'elastic' arteries comprising the aorta and the proximal part of some of the larger branches draining from it. When it was realized after careful investigations of the physical properties and structures of the arteries that the distinction between elastic and non-elastic arteries was not so clear-cut as originally thought many experiments were devised to determine the extent of the Windkessel. Thus, the very large paper of Wezler and Böger (1939) is devoted to this problem. This arose because with the powerful new instrument, the Frank manometer, a large amount of invaluable new data had been accumulated on the form of the arterial pressure pulse as it travelled through the arterial tree. In the initial formulation of the Windkessel theory the pressure pulse was thought of as an isolated event, i.e. that the system had returned to rest before the next heart-beat. The rapid rise to a dome-like peak (e.g. see Figs. 6.3 and 12.12) during the ejection phase, systole, was conceived as due to the filling of the Windkessel, followed by a drainage period following the closure of the aortic valves when the pressure was approximated by an exponential decay. With investigation of the pressure wave in the so-called 'drainage' arteries it was realized that the pressure swing there was often greater, the systolic portion was peaked and a secondary pressure wave, called the dicrotic wave, developed during diastole (e.g. Figs. 6.1, p. 119 and Fig. 12.12, p. 332). This led to modification of the original simple Windkessel analogue; the pressure changes due to ventricular ejection were assumed to be transmitted instantaneously through the reservoir, i.e. that the wave-velocity was infinitely high. Then to explain the change in wave form it was postulated that reflected waves were set up in the peripheral arteries which interacted with the pressure wave in the central reservoir with the formation of pressure nodes and antinodes at specific fractions of a wave-length. This was of itself somewhat anomalous because the initial pressure wave was assumed to be transmitted instantaneously at the beginning of the cycle but was followed by orthodox wave-transmission at a finite velocity determined by its elastic properties as investigated in the earlier work of the Webers and of Moens. Later workers were much taken with this analysis in terms of a resonance of the system although in a cycle of say 0·5 sec, in a system which is assumed to be wholly at rest by the end of this period, it gives rise to difficulties that were not always faced in any clear-cut manner. One confusion here seems to have arisen from Frank's original terminology. The appearance of the dicrotic wave in arteries like the femoral was early appreciated and Frank defines a term describing this sort of phenomenon in terms of the '*Grundschwingung*' of the Windkessel. Later workers (especially in the English-speaking countries) would translate this as 'resonance'; but, in fact, Frank also uses the term '*Resonanz*' and makes a clear distinction between them. The period of the '*Grundschwingung*' is apparently judged by the period between the systolic pressure peak and the dicrotic wave and is probably to be thought of as a 'natural oscillatory period' of the system.*

In spite of these criticisms of the theory, there is no doubt that it was very successful in predicting the stroke volume ejected by the ventricle and greatly increased our knowledge of the forms of the pressure pulse and of the elastic properties of the arteries. The criticisms advanced here are really aimed at the somewhat unwieldy mathematical edifices erected on the initial simple analogue model, by later followers of Frank, and the conflicting basic assumptions that had been added were quite overlooked. McDonald and Taylor (1959) give a fuller account than this sketch but not many reviews are in English. That of Apéria (1940) is of considerable interest because he tries to effect a compromise between Windkessel formulations and the standard physical analysis of wave transmission. In this one review he was not entirely

---

* *Grundschwingung* was apparently a neologism created by Frank and many of my German colleagues admit that they have difficulty in defining it or distinguishing it from resonance.

successful and his unfortunately premature death prevented him from pursuing the subject.

The main developments since 1950 have been in terms of treating the whole arterial system as being in a steady-state oscillation produced by the regularly repeated beat of the heart. This describes the pressure pulse as a collection of sinusoidal waves of frequencies determined by the harmonic, or Fourier, series. This approach was first used in a creative way by Womersley when he and I first met and collaborated in 1952 (Womersley, 1955b; McDonald, 1955a). Its formulation was relatively simple and straightforward and its basic assumptions clearly, and compatibly, defined. It was probably fortunate that I was completely ignorant of the literature on the Windkessel theory so that we never attempted to make a compromise hybrid theory between the two different approaches that Apéria (1940) had attempted to do and which made his conclusions difficult to interpret. As this book is an account of the work that developed from this beginning there is no need to enlarge upon it here. There was a fair amount of opposition to its introduction but this may largely be attributed to two reasons: firstly, the instinctive opposition to any new and unfamiliar approach (new, that is, to physiology, for the line transmissions equations were quite traditional to physics); secondly, the rather tedious calculations required to derive the harmonic components of the pulsatile waves. However, by the time the first full account of the steady-state oscillation approach to the circulation appeared in the form of the original *Blood Flow in Arteries*, in 1960, digital computers were becoming widely available in physiological laboratories. It was this fortunate coincidence that greatly accelerated the spread of this conceptual approach. In addition, by the 1960s, good flowmeters were becoming generally available and we were able to take an analytical approach so that flow calculated from the theoretical equations could be tested by the actual measured flows, a possibility that was denied to Frank and his followers. As experimental results showed that the original theory was not entirely adequate because of the existence of the reflected waves the theory was enlarged, notably by the powerful analyses of Taylor (1957a, b) using the standard telegraph equations of electrical wave transmission practice. Here again, Taylor kept to simple analogue models and checked all his results with experiments in hydraulic models and in animals.

Electrical circuits, however, are very easy to build and very soon we had several workers building electrical analogue models of the whole of the arterial tree (e.g., Jager et al., 1965; Noordergraaf et al., 1964). Based as they were on the Womersley equations initially these analogue models were instructive and useful. But once one starts working entirely with analogue electrical models it is all too easy to forget that they are not the hydraulic system that we are really concerned with. However elegant the electrical transmission, we cannot avoid the elementary truism—electricity is not water (or blood). As early as 1959 Taylor published a detailed paper demonstrating that the precise requirements of the hydraulic system could only be represented in a transmission line model by a single harmonic frequency at one time and therefore could not precisely represent a pulse wave compounded of a number of different harmonic frequencies. The building of an analogue of the whole arterial tree necessitates postulating a whole array of properties of the smaller vessels that were completely unknown by the biologists. The technical difficulties of working in the smaller vessels have always been a source of paucity of physical data that is a major block to the fuller development of haemodynamics. By contrast, the building of electrical analogues is relatively easy but only where their predictions have been checked by experiments in animals have they been reviewed in this book.

The situation with regard to mathematical developments of the wave-transmission equations in terms of a variety of postulated structural models is often worse because not only have they not been tested experimentally but parameters are often used which cannot be transformed into physical constants applicable to the arterial wall. There are some honourable exceptions to this, as in the papers by Cox (1968, 1969, 1970a, b) in which he has extended the initial thin wall model used by Womersley to cover walls of a finite thickness that correspond to the actual arterial wall. After several years of mathematical development in a complex set of equations his experimental tests of the two theories show that the results are only of the order of 6–7 per cent different, a difference which is barely detectable with the accuracy of our present instruments.

This problem of the precision of the accuracy of the instruments we have available can bring us back to the consideration of the scientific method that was discussed above (p. 3) and which we can illuminate a little from the points noted in the brief historical overview that we have made.

First, in terms of the emphasis on the importance of measurement that was made by Lord Kelvin, we can see how important this has been at each stage of the development of haemodynamics and shows why Stephen Hales deserves his honoured place in the physiology of our time. This need for more and better measurement all the time and the rapid expansion of haemodynamics since World War II has greatly depended on the great sophistication in instrumentation, especially of the miniaturized forms which physiology so badly needs. This has been made possible by the skills arising from the sophistication of armaments and of the machines required for the space programme. In certain schools of biomedical engineering there was often a feeling among the younger members that development of new theories was somehow superior to work as a mere instrument maker. In fact, the improved measurements we can make with improved instruments is absolutely vital to the development of an experimental discipline. Computers may be considered as instruments in this sense for a far from inconsiderable advantage of the use of the Fourier series was that, for the first time, we were able to describe a compound wave in quantitative terms in place of the large vocabulary of descriptive terms that had arisen to describe the pulse wave.

Measurement may not proceed any further than the collection of quantitative data. As such, it is usually regarded as hardly qualifying as research. But, as we have seen, we are urgently in need of a lot of accurate data on such simple things as the thickness of the arterial wall or the elastic properties of arteries. To a physicist or engineer all this sort of data about the materials he uses were determined so long ago that they are taken for granted and he has difficulty in conceiving of the fallibility of theoretical analyses of the performance of living systems.

From the acquisition of the data the need to develop hypotheses becomes evident. In an excellent and stimulating article, Platt (1964) has pungently pointed out the rapidity with which those sciences grow where the proper intellectual effort is given to making clear-cut hypotheses. He makes powerful use of the truism that 'a hypothesis that cannot be disproved is useless'. That is, the essence of scientific proof is the successive demonstration that alternate theories are not possible. The examples that Platt gives are almost entirely from molecular biology and of hypotheses to which a clear-cut 'Yes' or 'No' answer can be given. In many other fields, this is not too easy to achieve for the distinction between two alternative haemodynamic hypotheses may be a quantitative one. An example was given in the case of the theory developed by Cox (1970a) as an alternative to Womersley (1955c) where the proof or disproof of one or the other rested on the precision of our measurements. Nevertheless, there would be considerably less confusion in current haemodynamics if the exhortations of Platt (1964) or of other writers who have devoted their thoughts to the processes of scientific investigation such as Beveridge (1957) were heeded. The design of haemodynamic experiments often leaves much to be desired.

The successive steps in reformulating our hypotheses in the light of experimental test data needs no emphasis. The situation in haemodynamics is, however, not easy to define here. The system of branching tubes with which we have to deal is of such a complexity that it often appears overwhelming. The situation is usually met by making limiting assumptions, a virtual necessity when dealing with a system of non-linear anistropic visco-elastic tubes. A lot of progress has been made by treating the wall as linear in its elastic properties in that it is linear over the small range of strains that it undergoes in any given steady-state oscillation and also that it is not far from isotropic behaviour under normal physiological stresses. The viscous properties are also very important in that they play a big part in determining the dissipation of energy and the attenuation of the travelling wave. In a system where only short lengths of homogenous arteries are available this is difficult to measure and it is all too human to tend to disregard it in more complex theoretical treatments. Thus, there have been several papers dealing with the anistropy of the arterial wall and also its non-linear behaviour in terms of the theory of large elastic deformations—but the intellectual advances they achieve to me are more than balanced out in that the viscous properties are neglected. And some treatments tend to forget the fundamental assumptions on which they are based—the most obvious are the most easily forgotten. Thus, all classical elasticity theory deals with materials that are completely homogenous in structure whereas the arterial wall is a matrix of elastic fibres loosely held in a watery material (70 per cent of the arterial wall by weight can easily be removed by desiccation overnight).

The method of characteristics is also being introduced as a method of improving our analysis of our non-linear system but has not yet undergone any severe experimental testing. Intellectually, these investigations into non-linearity are greatly to be commended. That they receive very little consideration in this book is not because I regard them as negligible but, quite apart from considerations of space, because my emphasis throughout has been on experimental findings. As an experimental scientist, I work on the pragmatic dictum that, for my purposes, 'anything that we cannot measure must be regarded, for the present, as not existing'. This does not mean ignoring them; for example, even the most pragmatic of us would not deny the value of the Poiseuille equation in understanding the circulation, but, as we see in Ch. 2, there is no situation in the vascular tree where it can satisfy all the assumptions on which it is based—and in the closest situations to this requirement the vessels are so small and inaccessible that we cannot even determine their dimensions accurately.

Nevertheless, in the plethora of theoretical treatments that have been presented in the last decade or so, two scientific principles have often been overlooked. The first is that known as Occam's razor which was tersely set out in Latin as '*Entia non sint multiplicande praeteriter necessitatem*' which may be freely interpreted as 'Do not multiply your working hypotheses more than is necessary.' The second is the dictum that no mathematical equations can be more valid than the assumptions on which they are based. If the assumptions are incorrect then if the mathematics are without error the result must, of necessity, be incorrect also. In this respect pitfalls most commonly occur when there are basic assumptions which are implicit to the analysis without being consciously stated, because they have been used in previous work over a long period of time.

Examples of this type are penetratingly analysed in the field of classic hydrodynamics by Birkhoff (1960). The Euler equations of fluid motion have always been regarded as so complete that several great mathematicians such as Lagrange have stated that, starting with them, all systems of fluid flow can be derived. Yet he quotes Sir Cyril Hinshelwood (Lighthill, 1956) as saying that 'fluid dynamicists in the nineteenth century were divided into hydraulic engineers who observed what could not be explained and mathematicians who explained things that could not be observed' to which Birkhoff adds, 'It is my impression that many survivors of both species are still with us.' He then goes on to analyse several well-known paradoxes in mathematical hydrodynamics in terms of six hidden but plausible assumptions that have been accepted without question, or indeed without being aware of their existence.

Occasionally, one will find that some basic assumptions may be made too restrictively; an example of this sort was in the rigid separation between Windkessel theory, in which each pulse had to be regarded as a transient, and the wave transmission analysis that had to assume a steady-state oscillation. In fact, the attenuation in the arterial system is so high that we realize that the whole system may well come to rest within the period of the cardiac cycle. To illustrate this point, in the paper by Kouchoukos, Sheppard and McDonald (1970) where a Windkessel formula was being used to estimate stroke volume I found that it was possible to derive the formula as an approximation by starting from the Womersley equations (Ch. 15). In the same way we occasionally find that new formulations which have been advanced as refutations of earlier ones may, in fact, be essentially the same when analysed down to their basic components.

In the same way, by dissecting haemodynamics into its component parts, and synthesizing the whole from analyses of pulsatile pressure and flow in single arteries we find that the analysis of the whole complex system of the vascular tree may prove to be a lot simpler than a first view suggests. It is in the hope that this view can be transmitted to men entering the field that this book has been written.

2
Steady Flow of a Liquid in Cylindrical Tubes

In considering the circulation, we are naturally concerned with the laws governing the flow of liquids in cylindrical pipes. The simplest example is that of a long straight tube with a constant rate of flow (steady flow) along it. To maintain such a steady flow there must be a constant pressure applied to the liquid because of its viscosity or 'internal friction'. Flow in a cylindrical tube is described by the well-known Poiseuille equation which states that the pressure drop is directly proportional to the length of the pipe, to the rate of flow, and to the viscosity and is inversely proportional to the fourth power of the radius. If dye is injected into liquid flowing in under these conditions it is seen that the liquid in the axis of the tube is moving much faster than that near the wall and the front of the dye assumes a parabolic shape. The explanation for this is that the particles of liquid are flowing in a series of laminae parallel to the sides of the tube and the fluid actually in contact with the wall is stationary and each successive lamina is slipping against the viscous friction of the lamina outside it. When flow occurs in such parallel laminae it is called 'laminar'. If two tubes join to form a trunk and dye has only been injected into one of them it will be found that there is no mixing transversely across the tube and the streams remain distinct and are seen to flow side by side in the main trunk; this phenomenon is called streamlining. Hence laminar flow is often called 'streamline' flow. Alternatively, it may be called 'Poiseuille-type' flow because it obeys the Poiseuille equation.

If the rate of flow through a tube is continuously increased there comes a point when the resistance to flow increases quite sharply and the Poiseuille relation no longer applies. Dye injected at this stage into the stream shows that the fluid is mixing across the tube and that the particles of dye, and hence of the liquid, are no longer moving regularly in the line of flow but are following more or less random paths across the tube in addition to their main movement along the tube. The flow is then said to be 'turbulent'. The pressure–flow relationships of turbulent flow are not predictable with precision, so that for this reason alone it is important to know whether any flow being studied is laminar or turbulent. It should be emphasized, however, that this classical distinction of types of flow is only correctly defined for steady flow in rigid

17

tubes and there are intermediate stages of instability in the liquid which become of importance in the irregular flow systems of the living animal and which will be considered in Ch. 4.

LAMINAR FLOW IN VISCOUS LIQUIDS

The concept of viscosity is quite inseparable from the consideration of the way that liquids flow. Stated in its most general way we can say that if a force is applied to a portion of a mass of liquid it will begin to flow but that if the force is removed the movement will be brought to rest. On the other hand, if a similar portion of a body of liquid is kept moving, the movement will be communicated to the rest of the fluid. This property is clearly analogous to that of friction between solid bodies and hence was termed 'internal friction' by the earlier workers on the subject. Hatschek (1928) gives an interesting account of the development of these concepts from which the following account is derived.

The first theoretical consideration of the subject was made by Newton in the *Principia Mathematica* (Proposition LI, Theorem XXXIX) in which he considered the motion imparted to a large volume of fluid by the rotation of a long cylinder suspended in it. The hypothesis on which he based his derivation was 'that the resistance which arises from the defect of slipperiness of the parts of the liquid, other things being equal, is proportional to the velocity with which the parts of the liquid are separated from one another' (Hatschek's translation). 'Defect of slipperiness' (*defectus lubricatitis*) was the term used to describe what we now call viscosity. This hypothesis emphasizes immediately that in a fluid moving relative to a surface there are laminae slipping on one another and so moving at different velocities. There is thus a velocity gradient in a direction perpendicular to the surface. This gradient is usually called the rate of shear.

In modern terms, the velocity gradient is written as dv/dr where r is the distance from the axis. The force, or stress, τ, is defined by

$$\tau = \mu \cdot \frac{dv}{dr} \qquad \qquad \textbf{2.1}$$

where μ is the coefficient of viscosity (Fig. 2.1).

Although the concept of 'internal friction' of a liquid brings analogies with solid, sliding friction to mind, it should be noted that there are important differences between the two. Friction between two solid bodies is a function of the pressure exerted at the surface but this plays no part in the assumed friction between liquid particles. Solid friction requires a finite force to initiate movement and the force thereafter is independent of the velocity of the motion; in Newton's hypothesis any force will initiate flow and the force required thereafter varies with the velocity. With no experimental evidence as a guide, the definition of viscosity can only be regarded as a gigantic feat of intuition by Newton. Indeed to this day it remains unproven in terms of molecular forces although amply supported by the pragmatic justification 'that it works'.

Apart from this one theorem, Newton did not pursue the subject very far, although in the corollaries to the theorem he did consider the case of the flow

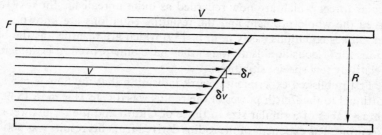

Fig. 2.1. Diagram showing the development of shear when a plate is moved at velocity, V, at a distance, R, from a fixed plate. It can be seen that the rate of shear will be $\delta v/\delta r$.

between two concentric cylinders. Nor was the problem studied again for more than a century. Nevertheless, this first contribution is commemorated in the use of the term Newtonian fluid for simple viscous fluids. The requirement for a Newtonian liquid is one whose viscosity does not vary with the rate of shear, that is to say, remains constant at varying rates of laminar flow.

The eighteenth century produced many outstanding mathematicians (Bell, 1965). Of these, the greatest was Euler, who, with Daniel Bernoulli devoted much attention to the analysis of liquid motion and so founded modern theoretical hydrodynamics. Nevertheless, they only dealt with the case of 'ideal' liquids, that is, fluids without viscosity which are incompressible. The first assumption may seem a large one (but water is a liquid of low viscosity) and it is still used in a lot of hydrodynamic analyses, which are based on Euler's equations of motion. Birkhoff (1960) has described these equations as 'being still the main tool of practical fluid mechanics'. It has been found possible to apply relatively little of this aspect of hydrodynamic theory to the blood circulation so that it is not usefully pursued here.

In terms of experimental work, Coulomb (1798) studied the damping of the oscillations of a disc suspended in liquids of different viscosities and made the important observation that the smoothness or roughness of the surface of the disc did not greatly influence the drag of the liquid. The first work on flow in cylindrical tubes appears to be that of Girard (1813) using brass tubes of from 2 to 3 mm in diameter. He obtained the relationship $Q = K.D^3P/L$ where Q is the volume flow per unit time, K is a constant, D the diameter, P the pressure drop along L, the length of the tube. Thus, he observed that the flow varied directly with the pressure and inversely with the length, but thought that it varied with the cube of the radius. Ten years later Navier made the first deductions of the theoretical equations for flow of viscous liquids in cylindrical tubes but obtained the incorrect result, already apparently confirmed by Girard's experimental results, that the flow was proportional to the cube of the radius.

The theoretical work of Navier (1827) was not, as we see, wholly successful and was developed by Poisson (1831), but both used assumptions of inter-molecular forces which are now regarded as quite unrealistic. Stokes (1845) reworked the whole problem and the resulting equations are known as the Navier–Stokes equations (see Ch. 6, p. 139) which are regarded as the basic equations for viscous liquids although they have only proved to be integrable in a relatively few special situations.

The first published experimental work indicating that the flow is probably proportional to the fourth power of the radius was due to Hagen in 1839. He used brass tubes of a similar size to those of Girard and the results were not very accurate. The exponent of the radius derived from his results was actually 4·12 and he assumed that the real value must be 4·0. Poiseuille published his first results in 1842 although there was not a full paper until 1846. On account of Hagen's priority of publication, some reference works use the name 'the Hagen–Poiseuille law'. Poiseuille's work, however, was much more detailed and precise (Joly, 1968) and it is generally agreed that it is just to name it Poiseuille's law. Poiseuille (1799–1869) had long been investigating the hydrodynamics of the capillary circulation; for example, he was the first to appreciate that the velocity profile was the reason for the varying velocities of individual red corpuscles. Herrick (1942) gives a most interesting account of the physiological observations Poiseuille made on the circulation before he turned to his classic work on the flow of liquids.

Poiseuille may be regarded as fortunate in two respects. In the first place, although he had training in physics he was also a physician who wanted to apply the results of his investigations to the understanding of the blood circulation. Hence, he worked with glass tubes of capillary size where his predecessors had been engineers and worked with much larger pipes. The use of minute tubes more easily maintains laminar flow and also greatly facilitates accurate measurement. In the second place, he was deflected from his original intention of using blood as a test liquid because no satisfactory way of rendering it incoagulable was known and he was compelled to confine his investigation to water. Blood flowing in capillaries shows anomalous viscous properties (Ch. 3) that would have introduced great complications in these pioneer studies.

Poiseuille used capillary tubes varying in internal diameter from 0·14 mm to 0·03 mm and his measurements were carried out with an accuracy and completeness that thoroughly deserve the regard which they have been accorded. His results were expressed by the formula

$$Q = \frac{K.P.D^4}{L} \qquad\qquad 2.2$$

where, as above, Q, P, and L are volume flow, pressure drop along the tube, and length of tube, respectively; D is the tube diameter and K is a constant.

The value of the constant K was determined under various conditions and shown to fall with decreasing temperature. This constant is clearly a measure of the viscosity but by purely experimental work it is not possible to define it other than empirically in this way.

The form of Poiseuille's law with which we are familiar is, in fact, dependent on the theoretical solution of the problem. Navier's early work on the equations of motion for viscous liquids were amplified and corrected by Stokes in the 1840s and the Navier–Stokes equations are the general solution of this problem. Stokes, however, did not tackle the particular case of the flow in a tube. The solution of this case was made independently by Wiedemann in 1856 and Hagenbach in 1860 who both produced the result that

$$Q = \frac{(P_1 - P^2)\pi R^4}{8\mu L} \qquad \textbf{2.3}$$

where μ is the viscosity so that it can be seen that Poiseuille's constant

$$K = \frac{\pi}{128\mu} \quad \left(\text{as } R^4 = \frac{D^4}{16} \right) \text{ or } \mu = \frac{\pi}{128K}$$

Hagenbach calculated μ from Poiseuille's data and obtained the result in modern units of $\mu = 0 \cdot 013084$ poises at $10°C$ (modern values $0 \cdot 013077$ P, see Bingham and Jackson, 1918; Barr, 1931).

The method of derivation of the solution used by Hagenbach was a simple one and it seems odd to us today to think that it should have taken so long to produce. Compared with the advances made in pure mathematics by the middle of the nineteenth century this is a very elementary problem in applied mathematics and furthermore a problem which had been subjected to experimental investigation for over forty years.

The basic assumption made for this solution, essentially that made by Newton, is that every particle of liquid is moving parallel to the axis of the tube with a constant velocity, v, and the force opposing the flow over unit area is proportional to the viscosity and the velocity gradient in the liquid. In a cylindrical tube the particles travelling at the same velocity will be symmetrically arranged as cylindrical laminae.

In a tube of radius R let us consider a cylindrical unit of liquid of length L and of radius r (Fig. 2.2A). The viscous force retarding its motion will be the area of its surface $(2\pi rL) \times$ (its viscosity, μ) $\times$ (the velocity gradient across the tube, dv/dr).

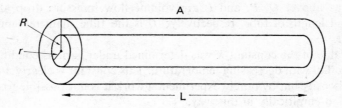

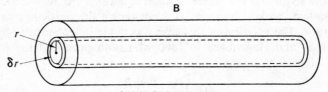

Fig. 2.2. Diagrams to illustrate the derivation of Poiseuille's law.
A. The first method (Hagenbach) when a small cylinder of liquid in the axis is envisioned.
B. The second method (Lamb) postulating an annulus of liquid of thickness, δr.

$$F_{visc} = 2\pi r \mu L . \frac{dv}{dr}$$

The force exerted by the pressure on the end of the cylinder is pressure $\times$ cross-sectional area less the force on the far end, so that

$$F(p) = \pi r^2 (P_1 - P_2)$$

where P_1 and P_2 are the respective pressures at either end of the length (L) of the cylinder considered. The pressure difference per unit length $(P_1 - P_2)/L$ is termed the pressure-gradient.

These forces are equal and opposite

$$\pi r^2 (P_1 - P_2) = -2\pi r . L\mu \frac{dv}{dr}$$

or

$$r(P_1 - P_2) = -2L\mu . \frac{dv}{dr}$$

so that the velocity-gradient is

$$\frac{dv}{dr} = \frac{-r(P_1 - P_2)}{2L\mu}$$

By integration we find that the velocity at radius, r, is

$$v = \frac{-r^2(P_1 - P_2)}{4L\mu} + C \qquad\qquad \textbf{2.4}$$

To determine the value of the constant of integration, C, it is necessary to make a further assumption of the boundary conditions. This is that the lamina in contact with the wall is at rest (an assumption made by Newton), i.e. when $r = R$, $v = \mathbf{0}$.

With substitution of these values we see that

$$C = \frac{R^2(P_1 - P_2)}{4L\mu}$$

so that

$$v = \frac{-r^2(P_1 - P_2)}{4L\mu} + \frac{R^2(P_1 - P_2)}{4L\mu} = \frac{(P_1 - P_2)}{4L\mu}(R^2 - r^2)   \qquad \textbf{2.5}$$

This is the equation for a parabola where $v = 0$ when $r = R$ and is a maximum when $r = 0$, i.e. at the axis of the tube (Fig. 2.3).

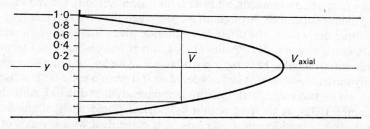

Fig. 2.3. A diagram of the velocity profile in steady laminar flow. This is a parabola whose equation is

$$V = \frac{(P_1 - P_2)(R^2 - r^2)}{4L\mu}$$

The actual equation of the curve shown is $V = 10(1 - y^2)$ where $y = r/R$ or the ratio of the radius of the lamina considered to the radius of the pipe.

The average velocity across the pipe ($\bar{V}$) can be shown to be half the axial velocity (see eqns. 2.5 and 2.6).

To obtain the volume of flow it is necessary to determine the volume of the paraboloid which has this parabola as its profile. That is, we must determine the volume of the solid of revolution of this parabola.

This volume is

$$Q = \int_0^R 2\pi v . r dr$$

or, substituting the value for v above (eqn. 2.5)

$$Q = \frac{2\pi(P_1 - P_2)}{4L\mu} \int_0^R (R^2 - r^2) r dr = \frac{(P_1 - P_2)\pi R^4}{8L\mu}   \qquad \textbf{2.6}$$

This is commonly referred to as the Poiseuille equation.

The average velocity ($\overline{V}$) across the tube is given by dividing the volume flow (Q) by the cross-sectional area (πR^2), so that we obtain, from eqn. 2.6,

$$\overline{V} = \frac{(P_1 - P_2)R^2}{8\mu L} \qquad\qquad \textbf{2.7}$$

The maximum velocity is at the axis of the tube so that from eqn. 2.5, by substituting $r = 0$, we obtain

$$V_{\text{axial}} = \frac{(P_1 - P_2)R^2}{4\mu L} \qquad\qquad \textbf{2.8}$$

Thus, the average velocity is half the axial velocity (Fig. 2.3). The lamina flowing at this velocity is the one of radius, r, such that $(R^2 - r^2) = R/\sqrt{2}$ or $r = 0.707R$. (The term 'average' velocity is used in the sense of the average across the pipe at any moment, and the term 'mean' velocity for the mean of time-dependent variations throughout a cycle when the flow is pulsatile.)

The simple derivation of Poiseuille's equation given above is often treated as the standard one, e.g. Kaufmann (1963), but is unsatisfactory in terms of the infinitesimal calculus because it postulates a 'cylinder' of finite size, and is physically unreal because this is considered as if it were a solid with a viscous drag only on its surface. A better method, apparently first due to Lamb about 1890 (Lamb, 1932), is to treat a thin cylindrical liquid shell of thickness, δr, inner radius, r, and length, L; its axis, z, is coincident with the axis of the tube and the velocity (v) is everywhere parallel to the axis, and a function of the distance (r) from this axis (Fig. 2.2B). The normal pressure on the end is now

$$F_p = (P_1 - P_2)2\pi r . \delta r \qquad\qquad \textbf{2.9}$$

The retarding force on the *inner* surface will be written as before but we are concerned with the differences between the two surfaces which will be the rate of change across the thickness, or

$$F_{vise} = \frac{-\partial}{\partial r} (\mu \ . \ \frac{\partial v}{\partial r} \ . \ 2\pi r L)\delta r \qquad\qquad \textbf{2 10}$$

Equating these, we obtain

$$\frac{\partial}{\partial r} \left(r . \frac{\partial v}{\partial r} \right) = -\frac{(P_1 - P_2)}{\mu L} . r \qquad\qquad \textbf{2.11}$$

Integrating once we obtain

$$\frac{\partial v}{\partial r} = -\frac{(P_1 - P_2)}{2\mu L} . r + \frac{A}{r} \qquad\qquad \textbf{2.12}$$

where A is the constant of integration.

Since flow is symmetrical at the axis then when

$$r = 0, \frac{\partial v}{\partial r} = 0 \quad \therefore \quad A = 0$$

and

$$\frac{\partial v}{\partial r} = -\frac{(P_1 - P_2)}{2\mu L} \cdot r$$

Alternatively, Lamb (1932) writes the solution of 2.11 as

$$v = -\frac{(P_1 - P_2)}{4\mu L} \cdot r^2 + A \ln r + B \qquad \qquad 2.13$$

and points out that, since the velocity must be finite at the axis, then we must have $A = 0$. The solution for $B = 0$, due to zero velocity at the wall, is as for C in eqn. 2.4. Equation 2.11 may also be written in the form

$$r \cdot \frac{\partial^2 v}{\partial r^2} + \frac{\partial v}{\partial r} + \frac{(P_1 - P_2)}{\mu L} \cdot r = 0 \qquad \qquad 2.14$$

or

$$\frac{\partial^2 v}{\partial r^2} + \frac{1}{r} \cdot \frac{\partial v}{\partial r} + \frac{(P_1 - P_2)}{\mu L} = 0 \qquad \qquad 2.15$$

and we shall later find this form in Womersley's derivations in Chs. 5 and 6. (In the later usage the symbol w is commonly used in place of v; this convention is explained in Ch. 5, p. 101.)

To evaluate Poiseuille's equation (2.6) all units must be consistent. Thus, in the CGS system $Q = cm^3/sec$ and R and L are in cm while $P = dyn/cm^2$. The conversion of P into mm Hg, so commonly used in physiology, is effected by multiplying by $1/10$ to convert to cm Hg and then multiplying by the density of mercury, 13.6 g/cm^3, and the gravitational constant, g (approx. 980 cm/sec^2), i.e. 1 mm Hg $= 1.33 \times 10^3$ dyn/cm^2.

The CGS unit of viscosity is the poise (P) and is named in honour of Poiseuille. It is the force required to move a unit area through a liquid to create a unit velocity gradient and is thus defined as 1 dyn sec./cm^2 or 1 g cm^{-1} sec^{-1}. For convenience the centipoise (cP) is often used; the viscosity of water is very close to 0.01 P (1.0 cP) at 20°C (more precisely it is 1.00000 cP at 20.2°C (Bingham and Jackson, 1918). The value taken for blood with a haematocrit of 45 per cent in most calculations in this book is 0.04 P (4.0 cP) at 37°C. There have been a variety of values for blood viscosity published in the literature; for that reason a survey of measured values is given.

The viscosity of blood

Because whole blood behaves as a non-Newtonian liquid and the rate of flow and the size of tube influences the apparent viscosity of blood, attention should be paid to the method of measurement when comparing published values. The viscosity also varies with the red cell concentration. The anomalous viscous behaviour of blood is considered in detail in Ch. 3.

The viscometers used in most measurements of blood viscosity have been some form of capillary viscometer; in these the rate of flow through a standard capillary tube under a measured pressure-head, is recorded. To minimize the determination of instrument characteristics, such as corrections for inlet length (p. 28), a direct comparison of the time for a standard volume of blood to flow through is made with the time taken by the same volume of water under the same pressure. The viscosity is then expressed as the relative viscosity with respect to water. As the apparent viscosity increases at low rates of flow, i.e. low rates of shear (a phenomenon first clearly described by Hess, 1911), a viscometer capable of high rates of flow should be used. The capillary should not be smaller than 1 mm in internal diameter. Hess himself designed an instrument that is excellent and still in common use. For precise viscometry the Couette or concentric cylinder is often preferred. In the usual pattern the liquid under test is placed in the space between two cylinders; the outer one is rotated and the torque on the inner cylinder is measured at given rates of rotation of the outer cylinder. If the gap between the cylinders is small compared to their radii the velocity-gradient is virtually constant. The cone-and-plate viscometer also subjects the liquid to a uniform shear (details of design and operation are given by standard works such as Hatschek, 1928; Barr, 1931, and Whitmore, 1968). The very sensitive concentric cylinder viscometer built by Gillinson, Dauwalter and Merrill (1963) has been used in recent years by Merrill's group, but principally to study anomalous viscous behaviour.

Relative viscosities given below are commonly regarded as being the same in magnitude as the true dynamic viscosity in centipoises because the viscosity of water at 20°C is 1·0 cP. If the temperature coefficient of blood is the same as water the relative viscosity would not vary with temperature. There is evidence, however, that the viscosity of blood falls about 1·1 times faster than the viscosity of water with a change of temperature from 20°C to 37°C. The relative viscosity at 37°C would thus be about 90 per cent of the relative viscosity at 20°C.

The relative viscosity of blood is reported as being between 2·5 and 4 (Green, 1944) but most reference books give a higher figure, 4·7 at 38°C for man and dog (Albritton, 1952), 4·8–5·2 (Whitby and Britton, 1950), 3·9–5·3, mean 4·7 for males, 4·4 for females (Bazett, 1941), 3·5–5·4 (mean 4·6) (Wintrobe, 1967). In absolute units, at 37°C this gives values from 0·017 P to

0·0371 P. A mean value of the relative viscosity for human blood of 4·6 is supported by the large series of measurements by Hess (1908) and Nygaard, Wilder and Berkson (1935) 4·64 + 0·025. With dogs' blood Coulter and Pappenheimer (1949) made careful observations on the apparent viscosity in absolute units at varying haematocrits but unfortunately the different experiments were performed over a wide range of temperatures. Calculating the relative viscosities for the experiments with haematocrit values between 40 and 45 per cent their values range from 5·62 to 6·38 which correspond to absolute viscosities of 0·039 P to 0·044 P at 37°C. These were all measured at high rates of laminar flow but before the onset of turbulence. It will be seen that they are rather higher than the textbook values quoted above.

It is seen that there is no great measure of agreement between various observers concerning the precise value of the viscosity of whole blood. In an animal such as the rabbit with a low haematocrit (Wintrobe, 1967), I have assumed the viscosity at 37°C to be 0·017 P, at the lower end of the range quoted. For dogs and human beings the value would appear to lie between 0·03 and 0·04 P, in tubes of radius greater than 0·01 cm, and such values will be assumed for calculations involving the large vessels.

The viscosity of serum and plasma is lower but in spite of the lack of complication due to the presence of corpuscles there is no very great measure of agreement. Bircher (1921) found the relative viscosity of human serum in the range 1·7–2·0, with whole plasma having values 0·2 to 0·3 higher. Nygaard *et al.* (1935) give the value 1·96 ± 0·004 for serum. Bazett (1941) gives 1·5–1·7 for human plasma. Recent determinations by Merrill *et al.* (1963), with the concentric cylinder viscometer, of the viscosity of normal plasma give a relative value of 1·6. This gives good agreement with the range quoted by Bazett.

THE APPLICABILITY OF POISEUILLE'S EQUATION TO THE CIRCULATION

The conditions under which Poiseuille's equation applies precisely are implicit in the method by which it is derived theoretically. In view of its importance in the hydrodynamics of the circulation these conditions should be considered in more detail. They are as follows:

(*1*) *The fluid is homogenous and its viscosity is the same at all rates of shear.* Blood is, of course, a suspension of particles but it has been shown that, in tubes in which the internal diameter is large compared with the size of the red cells, it behaves as a Newtonian fluid. In tubes with an internal radius less than 0·5 mm, changes in apparent viscosity occur. This is important in the study of flow in small vessels and is discussed more fully below in Ch. 3. In the larger arteries and veins, however, blood may be considered as a homogenous fluid with a viscosity that is independent of the velocity-gradient.

(2) The liquid does not slip at the wall. This was the assumption that $v = 0$ when $r = R$ which was made in evaluating the constant of integration in the equations on p. 23. As Poiseuille's law would not be valid if this were not true, the law may be used as a test for the assumption; it is held to be universally true for liquids (Kaufmann, 1963; Birkhoff, 1960). Even when gas flows over a solid surface there appears to be no appreciable slip under normal conditions though it may have to be considered with a rarefied gas. These conclusions are derived from the detailed review by Goldstein (1938).

This point is of some importance as it has occasionally been suggested that some of the anomalous flow properties of blood in blood-vessels may be due to non-wettable properties of their endothelial lining with a consequent slip at the wall. Even if the endothelium were shown to be non-wettable the conclusion, that slipping would result, is unjustifiable. For example, Poiseuille's law holds for the flow of mercury in a glass tube so that there must be zero velocity at the wall.

The appearance in flowing blood of a narrow but cell-free zone at the walls of the tube has led some workers to treat this lower viscosity zone as a region of 'slip'. This can be convenient as a mathematical device but should not be taken as a physical reality. The point is discussed well by Whitmore (1967) and is elaborated in Ch. 3 (p. 66).

(3) The flow is laminar, that is, the liquid at all points is moving parallel to the walls of the tube. At rates of flow above a critical value this is no longer true and the flow is turbulent. The deviation from Poiseuille's law that this causes is discussed in the next section (p. 30). Turbulent flow may occur in the largest blood vessels but as the flow here is also pulsatile, condition (4) below is not satisfied so that Poiseuille's law cannot be applied. The evidence available on the occurrence of turbulent flow in the circulation is reviewed in Ch. 4 where it will be seen that laminar flow is almost certainly present in all the vessels where flow is sufficiently steady to consider applying Poiseuille's law.

(4) The rate of flow is 'steady' and is not subjected to acceleration or deceleration. If the velocity is altered the pressure-gradient is utilized partly in communicating kinetic energy to the liquid and the equations do not apply. As the flow in all large arteries and the intrathoracic veins (Brecher, 1956) is markedly pulsatile, it is clear that Poiseuille's law cannot be applied to them. The velocity profiles and the pressure–flow relationship of flow under these circumstances is considered below in Chs. 4, 5 and 6.

(5) The tube is long compared with the region being studied. Close to the inlet of a pipe the flow has not yet become established with the parabolic velocity profile characteristic of laminar flow. The distance required to establish the steady form of flow is known as the 'inlet length' and here Poiseuille's law does not apply. Within the inlet length the assumption made in the derivation that there are no accelerations along the axis of the tube is not true. It is,

therefore, a special case of the steady flow condition discussed in (4) above. In viscometers where a flow from a reservoir through a narrow tube is measured a correction for this effect must be applied (Newman and Searle, 1957).

The transition from a flat velocity distribution, at the entrance of a tube, to the fully-developed parabolic velocity profile is illustrated in Fig. 5.6 and discussed on p. 109. This distance over which the transition takes place is called the 'inlet' or 'entrance' length and a correction factor to the measured length of the tube is made. A second phenomenon that also affects the energy expenditure is the kinetic energy involved in transition from a flat to a parabolic profile.

The corrections for inlet length arise from two closely-related sources. They are discussed, and illustrated, on p. 110. From a large reservoir the profile at the origin of the tube is virtually flat; viscous drag has its first effect at the boundary layer at the wall and this involves more and more layers up to the axis; the 'boundary' layer may then be regarded as filling the tube. The velocity profile is then the Poiseuille parabola, and the flow is said to be 'established.'

For the length correction the value L is increased by a factor $K_1 \cdot R$, where K_1 may be taken as 1·64 in all cases. Thus, for L write $(L + 1\cdot64R)$ where R is the radius of the tube.

The other term (kinetic energy) can be corrected by using an adjusted term $(\Delta P')$ for the pressure-drop:

$$\Delta P' = (P_1 - P_2) - \frac{Q^2 \rho}{\pi^2 R^4} \qquad \textbf{2.16}$$

For very precise work the second term on the RHS should be multiplied by another constant K_2 which empirically depends on the design of the apparatus but is usually very close to 1·0.

The practical form of Poiseuille's equation for a relatively short tube then acquires the formidable appearance of

$$Q = \frac{(P_1 - P_2) - \dfrac{Q^2 \rho K_2}{\pi^2 R^4} \cdot \pi R^4}{8\mu\,(L + K_1 R)} \qquad \textbf{2.17}$$

where $K_1 =$ approx. 1·64 and $K_2 =$ approx. 1·0.

These corrections are important in relation to accurate work with viscometers or if using Poiseuille's law in short tubes such as hypodermic needles.

In the circulation there is never this condition of a stationary reservoir leading to steady laminar flow so that this correction does not apply. This special problem of the inlet length with pulsating flow in relation to the proximal aorta is discussed below (Ch. 5, p. 112).

(6) *The tube is rigid; the diameter does not vary with the internal pressure.*

Blood vessels are elastic structures and distend with increasing internal pressure (Ch. 10). The flow will not then be solely determined by the pressure-gradient. This distensibility is much less in the small vessels and is less predictable because the wall is largely composed of smooth muscle. This commonly constricts in response to an increase in the internal pressure (Bayliss, 1902; Folkow, 1964). It is only in such small vessels that the flow is sufficiently steady to apply Poiseuille's equation.

Wezler and Sinn (1953) considered radius to be a function of pressure and derived a pressure–flow relationship in vascular beds on this basis (a situation mathematically analogous to deriving Poiseuille flow for a compressible fluid, such as air). It has found little application by subsequent workers. Levy and Share (1953) and Levy et al. (1954), for example, found linear pressure–flow relations under a wide variety of conditions.

The assumptions underlying the Poiseuille equation which are discussed above can be seen to apply only approximately, at best, in the living circulation. Succeeding chapters (3–5) will examine the degree of these approximations in more detail. It must be admitted that using the steady flow criterion alone the equation is only directly applied, in the arterial tree, to vessels which are so small, numerous, and inaccessible that even their dimensions can only be roughly measured so that no hydrodynamic sophistication is possible. Nevertheless, there is no question that the understanding of the Poiseuille equation is fundamental to haemodynamics.

Baez, Lamport and Baez (1960) found that the diameter of capillaries and other minute vessels varied very little with changes of internal pressure in the range of 20–100 mm Hg. So rigidly did the capillaries (which have no smooth muscle) appear to behave that Fung, Zweifach and Intaglietta (1966) were led to postulate that the extracellular fluid has a gel-like structure which effectively strengthens the wall. Within the limits of accuracy of determination of such vessel dimensions under experimental conditions, it would appear that changes in internal pressure do not produce significant changes in size in very small vessels. The changes in arterial diameter with pulsatile pressure are discussed in Ch. 10.

TURBULENT FLOW

It was observed both by Hagen and by Poiseuille that the law relating pressure and flow ceased to be kept when there was a high rate of flow. This was rightly attributed to the breakdown of laminar flow and the onset of turbulent flow. It was not, however, until the work of Osborne Reynolds in 1883 and subsequently that the conditions determining the transition from laminar to turbulent flow were described precisely. Reynolds injected a filament of dye in the axis of a tube in which all irregularities at the inlet and of the wall had been eliminated. At low rates of flow, the motion of the fluid, as shown by the dye, was smooth and regular. Any disturbance introduced into the fluid was soon damped out. At higher rates of flow the liquid became more sensitive to disturbances. At a critical point a stage was reached when smooth flow could no longer be maintained and 'the motion of the fluid becomes wildly irregular and the tube appears to be filled with interlacing and constantly varying streams, crossing and recrossing the pipe' (Lamb, 1932).

The critical point was found to be dependent on the diameter of the tube, the mean velocity of the flow and the density and viscosity of the liquid. This was expressed as a dimensionless quantity, known as the Reynolds number which, when applied to flow in a circular pipe, is

$$Re = \frac{\bar{V}D\rho}{\mu} \qquad \textbf{2.18}$$

where $\bar{V}$ is the average velocity of flow across the pipe, D is the diameter of the tube, ρ is the density of the liquid and μ its viscosity. The fraction μ/ρ is known as the kinematic viscosity, written as ν. The CGS unit of kinematic viscosity is the *stokes* (cm^2/sec).

Reynolds formula is thus often expressed as

$$Re = \frac{\bar{V}D}{\nu} \qquad \textbf{2.19}$$

It will be seen that not only does an increase in average velocity cause turbulence, but also that at a given velocity of flow, turbulence will occur in large tubes before it will in small ones.

The fact that the characteristic property of the fluid concerned in determining the stability of laminar flow is the kinematic viscosity, gives rise to some apparently surprising results. Thus, a gas like air might appear to be more easily disturbed than blood, or even water, but is actually more stable. Its absolute viscosity is, of course, much less than water (at 20°C, air, 0·0181 cP; water, 1·00 cP) but because the density of air is proportionately lower its kinematic viscosity is actually some 10 times as great as water at 20°C (air, $10·5 \times 10^{-2}$; water, $1·007 \times 10^{-2}$ stokes). Furthermore, as the viscosity of gases increases with temperature while that of liquids decreases the difference is greater at body temperature. The kinematic viscosity of blood at body temperature (38°C) is about $3·8 \times 10^{-2}$ stokes and that of water is $0·686 \times 10^{-2}$ stokes, while that of air (at 40°C) is $16·9 \times 10^{-2}$ stokes (Goldstein, 1938). Thus, at body temperature a steady laminar stream of air in a bronchus, for example, would be stable at a velocity four times greater than that of blood in a blood vessel of comparable size. This also serves to emphasize that in terms of hydrodynamics both blood and water are thought of as liquids of low viscosity.

A certain amount of confusion arises in physiological literature by the use of radius in place of diameter in this equation, especially as quoted figures are often compared without reference to different ways of computing the figures. The general formula for Reynolds number for a channel of any shape is

$$Re = \frac{4m\overline{V}}{v} \text{ (Goldstein, 1938)} \qquad \textbf{2.20}$$

where m is the 'mean hydraulic depth' which is defined as the cross-sectional area divided by the perimeter. Thus, for a circle

$$m = \frac{R}{2} \text{ and } 4m = \text{Diameter}$$

Hence, this formula (eqn. 2.18 or 2.19) is used throughout in the present work in order to conform to standard hydrodynamic practice and the values of other workers are converted, where necessary, to comparable values.

(In the literature of hydrodynamics the use of what may be termed 'local' Reynolds, numbers at the surface of suspended particles, etc., will also be found. The formula is of the general form $Re = Vd/v$, where V is defined as the free stream velocity and d may be the diameter of a sphere or a cylinder; it may also be defined as the distance along a boundary layer, as in an inlet length (p. 108), or even the thickness of a boundary layer (Kaufmann, 1963, p. 277). The detailed development of such problems in flow stability in relation to irregularities of the wall is beyond the scope of this book but some practical applications are discussed in Ch. 4, p. 90).

The critical value of the Reynolds number in a pipe is usually stated to be 2,000 (a later value of 2,300, due to Schiller, is thought to be more general). This, however, is an experimentally determined value and is very dependent on the conditions of the experiment. Reynolds called it the 'lower critical value.' With very carefully controlled flow from an undisturbed reservoir into the tube, Reynolds himself was able to maintain laminar flow up to a value of 12,000 and much higher values (up to 40,000—Birkhoff, 1960) have been attained. A value close to 2,000 for the lower critical Reynolds number in blood (when calculated from diameter) has been determined by Coulter and Pappenheimer (1949).

The standard critical Reynolds number of 2,000 is obtained when there are disturbed conditions in the reservoir. With such conditions it is difficult to cause turbulence in a regular tube at figures below this value. Other disturbances are found, however, at lower values. The period of laminar flow has been described by Schiller (see Goldstein, 1938, Ch. 7) as falling into three regimes. The first is the period of completely undisturbed flow with the streamlines running parallel to the sides of the tube. These streams begin to exhibit a wavy motion at higher Reynolds numbers which is described as the second regime, and these oscillations get larger and vortices start forming at the border and are carried down the tube. The third regime is that with vortex formation, and as they become larger and more frequent this merges into a condition of turbulence. The stage at which these conditions of disturbed flow, heralds of approaching breakdown of the flow pattern, appear, depends on the degree of disturbance in the reservoir or on roughnesses at the entry of the pipe. Naumann recorded a Reynolds number of 280 for the beginning of the second regime with a sharp entrance orifice in the pipe, and White and Davis a similar value with a very disturbed reservoir. The third regime usually begins at $Re = 1,600$ but may be considerably earlier with these other disturbing factors at work. This vortex regime at Reynolds values below 2,000 is of considerable importance in the living animal because of the variety of disturbing effects on flow (which are discussed in Ch. 4).

The mere evaluation of the Reynolds number is not, of itself, a proof of the existence of laminar or turbulent flow. The best way to demonstrate turbulence is to measure the pressure–flow relationship and demonstrate that this deviates from that of laminar flow. Whereas with unvarying laminar flow the pressure drop per unit length (pressure-gradient) varies linearly with the rate of flow, when turbulence is present it varies approximately with a higher power of the rate of flow. In a pressure–flow diagram this shows as a discontinuity (Fig. 2.4). In other words, a greater pressure-gradient is required to maintain turbulent flow than is required for laminar flow. The conditions for

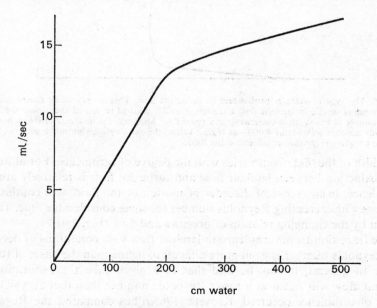

Fig. 2.4. The relation between pressure-gradient and flow in a pipe. At low rates of flow there is a linear relationship and the flow is laminar. The inflection in the curve indicates the onset of turbulence; turbulent flow requires a larger pressure-gradient than the equivalent laminar flow.

turbulent flow have not been precisely determined in hydrodynamics (Ch. 1) because it is not possible to give a precise description of the motion of the liquid. The fluid particles in addition to flowing along the line of the tube pursue random pathways in other directions and small eddies or vortices are formed. Thus extra energy is required to maintain the increased movement of fluid that does not directly contribute to the forward flow; that is, an increased pressure is required to maintain it. Whereas in laminar flow $Q \propto \Delta P$, when the flow becomes turbulent, the relation becomes $Q^n \propto \Delta P$ where n is greater than 1, and increases to 2 with increasing Reynolds number (Goldstein, 1938). Thus, the term 'turbulence' does not specify the flow condition exactly in the way that the term 'laminar flow' does, but indicates a class of regimes which are spoken of as having varying degrees of turbulences.

Where measurements of the pressure-gradient and flow are not practicable the type of flow may be observed from the distribution of injected dye, as Reynolds did in his pioneer experiments. Whereas such dye will be distributed in a parabolic velocity profile in steady laminar flow, in turbulent flow the dye is seen to be mixed across the tube, although there will still be a region of shear near the wall (Fig. 2.5). The extent to which this region of shear extends and

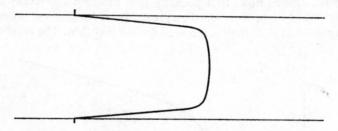

Fig. 2.5. The type of velocity profile seen in turbulent flow. This is very much flatter than the corresponding profile in laminar flow but there is still a marked region of shear near the walls. This example is based on a cinematograph record by McDonald and Helps (1954) where the Reynolds number was about 4,000—at higher values the velocity distribution would doubtless become progressively more equal across the tube.

the width of the 'flat' front varies with the degree of turbulence. For although the distinction between laminar flow and turbulent flow is relatively abrupt, turbulence, in the sense of disorder of motion of the fluid, will continue to increase with increasing Reynolds number for some considerable time. This is shown by the changing relation of pressure and flow (Fig. 2.4).

The transition from turbulence to laminar flow with conditions of decreasing Reynolds number is even more difficult to define than the onset of turbulence. In general, it may be said that in a given tube the restoration of laminar flow will occur at a lower Reynolds number than that at which the onset of turbulence occurred. Krovetz (1965a) has compared the Reynolds number at transition, with both increasing and decreasing flow velocities. A typical pair of values was Re = 2,400 for transition from laminar to turbulent flow and 2,100 for transition back to laminar (using dye pattern as the criterion). As variation in the rate of flow is found in all blood vessels in which the Reynolds number is in the critical region, this point is of considerable interest. As stated above, disturbances generated in truly laminar flow will be damped out and this is commonly used to define turbulence as the condition of steady flow where a disturbance, once started, will increase in size until it involves the whole body of the liquid. The consideration of turbulence in pulsating flow such as is found in arteries and the larger veins is, therefore, somewhat difficult. If a disturbance in the flow is short-lasting one cannot know whether its transient character is due to a regime of instability that is too brief to produce turbulence throughout the liquid, or whether the flow is inherently stable and hence has damped out the disturbance.

The problem of definition of turbulence in pulsatile flow arises because the accepted definition in hydrodynamics is in terms of steady flow. This definition states that a flow is turbulent if any initial disturbance that is created increases with time until it involves all the flowing fluid; conversely, if such a disturbance decays with time then the flow is stable. In pulsatile flow in blood vessels, large vortices are often seen which may cause a disturbance across the whole lumen, as indicated by dye-dispersion. With a change in flow rate, the vortex will disappear but the dispersion of dye remains. Helps and McDonald (1954a) proposed that the term 'disturbed' flow should be used for situations where the flow is neither clearly laminar nor clearly turbulent. This term has also been adopted by Yellin (1966) in a detailed study of the transition process between laminar and turbulent flow under pulsatile conditions. The prevalence of various flow-patterns in the circulation is discussed in Ch. 4.

From the practical point of view in studies of the circulation the importance of determining whether flow is turbulent or laminar will be considered under the following heads in subsequent chapters. First, the mixing effect of turbulence, or related disturbances of flow, is relevant to the question of the composition of blood samples as representative of the blood in the vessel or heart chamber from which they are withdrawn. Second, the applicability of hydrodynamic equations relating pressure to flow is diminished if the flow is not laminar. This deviation may not be as great in pulsatile flow as in steady flow (see Chs. 5 and 6), but is clearly of some importance in detailed hydrodynamic studies. Third, the energy dissipated in disturbed, or turbulent, flow will appear in part as acoustic energy and thus becomes significant in assessing the causation of heart sounds and cardiovascular murmurs (p. 82).

BERNOULLI'S THEOREM

Up to this point we have concerned ourselves with the behaviour of viscous liquids. It was mentioned briefly that Daniel Bernoulli (1700–82) developed the theoretical behaviour of 'ideal' fluids, ignoring the forces of viscosity. One theorem he developed is of importance in the hydrodynamics of the circulation and must be considered briefly here.

Bernoulli's theorem may be deduced from the principle of the conservation of energy (Newman and Searle, 1957). If we image a section AB of a tube of changing diameter with a flow of liquid passing through it, then the amount passing into the section of the tube at A must be equal to that passing out at B. If the cross-sections of the tube at the two ends are A_1 and A_2 and the velocities are V_1 and V_2 respectively, then the volume entering per unit time is A_1V_1 and

$$A_1V_1 = A_2V_2$$

If the pressure at either end is p_1 and p_2 then the work done on the fluid entering AB per unit time is $p_1A_1V_1$, and on that leaving is $p_2A_2V_2$. The fluid also has kinetic energy (which is $\frac{1}{2}mV^2$). At the point A

$$m = \rho A_1 V_1 \ (\rho = \text{density})$$

so that the kinetic energy at the point of entry is

$$\tfrac{1}{2} \cdot V_1^2 \cdot \rho \cdot A_1 V_1$$

If there is a difference in height between the two ends there will be a net external gravitational force acting on the mass of fluid; for heights, h_1 and h_2, this will be $g . \rho . A_1 V_1 h_1$ and $g . \rho . A_2 V_2 h_2$ respectively.

The total energy at the entry will be equal to the energy at the outflow so that

$$p_1A_1V_1 + \rho A_1V_1(\tfrac{1}{2}V_1^2 + g \cdot h_1) = p_2A_2V_2 + \rho A_2V_2(\tfrac{1}{2}V_2^2 + g \cdot h_2) \qquad \textbf{2.21}$$

which can be reduced to

$$(p_1 - p_2) + \tfrac{1}{2}\rho(V_1^2 - V_2^2) + \rho . g . (h_1 - h_2) = \text{constant}$$

which can be simplified, by dividing through by the density, to

$$\frac{p}{\rho} + \frac{V^2}{2} + gz = C \qquad \textbf{2.22}$$

where z is the difference in height $(h_1 - h_2)$ and is commonly zero when considering a horizontal tube; $V^2 = (V_1^2 - V_2^2)$ and $p = (p_1 - p_2)$. The energy thus consists of three parts; the pressure energy, p, the kinetic energy $\rho V^2/2$ and the potential energy in a gravitational field, ρgz.

It can be seen that if the velocity is increased in a horizontal tube then the lateral pressure must be correspondingly decreased. This effect is particularly apparent at a constriction in a vessel, and is applied in devices as various as the common laboratory water-pump and the orifice, or Venturi, meters that have been used for measuring blood flow. Provided that the conditions of applying the theorem are such that the changes in kinetic energy are large compared to the viscous forces the latter may be neglected. With steady flow in a tube system whose geometry is known the pressure head representing the viscous losses can be calculated from the Poiseuille equation and allowed for when measuring the pressure energy.

The inverse of the situation in the meters mentioned above occurs when a solid obstruction is placed in the flowing liquid. At one point on the front surface the velocity will be zero and this is called the 'stagnation point'. Here the pressure will be increased by the amount of the kinetic energy, and the increase is called the 'stagnation' pressure. The actual pressure recorded is the 'total' pressure, p_t; thus

$$p_t = p + \tfrac{1}{2}\rho V^2 \qquad\qquad \textbf{2.23}$$

where V will be the velocity of the lamina or streamline of flow which is brought to rest. It will, therefore, vary according to the position of the stagnation point in respect of the velocity profile. This is the principle of the Pitot tube (p. 231). It is also the source of error in measuring arterial pressure with a catheter orifice facing in the direction of the flow (p. 232).

Bernoulli's theorem can be applied to unsteady flows. The expression is derived from the general case by considering the fluctuations of flow as variables in respect of position s along a streamline in respect of time (Kaufmann, 1963) written as

$$\frac{\partial}{\partial s}\left(\frac{V^2}{2} + \frac{P}{\rho} + gz\right) + \frac{\partial v}{\partial t} = 0$$

By integrating along the streamline at constant t we obtain

$$\frac{V^2}{2} + \frac{p}{\rho} + gz + \int_0^S \frac{dv}{dt}\cdot ds = \text{constant} \qquad\qquad \textbf{2.24}$$

The use of the theorem is not common in haemodynamics; although viscous effects can be incorporated, as pointed out above for steady flow, it has been preferred to derive non-steady flows from the general form of eqn. 2.15—see eqn. 5.1. These derivations are set out in Chs. 5 and 6.

THE EFFECT OF CHANGE IN THE SIZE OF THE VASCULAR BED

We have already considered the relations between the pressure-gradient, rate of flow and internal lumen for steady flow in a straight tube. Changes in lumen of arteries, however, are virtually all associated with the occurrence of branches. These branches are, individually, narrower than the parent trunk but the total cross-sectional area nearly always increases when branches are given off. It is, therefore, of interest to see how a change in the size of the channel due to the occurrence of branches will affect the rate of flow, the Reynolds number and the pressure-gradient. This can be simply derived for steady flow but, of course, this makes it of somewhat academic interest in a consideration of the larger arteries because pulsatile flow has quite different pressure–flow relationships. Using analogous electrical terms we are here calculating the changes in *resistance* in the vascular network, whereas we really need to know the changes in *impedance*. The latter problem is more difficult so that it is worth considering the simplest conditions first. These conditions apply in general throughout the venous system and also approximately in small arteries (Ch. 6). The change in impedance at points of arterial branching is considered in Ch. 12.

Take a main vessel, cross-sectional area A_1, that divides into n branches of equal size and each of cross-sectional area, A_2 (Fig. 2.6). If the total vascular

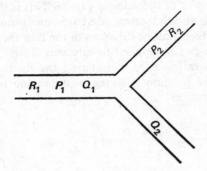

Fig. 2.6. A junction with two equal branches.

bed changes by a factor d, i.e. $dA_1 = (n \times A_2)$ we can describe the behaviour of the bed in terms of the ratio d without considering actual cross-sectional areas.

Let the pressure-gradient, $(P - P')/L$ or ΔP, in the main trunk be P_1 and that in the branches P_2, similarly Q_1 and Q_2 the respective volume rates of flow, R_1 and R_2 the radii, and V_1 and V_2 the average linear velocities of flow.

The only determining condition is that the rate of flow into and out of the system must be equal or

$$Q_1 = nQ_2$$

Since the rate of flow is the mean velocity times the cross-sectional area of the tube

$$Q_1 = V_1 \pi R_1^2 = nV_2 \pi R_2^2$$

or

$$\frac{V_1}{V_2} = \frac{nR_2^2}{R_1^2}$$

By definition,

$$d = \frac{n\pi R_2^2}{\pi R_1^2}$$

$$\therefore \frac{V_1}{V_2} = d \qquad \textbf{2.25}$$

that is to say, that the mean velocity of flow in the branches will be less by a factor of d whatever the number of branches.

If the velocity of flow and the radius are both less in the branches obviously the Reynolds number will decrease if the vascular bed increases.

$$Re_1 = \frac{2R_1 V_1}{v} \quad \text{and} \quad Re_2 = \frac{2R_2 V_2}{v}$$

or

$$\frac{Re_1}{Re_2} = \frac{R_1 V_1}{R_2 V_2} = d \cdot \frac{R_1}{R_2} = d\sqrt{\frac{n}{d}}$$

$$= \sqrt{(nd)} \qquad \textbf{2.26}$$

As n is always greater than 1 the Reynolds number will remain unchanged only if there is a narrowing of the bed so that $d = 1/n$.

The same reasoning applied to a constriction in an unbranched tube, i.e., $n = 1$ and $d < 1$ the Reynolds number will increase continuously as the tube gets narrower *provided* there is a sufficient head of pressure to maintain a constant rate of flow. In the circulation the maximum pressure drop across the constriction is determined by the arterio-venous pressure difference. When this maximum is reached further constriction will cause a reduction in flow. The Reynolds number thus rises at first and then begins to fall—an effect well demonstrated by Dawes, Mott and Widdicombe (1955) during constriction of the ductus arteriosus.

In a similar way, from Poiseuille's equation, we may compare the pressure-gradients in the main trunk and the branches

$$Q_1 = \frac{P_1 \pi R_1^4}{8\mu} = nQ_2 = \frac{nP_2 \pi R_2^4}{8\mu}$$

so that

$$\frac{P_1}{P_2} = \frac{nR_2^4}{R_1^4}$$

and as

$$\frac{R_2^2}{R_1^2} = \frac{d}{n}$$

$$\frac{P_1}{P_2} = \frac{d^2}{n} \qquad \textbf{2.27}$$

from which we see the interesting result that for steady flow the pressure-gradient (the 'vascular resistance') remains the same only if

$$d = \sqrt{n} \text{ and increases when } d < \sqrt{n}.$$

As the minimum value of $n = 2$, the pressure-drop will be greater in the branches of a bifurcation unless the cross-sectional area of the vascular bed increases by a factor of more than 1·414.

The average value for d that is often quoted is 1·26 at a major arterial bifurcation, and this appears to originate from the work of Blum (1919) and was used by Hess (1927). In this situation, we can see that the velocity in the branches (eqn. 2.25) will be 1/1·26, or 0·8, of that in the parent trunk; the Reynolds number will also decrease (eqn. 2.26) by the factor $1/(2 \times 1·26)^{1/2}$, or 0·63; the pressure-gradient on the other hand will increase by the factor $2/1·26^2$, or 1·26.

The relation between pressure-gradient and flow is commonly expressed as the fluid resistance (see following section); if the resistance is expressed as the ratio of pressure and volume flow (eqn. 2.30), i.e. P/Q and is indicated by K, then $K_1 = P_1/Q_1$, and from eqn. 2.27

$$\frac{K_1}{K_2} = \frac{P_1}{P_2} \cdot \frac{Q_2}{Q_1} = \frac{d^2}{n} \cdot \frac{1}{n} = \frac{d^2}{n^2} \qquad \textbf{2.28}$$

If the resistance is expressed in terms of the average flow velocity and indicated by k we have $k_1 = P_1/V_1$ and from eqns. 2.25 and 2.27 we obtain

$$\frac{k_1}{k_2} = \frac{P_1}{P_2} \cdot \frac{V_2}{V_1} = \frac{d^2}{n} \cdot \frac{1}{d} = \frac{d}{n} \qquad \textbf{2.29}$$

Therefore, the fluid resistance will remain unchanged in an individual branch beyond a subdivision only if the total cross-sectional area of the branches is larger than that of the parent trunk by a factor that is the number of branches—which at a minimum is two. This applies equally whether the resistance is measured in relation to the volume flow or to the flow velocity. As no one has ever observed an increase in the size of the vascular bed by as large a factor as 2, at any bifurcation, it follows that the vascular resistance measured in each branch will always increase.

If, however, the vascular resistance of all branches is taken together then the volume flow is the same on either side of the junction and the corresponding resistance will vary as the pressure-gradient (eqn. 2.29). As pointed out above this means that at a bifurcation the cross-sectional area must increase by a factor of $\sqrt{2}$ for the resistance (in terms of volume flow) to remain unchanged.

It is interesting to note that, in all the relations worked out above, the only one that is determined by the total cross-sectional area of the bed alone is the velocity of flow. The measurement of the mean velocity on either side of a vascular subdivision could therefore be used as a measure of the change in the size of the vascular bed in the living animal. The dimensions of the vessel in the living animal is the subject of considerable controversy and is discussed at the end of this chapter. In a more general way, the changes in mean velocity can be used to indicate where the main changes of size of the bed occur. For example, in the dog the mean velocity in the proximal aorta is usually 15–20 cm/sec and in the femoral artery is about 10–12 cm/sec. This implies that the vascular bed measured at arteries of the same order as the femoral has increased by about 50 per cent compared with the aorta. In the capillaries, however, where the mean velocity is about 0·05 cm/sec there must be an increase of the vascular bed to 300–400 times that of the aorta. Such generalizations are, of course, only approximate as they imply an equal degree of arteriolar constriction in all the main vascular beds so that blood flow is not being shunted preferentially through any one of them.

The consideration of the division of flow between unequal branches cannot be satisfied in such a general way because there are a different set of pressure-flow relations for each (Fig. 2.7). As before, $Q_1 = Q_2 + Q_3$, and from Poiseuille's law we can see that

$$\frac{Q_2}{Q_3} = \frac{P_2 R_2{}^4}{P_3 R_3{}^4}$$

P is the pressure-gradient, that is, the fall in pressure per unit length and unless we know the length and fall in pressure-gradient in both channels the

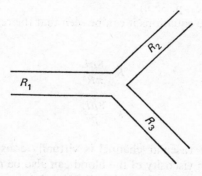

Fig. 2.7. A division into unequal branches.

flow down each branch cannot be predicted. It is usual to assume that as the pressure in each branch will fall to the same capillary pressure, $P_2 = P_3$, but this makes the further assumption that the overall lengths of the two branches are the same. If P_2 is equal to P_3 the relative flows in the branches will, of course, be proportional to the fourth power of their radii, R_2 and R_3.

THE MEASUREMENT OF PERIPHERAL RESISTANCE

The application of Poiseuille's formula (eqn. 2.6) to any set of blood vessels, in the way it was used in the preceding section, requires a knowledge of the dimensions of those vessels. When considering the vascular system of the body, or of one of its regions, we do not have this information. The formula can, however, be simplified by writing

$$P_1 - P_2 = KQ = k\overline{V} \qquad \textbf{2.30}$$

and from analogy with Ohm's law the terms K, or k, are called the fluid resistance because the pressure-drop is analogous with the potential difference and the blood flow with the current. It is usual to calculate the resistance in terms of volume flow; but, as was seen in the previous section, it is often more illuminating to compare the velocity of flow in various vessels, so that we will also consider the 'velocity resistance'. Pursuing the analogy, the Poiseuille formula only applies to steady flow, the equivalent of direct current. In arterial channels where the flow is pulsatile this might be thought to be inapplicable. Pulsatile arterial flow, however, always has a steady flow component—the mean flow—and it is possible to apply the direct current concept to this mean flow. The corresponding pressure–flow relation for the oscillatory flow is, using alternating current theory, called the fluid impedance (see Ch. 6). (In the wider implications of this analogy it is often more useful to take velocity as the analogue and so, at the risk of confusion, it is here also applied to resistance; the convenience of this measure is more apparent in comparing impedances, p. 355.)

From the Poiseuille equations it can be seen that the resistance in eqn. 2.30 is expressed by

$$K = \frac{8\mu L}{\pi R^4} \qquad \textbf{2.31}$$

$$k = \frac{8\mu L}{R^2} \qquad \textbf{2.32}$$

The length of any vascular channel is virtually constant for anatomical reasons and the mean viscosity of the blood can also be regarded as constant (although as will be seen in Ch. 3 the viscosity does vary with the radius in small vessels). The vascular resistance is thus very largely determined by the radius of the vessels. In the complete vascular bed of, say, one limb, the total fluid resistance may be regarded as the resistances of, respectively, the arteries, the arterioles, the capillaries and the veins in series. As the resistance is proportional to the drop in mean pressure it is apparent that the resistance of the arterioles constitutes the largest proportion of the whole. Thus, the mean arterial pressure is about 100 mm Hg and has fallen very little in the smallest arteries in which it has been measured. In the capillaries it is generally agreed to be about 30–34 mm Hg at the proximal end and 12–15 mm Hg at the distal end; most of this fall (up to 60 mm Hg) will occur in the 5 mm or so immediately proximal to the capillaries. The pressure in the large veins will only be a few mm Hg so that of a total pressure drop of 100 mm Hg, up to 60 per cent may occur in the arterioles, about 15 per cent both in the capillaries and in the veins (totalling 30 per cent) and about 10 per cent in the arterial system. The total peripheral resistance is thus dominated by the calibre of the arterioles but the other components of the vascular bed are by no means negligible. The fact that the arterioles can be actively altered in size by physiological mechanisms has focused special attention on their contribution to the peripheral vascular resistance. Indeed, under controlled conditions, the measurement of the resistance is a useful and simple way of studying vasomotor activity. Nevertheless, it is regrettable that the term 'peripheral resistance' has so often been used as if it were synonymous with 'arteriolar resistance'.

The value of the concept of peripheral, or vascular, resistance, has been questioned by some authors. The basis of most of their comment has been due partly to the somewhat slipshod way that approximations have been introduced without assessment of the consequent errors, and partly to verbal short cuts such as regarding the arteriolar vessels as the whole of the peripheral resistance. In addition, it has been criticized as being an artificial, or abstract, idea, useful only for manipulating experimental data. To some extent this is true but only to the extent that the concept of electrical resistance is abstract—for it also only expresses the relationship between the current and potential drop in a circuit. Similarly the measurement of changes in the resistance of a circuit can only give net, or overall, effect and cannot distinguish changes of individual components.

The measurements that need to be made are basically the same in all cases— the mean pressure at the beginning and the end of the vascular bed to be studied and the total flow. For the total vascular resistance of the body this means that in place of eqn. 2.30 we can write

(Mean aortic pressure – mean right atrial pressure) cardiac output = total peripheral resistance

As the pressure in the great veins is very small in comparison with the aortic pressure it is usually taken as zero, and the formula is often rendered as

$$ABP = CO \times TPR$$

In smaller regions of the systemic bed the approximation of taking the venous pressure as zero may introduce appreciable errors. In the pulmonary circulation the arterial pressure is much lower and left atrial pressure probably higher; it is then very inaccurate to estimate vascular resistance without measuring the atrial pressure.

The units in which the peripheral resistance is expressed have varied with different authors. The Peripheral Resistance Unit (PRU) introduced by H. D. Green is in the empirical units of mm Hg per ml/min; in practice, this works out in numbers of convenient dimensions in regional vascular beds, but as with all arbitrary units, is difficult to convert or correlate with other dimensions. In standard physical units the corresponding units are dyn sec/cm^5 if volume flow is used, or dyn sec/cm^3 if flow velocity is used.

Taking some average figures for the human subject we can calculate some representative values.

(a) *Total peripheral resistance.* If the cardiac output is 4·5 L/min (75 cm^3/sec), the mean arterial b.p. 100 mm Hg and the mean velocity of flow is 15 cm/sec (i.e. R is c. 1·25 cm)

$$\text{then } K = \frac{100}{4,500} = 0.022 \text{ PRU}$$

$$\text{or } K = \frac{10.0 \times 13.6 \times 980}{75} = 1.78 \times 10^3 \text{ dyn sec/cm}^5$$

$$\text{or } k = \frac{10.0 \times 13.6 \times 980}{15} = 8.89 \times 10^3 \text{ dyn sec/cm}^3$$

(b) *Peripheral resistance of femoral vascular bed.* If volume flow is 225 cm^3/min (3·75 cm^3/sec) and the mean velocity is 12 cm/sec

$$\text{then } K = \frac{100}{225} = 0.44 \text{ PRU}$$

$$\text{or } K = \frac{10.0 \times 13.6 \times 980}{3.75} = 3.55 \times 10^4 \text{ dyn sec/cm}^3$$

$$\text{or } k = 11.1 \times 10^3 \text{ dyn sec/cm}^3$$

(c) *Vascular resistance of a single capillary.* Taking the following values for a typical capillary we may obtain comparative values for the smallest vessels: pressure 30–15 mm Hg, mean velocity 0·5 mm/sec and a diameter of 10 μm.

$$K = 5 \times 10^{11} \text{ dyn sec/cm}^5$$

and
$$k = 4 \times 10^5 \text{ dyn sec/cm}^3$$

(From the same figures it may be computed that there must be a total of 2×10^9 capillaries of this size and that their total surface area is 32 m^2. The femoral artery values taken above are scaled up proportionately from values observed in the dog.)

Thus, the vascular resistance may be estimated for a single channel or for the whole vascular bed (from the point of measurement of arterial pressure to the point in the veins where the pressure was zero, i.e. atmospheric).

The contribution of the various grades of vessels to the peripheral resistance has been studied by various workers. The estimate given above (p. 42) is, of course, very approximate and the pressure-drop across various sections will vary considerably with vasomotor activity. It is also of interest to know whether a change in mean pressure can alter the peripheral resistance by causing a passive change in the calibre of the small vessels. Read, Kuida and Johnson (1958) measured the total peripheral resistance in dogs that were being perfused by a pump so that the total flow was accurately known and found that a rise in venous pressure consistently caused a fall in the resistance. At its largest this was about 20 per cent change in PR for an increase of 20 mm Hg in venous pressure and a fall of some 60 per cent with a rise in venous pressure to 60 mm Hg. This is thought to be mainly due to a dilatation of the small venous channels although the arterial pressure increased a corresponding amount. Levy, Brind, Brandlin and Phillips (1954) used the Fick principle to measure the cardiac output and found that, when the baroreceptors were denervated, the peripheral resistance remained constant with changes in mean arterial pressure. This suggests that the arterioles do not distend passively with an increase in pressure. When the baroceptors' reflex pathways were intact a rise in arterial pressure caused a marked fall in resistance indicating arteriolar dilatation. In the vascular bed of a leg that was being perfused Phillips, Brind and Levy (1955) measured the resistance when both arterial and venous pressures were changed so that the pressure-gradient remained the same but the transmural pressure, i.e. the distending pressure, was altered. They found evidence that increase of transmural pressure caused a fall in resistance. In a later paper Levy (1958) found that this change was much more marked when arterial pressures were changed than when the changes were on the venous side. This finding seems to be at variance with the previous findings of Levy et al. (1954) that changing arterial pressure did not alter the total peripheral resistance. It also differs from the results of Read et al. (1958) where a rise in venous pressure consistently caused a distinct fall in resistance. It is possible that the vascular beds of various regions differ in this respect. Final agreement is far from being reached on this topic as other workers, notably Folkow (e.g. Folkow and Löfving, 1956) have produced much experimental evidence that a rise in arteriolar pressure causes vasoconstriction because of the myogenic response of the smooth muscle in the wall (Folkow, 1964).

Measurement of the peripheral resistance is not, therefore, a very good analytical method for distinguishing the behaviour of individual sections of a vascular bed. For separating the effects of changes in flow or vasomotor activity, however, it is simple and direct. As an example some results of Leusen, Demeester and Bouckaert (1954) may be used. In a series of dogs a fall in the pressure of their isolated carotid sinuses caused an increase in mean arterial blood pressure from 125 to 194 mm Hg (55·2 per cent). At the same time the cardiac output increased from 3·3 to 4·3 l/min (30·3 per cent) and the total peripheral resistance from 3,140 to 3,750 dyn sec/cm^5 (19·4 per cent). It is clear that the increase in cardiac output played a greater part in increasing the blood pressure than vasoconstriction did. After a haemorrhage of 10 per cent of their estimated blood volume the corresponding increases were: arterial pressure, 72·5 per cent, cardiac output, 26·3 per cent, and peripheral resistance, 38·5 per cent. The rise in pressure was then due more to vasomotor activity than to the increase in cardiac output. These figures alone, however, cannot give any information as to which parts of the vascular bed have constricted. From general knowledge it is assumed that it will largely be in the arterioles, but venous constriction may well play a part in the response to sinus hypotension. Such constriction would cause an increase in cardiac output but would also increase the total resistance, although there is little information on which we can estimate what proportion of the total increase this would be.

THE DIMENSIONS OF THE ARTERIAL TREE

Nothing demonstrates the difference between applying hydrodynamics to a man-made system and to the living array of arteries so dramatically as the uncertainty about the size of the lumen of blood vessels, the thickness of their walls, and, in the smaller vessels, their length; in inanimate tubes these dimensions are known with great precision. The problems arise, in part, from the range in size of individuals of a species and also from the fact that functioning arteries are elastic tubes subject to a distending pressure. The first factor requires the measurement of as many vessels as possible in the same individual and this is most easily done after death; this, however, removes the distending pressure with a consequent diminution in size. As the elastic properties of the wall are non-uniformly distributed (Ch. 10) this, in turn, will alter the ratios of the cross-sectional areas at each point of branching. The use of controlled-setting plastics (or resins) in the past ten years (which has provided a means whereby internal casts of the arterial tree can be made) has improved the situation. Ideally they can be injected after death at a normal arterial pressure which is held steady until the casting material is set and measurements of the internal bore made on the complete cast. To date, few such studies have been made and the measurements (considered below) have been confined to the major arteries. For all the smaller branches down to the capillaries their small size and dispersal within the tissues has made us rely on painstaking measurements on histological sections using a microscope. Radiology with injected contrast media has been used by a few workers, e.g. Reynolds et al. (1952) and, in the cat, by Arndt, Stegall and Wicke (1971). The large numbers of X-ray arteriographs that are made annually in all major medical centres would suggest a large source of data which has not, to my knowledge, been systemically organized.

In view of the complexity of the vascular network it is necessary to be selective. The overall pattern of branching with considerations of total cross-sectional area, pressure drop, resistance and flow rates was considered in detail by Hess (1927), largely based on the extensive German literature up to that time. The total cross-sectional area has long been known to increase greatly by the time the level of the capillaries has been reached; this was shown above (p. 41) in relation to the fall in flow velocity and the rise in resistance in a number of parallel channels. An approximate curve of this change in the aorta and its arterial branches is shown in Fig. 2.8 which was

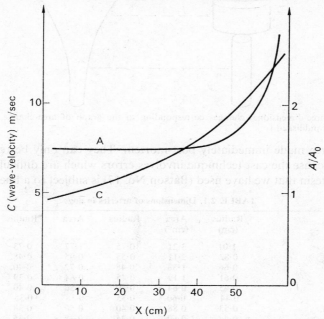

Fig. 2.8. Diagram to show the relative change (A/A_0) in cross-sectional area in the arterial tree with distance measured from the aortic valves. The line marked C shows the change in wave-velocity that occurs. (Gessner, unpublished.)

drawn by Gessner (unpublished); on the same graph the progressive increase of wave-velocity indicating a decrease in distensibility (Chs. 10 and 14) with distance from the heart is also indicated. Many of the wave-velocity values here have, indeed, been derived from distensibility measurements made with strain-gauge calipers (Ch. 10). In terms of a model analogue Gessner showed that, three-dimensionally, this looks like a loudspeaker horn, and, being Swiss, he named it the 'Alpenhorn' model (Fig. 2.9). Because it is made up of parallel arrays of small tubes the flow resistance also rises in a similar fashion to the increase in area. It was introduced as a corrective to many electrical analogue models which treat the aorta as a tapering tube (in the sense of getting progressively narrower) which, as will be seen below, is only true if the branches are ignored. A detailed numerical survey into the cross-sectional area data down to the smallest vessels has been made by Iberall (1967) which is discussed below.

The data on aortic and major arterial dimensions which is considered here is from the excellent paper of Patel *et al.* (1963) and from unpublished results from my own laboratory. These measurements were made on casts of the

C

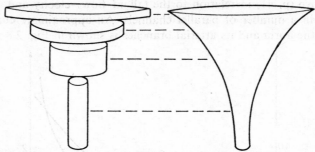

Fig. 2.9. Three-dimensional changes corresponding to the graph of area-change in Fig. 2.8. (Gessner, unpublished.)

arterial tree made immediately post-mortem. They can only be regarded as guides because the cast technique involves errors which are difficult to allow for. The resin that we have used (Batson No. 17) is subject to a linear shrink-

TABLE 2.1. Dimensions of arteries in dogs

Artery	Radius (cm)	Area (cm²)	Radius	Area	Radius	Area
Asc. aorta	1·01	3·21	0·75	1·77	0·73	1·77
Thor. A I	0·82	2·11	0·55	0·95	0·48	0·78
Thor. A II	0·66	1·38	0·48	0·72	0·40	0·52
Thor. A III	0·61	1·19	0·45	0·64	0·39	0·51
Abd. A I	0·45	0·64	0·40	0·50	0·40	0·52
Abd. A II	0·44	0·60	0·35	0·38	0·35	0·39
Brach. ceph.	0·53	0·88	0·40	0·50	0·38	0·49
L. Subcl.	0·44	0·60	0·35	0·38	0·35	0·41
Coeliac	0·29	0·27	0·23	0·17	0·25	0·21
Sup. mes.	0·34	0·35	0·23	0·17	0·23	0·18
Renal (2)	0·19	0·12	0·15	0·07	0·19	0·12
Iliac (2)	0·23	0·17	0·24	0·18	0·23	0·13
Sacral	0·23	0·17	0·20	0·13	0·18	0·10
Int. cost. (20)	0·09	0·029	0·06	0·01	0·06	0·01
Inf. mes.	——	——	0·10	0·03	0·12	0·05
Lumbar (8)	——	——	0·10	0·03	0·08	0·02
Comm. carot.	——	——	0·20	0·13	0·25	0·20
Vertebral (2)	——	——	0·12	0·05	——	——
R. subcl.	——	——	0·28	0·25	——	——
Axillary	——	——	0·20	0·13	——	——
Femoral	——	——	0·15	0·07	——	——

Average values of the radius and internal cross-sectional area for three sets of data measured in dogs. The left-hand set is taken from Patel *et al.* (1963) and is based on external measurements made with strain-gauges combined with casts of the vessels. The other two sets are from two different series of plastic casts, previously unpublished; the central sets were made in collaboration with Dr. E. O. Attinger and his colleagues in Philadelphia and the right-hand set with the controlled pressure device, described in the text, in Alabama with the collaboration of Mr. J. E. Webster. (In these sets areas were calculated in each animal and then averaged, rather than calculated from the average radius.)

The locations of Th. A I, II, III and Abd. A I, II are marked on the thoracic and abdominal aorta in Fig. 2.10; the locations are designed to permit comparison with the measurements of Patel *et al.* (1963). Asc. A, Th. A. and Abd. A. connote ascending, thoracic and abdominal aorta; Br. ceph.—brachiocephalic; L and R subcl.—left and right subclavian; Sup. and Inf. mes.—superior and inferior mesenteric in human anatomical nomenclature; Int. cost.— Intercostal; Comm. Carot.—common carotid.

age of at least 10 per cent on setting; Patel *et al.* used 'Jeltrate' which sets into a rubbery material in which contraction (personal communication) is very small. We have attempted to inject the liquid resin, which flows easily through the capillaries, at a sustained pressure of 100 mm Hg. Once setting begins, because of shrinkage, the effective distending pressure is not known; in the earlier experiments the injecting pressure was not well controlled and the distending pressure was almost certainly less than 100 mm Hg. Patel *et al.* (1963) do not mention at what pressure they injected but say that the cast measurements were adjusted in the light of the external diameters determined in the living animal.

Figure 2.10 is a diagrammatic scale drawing of a large part of the arterial tree; the dimensions of selected vessels are given in Table 2.1. The relative sizes of other vessels may thus be determined approximately. The values for the radius are all rather smaller than those of Patel *et al.* 1963, also given in the table. This difference may be due, in part, to the smaller size of our dogs and in part to the adjustments of size to the living artery mentioned above. It certainly indicates that there is a considerable individual variation in these laboratory animals.

TABLE 2.2 Changes in area over major arterial regions

Segment	Area Ratio	Length (cm)	Area Ratio	Length	Ratio	Length
Asc. A–Th. A I	1·12	6·5	1·03	7·0	0·95	5·0
Th. A I–Th. A II	0·79	9·5	0·87	10·0	0·84	7·8
Th. A II–Th. A III	1·07	6·0	1·04	7·6	1·00	6·9
Th. A III–Abd. A I	0·77	6·0	1·05	4·2	1·43	5·8
Abd. A I–Abd. A II	1·86*	7·5	2·20	11·4	1·96	9·0
Abd. A II–Term.	0·80*	4·0	1·29	0·8	1·19	5·6
Asc. A–Term.	1·16*	39·5	1·62	41·0	1·48	40·1
Asc. A–Th. A III	1·01	22·0	0·98	24·6	0·93	19·7
Th. A III–Term.	1·26*	17·5	2·30	16·4	1·98	20·4
Br. ceph.-subdiv.	——	——	1·00	3·2	——	——
L. subcl.-subdiv.	——	——	0·98	5·4	——	——

The area ratios and lengths of segments derived from the sets of data shown in Table 2.1. Area ratio is defined as the ratio of the summed lumen area of all branches arising from an arterial region, plus the area of the trunk leaving the segment, to the cross-sectional area of the trunk entering the segment. For example, the segment Ascending Aorta—Thoracic Aorta I, the ratio is between the sum of the areas of the brachiocephalic and left subclavian arteries and the lumen of Thor. A. I divided by the area of the Asc. A cross-section. Thus, it is a measure of the change in the total cross-section area of the bed into which the blood flows. Term.—distal termination of aorta.

In relation to the discussions in the literature regarding 'taper', the ratios of cross-sectional areas across various regions are interesting (Table 2.2). Considering the aorta from just beyond the arch (Thor. A.I.), the area just above the diaphragm (Thor. Aorta III) is 0·56–0·67 of the proximal section; the area just proximal to its terminal branching (Abd. A. II) is only 0·28–0·4. When the

* Omitting unnamed branches of abdominal aorta not listed in Patel *et al.*, 1963.

additional area of the origins of its branches is added the ratio between the
ascending aorta and the bed to the diaphragm is 0·93–1·00. This shows a slight
contraction (it is odd that such contraction as there is seems to take place in

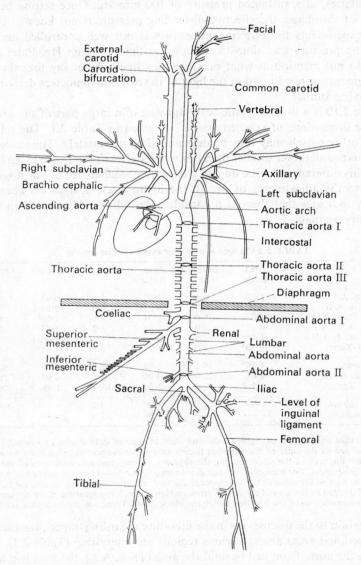

Fig. 2.10. A diagrammatic representation of the major branches of the arterial tree. The drawing is
to scale but the scale of the diameters is double the scale in lengths. The measurements are from
plastic casts of the vessels; the numerical values refer to the central set of numbers in Table 1.

The rings marked Th. AI, Th. AII, etc, show the levels at which the diameters and cross-sectional
areas are measured for the values in the table.

the first half of the thoracic aorta which is not wholly compensated by the bed expansion in the second half). In the abdominal aorta, by contrast, there is a considerable expansion of the vascular bed due to the branches of the abdominal aorta and the bed expands by a factor of 1·19–1·56. The change in area across the arch of the aorta is from 1·12 to 0·95 and from the ascending aorta along the whole aorta and its branches is from 1·16 to 1·62. Compared to the rapid expansion of cross-sectional area over short distances when the small orders of vessels are reached relatively close to the sites of major branches, this expansion is, over an approximately 40 cm length, small; hence, on the overall diagrams of areas (Figs. 2.8 and 2.11) it appears to be almost

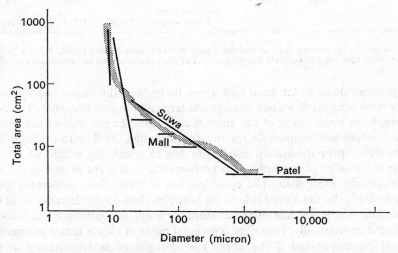

Fig. 2.11. A diagram showing the distribution of cross-sectional area of the total vascular bed based on the values under B on the right of Table 4 and are from Iberall (1967). The names inserted on the graph indicate the areas on the curve which are taken from the estimates of the authors quoted; thus, the large vessel values are from Patel *et al.* (1963) and the others from series of papers by Mall and Suwa, cited by Iberall.

invariant by comparison with the large change in area which occurs soon after.

One approach for a mathematical model to deal with the multiplicity of branches along the length of the aorta that has been suggested at various times is to make it analogous to a tube that is leaking along its length; this is a problem for which the analysis is known but the word 'leak' is used in its everyday sense of being small in proportion to the main flow. A consideration of the relative flow through branches shows that this is misleading. The values for man are more dependable than are available for the dog for these mean flow measurements through the principal organs are standard clinical diagnostic procedures. Representative values are given, for a man at rest, in Table 2.3. It can be seen that, of the flow leaving the ventricle, approximately

TABLE 2.3. Distribution of flow in humans at rest

Circulation	Blood Flow (ml/min)	(% total)	Flow into various regions (ml/min)	% total
			Upper body	
Splanchnic*	1,400	24	Brain and heart	1,000	
			Muscle and skin (est.)	500	
Renal	1,100	19	Sub-total:	1,500	26
Cerebral	750	13			
Coronary	250	4	*Trunk:* (4,300 ml/min enters Thor. Aorta, 74%)		
Skeletal muscle	1,200	21	Liver and intestine	1,400	
Skin	500	9	Kidneys	1,100	
Other organs	600	10	Muscle and skin (est.)	300	
	5,800	100		2,800	48
			Terminal aorta		
			Pelvic organs and legs	1,500	26

The values for the volume flow to various organs is taken from Milnor (1968, Table 8.2). The values were then used to estimate the proportions of the cardiac output to three main regions of the body.

25 per cent flows to the head and upper limbs (and the heart) and approximately 40 per cent flows out through the large abdominal branches. The flow through the termination of the aorta is only some 25 per cent of the whole. These values are comparable for the dog although the flow to the hind-legs is probably proportionately less in the dog in which the weight of muscle there is a smaller proportion of the body-weight than is the muscle in the legs of habitually erect man. The consideration of these flows illustrates more dramatically the functional role of the branches than do the dimensions of the branches. The direct line of the anatomical aorta unconsciously leads us to isolate it conceptually. From the functional point of view a better perspective would be maintained if the aorta was thought of as terminating at the diaphragm in a group of large branches supplying the important organs of the abdomen.

A corresponding set of values of flows with various regions in the dog is also given by Green (1950). He also prepared a table of a set of values for the dimensions, number of branches, etc., that is a standard reference. The only revision that might be desirable today would be to incorporate the measurements of the aorta and large arteries that have been reviewed above. For the smaller values reliance has long been made of measurements of vessels throughout the mesenteric bed by Mall (1888) although he also studied the vessels of the stomach, adrenal, spleen and liver (Mall, 1905). Attention was focused on Mall's early data by Schleier (1918) by an analysis of the haemodynamic factors implicit in his sets of dimensions of the branching system. Schleier's table was introduced into the textbook contribution of Bazett (1941), and repeated by Milnor (1968), so that it is easily available. A most

* Splanchnic: flow through hepatic vein, i.e. volume supplied to liver, intestines, and spleen.

TABLE 2.4. Estimated dimensions of the arterial tree

A. Level	Name	Int. Diam. (mm)	No. of tubes	Length	Total area (cm²)	B. Level	Diameter (mm) Entrance	Diameter (mm) Exit	Ave. Entr.	Total area (cm²)	No. of tubes
1	Aorta	10	1	40	0.8	1	20	7	20	3.2	1
2	Large arteries	3	40	20	3.0	2	10–18	1.8	3.2	3.4	20
3	Main branches	1	600	10	5.0	3	4.0–1.0	0.4	3.4	3.4	260
4	Secondary branches	0.6	1,800	4	5.0	4	2.0–0.4	0.4	0.8	4.0	800
						5	0.8–0.2	0.2	0.31	5	7×10^3
5	Tertiary branches	0.14	76,000	1.4	11.7	6	0.4–0.1	0.1	0.16	6	3×10^4
6	Terminal arteries	0.05	10^6	0.1	19.6	7	0.2–0.04	0.04	0.08	10	2×10^5
7	Terminal branches	0.03	13×10^6	0.15	91	8	0.1–0.025	0.025	0.032	16	2×10^6
8	Arterioles	0.02	4×10^7	0.2	125	9	0.06–0.015	0.015	0.02	25	8×10^6
						10	0.03–0.008	0.008	0.012	35	3×10^7
9	Capillaries	0.008	1.2×10^9	0.1	600	11	0.015–0.008	0.008	0.008	80	2×10^8

A. Values taken from Green (1950).   B. Values taken from Iberall (1967)

The enumeration, size of vessels, and total cross-sectional area of the arterial tree collated from various sources by Green (1950), Section A. and by Iberall (1967), Section B. Iberall classifies the tree in eleven levels of subdivision without giving them anatomical names so that the table is arranged to give approximate correspondences with the nine named levels used by Green.

The most remarkable difference between the two sets of values is in the estimate of cross-sectional area of the capillary bed, and indeed from the beds of the terminal arterioles and more distal levels. This is largely related to the differing estimates of the number of parallel channels. Iberall's estimate of 80 cm² for the area of the capillary bed is closer to the value commonly found in physiological textbooks; the larger value of 600 cm² may well be possible under conditions of tissue activity, when it is known that the number of capillary channels visible under the microscope increases greatly (especially in active muscle).

valuable paper by Iberall (1967) has drawn our attention to Mall's neglected work and also more recent work by Suwa (1963) in Japan. This latter work, in humans, has analysed the geometry of the circulations of the kidney, intestine, femoral bed, pancreas, heart, the cerebral cortex and the basal ganglia of the brain. From these Iberall has drawn an illustrative figure (Fig. 2.11). Part of his accompanying table is given in Table 2.4. In order to match work from various sources he has described eleven different levels of subdivisions; physiologists are more familiar with the nine levels characterized by Green (1950) so that these are also included in this table to make anatomical identification easier. It should be emphasized, however, that under normal living conditions the internal diameter of arterioles and capillaries varies widely under vasoconstrictor and dilator influences. From these values and the simple relations between total cross-sectional area and number of branches arising from each parent branch which were discussed above (p. 53) the changes in resistance and mean velocity can be easily derived. It is found that the resistance (and, hence, by implication the impedance) increased very rapidly over the very short distance between the tertiary arterial branches and the capillaries. It is on such considerations that it is postulated that the large rise of impedance in these vessels is the main site of wave reflection which is discussed in Chs. 12–14.

The large field of work covered by research into the special problems of the microcirculation cannot be adequately considered. From the physiological point of view the capillaries may be thought as the functional *raison d'être* of the circulation where the transport of oxygen, and other substances required by the tissue cells, and the removal of metabolic products, necessary to maintain the life of the cell of the body, takes place. This brief summary of the anatomical array of tubes supplying these capillary beds is given to put in perspective the role of the arteries in this distribution of blood, from the pump that is the heart, to the tissues of the body; the role of the veins in returning the blood to the heart is equally important, but for present purposes may be regarded as being arrayed in the same way as the arterial tree. It is through these complex arrays that we need to consider the flow of the blood.

3
The Viscous Properties of Blood

In the theoretical treatment of liquid flow (Ch. 2) pressure–flow relationships of a Newtonian fluid were analysed. A Newtonian liquid is, by definition, one in which the coefficient of viscosity is constant at all rates of shear. This is closely approximated by most homogenous liquids but suspensions of particles show deviations from it. As might be suspected, such anomalous behaviour becomes most apparent as the particle size becomes appreciably large in comparison with the dimensions of the channel in which it is flowing. Blood is essentially a suspension of erythrocytes in plasma and shows anomalous viscous properties.

These anomalies are of two kinds: (1) at low shear rates, the apparent viscosity increases markedly; indeed, it has now been almost certainly shown that it may cease to flow in the presence of a measurable stress, i.e. to possess a 'yield stress'; (2) in small tubes the apparent viscosity at higher rates of shear is smaller than it is in larger tubes; this progressive diminution with tube size begins to be detectable with tubes of less than 1 mm internal diameter, i.e. about 100 times the major diameter of the cells (which is c. 10 μm) and becomes marked in tubes of the order of 100–200 μ in diameter. Relatively little detailed quantitative work has been done on glass tubes smaller than 40 μm I.D. because of technical difficulties. At tube sizes of 10 μm or smaller the deformation of the cells will introduce more complicating factors.

These two types of anomaly may be referred to as the 'low shear' and 'high shear' effects. They have been the object of intensive research for many years and the literature on the subject is very large. This interest in part is due to the challenge of the very nature of viscosity, which, in turn, is allied to our inability to predict the properties of liquids in terms of their molecular properties. A full review of the literature would thus include such theoretical contributions as that of Einstein (1906). On the other hand, the hydrodynamic description of the circulation clearly requires a measurement of the viscosity of the blood as accurately as it may be achieved.

This second aspect is the one that is relevant to the present study. The brief review given here will emphasize the quantitation of anomalies that may introduce errors into the hydrodynamic analyses of blood flow which assume a Newtonian viscosity of blood. The 'high shear' or 'small tube' effect mentioned above clearly applies in a study of the small vessels. Nevertheless, in applying a physical equation such as that of Poiseuille (2.2) to a vessel of, say, 200 μm diameter we are faced not only with viscosity changes but with the fact that none of the parameters of the equation can be measured at all accurately in the living vessel. Even the dimensions are inaccessible except in a few regions, such as the mesenteric microcirculation; furthermore, the radius of small vessels normally appears to vary continuously. Nevertheless, some of the anomalies of blood viscosity are large and it is conceivable that they introduce systematic errors into physical analysis of blood flow.

Virtually all the work to be discussed has been done *in vitro*; to the non-specialist it is not always easy to compare the magnitude of the parameters analysed with those one might expect to find in the circulation. Haynes and Burton (1959) have given typical values they have calculated for the shearing stress at the vessel wall throughout the circulation and compare them with the values in tubes at which the 'low shear' anomaly is seen. They come to the comforting conclusion that normal values in the circulation are too high for it to have significance; this was also the opinion expressed by McDonald (1960) but more recent work has cast some doubt on this and it will be re-examined.

Reviews of the rheological properties of blood that are recommended for initial reading are Bayliss (1960, 1962) and more recent work is clearly covered in a briefer review by Wayland (1967). The more detailed review by Bayliss (1952) has long been a standard reference. The monograph by Whitmore (1968) provides an excellent coverage of the contents of this chapter without being too detailed. The review of Merrill (1969) is particularly thorough in considering the low shear behaviour of blood to which he and his group have made a big contribution; the review by Johnson (1969) on the other hand is more physiologically oriented towards work done in living capillaries.

THE DEFINITION OF VARIABLE VISCOSITY

In Ch. 2, the coefficient of viscosity (μ) in a flowing liquid was defined as the constant of proportionality between the stress applied (τ) and the velocity gradient, or rate of shear (dv/dr, sometimes indicated by γ) of the liquid laminae. This is expressed by the equation

$$\tau = \mu . \frac{dv}{dr} \qquad \textbf{3.1}$$

If the viscosity is measured in a concentric cylinder (Couette) viscometer or a cone-and-plate viscometer the rate of shear is approximately constant throughout the liquid and is measured directly, as is the applied stress.

Results on changes in viscosity with changing rate of shear are, thus, simply displayed by plotting the stress against the rate of shear as in Fig. 3.1.

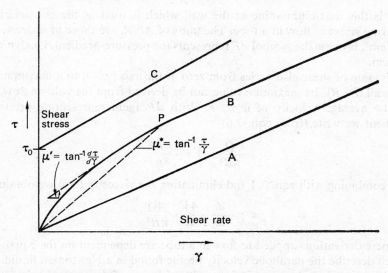

Fig. 3.1. A diagram to show different types of flow behaviour. Shear stress, τ, is the ordinate and shear rate, γ, is the abscissa.

A. A Newtonian fluid; the relation between stress and shear is linear from the origin onwards.

B. A non-Newtonian liquid with asymptotic Newtonian behaviour. Beyond the point P, at higher shear rates the relationship is linear but below that it is non-linear but the curve passes through the origin. The 'differential' viscosity, μ', is defined by the slope of the curve $\mu' = \tan^{-1} d\tau/d\gamma$. The 'generalized' viscosity, μ^*, is the ratio of the applied stress to the shear rate; thus, at point $P\mu^* = \tan^{-1}\tau/\gamma$. Wayland (1967) calls this the 'secant' viscosity.

C. A Bingham body; when stress is applied there is no flow until it exceeds a certain value τ_0. This value, τ_0, is called the 'yield stress'.

Most of the work on the subject has, however, been done in cylindrical tubes, a situation which is analogous to that of flow in blood vessels. In order to be able to compare results from the two methods directly it is necessary to define stress and rate of shear in terms of the variables pressure-gradient, rate of flow, and tube radius.

From eqs. 3.1 and 2.4 we can write

$$\tau = \mu \cdot \frac{dv}{dr} = \frac{-r(P_1 - P_2)}{2L} \qquad \textbf{3 2}$$

It is usual in these formulations to use ΔP as the pressure-gradient so that $\Delta P = (P_1 - P_2)/L$, so that (ignoring the sign which is irrelevant in this context) we obtain

$$\tau = \frac{\Delta Pr}{2} \qquad \textbf{3 3}$$

where r is the radius of a given lamina of liquid. The radius, r, is zero at the

axis so that the stress is also zero. The maximum stress is at the wall where
$r = R$ and

$$\tau = \Delta PR/2 \qquad \textbf{3.4}$$

It is this maximum value at the wall which is used as the characteristic
shearing stress of flow in a tube. The units of $\Delta P.R.$ are those of a stress, i.e.
dyn/cm², because the symbol ΔP represents the pressure-gradient, i.e. dyn/cm²
per cm.

The rate of shear also varies from zero at the axis ($\gamma = 0$) to a maximum at
the wall ($r = R$). Its maximum value can be derived from the volume flow, Q,
or the average velocity of flow, $\overline{V}$. With ΔP again representing pressure-
gradient we write (from eqn. 2.6)

$$\frac{Q}{\pi R^2} = \overline{V} = \frac{\Delta PR^2}{8\mu} \qquad \textbf{3.5}$$

and combining with eqn. 3.4 and eliminating the viscosity term we obtain

$$\gamma = \frac{dv}{dr} = \frac{4\overline{V}}{R} = \frac{4Q}{\pi R^3} \qquad \textbf{3.6}$$

These derivations applied to flow in a tube are dependent on the equations
which describe the parabolic velocity profile found in a Newtonian liquid. As
will be seen below, variations of viscosity with rate of shear cause a deviation
from this form, as will oscillatory flow, so that the evaluation of the rate of
shear and stress at the wall in this way is only approximate. Nevertheless, in
plotting results graphically the values calculated in this way are the clearest
way of demonstrating regions of deviation when flow behaviours in tubes of
different size are being compared.

When shear stress is plotted against shear rate the resulting line will express
the behaviour of the viscosity. Newtonian viscosity will give a straight line
passing through the origin (Fig. 3.1A). The behaviour of blood, however, is
represented by curve 3.1B in which, at higher shear rates, the line is essentially
straight and curves around to the origin at low shear rates. Another type of
flow is of a material represented by 3.1C where there is no flow up to a stress of
τ_0 and flows thereafter; the stress τ_0 is called the 'yield stress'. This type of
material is called a Bingham body (after Bingham, who first coined the term
'rheology'). Such a curve initially represents the behaviour of a solid for
stresses below the yield stress and thereafter the behaviour of a liquid.

In regions of the stress–shear rate curves that are linear the liquid is often
said to have a Newtonian viscosity. Wayland (1967) has emphasized, however,
that this is not correct, if the line does not pass through the origin when
linearly extrapolated. The viscosity as normally calculated from Poiseuille's
law will be derived from the ratio of the values of τ and γ at each point; a
more realistic value would be derived from the slope of the line, i.e. $d\tau/d\gamma$.
The former of these two viscosities Wayland calls the 'secant' viscosity and

the latter the 'differential' viscosity but the terms are not in general use. The distinction is, however, clear if the data are plotted in this way.

The experimental data on flow in tubes are often plotted in other ways. The direct plot of volume flux against the pressure drop along a measured length of tube will have the same form as that of the shear rate/stress for any given tube and is used by many authors. Another method often used is to calculate the apparent viscosity, μ', from the pressure–flow relations at each flow rate (Haynes, 1961) and plot this as the ordinate (Fig. 3.2). At high shear rates (or

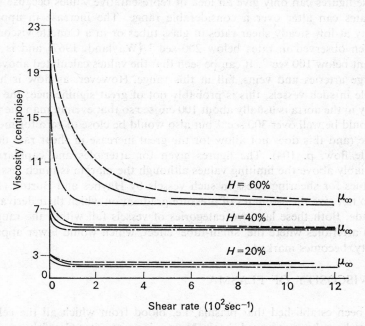

Fig. 3.2. The plot of measured viscosity in a small tube (747μ ID) as shear rate changes. The viscosity (in cP) is plotted as the ordinate against the shear rate on the abscissa. The relation of the measures of viscosity discussed in the text are shown. The upper dashed (– – –) curve, μ, the apparent viscosity calculated from Poiseuille's law, is not the most informative curve because it deviates the most from linearity at lower shear rates (see curves for $H = 60\%$ particularly). This shortcoming is much less present in the 'differential' viscosity, μ', which is proportional to the slope of the pressure–flow curve; indicated by dash-dot line (– · –). The solid line (——) is the 'generalized' viscosity, μ^*, which is proportional to the ratio of the applied stress to the shear rate at the wall.

Three sets of curves are shown for varying values of haematocrit ($H = 60\%$, $H = 40\%$, $H = 20\%$). At increasing shear rates they all approximate to a constant value which is called the 'asymptotic' viscosity ($\mu\infty$). (Redrawn from Haynes, 1961.)

high stresses) the viscosity reaches an asymptotic value (μ_∞); some authors prefer to plot the ratio μ'/μ_∞ as ordinate rather than the actual value of μ' in poises.

In order to put the shear rate in physiological perspective, it is useful to calculate a few typical values.

TABLE 3.1

Vessel	Radius (cm)	Mean flow velocity (cm/sec)	Shear rate at wall (sec^{-1})
Ascending aorta (man)	1·25	25	80
Ascending aorta (dog)	0·50	25	200
Inferior vena cava (man)	1·75	12	28
Arteriole (small artery)	0·01	1·0	400
Capillary	0·0005	0·5	400

These figures can only give an idea of representative values because mean flow rates can alter over a considerable range. The increase in apparent viscosity at low steady shear rates in glass tubes or in a Couette viscometer has been observed in rates below 200 sec^{-1} (Wayland, 1967) and is quite apparent below 100 sec^{-1}. It can be seen that the values calculated above, for the large arteries and veins, fall in this range. However, as flow is highly pulsatile in such vessels, this is probably not of great significance; the peak velocity in the aorta is usually about 100 cm/sec so that even in man the shear rate would be well over 300 sec^{-1} but also would be close to zero for most of diastole (and this does not allow for the great increase in shear rate due to pulsatile flow, p. 104). The figures given for arterioles and capillaries is appreciably above the limiting values although the margin is much less than the values for shearing stress in such vessels by Haynes and Burton (1959) who do not give the estimates of pressure-gradient on which their derivations are made. Both these last two categories of vessels fall within the range of human arterioles where the 'small-tube' effect, which would lower apparent viscosity, becomes marked.

THE VISCOSITY OF PLASMA

It has been established that plasma, i.e. blood from which all the cellular elements have been removed, has a Newtonian viscosity. Careful tests have been made in concentric cylinder viscometers (Cokelet et al., 1963) and in capillary tubes (Merrill et al., 1965a) over a range of shear rates from 0·1 to over 1,200 sec^{-1} and no significant departure from linearity was found. These authors report a viscosity of 1·6 relative to water. Other authors have reported plasma to be non-Newtonian in varying degrees but only when an apparatus is used which allows plasma–air interfaces to occur; it appears that the abnormal results are due to a denatured protein layer at the interface (Wayland, 1967). As plasma is a colloidal suspension of protein in an electrolyte solution (concentration 7–7·5 g/100 ml) it might be expected to show some deviation from the behaviour of a pure liquid. As Wayland (1967) points out, however, the longest dimension of any of the particles is the length of the fibrinogen molecule [c. 50 (nm) mμ]. Even in a capillary of 5μ bore this particle dimension would only be 1 per cent of the lumen. As noted above, deviations of viscosity are not seen until particle size is a much larger fraction of tube diameter. In certain pathological states there is some suggestive evidence that measurable non-Newtonian behaviour may be found in plasma. The deviations reported are small. Otherwise, all critical studies have shown plasma to have a Newtonian viscosity.

THE VISCOUS BEHAVIOUR OF BLOOD

If red cells are progressively added to plasma the viscosity increases. Marked non-Newtonian properties are not seen until the concentration of cells exceeds 10 per cent. If the viscosity is measured in a tube with an internal radius of about 0·5 mm (500 μm) or larger, and shear rates which are not less than 200–300 sec^{-1}, it will be effectively independent of tube size but will vary with the cell concentration.

(Cell concentration is expressed as the haematocrit value, which is the percentage volume of the blood in which the cells have sedimented by centrifugation; this packed cell volume includes a small volume of plasma 'trapped' between the cells but this is usually neglected unless specifically stated, when it is usually called the 'true' haematocrit. The difference is small but not negligible; a haematocrit of 45 per cent represents a true cell volume of about 41 per cent.)

The variation of viscosity with haematocrit is shown in Fig. 3.3; this is often

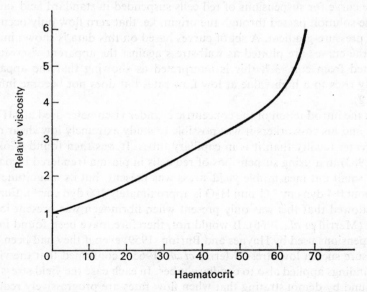

Fig. 3.3. The variation of viscosity with the haematocrit values. The ordinate is the asymptotic viscosity *relative* to that of *plasma* = 1. The abscissa is the packed cell volume or haematocrit. (Normal value for plasma viscosity = 1·6 cP). (Data taken from Whitmore, 1968.)

called the 'asymptotic' viscosity as it is the constant value which is reached at high shear rates. The values shown are based on those of Whitmore (1968) but they are in reasonable agreement with those derived from other authors such as Coulter and Pappenheimer (1949). For practical purposes, the viscosity may be regarded as varying linearly with cell concentration from 0 per cent (plasma) to a haematocrit of about 45 per cent. This covers most experimental or clinical conditions. The viscosity rises much more rapidly with cell concentration with values above this.

EFFECTS OF LOW SHEAR RATE

If the pressure–flow curve is recorded in a capillary tube, the curve is similar to that shown in Fig. 3.1B. A lot of earlier data did not extend to very low shear rates; when the linear portion of the pressure–flow curve was extrapolated it made a positive intercept on the pressure axis, often of several mm Hg. This was interpreted as indicating that blood was a semi-plastic body, of the kind first described by Bingham; a Bingham-body at rest will deform under an applied stress but will only begin to flow when the stress exceeds a limiting value, the 'yield' stress. This concept has been well set out by Lamport (1955). Careful studies by Kümin (1949) and Bayliss (1952) at low flow rates showed that the pressure–flow curve deviated towards the origin and probably passed through it. Later Haynes and Burton (1959) showed fairly conclusively that the curve for suspensions of red cells suspended in standard acid–citrate dextrose solution passed through the origin, i.e. that zero flow only occurred at zero pressure-gradient. A set of curves based on this data is shown in Fig. 3.4. If the curves are plotted as wall-stress against the apparent viscosity as calculated from eqn. 3.7, this is interpreted as showing that the apparent viscosity rises to a high value at low flow rates but does not become infinite (Fig. 3.2).

With the introduction of the concentric cylinder viscometer used at MIT by Merrill and his co-workers it was possible to study extremely low shear rates with greater facility than it is in capillary tubes. It was then found (Cokelet et al., 1963) that using suspensions of red cells in plasma (rendered incoagulable) a small but measurable yield stress was present, but its magnitude was only about 0·4 dyn cm^{-2} (1 mm H$_2$O is approximately 100 dyn cm^{-2}). Further study showed that this was only present when fibrinogen was present in the plasma (Merrill et al., 1966). It would not, therefore, have been found in the cell suspensions used by Haynes and Burton (1959) even if they had been able to measure such a low stress. Merrill et al. (1965a) confirmed that the viscometer findings applied also to capillary tubes. In each case the yield stress was only found by demonstrating that when flow rates are progressively reduced they become zero while there is still an applied stress. To date it has not been possible to demonstrate the inverse of the situation starting with blood at rest, which Wayland (1967) attributes to the fact that the red cells sediment in stationary blood.

The analysis of the low shear phenomena in blood has been especially

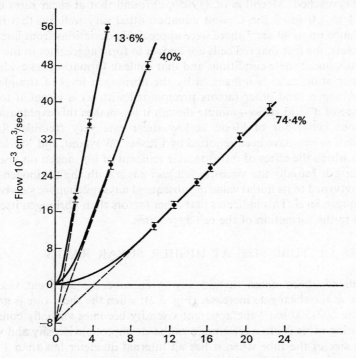

Fig. 3.4. Curves showing the simple relation of flow to pressure-gradient in a small tube (472μ ID). Curves are shown for haematocrit values of $13\cdot6\%$, 40% and 74% for suspensions of red cells. All curves are linear at the higher flow rates and when this linear portion is extrapolated backwards they all appear to coincide at a point of negative flow. The actual curves deviate from these lines and pass through the origin. This deviation is known in physiology as the Fahraeus–Lindqvist phenomenon. (Redrawn from Haynes, 1961, *Trans. Soc. Rheol.* **5**, 85, Fig. 2.)

studied by Merrill and his group (1963*a*, *b*; 1965*b*, *c*). They found that in this region the results fitted a form of the Casson (1959) equation

$$\tau^{1/2} = \tau_y^{1/2} + (K.\gamma)^{1/2} \qquad\qquad 3.7$$

where τ is the shear stress, τ_y the yield stress, and γ the rate of strain; K is a constant which, in the case of blood, is usually equal to the asymptotic or Newtonian viscosity, μ_∞.

This equation was originally proposed by Scott Blair but the basic equation was developed by Casson to explain the flow behaviour of printing inks. It assumes that at low shear rates the particles form aggregates which link into chains; the interactions of these chains are the cause of the yield stress. When this is exceeded the chains break and with progressive increase of shear the rate of breakdown of the aggregate exceeds that of recombination. The viscosity then falls until, when all the particles are separate, the asymptotic viscosity is reached. Merrill *et al.* (1965*b*, *c*) found that at shear rates in the range 0·1 to 1·0 sec^{-1} the Casson equation fitted very well but that in the further range up to 40 sec^{-1} there were appreciable deviations from linearity. Nevertheless, the fact that red cells are known to form aggregates in the form of rouleaux under these conditions and that rouleau formation (as evidenced by sedimentation rate) is influenced by the fibrinogen level of the plasma, while fibrinogen (and other factors precipitated with it) is essential for the occurrence of a yield stress—minute though it is—makes this explanation of the viscous behaviour of blood at low shear rate very credible. Recent experiments *in vivo* have been reported by Frasher, Wayland, and Meiselman (1968) in which the effect of intravascular removal of fibrinogen on viscosity was observed. Initially the viscosity fell *pari passu* with the fibrinogen level but was returned to its initial value in subsequent days much more slowly than the fibrinogen level. This indicates that other factors than fibrinogen itself are involved in the formation of the cell aggregates.

EFFECTS OF TUBE SIZE AT HIGHER SHEAR RATES

It has already been noted that in any given tube the apparent viscosity decreases as the shear rate increases (Fig. 3.2); when the shear rate is greater than some 200–300 sec^{-1} the apparent viscosity becomes virtually constant. This limiting value is often referred to as the 'asymptotic' viscosity and varies with the size of the tube when it has an internal diameter less than 1 mm. Above that size of tube there is no measurable change with the lumen and this value is also referred to as the 'asymptotic' viscosity and designated as μ_{∞}. The form of the curve shows that the term 'asymptotic' viscosity is more properly given to this second meaning and the term 'apparent' viscosity to the values dependent on the dimensions of the tube. With a tube of 300 μm diameter the viscosity has reached some 93–95 per cent of its final value. In a tube of 20 μm diameter the viscosity is only 50 per cent of its final value.

This effect was first described by Fahraeus and Lindquist in 1931 and is often known by their names. That the effect occurs in the living vascular bed was demonstrated by Whittaker and Winton (1933) who showed that blood perfused through a hind-limb had a viscosity relative to saline of 2·2; when measured in a high-velocity viscometer the relative viscosity was 4·0. Fahraeus and Lindquist also found that if the blood flowing in a small bore tube was trapped and the cell concentration was measured this concentration was lower than that of the blood in the reservoir. This lowering of the 'dynamic' haematocrit has been frequently confirmed. It is due to the fact that the regions close to the wall of the tube are relatively deficient in cells. Such a region can be easily observed with a microscope in both glass capillaries and living ones. The ease of observation is, however, somewhat illusory because refraction of light at the sides of a cylindrical tube will have a similar appearance. For this reason most of the evidence before Bayliss' critical review of 1952 can be discounted.

One of the first critical measurements of the size of the 'cell-free' zone was that of Taylor (1955) who studied the variations in optical density from the wall to the centre of suspensions of red cells flowing in glass capillaries. A careful study by Bayliss (1959), using a photographic method, produced results which were in agreement. The cell-free zone was considerably smaller than was generally supposed and in a tube of 100 μm diameter was not greater than 2–5 μm wide although the optical density was reduced over a zone varying from 5–20 μm. These results were extended in a last paper (Bayliss, 1965). The cell-free zone is virtually independent of tube size but of course is relatively larger and more obvious in very small tubes. A dynamic study of this zone has been made by Bugliarello and Hayden (1962) using high-speed cinematography at speeds up to 3,000 frames/sec. The tube was orientated vertically so that sedimentation would not cause cell-movement towards the wall. It was seen that even the region close to the wall was not truly 'cell-free' for individual cells would move in and out of this zone. The cell-free zone is thus, in effect, a statistical concept, but nevertheless a real entity. The width of the zone appears to increase slightly as the haematocrit falls; the values quoted are for cell concentrations of the order of 35–45 per cent.

A corollary of a cell-deficient region near the wall is that more of the cells are in the central region of the tube. This is also the region where flow velocity is higher and hence the cells of blood will traverse at a higher net velocity than the plasma. This has been found to be the case in the whole circulation by Groom *et al.* (1957), Rowlands, Groom and Thomas (1965), Thomas *et al.* (1965) and Rowlands (1966), who labelled cells and plasma with different radioactive markers and demonstrated the different transit times directly. Another result of this is that the ratio of total red cell volume to total circulating plasma is lower (the 'total blood haematocrit'). In accurate determinations of blood volume it is thus necessary to measure both cell volume and plasma volume rather than measure only one of these volumes and predict the blood volume from the haematocrit value of a single sample.

The effective size of the cell-free (or 'plasmatic') zone can be indirectly calculated from the relative transit times and gives values of the same order of magnitude. Thomas (1962) has also shown that the same results derive in tube models whether flow data or concentration measurements are used.

THE CAUSE OF THE REDUCED APPARENT VISCOSITY

The presence of a low cell concentration in the regions close to the wall will result in a lowered viscosity, approximating to that of plasma, in this region. As this region forms a greater proportion of a narrow tube than of a wider one the lowering of the overall viscosity will be more marked. Detailed calculations are given by Bayliss (1962) and Thomas (1961, 1962) and it is generally accepted that this is not only the simplest but also an adequate explanation of the 'wall' effect, i.e. the reduction of the 'apparent' viscosity of blood in small tubes.

The phenomenon of viscosity dependence on tube diameter is present not only in blood but in all suspensions and it has been named the 'sigma' phenomenon by Schofield and Scott Blair in 1930. The analysis of this was especially developed by Dix and Scott Blair (1940). The presence of solid particles of finite size will cause regions of flow that are unsheared so that the normal integration of flow in infinitely thin layers (Ch. 2) is invalid but should be a summation of a series of layers of finite thickness. (Contrary to some accounts the name 'sigma' phenomenon does not derive from the capital Greek letter symbol used to indicate such a sum but from a special early use of the symbol sigma by Schofield and Scott Blair.) This analysis in these papers gives results similar to those derived from the 'wall' effect alone. Klip (1961), however, has challenged this and demonstrated mathematically that, in the presence of a marginal cell-free zone, unsheared layers in the more central regions would produce an *increase* in apparent viscosity. Thus, there is no final agreement on the precise analysis of the causes in the variation of viscosity but all workers agree that the major cause is due to the presence of a marginal region of low viscosity (the 'cell-free' zone). This phenomenon of high shear near the wall may be approximated mathematically by assuming a constant viscosity for the central red cell region and allowing it to 'slip' at the wall. Slipping is analogous to the friction of one solid mass sliding on another and there is neither evidence for this, nor any hydrodynamic reason why plasma at the wall should behave like this, as has been pointed out by Whitmore (1967). Nevertheless, the use of the mathematical device has led some writers to treat it as if it actually occurred. True 'slip' has never been demonstrated between a liquid–solid interface, certainly not under any conditions comparable to flow in capillaries (see Ch. 2, p. 28).

THE CAUSES OF A FREE-CELL ZONE AT THE WALL

The simplest explanation for low concentration of cells in the region next to the wall has been named the 'wall-exclusion' principle (Bayliss, 1959). Let us assume a suspension of particles of finite size, in which the concentration is uniform throughout a large volume of fluid. This may be considered mathematically as a distribution of points representing the centres of the particles. If a solid wall is placed in this liquid all such points will be excluded up to a distance equal to the mean radius of the particles because they cannot approach closer than being in contact with the wall. If we regard the radius of the red cells as being 5 μm it can be seen that this approximates closely to the measured width of the zone found to be deficient in cells. When the cell concentration is high, as in normal blood, there seems little doubt that this simple principle is almost the sole determinant of the marginal plasmatic zone.

The forces that may act on particles to move them transversely in a flowing stream has been a fascinating, if controversial, subject for many years. Because a central stream of cells is so apparent to the eye when viewing a capillary through a microscope, physiologists commonly regard it as self-evident that physical forces drive the cells into the axial stream. One analogy that has been used is that of a ping-pong ball supported in the centre of a jet of water, to be seen in any fairground. Quite invalid applications of Bernoulli's theorem have been invoked, but need not be considered. The Magnus effect, which causes a spinning tennis ball to swerve, has also been suggested but does not constitute a satisfactory solution. The actual analysis of the physical forces is complex; Saffman (1956) showed mathematically that an axially-directed force, although of small magnitude, would be exerted on spherical particles suspended in a flowing liquid. Segré and Silberberg (1961, 1962), Segré (1965) and Silberberg (1965) demonstrated that such particles do, in fact, move away from the wall; surprisingly, however, particles initially in the axial stream moved towards the wall and the equilibrium position was in a paraxial annulus. This was named the 'pinch' effect. Goldsmith and Mason (1961) found that the migration only occurred above a limiting particle Reynolds number (p. 31) and was more marked if the particles were not rigid but deformed in the flow. Both are agreed that the effect can only be observed at low concentrations, certainly well below 10 per cent. When the concentration is not very low interaction between the particles appears to produce a counter-force which arrests the migration. A close analogy to events in a cylindrical tube is probably made by the experiments of Brandt and Bugliarello (1966) in which a channel which was very wide in comparison to its depth was used to study the flow of a suspension of particles. This demonstrates the formation of a marginal zone initially although the pattern develops instabilities at great distances from the entrance (they were using concentrations of 5 per cent or less). The study of concentrations in the physiological range is extremely difficult because of the large number of particles. Goldsmith and Mason (1964, 1966) have made an ingenious model with such high concentrations of transparent plastic spheres of which a small percentage are coloured so that they may be observed, a technique, especially valuable in demonstrating the form of the velocity profiles. The present experimental evidence indicates that, at cell concentrations equivalent to that in normal blood, the transversely acting forces (which are always small) produce very little net effect because of particle interaction. They probably account for the increase in width of the marginal clear zone at low haematocrit values, i.e. when this zone is wider than can be accounted for by the wall-exclusion effect.

The *velocity profiles* of steady laminar flow in a particle suspension will deviate from that of the parabolic profile of homogenous liquid flow. The marginal plasma zone will have a lower viscosity than the central region; this would be expected to lead to a flattening of the profile in the central regions. If it is assumed that the viscosity varies as a mathematical function of the distance from the wall then the prediction of the profile is relatively simple; two cases where the viscosity varied as a power function of the distance from the wall were calculated by Womersley and are illustrated in Fig. 5.5. Several authors have recorded the profiles in model experiments but the ones recorded by Bugliarello's group (Bugliarello, Kapur and Hsiao, 1965, provides a summary; Bugliarello and Sevilla, 1970, results in tubes 40–70μ) on blood in glass capillaries are the most detailed. From high-speed cinematograph films they used the red cells themselves as velocity markers and were thus able to plot, directly, the velocity in the successive laminae. The deformation of the parabolic profile varies with the haematocrit, the velocity of flow, and tube diameter (which ranged from 35 to 84 μm) in a way that is difficult to summarize without reference to the original figures. In general, none of the recorded profiles are as flat in the central regions as the predicted curves shown in Fig. 5.5.

An ancillary derivation by Bugliarello *et al.* (1965) was the 'viscosity profile', calculated from the observed velocity gradient at each point on the profile. Unexpectedly, in the view of the behaviour of blood at low shear, the maximum viscosity was not recorded on the axis of the tube but in the region lying approximately midway between the axis and the wall. This cannot be explained in terms of the relatively simple analyses of the viscosity of blood which have been surveyed above. It does, however, suggest a parallel to the observations of optical density which Taylor (1955) made in red cell suspensions flowing in glass capillaries. The low optical density he found in the marginal zone has already been noted (p. 65); on traversing inward it was found that the maximal optical density was in the paraxial region and fell to a lower value in the axial region. Bayliss (1959) recorded similar results. Taylor suggested that in the region of higher shear the cells were more constantly oriented in the line of flow and hence allowed a greater transmission of light. This was a difficult interpretation but would also provide a possible explanation of the viscosity profiles found by Bugliarello, although his films do not appear to show any preferred orientation. Other studies have been made (Wiederhielm and Billig, 1968) in which flowing blood in a vessel was arrested by quick freezing. These show that the cells in the region closer to the wall are relatively well-orientated and that light transmission in the axial region is much higher than in the paraxial region. The vessels studied were larger than the glass tubes used by Bugliarello; no significant change in cell concentration across the tube was seen except in the marginal zone. The orientation of cells was more marked in blood vessels than in glass tubes.

BLOOD VISCOSITY IN OSCILLATORY FLOW

All the detailed studies on blood viscosity discussed above have been concerned with steady flow. In a large part of the circulation the flow is, however, highly pulsatile. In many vessels there is a reversal of flow for some part of the cycle so that the maximum shear rate will be momentarily zero. Furthermore, as shown in Ch. 4, in oscillatory flow with a Newtonian liquid the axial region of the velocity profile is much flatter than in steady Poiseuille flow so that very low shear conditions will be transiently present over greater regions. The change in profile will also cause much greater shear rates to be found close to the wall than for the same mean flow rate in Poiseuille flow. Prediction of the precise viscous behaviour of blood in oscillatory flow is difficult if the determining factors are time-dependent, e.g. if the formation of cell-aggregates is the cause of the high viscosity at low shear-rates as postulated above (p. 64) they may take longer to form than exists in a situation where the flow is reversing rapidly.

Taylor (1959a) made a detailed theoretical investigation of the effects of shear-dependence of blood viscosity in pulsatile flow. In terms of the Womersley equations (see Chs. 5 and 6) and the viscosity data of Kümin (1949) he concluded that, in all the larger arteries, the use of the asymptotic viscosity, μ_∞, would at most lead to an error of about 2 per cent in the calculation of flow from a pressure-gradient.

Kunz and Coulter (1967) have made experimental studies of sinusoidally varying flows of blood in a glass tube of I.D. 0·34 cm. The pressure–flow relations were analysed in terms of the Womersley equation (6.4) and were compared with that of water and a 60 per cent glycerol solution. The water and glycerol solution, both Newtonian liquids, fitted the curve predicted by the equation well. With blood of a haematocrit up to 40 per cent the viscosity behaviour was essentially Newtonian at frequencies above 1 Hz; for a haematocrit of 64 per cent it was stable above 3 Hz but with a haematocrit of 85 per cent no linear plot of impedance (see Ch. 6) was found up to 8 Hz. Below the frequencies cited the viscosities rose although the effect was not marked with haematocrits below 64–68 per cent. With a haematocrit of 47 per cent a reasonably good fit for the oscillatory pressure–flow curve over the whole range could be made by taking the viscosity as approximately 0·03 P throughout the frequency range.

As will be seen in Ch. 6, the parameter determining the kinetic similarities of oscillatory flow is $\alpha = R(\omega/\nu)^{1/2}$ where R is the tube radius, ω the angular frequency and ν the kinematic viscosity of the liquid. The value of α at the 1·0 Hz frequency in the experiments quoted above is about 2·5 which is analogous to, but usually smaller than, that of the fundamental harmonic of pulsatile flow in the superficial femoral artery of a dog. Satisfactory measurement of a pressure-gradient in a vessel smaller than this has not, so far, been achieved. With an increase of α the inertial term becomes much greater than the viscous resistance term so that the pressure–flow relation is not sensitive to small changes in viscosity. To this extent the theoretical predictions of Taylor are borne out by the experimental work of Kunz and Coulter described here. Important as this study has been, it would be interesting if it could be extended in terms of the detailed theoretical analyses that have been used for steady flow studies of viscosity, and that the investigations be extended into smaller tubes. Nevertheless, for practical purposes, the tube size used is more relevant to conditions in arteries where the equations for pulsatile flow find their main application.

This account can only be a selective summary of work in a field which has been extremely active. The symposium volumes edited by Copley (1965, 1968, 1971) provide excellent surveys of current work. The papers of Charm, Kurland, and their colleagues, Dintenfass and Oka (especially on flow in tapered tubes) have not been discussed but some are included in the references. Work in living capillaries, in which workers such as Bloch and Branemark have made many contributions, has led to the foundation of a new journal (*Microvascular Research*) to which reference should also be made.

4
Turbulence and Disturbed Flow Patterns in the Circulation

When flow is steady the criteria which distinguish turbulent from laminar flow are well defined and have been discussed in Ch. 2. Although blood has anomalous viscous properties (see Ch. 3) due to the fact that it is a suspension of cells in a colloid solution the available evidence indicates that it behaves like a homogenous liquid in the laminar–turbulent transition process.

Early work on the critical value for Reynolds number (eqn. 2.18) has been reviewed by Bayliss (1952, 1962) but the most clear-cut work was that of Coulter and Pappenheimer (1949). They studied the steady flow of blood (with samples of varying haematocrit values) in a long tube of 2·52 mm internal diameter. By the orthodox method of recording the discontinuity in the pressure–flow graph (Fig. 2.4) they recorded the onset of turbulence at a Reynolds number of 1960 ±160. (They used the radius in their formula and actually reported a value of 980 ±80.) This is sufficiently close to the accepted value of the lower critical number for other liquids to show that blood does not behave anomalously in this respect.

Some confusion has resulted from speculations they made, on the nature of the apparently turbulent flow, based on measurements of the longitudinal electrical resistance. They found that this did not alter at the onset of turbulence. The electrical resistance was assumed to be a measure of the orientation of the cells along the line of flow so that they deduced that the turbulence, which caused an increase in fluid resistance, was confined to the plasma sleeve; the red cells that aggregated in the more axial streams were presumed to remain oriented and so maintain laminar flow in the centre of the tube. The evidence reviewed in Ch. 3 shows that the plasma 'sleeve' is only a few microns thick which, as Taylor (1959a) has pointed out, makes it difficult to conceive as a model which requires turbulence to be limited to this region. The consideration of Taylor's and Bugliarello's experiments (p. 68) has also shown that cell orientation, which is almost certainly a function of rate of shear, is far from uniform across a tube. The most probable explanation of the failure to find a change in electrical resistance is that advanced by Taylor (1959a). That is, that the cells in the axial region of low shear are far from being well orientated in laminar flow; in early turbulence this will be the

71

region mainly involved but will not produce sufficient change in the existing disorder of the cells to affect the electrical resistance. The rates of flow studied did not extend the Reynolds numbers much beyond the transition point and the effect of high degrees of turbulence on the electrical resistance is, therefore, not known.

In the circulation the existence of markedly pulsatile flows complicates the picture and is considered in detail below. Otherwise, in terms of hydraulics the circulation is made up of very small tubes; if the flow was steady throughout the system (cardiac output remaining the same) the Reynolds numbers would virtually all be below the critical value. From Table 4.1 (p. 83) it can be seen that for the mean flows in an average-sized dog a value of 2,000 is not transcended even in the ascending aorta although in the human it probably would be over a short region of the proximal aorta. In larger mammals the distribution of higher Reynolds numbers will extend still further into the arterial and venous systems* but the situations in vessels that are the site of the main components of the flow resistance will not be affected.

In only a relatively small part of the circulation can the flow be regarded as steady. The flow in the large arteries is highly pulsatile but the flow oscillations are progressively diminished with the branching of the system. Capillary flow in the systemic bed is normally steady; many ciné-films have been made of capillary networks to support this generalization provided minor variations in flow rate are neglected. In the arterioles proximal to the capillary beds marked oscillations of flow are usually seen. This transition between the arteriolar pulsations to steady capillary flow seems to occur in the small arterioles. The lumen of arterioles varies greatly with changes in the state of contraction of the muscle in the wall and with vaso-dilatation the capillary can become visibly pulsatile. In the capillaries of the pulmonary circulation flow is markedly pulsatile and there is an appreciable amount of transmission of flow and pressure oscillations into the small veins.

Flow in peripheral veins is regarded as steady. In an organism at rest the appearance of non-steady flow conditions is related to the fluctuation of intrathoracic venous pressure with respiration. In the study of venous flow patterns in the rabbit, Helps and McDonald (1954a) found marked variations of flow velocity in the distal abdominal vena cava and the veins of the neck; even more marked changes were observed in the portal vein flow due to movement of the diaphragm. Oscillations of a cardiac rhythm were seen in the vena cava but they were small.

Close to the heart, within the thorax, venous flow becomes highly pulsatile. Extensive studies by Brecher (1956) using a bristle flowmeter show that the pattern is somewhat complex with respiratory and cardiac rhythms super-

---

* John Potter investigated, in 1950, the specimens of whole aorta in the Natural History Museum in London. This led us to the conclusion that flow in the thoracic aorta of a medium-sized blue whale would be turbulent whenever the linear velocity exceeded 3–4 cm/sec.

imposed. Similar effects would undoubtedly occur in the pulmonary veins. As pulmonary capillary flow is pulsatile we can assert that no regions of steady flow will occur in the pulmonary circulation.

As the concept of the critical Reynolds' number distinguishing laminar from turbulent flow is based on steady flow studies, its application to the steady flow regions of the circulation is valid. Helps and McDonald (1954a) observed the flow patterns of dye injected into veins (by arranging remote injection sites, disturbances due to the presence of catheters, or to the act of injection, were avoided). They found stable laminar flow patterns in most veins of the rabbit, with the thoracic vena cava and the portal vein being the main exception. The Reynolds numbers they recorded (see Table 4.1) were below 400 in all these veins. These values were calculated in the rabbit; assuming that the linear velocity of flow is much the same at any given anatomical site in all mammals studied (comparable values for the rabbit, dog and human are given in Table 4.1) the Reynolds number at any given site will vary directly with the internal diameter, if the viscosity of the blood is the same. Information on this last point is sketchy but probably shows considerable species variation. The value for rabbit blood that was taken in all values quoted in Table 4.1 was 0·017P, which is probably low for any type of mammalian blood so that the Reynolds numbers given are probably in excess of true value.

Stable laminar flow in small veins produces striking streamline patterns. Franklin (1937), for example, saw bright red streams of well-oxygenated blood entering the vena cava from the uterine veins and followed them towards the heart. His interest had been aroused by an account by Claude Bernard of a similar bright streamline in the blood flowing from an active submandibular salivary gland following stimulation of the chorda tympani nerve. Similar streams of blue dye can be followed from peripheral branches along the vena cava; or they can be traced from a radical of the mesenteric vein through to the portal vein, keeping their identity as they negotiate junctions and running parallel with other streams from other branches. These have been recorded on film by McDonald and Helps (1954b). With very quiet respiration the dye would maintain some sort of identity through the portal vein and stain a localized region of the liver.

Observations of this kind have led to the suggestion that streamline flow may determine the regional distribution of blood from certain organs. Thus Copher and Dick (1926) suggested that a tendency of splenic blood to go to the left lobe of the liver in their observations, might be a cause of yellow atrophy of the liver mainly affecting the left lobe. Helps and McDonald (1954a) found that slight movements of the stomach would radically alter, or even destroy, the streamline pattern in the portal vein, even when respiratory movements did not break it up. This would suggest that in an intact mobile animal it would be very unlikely that a stable pattern would be maintained, especially in a larger animal. This doubt was borne out by the studies of Dreyer (1954) who injected radiopaque material into the spleen; he found evidence of streamline flow in the portal vein in only one out of fifteen patients and in two out of five dogs. The chance of coherent streams surviving through the heart seems non-existent but has been suggested by a few authors and is discussed separately (p. 86).

In *capillaries* there would appear to be no question as regards the presence of normal laminar flow because the Reynolds number is so minute, of the order of 0·001–0·005. Taylor (1955), however, questioned whether the size of the red cells in relation to the lumen, especially when they rotated, would not cause conditions somewhat like turbulence. Prothero and Burton (1961) discussed the subsidiary flows between cells in relation to increasing diffusion rates, and they have been the subject of more precise hydrodynamic formulation by Bugliarello *et al.* (1968) and by Bugliarello and Hsiao (1970). There would appear to be no question that the flow is laminar although it forms subsidiary vortex-like flows between cells.

STABILITY OF PULSATILE FLOW

All the evidence above indicates that wherever there is steady flow in the circulation the flow is laminar. This is in spite of the fact that factors such as branching and the presence of valves tend to cause instability. The evidence, however, is not very informative about the stability of blood flowing in vessels because the Reynolds number in all cases is far below the critical number.

In all vessels with a higher Reynolds number the flow is also markedly pulsatile. Where a breakdown of an observed laminar flow pattern is observed over only one part of a cycle it is difficult to define the flow as laminar or turbulent and the term 'disturbed' flow is used (p. 34). Some description of disturbances that have been seen in pulsatile blood flows will indicate the range of the phenomena. Examples are chosen which are manifestly not due to valves or other well-defined sources of a disturbance.

Helps and McDonald (1954a) observed that vortex rings were formed in the thoracic vena cava when flow reversed, but that they were damped out when forward flow was re-established. This was not considered as true turbulence because the Reynolds number was well below the critical value throughout the cycle and furthermore the disturbance occurred at a time when flow velocity was minimal. In addition, the vortex rings did not involve all the blood in the vein. In the rabbit aorta, McDonald (1952b), using high-speed cinematography, showed that, while laminar flow with a parabola-like profile could be seen in early systole, the dye pattern was disrupted completely during the peak systolic ejection and the flow appeared to be turbulent (Fig. 4.1). A laminar flow pattern was re-established in diastole although it was impossible to determine at what point it started and streams could not be clearly seen until well into diastole when the flow velocity was very low. In this case it may be more justifiable to call the flow 'turbulent' because the

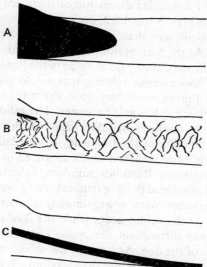

Fig. 4.1. Successive patterns of distribution of injected dye in the rabbit abdominal aorta—traced from single frames of a high-speed cinematograph film.

A. In early systole, the front is approximately that of a parabola such as that found in pulsating laminar flow.

B. There is a scattering of dye throughout the vessel due to turbulence during the period of peak velocity.

C. A stream of dye reformed during the period of backflow after the end of systole.

disturbance spread right across the artery and was initiated at a time of high flow velocity. The 'turbulent' phase was very brief, however, and probably did not persist for more than 50 msec. Evans (1955), furthermore, has pointed out that the dye appears to be disposed in the form of helical vortices and is not randomly distributed, but he regards this as a usual phenomenon in early turbulence. The Reynolds number in this case, calculated from the peak flow velocity, was at most 1,000 and so considerably below the usually accepted critical value of 2,000.

The first example described above (the thoracic vena cava) may, therefore, illustrate one group of causes of disturbed flow. This type is due to conditions, in this case probably a rapid reversal of flow, that create large vortices which are damped out by the inherent stability of the flow. The second example (the rabbit aorta) would then fall into a second group where a very rapid acceleration may produce a period of true instability that is short-lived because the high velocity is only maintained for a very short time.

From these observations there seems little doubt that oscillatory flow can become unstable at Reynolds numbers that are considerably below 2,000, even when these are calculated from maximum flow velocities which are only reached momentarily. Attempts have been made to relate the relative stability of steady and oscillatory flow to the differences in velocity profiles between these types of flow. For a detailed discussion of oscillatory flow profiles see Ch. 5. As can be seen in Figs. 5.1 and 5.2, the maximum rate of shear close to the wall is higher in oscillatory than in steady flow. Hale, McDonald, and Womersley (1955) made the assumption that the critical Reynolds number was simply related to the maximum rate of shear in the liquid. They calculated the equivalent steady flow average velocity that would give the same maximum rate of shear as a given oscillatory flow. From the equivalent velocity they could derive an effective Reynolds number. The ratio between effective and orthodox Reynolds numbers was dependent on the parameter α (eqn. 5.1), that is, it was a function of the frequency of oscillation as well as diameter. The only experimental evidence which appeared to support the hypothesis was that the maximum Reynolds numbers, calculated in the normal way in both the rabbit aorta and the dog femoral artery, were about 1,000, for flow velocity and diameter were approximately the same. Yet transient 'turbulence' was seen in the rabbit aorta while the flow in the dog femoral artery appeared laminar throughout the cycle. The rabbit's heart-rate was much higher than that of the dog. As a result, the 'effective Re' for the rabbit was almost 2,000 whereas that for the dog was only 1,300. Following this initial 'success' the hypothesis has not acquired any further evidence to support it. Its predictions were attractively quantitative but there is no hydrodynamic evidence to suggest that maximum rate of shear is the only determinant of stability. The experimental evidence that the frequency of oscillation is an important factor probably has significance.

Other features of the velocity profile have been considered. Prandtl (1952) quotes some theoretical work of Lord Rayleigh which indicated that re-entrant angles in a velocity profile were points of instability, and in more recent work, Tollmien has shown that S-shaped inflexions in the profile are, in fact, the points were stability breaks down. Prandtl suggests that it is the production of such inflexions by small irregularities in the wall that initiate turbulence in steady flow. Certainly in a glass model reversal of flow easily causes vortex rings to appear at the points of backwards inflexion that can be seen in the profiles illustrated in Figs. 5.1 and 5.2. The vortex rings that Helps and McDonald (1954a) observed in the inferior vena cava of the rabbit occurred at this situation during reversal of flow. The rate of shear is, of course, zero at the apex of such an inflexion. Evans (1955) has suggested, on the basis of Theodorsen's work, that turbulence originates in such vortices. Yellin (1966), however, states the point of inflexion criterion has only been studied in flat plate flow and not in tube flow. Also against this must be set the fact that in the rabbit aorta the instability of the flow developed during the rapid acceleration phase in systole apparently before any reversal of flow took place, and when the rate of shear would be maximal. This suggests that both high rates of shear and inflexions in the velocity profile may cause instability in oscillating flow when the Reynolds number is relatively high. From the consideration of the probable value of the Reynolds numbers found in the circulation detailed below, it seems likely that transient turbulence during systole will be found in the larger arteries, but that laminar flow should be found in, at least, the greater part of diastole.

In terms of the circulation, it is clear that the presence of oscillatory flow does not prevent the occurrence of stable laminar flow. Thus, McDonald and Potter (1951) showed that flow in the basilar artery of the rabbit (formed on the base of the brain by the fusion of the two vertebral arteries) was laminar. Dye injected into one vertebral artery remained on its own side of the basilar artery and was distributed only to branches arising from the same side (Fig. 4.2). The vessel was only 0·6 mm in diameter yet flow varied from c. 5 cm/sec

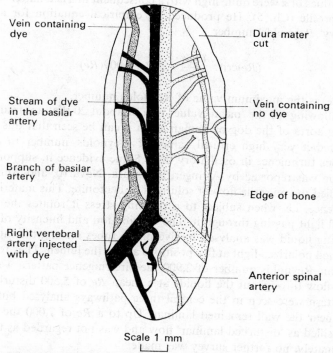

Vein containing dye

Dura mater cut

Stream of dye in the basilar artery

Vein containing no dye

Branch of basilar artery

Edge of bone

Right vertebral artery injected with dye

Anterior spinal artery

Scale 1 mm

Fig. 4.2. Streamline flow pattern in the basilar artery of a rabbit shown by injection of dye into one vertebral artery. The unilateral distribution persists through the regions of supply for it is seen returning in the vein of the same side. The peak value of the Reynolds number here was less than 100; this low value is the main reason for the stability of laminar flow at this junction compared with that shown in Fig. 4.6.

This figure is a tracing of a still photograph; the phenomenon was also recorded on a colour cine-film (*Blood streams in the basilar artery*—now available from the Wellcome Foundation, London, N.W.1). This film also shows the changes in pattern with partial and total occlusion of the contralateral vertebral artery.

in diastole to a peak of c. 35–40 cm/sec in systole. The peak Reynolds number was less than 100. Flow in other small arteries and in all arterioles is, therefore, almost certainly laminar. In larger vessels, Helps and McDonald (1954a) showed discrete streams of dye in the abdominal inferior vena cava of the rabbit, in which the flow was oscillatory, with peak Reynolds numbers of 300–400.

In model studies, Kunz and Coulter (1967) found no discontinuity in the oscillatory pressure–flow relation of glycerine–water mixture up to a maximum Reynolds number of 2,040.

If turbulence is defined in oscillatory flow as it is in steady flow, i.e. a condition where disturbance involves all the liquid throughout the cycle, then oscillatory flow may be stable to higher Reynolds numbers than is steady flow. Cotton (1960) studied the onset of continuous turbulence in a model using injected dye. His glass tube was wide but the frequencies were low so that the values of α were quite high with a consequent marked flattening of the velocity profile (Ch. 5). He produced an empirical equation for a critical 'oscillatory' Reynolds number

$$(Re)\text{crit} = \frac{(Re)}{\alpha} \times 532 + 0\cdot009(Re) \qquad\qquad \textbf{4.1}$$

where (Re) is the maximum value of Reynolds number.

Even allowing for the 'mean' values of α of about 20 that are found in the ascending aorta of the dog or human aorta it can be seen that this formula would predict very high critical values of Reynolds number to establish continuous turbulence in oscillatory flow. Some evidence in support of this contention was reported by Attinger, Sugawara, Navarro, and Anné (1966) who studied the pulsatile flow of solutions of bentonite. This material shows birefringence, i.e. when subject to a shearing stress it rotates the plane of polarized light passing through it. The distribution and intensity of shear in the flowing liquid was analysed by five photo tubes sensing the intensity of transmitted polarized light at five positions across the lumen. They found that at a mean Reynolds number of 2,900 the birefringence pattern was that of laminar flow throughout the liquid; at a mean Re of 5,500 disturbances of flow pattern were seen in the central three pathways analysed but the two regions near the wall remained laminar. Up to a Re of 7,000 the flow was still classified as 'disturbed laminar' flow and was not regarded as turbulent. Unfortunately, no further survey was made.

Yellin (1966) has also used bentonite to make a detailed survey of the laminar–turbulent transition in pulsatile flow imposed on a steady flow. Although the physiological implications are well discussed, the experimental situation always had a pulsatile flow which was relatively small compared to the steady component. The largest pulsatile flow was one-third the amplitude of the steady flow and was often only one-tenth; in arteries the oscillatory component commonly has an amplitude of at least five or six times the steady flow (see Ch. 10) and in the smallest arteries recorded it is at least of the same magnitude. The flow of the dilute bentonite solution was observed and photographed through crossed polaroid filters. With the onset of instability short regions, or 'slugs', of apparently turbulent flow would appear and travel with the flow. (By 'slug' Yellin seems to be describing periodic shedding of vortices.) With increasing Reynolds number their frequency of formation and rate of growth would increase; these two factors were plotted as criteria of instability. In steady flow no disturbances were observed up to a Reynolds' number of 2,270; between 2,270 and 2,450 a few 'slugs' were formed but propagated without change in size but above 2,450 they grew with a characteristic velocity and appeared with increasing frequency. When oscillatory flow was superimposed there was no significant growth rate to an Re of 2,450 and thereafter tended to be slower. The frequency of appearance, on the other hand, tended to increase above an Re of 2,800. The growth-rate was lowest when the frequency was lower and the oscillatory amplitude larger. An explanatory hypothesis was developed from the consideration of the viscous forces that would tend to dissipate any disturbances initiated near the inlet. (Yellin takes the view that the genesis of turbulence is entirely due to the growth of small disturbances present in the reservoir and in the entrance length.) He postulates that viscous forces only dominate inertial forces while the Reynolds number is below its critical value during the cycle. From this he defines a dimensionless relaxation 'time' τ given by

$$\tau = \theta v (Re_c - Re)/2r^2 \qquad\qquad \textbf{4.2}$$

where Re_c is the critical Re and Re is the minimum Re of the cycle; θ is the time during the sinusoidal cycle when the Reynolds number is less than critical, v is the kinematic viscosity of the liquid and r is the radius of the tube.

This dimensionless parameter is clearly dependent on the frequency of oscillation although no limiting values are proposed. In a qualitative way it is in agreement with the obervation noted above (p. 76) that disturbances in arteries are more commonly observed at faster heart-rates.

Certain subsidiary observations made are also of interest: (1) Disturbances were always seen at the time of flow reversal; this has been observed in flow in the vena cava (p. 74); (2) acceleration of flow appeared to be very stable in a simple tube but was far more unstable at a source of disturbances. This latter point might be relevant to the role of the aortic valves and is discussed below (p. 95). In the model, deceleration of flow appeared to be more often associated with the growth of disturbances than did acceleration of flow. This would appear to be contrary to the arterial observations illustrated in Fig. 4 but the origin of the renal arteries may be a source of disturbances in this

D

situation. Reference to Fig. 1 in McDonald, 1952*b*, however, shows that the actual situation is quite similar in that the break-up of the flow pattern began at peak-velocity and continued on in the deceleration phase.

Most recently, studies have been made of the flow pattern within the aorta with the technique of hot-film anemometry (Schultz *et al.*, 1969). Thin metal films on small probes are heated above blood temperatures by electric current; the flow in contact with the probe cools it proportionately to the rate of flow. A feedback circuit varies the heating current to keep the film temperatures constant; the variations in the current measure pulsatile flow. By varying the position of the probe across the artery the velocity profile has been recorded (Ch. 5). In addition, any major disturbance in flow pattern at any time in the cycle will show up as rapid oscillations on the flow record.

Such oscillations are, in fact, seen in some of the records. The studies are far from exhaustive yet but two conclusions seem quite clear. First, that the onset of disturbed flow or turbulence occurs at, or very shortly after, the peak velocity and was predominant during the deceleration phase (Fig. 4.3)—

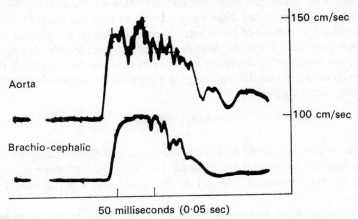

Fig. 4.3. Recordings of arterial flow pulses recorded with heated film probes. Upper trace—ascending aorta; lower trace—proximal brachiocephalic artery. The onset of flow disturbances marking transient turbulence of the flow can be seen. A typical pattern when this occurs only in the deceleration phase following peak velocity is seen especially in the brachiocephalic artery. In the aorta the turbulence persists for a greater proportion of the ejection period. (Figure by courtesy of Dr. D. Schultz.)

provided no valvular disease at the aortic orifice was present. This is similar to the findings in Yellin's model discussed above. Second, these phases of turbulence were found in the human only when the Reynolds number exceeded about 7,500, whereas in the dog they were observed with Reynolds numbers of the order of 2,500. These are important observations for they show that the flow in the rapidly accelerating phase of ejection is always essentially laminar. Certainly more so than McDonald (1960) had presumed or was indicated by the flow patterns illustrated in glass models of the aortic arch by Meisner and Rushmer (1963*a*) with bentonite solutions. In the first place, the vortices arising from the free edges of the valve cusps (which appeared to be likely from the films of McMillan, 1952) seemed to have been confined to the aortic sinuses behind the cusps and were not shed into the main stream. Flow around the valves is discussed below (p. 95). Secondly, the ejection pattern in the outflow tract of the ventricle is apparently more nearly laminar than would be predicted from the outflow from a reservoir in a model. This may well be due to the movement of the wall inwards as the ventricular volume decreases, a situation that can greatly increase the stability of the flow (Schultz, personal communication).

Some reservation must be made in this account as to whether the oscillations recorded in the unusually fast ejection curves are the sole indication of the occurrence of turbulence. Direct observation with high-speed cineradiography shows flow patterns which cannot be simply described as laminar; Lynch and Boye (1968) describe 'both axial and radial movements of the fluid as it is forced along the aorta'. Ohlsson (1962) also has observed disturbed flows in the aorta with a similar technique. The size of the fluctuations recorded as 'turbulent' by the anemometer suggests that fairly large eddies were present. There is probably no serious doubt, however, that disturbances too small, or too transient (the frequency response of the device is at least 200 Hz) to be detected will not make a large contribution to the disturbance of the flow pattern. That the eddies are not large enough to be synchronous across the aorta, is indicated by the fact that they are not recorded by electromagnetic flowmeters which record an integrated average of velocities across the whole tube when an external probe is used. In the case of the intravascular electromagnetic flow probe (Mills and Shillingford, 1967, Ch. 9) the averaging is over a less well-defined part of the total cross-section which is defined by the range of the magnetic field of the probe.

The difference between the Reynolds number at which flow stability breaks down in the human and dog aorta suggests that, in rapidly time-variant flows such as are present here, a further scale factor for vessel size in addition to the Reynolds number is involved. The most probable one, discussed by Bellhouse and Reid (1968) and Bellhouse and Bellhouse (1968) in relation to vortex formation at the valves, is the dimensionless Strouhal number, *St*. This is defined as

$$St = \frac{f \cdot R}{\overline{V}} \qquad\qquad \textbf{4.3}$$

where f is the frequency, R is the radius, and $\overline{V}$ the average velocity across the pipe. In essence, it determines the time available for vortex formation to occur and numerical examples are discussed in relation to the action of the aortic valves (p. 97).

It is interesting to note that the dimensionless parameter α which plays such an important role in the pressure–flow relations of oscillatory flow (eqn. 5.1 and on) is related to the Reynolds and Strouhal numbers:

$$\alpha^2 = R^2 \cdot \frac{2\pi f}{v} = \pi \cdot Re \cdot St \qquad \textbf{4.4}$$

(if the Reynolds number is calculated from the radius instead of the diameter the expression on the RHS is $2\pi \cdot Re \cdot St$). This indicates a line of investigation of the empirical relation for the critical conditions of the onset of turbulence in oscillatory flow derived by Cotton (eqn. 4.1). He incorporated the ratio Re/α. It would be interesting to test the applicability of the ratio Re/α^2, i.e. a factor of the Strouhal number, to his result.

The evidence, at present available, thus leads to no definite conclusions. At present there are no generally agreed critical values for Reynolds number above which laminar flow is completely unstable although anemometry techniques hold great promise. On the other hand, transient disturbances of all the flowing liquid can occur at low local Reynolds numbers, even at moments of zero flow when flow reverses. Whether or not such disturbances can usefully be classified as turbulence depends on considerations of energy dissipation. Attinger et al. (1966) reported that the energy losses when disturbances occurred in the central regions (p. 78) were little different from those in laminar flow and the disturbed high-frequency components contributed less than 5 per cent of the total dissipation; pressure–flow relationships were not, however, a primary object of their study in terms of critical evaluation.

The existence of audible sounds (the heart sounds and murmurs when present) indicates that acoustic energy is being dissipated over and above viscous losses. Sources of cardiovascular sound generation are too controversial to be considered fully here; while it is highly unlikely that they are due to turbulent flow alone, but also involve vibration of solid structure, the generation of sound is incompatible with stable laminar flow.

Finally, it is, for many purposes, sufficient to establish that there is enough disturbance of flow at some part of each cycle to cause complete mixing of the blood in the heart chamber or blood vessel that is being studied. Such evidence as was presented above shows that this can occur at much lower Reynolds number than is necessary to create a condition resembling turbulence throughout a cycle.

REYNOLDS NUMBER IN THE CIRCULATION

While the evaluation of the Reynolds number in a given region is insufficient to characterize the nature of the flow it is a useful guide to the relative stability of the flow. Against the background of this information it is easier to

TABLE 4.1 Estimated Reynolds numbers in the circulation

Species	Vessel	Diameter (cm)	Velocity (cm/sec)	Reynolds no.	Authors
Human	Ascending aorta	2·30–4·35	21·3–87·4 (mean systolic)	5,000–12,000	Prec et al. (1949)
Human	Pulmonary trunk	2·32–3·50	33·1–63·5 (mean systolic)	5,000–10,000	
Dog	Ascending aorta	1·0	40 (mean systolic)	2,360	Green (1944)
Dog	Prox. thor. aorta	1·0	112 (peak)	3,000–3,500	Spencer and Denison (1956)
Dog	Distal thor. aorta	0·77–0·82	114–128 (peak)	2,450–2,590	
Rabbit	Abdominal aorta	0·53–0·61	106–141 (peak)	1,710–1,970	
Dog	Abdominal aorta	0·3	60 (peak)	1,960	Hale et al. (1955)
Dog	Femoral	0·3	100 (peak)	1,300	
Dog	Saphenous	0·1	30 (peak)	80	McDonald (1960)
Rabbit	Basilar	0·06	40 (peak)	100	McDonald and Potter (1951)
Lamb	Ductus arteriosus	0·24	60 (mean)	750	Dawes et al. (1955)
Dog	Small mesenteric artery	0·005	2·1	0·28	
Dog	Arteriole	0·0025	0·28	0·018	from Schlier (1918)
Dog	Capillary	0·0008	0·05	0·001	
Rabbit	Small mesenteric vein	0·01	1·0	0·6	
Rabbit	Abdominal vena cava	0·34	18·0 (peak)	360	
Dog	Abdominal vena cava	1·0	15·0 (peak)	930	Helps and McDonald (1954a)
Rabbit	Thoracic inf. v. cava	0·6	18·0 (peak)	660	
Human	Thoracic inf. v. cava	2·0	10·7–16·0 (mean)	1,320–1,980	

From direct velocity measurements using a heated film probe Schultz et al. (1969) conclude that peak Reynolds number in dogs may well reach 4,500–5,000 and in man as high as 12,000. These are well above values at which stable laminar flow might be expected but virtually undisturbed flow was observed at Reynolds numbers as high as 7,800 in man and 2,300–2,800 in dogs. The effect of diameter of vessel on the time taken to the onset of turbulence is discussed in the text.

assess the effect of other factors which cause disturbances of flow such as valves, presence of branches, and so on.

The values of Reynolds' number that have been estimated in the circulation are shown in Table 4.1. Only values to be found in systole are given for arteries as diastolic values are rarely quoted. As there always appears to be zero flow at some point during the cycle in all large arteries, and hence a Reynolds number of zero, it can be seen that its fluctuations are very great. It should be emphasized that the conditions determining the onset of turbulence at a critical Reynolds number have been determined experimentally only for steady flow. The application of this work to pulsating blood flow should be interpreted with reserve in the light of the discussion above.

MIXING OF BLOOD

In vessels

From the practical point of view the degree to which disturbances in the flow pattern cause mixing of the blood is most important in physiology and medicine. We know that the composition of venous blood varies considerably according to the metabolic activity of the organ from which it drains, so that it is important to know if a sample of blood from a vein is representative of all the blood in it or whether its composition is dependent on the drainage through one or more of its tributaries. The extent of the mixing of dye is also important in indicator-dilution methods for estimating blood flow. The easiest way to observe the mixing is to inject a dye into a tributary and watch its flow in the larger vessels. Unfortunately this direct method is only easily applicable to small vessels and we have seen from the evaluation of the Reynolds number (Table 4.1) that these are almost certainly laminar. Observations have amply borne out this prediction. Franklin (1937) reviews a considerable body of evidence in the smaller veins and Helps and McDonald (1954a) confirmed that there was almost total absence of mixing in veins as large as the rabbit abdominal vena cava where the Reynolds number was about 350. Even so, the streamline pattern is easily disturbed and it is probable that inserting a needle or catheter to take a sample would, of itself, cause a certain amount of mixing. An attempt to assess this effect quantitatively is made below (p. 86).

When the flow becomes subject to pulsatile changes as in the great veins of the thorax, the maintenance of clear-cut streams is very much more difficult. The effect of pulsation on stability of flow has already been discussed, but in a situation like the inferior vena cava, while we can say with certainty on the evidence that considerable disturbance of flow exists (Helps and McDonald, 1954a), it is quite different to assert that *complete* mixing occurs. Even in a condition of turbulence physical admixture will take a certain amount of time to occur, so that near the entry of a large tributary, like the hepatic vein for example, there might well be a difference in composition compared with the blood, say, in the right atrium. Ultimately, the evidence from sampling must determine our views on the reliability of such a sample, and general considerations can only act as a guide.

It is unfortunate that the sites where we should most like direct observational evidence mainly concern the large veins and arteries, and that the thickness of the walls makes such direct observations difficult or impossible. A certain number of investigations have been made with cineradiography and these have been very valuable and should be extended. The interpretation of the results is a little limited by the lack of detail in the pictures. Also to obtain better contrast it is usual to inject the radiopaque substance rapidly and this, of itself, will tend to change the normal flow very greatly.

The widespread use of indicator-dilution methods to measure blood flow also makes it necessary for us to know the characteristics of the flow in the regions where they are applied. It is not possible here to cover the many modifications and application of the technique; the details and theoretical basis of these methods have been lucidly set out by Meier and Zierler (1954) and by Zierler (1962a, b) and the extension to the measurements of vascular volumes has also been treated theoretically by Grodins (1962). An earlier review by Dow (1956) is also valuable in treating some problems of interpretation which tend to be overlooked. Rossi, Powers, and Dwork (1953), on the basis of experiments with models, showed that the technique would be in error if the flow is laminar and inadequate mixing occurs. (Caro (1966) has shown that in perfect laminar flow in a tube the wash-out curve would not be exponential.) If, however, there is a region in the system between the point of injection and the point of sampling where there is turbulence, or complete mixing from any cause, then the standard formula will apply. The concentration of indicator is then uniform across the outflow side of the network and sampling from any portion will be representative of the whole. Rossi *et al.* did not pursue the implications of this comment but insofar as the method is applied to the measurement of cardiac output the heart is clearly the region where such complete mixing is likely to occur. As is seen in the discussion in the next section, all the evidence suggests that normally blood is completely mixed on passage through the heart so that the technique is valid. Conversely, the general experience of the accuracy of indicator–dilution methods is further evidence for the complete mixing of blood in passing through the heart.

When an indicator–dilution technique is used in a peripheral vascular bed the situation is rather different, for the Reynolds number may be below the critical value (Table 4.1) and doubts are raised about the degree of mixing. The mixing problem was specifically studied by Zierler and his colleagues (Andres *et al.*, 1954) in measuring blood flow in the arm. The efficiency of jet-injection into the brachial artery was compared to injections at a lower rate by sampling from both radial and ulnar arteries. In fact, fairly complete mixing was achieved without special precautions and was not much improved by jet-injection (which tended to cause haemolysis). This further indicates that the disturbances in the circulation, whether they be due to pulsation, the origin of branches, or the other causes that are discussed in this chapter, will always cause a considerable degree of mixing. The actual act of injecting, or sampling, with a needle or catheter in a vessel is itself a potent cause of eddy formation and hence of mixing. With withdrawal rates of, for example, 2·0 ml/sec, as are commonly used in indicator–dilution studies, the concentration measured will be the average for all the dye in the volume in terms of the time-constant of the recording device used. Even when more rapid recording devices, such as thermistors in thermo-dilution methods, are used without withdrawal of blood, there will still be some averaging effect so that small variations in mixing will not be of practical importance.

In the heart

In terms of a hydrodynamic model the heart may be regarded as the reservoir supplying tubes emerging from it. As the standard description of the critical Reynolds number requires disturbed conditions in the reservoir, there is no doubt that this condition is satisfied but is of little consequence in view of the uncertainties underlying the application of the Reynolds number concept to the pulsating flow in arteries. The only real concern is with the degree of mixing of the blood passing through it that occurs. Treating the heart as a wide channel we can see from comparison with the large vessels that high Reynolds numbers must be found there during ejection. During inflow into the ventricle the presence of the tricuspid and mitral valves and the irregular shape of the interior of the ventricle with the presence of the chordae tendinae and trabeculae will all create a swirling motion of the blood which will promote mixing. The outward movement of the walls of the distending ventricle will add to this but it is possible that inflowing blood will not complete mixing with all the blood remaining in the heart from the previous systole, especially in the crevices of the trabeculae. The high-speed radiography films (540 or 270 frames/sec) of Lynch and Bove (1968) in which contrast material is injected into the left atrium provide excellent evidence on these points (Fig. 4.4). They describe the flow into the ventricle in these words, 'The shape of the contrast front is quite flat but expands as it moves towards the opposing wall. . . .' The valve cusps trailing into the moving stream will naturally cause eddies to form. Initially, small eddies form as the contrast medium falls towards the opposing ventricular wall. When the material reaches this wall, large eddies develop and a swirling motion is easily seen in the lateral projection. The predominant eddy involves the entire ventricular cavity, mixing the contrast medium in a rotation towards the outflow tract. Bellhouse (1972) has also observed similar large eddies involving an artificial ventricle caused by the mitral valve. During ejection the studies made with hot-film anemometers in the aorta and discussed above (p. 80) suggests that flow is essentially laminar in the outflow tract but from the foregoing descrip-

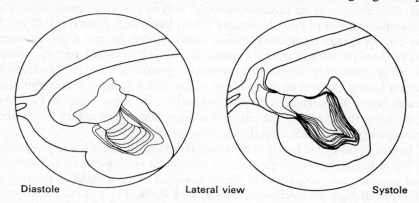

Diastole   Lateral view   Systole

Fig. 4.4. These figures are made up of tracings of the front of radiopaque dye filmed by high-speed radiography. The drawing on the left shows inflow through the mitral valve in diastole and the whole ventricle seems to fill evenly except for small regions on either side of the cusps of the valve.

In the second drawing successive outlines are drawn during systole when ejection into the aorta is occurring. The dye fills the ventricle evenly; in the aorta the velocity profile is seen to be markedly skewed on the inside of the bend around the arch. (From Lynch and Bove, 1968.)

tion mixing is already achieved. More direct evidence of flow pattern within the heart by means of these anemometers would be very helpful in amplifying our knowledge. But no one who has attempted to demonstrate laminar flow in models is likely to have any illusions about the difficulty of demonstrating continuous streamlines through the chambers of the heart. Cineradiographic films of the flow of lipiodol in the dog's heart (Rushmer, 1970) show the swirling motion of the blood in the ventricles very clearly.

With the introduction of image intensification, the use of such films has become, in some clinics, a standard procedure for the measurement of ventricular volume (Dodge *et al.* 1960, 1962). The usual rate of filming has been at 60 frames/sec but high-speed filming (c. 500 frames/sec, Lynch and Bove, 1969) has also been done. These records are essentially similar to those previously reported in the smaller dog heart and there can be no doubt that any streamline pattern there might be in the atria flowing into the ventricles is thoroughly broken up, even when allowance is made for the effect of the injection of the radiopaque substance.

On the question of mixing of blood in the heart there is also a great deal of evidence derived from the standard practice of using an intracardiac catheter to sample mixed venous blood for determinations of the cardiac output by the Fick principle. This evidence can only be summarized briefly here. It is generally agreed that blood is thoroughly mixed, in a normal heart, by the time it reaches the pulmonary artery. In many clinics this is the standard site for sampling. The catheter is less commonly left in the right ventricle for fear of causing ectopic beats, but here again complete mixing is regarded as occurring (e.g. Warren, 1948). In the atrium, however, some workers have suggested that differences between successive samples may be due to the persistence of a streamline pattern of flow. Cournand (1948) has stated, however, that in 75 per cent of catheterizations successive atrial samples do not differ by more than 0·2 vol per cent in oxygen content. Gorlin (1958) gives larger variations as being commonly found. My personal opinion is that the inadequate mixing is only likely to be in the region of the orifice of the coronary sinus (in hearts where the atrium is beating normally). In the atrium, in fact, the sampling catheter is near the entry of a large vein, the coronary sinus, and incomplete mixing is not a good indication of laminar flow.

In greatly distended hearts in advanced failure where there is a large volume of blood left at the end of systole, even ventricular mixing may be incomplete, and variation may also occur in the composition of the samples in the region of septal defects (Wiederhielm, Bruce, and John, 1957). Lynch (personal communication) also reports poor mixing in ventricular aneurysms. This is due to the fact that, even with fully developed turbulence the mixing of two volumes of liquid can never be instantaneous.* Such mixing cannot be predicted theoretically and the determination of the size of the zones of unmixed, or partially mixed, blood can only be determined experimentally.

Even in the case of the normal heart, the criteria for which mixing is considered need to be carefully evaluated. The discussion above indicated that blood flowing into the heart is normally thoroughly mixed before it is ejected. The composition of the inflow does not suddenly change. In techniques that have been developed to measure diastolic and end-systolic volumes by indicator–dilution methods the demand is more stringent. Here a small amount of indicator is rapidly injected and the dilution distribution during subsequent systoles is recorded. In the original method (Holt, 1956) saline was used and changes in conductivity in the outflow measured, but dye (recorded photoelectrically in blood drawn through a cuvette) or cold liquid (recorded with a catheter-tip thermistor) has also been used. Results currently recorded do not correlate very well with volume measured by other techniques such as radiography. The subject has been reviewed in detail by Holt (1966).

* *Geographical footnote*: In this respect, it is interesting to draw an analogy even though it is on a somewhat larger scale, with the distinct 'streams' seen in rivers. Where one tributary has clear water, while another is muddy, the waters when they join can be followed distinctly—often for several miles. In former days, the examples most quoted were of the Rhone, or the Danube at Vienna; nowadays, when our academic colleagues travel further afield, I am told of the same appearance at the junction of the Blue and White Nile at Khartoum, and also in rivers in New Zealand. Unfortunately, these are not examples of streamlines in laminar flow as seen in veins for, with Reynolds number of the order of millions, these rivers are all turbulent. They are, however, a reminder that even with fully developed turbulence the mixing of large volumes takes a long time. I am indeed sorry to have to demolish this piece of haemodynamic folklore but at least it shows how important scale is in drawing analogies between different systems.

The discrepancy is commonly attributed to failure of even distribution of indicator throughout the diastolic volume, though in some methods it is questionable whether the recording system follows the concentration in the ejected blood sufficiently rapidly. When sampling from the aorta it is a common finding that the end-diastolic volume is over-estimated; an analysis by Carleton, Bowyer, and Graetinger (1966) used ascorbic acid as an indicator detected polarographically (nevertheless the time to teach 95 per cent of full response was 0·6 sec). From detectors placed in the ventricle they suggest that blood entering through the mitral valve is preferentially displaced towards the outflow tract without thorough mixing with blood in the cavity of the ventricle. This concept was first suggested by Swan and Beck (1960) in radiographic evidence, though the study of high-speed angiographic film by Lynch and his colleagues has failed to see this effect (Fig. 4.4). This point should be studied more critically with detectors more precisely located than electrodes on the end of a free catheter can be.

The mixing in the ventricle required in the indicator-dilution technique requires an initial fast dispersion of injected indicator throughout the ventricle during diastole; in subsequent cycles it requires rapid mixing of inflowing blood with the previous end-systolic volume. This is a more stringent requirement for the mixing of blood across a vessel than in a normal ventricle. This has recently been carefully investigated by Dr. Lloyd in my laboratory. Lloyd (1971) and Lloyd and McDonald (1971) built an apparatus which activates an isolated left ventricle (with intact mitral and aortic valves) at controlled frequencies and rates of ejection. In successive identical runs the temperature was monitored at 16 different sites in the ventricular cavity. Initially a small injection of cold saline (1·5–2·0 ml at 25°C) was made in early diastole. The mixing of the first injection was found to be poor during the cycle in which it was made. Following the mitral inflow at the next and subsequent beats the mixing was greatly improved and the thermistor monitoring the temperature in the root of the aorta showed that mixing was much improved there. Nevertheless the ventricular volume estimated did not correlate with the statically measured volume to make it a reliable estimate. The method did, however, show most interesting maps of the mitral inflow into the ventricle.

The *fetal heart* may be likened to the adult heart with a congenital septal defect in the neighbourhood of which mixing may be incomplete. Barclay, Franklin, and Prichard (1944) produced evidence that the blood from the inferior vena cava of the fetal lamb passed through the foramen ovale without mixing much with blood from the superior vena cava. Oxygenated blood from the placenta thus went to the left side of the heart and so preferentially to the head. The venous blood from the superior vena cava would be distributed to the hind part of the body via the pulmonary artery and ductus arteriosus. In a small heart such incomplete mixing in the atrium might well occur though the separation of the two streams is likely to be far from complete. The phenomenon has been disputed by Dawes, Mott, Widdicombe and Wyatt (1953) who found no significant difference between the oxygen content of blood from the carotid and that from the distal aorta.

The only hearts in which laminar flow phenomena have been seen are those of some small amphibia such as the frog (Simons and Michaelis, 1953). The conditions here, however, are markedly different from those in the mammal owing to the very small size of these hearts with a low flow rate and low pulse frequency in addition to the anatomical peculiarity of the spiral valve. The flow patterns in vertebrates with a single ventricle are reviewed by Johannsen and Martin (1965).

In the mammal, especially the human, the evidence about the mixing in the emerging great vessels constitutes the last stage in the consideration of the effect of the heart on the flow patterns in the circulation. Reference has already been made to the results of sampling in the pulmonary trunk. In the systemic circulation sampling is often done much further peripherally so that we need to consider also the effects of the curvature of the arch of the aorta, the origins of branches and of valves.

CURVES IN A TUBE

The effect of curving a pipe is to increase the stability of flow. The critical Reynolds number increases quite markedly and a lower critical number of 7,000 is quite easy to obtain. The magnitude of the effect depends on the ratio of the radius of curvature to the radius of the tube (Goldstein, 1938). The arch of the aorta is the best example of a curved tube in the circulation, but in view of the presence of large branches in it and the proximity of the heart, a simple application of hydrodynamic theory cannot be made with any precision.

Liquid in a curved tube sets up *secondary flows* that cause a streamline of dye to follow a helical course in place of the path parallel to the wall that is seen in a straight tube. This can be most simply explained in terms of the centrifugal force associated with motion in a curve. This force is greatest in the axial streams because they are moving fastest, and least in the liquid near the wall which is moving slowly. Therefore, the liquid in the middle of the stream creates a secondary flow towards the outer wall of the curve; this forces the liquid nearer the wall to flow towards the inner wall. Thus, there are two minor circulations set up within the tube separated by the medial plane in the line of the radius of curvature (Fig. 4.5).

In terms of a velocity profile that would otherwise be 'flat' across the lumen of the tube—as would be expected in pulsatile flow in a vessel the size of the aorta (Ch. 5)—this results in a skewing of the profile with higher velocities on the outer side of the curve than on the inner side. Such an asymmetry of the velocity profile has been found in the proximal aorta by Schultz et al. (1949).

The fact that some such effect is detectable even in the ascending aorta indicates that the line of flow from the outflow tract of the ventricle into the aorta is somewhat curved. The asymmetry of the velocity profile in the

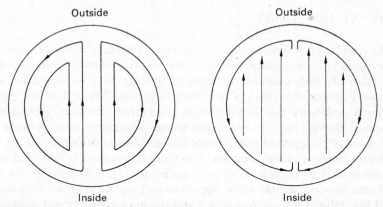

Fig. 4.5. Diagrams of secondary flows which develop in a pipe at a bend. The outside of the bend in both cases is at the top of the diagram, and flow in the centre of the pipe moves centrifugally and then circulates more slowly back around the circumference. The drawing at the right shows the change that occurs when the radius of the bend gets smaller; in a tighter bend more of the central region is flowing centrifugally. Both these cases are for steady flow with a parabolic profile.

With pulsatile flows the central region tends to become a region of vortices with the secondary flows becoming more confined to the region nearer the wall.

proximal ascending aorta is a source of error in the measurement of flow at this site with an electromagnetic flowmeter (which assumes a symmetrical velocity profile, Ch. 9). In fact, the asymmetry recorded by Schultz and his colleagues (1969) in the descending aorta is not much greater than they found at the mid-point of the arch (their Fig. 10) so that the potential error due to this cause may be small. The apparent secondary flows they found are smaller than would be expected after flowing around rather more than a half-circle. This may be due to interaction with subsidiary secondary flows at the origin of the large branches on the arch (see below).

Helical flow paths of radiopaque droplets as they move around the aortic arch during systole are reported by Lynch and Bove (1968) from high-speed films. With water-soluble contrast material they also show essentially flat profiles. The asymmetry seen is marked in the arch in the region of the branches but velocities are highest on the inner side of the curve; this emphasizes the complicating effect of these branches on arch flow patterns.

A more detailed set of velocity profiles with a skew asymmetry are reported using bentonite flows in a model by Attinger *et al.* (1966). McDonald (1968*b*) has suggested that these are due to secondary flows resulting from bends that were necessarily present in the set-up of the model; if so, they constitute the most detailed study of the velocity profiles in oscillatory flow with secondary flows present that have been published.

Illustrations of the appearance of secondary flows in models of the aorta and its branches have been made by Timm (1942, using dye) and by Meisner and Rushmer (1963a, using the birefringence of bentonite).

FLOW AT JUNCTIONS

As the circulation is functionally a distributing system of pipes, junctions are a very predominant feature. Yet orthodox hydrodynamics appears to have paid relatively little attention to them so that we have no sound basis for discussing the possible effect of branching in the stability of flow in a pipe. It is complicated by the fact that the origin of a branch introduces a bend of the streamline flowing into it and hence causes secondary flow. Barnett and Cochrane (1956) reported experiments on the division of flow in steady flow in various types of model junction. The types of junction to be found in the circulation may be considered in three main types. (1) The division of a main trunk into two, or possibly more, approximately equal branches. This may be called the 'bifurcation' or λ-junction and the most characteristic example is the bifurcation of the abdominal aorta into the two iliac vessels. (2) The reverse condition where two or more branches of equal size joint to form a single trunk. This may be called the fusion junction or λ-type. This type is almost exclusively found in the venous system, the only arterial example of note being the fusion of the two vertebral arteries to form the basilar artery on the medulla. (3) The 'side-branch' where a single branch, usually of much smaller dimensions, leaves the parent trunk at an angle which depends on the anatomical position. In the larger vessels, this is the most common group for it contains so many variations.

In the case of the first and third groups the blood is flowing from a region of higher Reynolds number to one of lower Reynolds number. It is well established that the total size of the vascular bed increases at each subdivision and the effect of this in decreasing the Reynolds number has been demonstrated above (eqn. 2.12). The first effect of this will be to increase the stability of flow and conditions of laminar flow are most easily demonstrated in the smaller branches away from the heart. At the point of junction, however, there is a discontinuity in the wall and the effect of this is probably akin to a physical obstacle in the flow, which causes a sudden deflection in the motion of the liquid.

The most striking demonstration of this was shown in a high-speed film (McDonald, 1952b) made of flow at the bifurcation of the aorta in a rabbit (Fig. 4.6). The axial stream of the aortic blood could be seen to impinge on the wall joining the two iliac vessels and rebounded from it so that eddies were set up near the orifices of the two branches. The dye nearer the walls of the aorta flowed more smoothly around the bend into the branches. In the rabbit ((Re) less than critical) these eddies only persisted through systole and died out early in diastole, but in a larger animal would be expected to persist for much longer. In Fig. 4.6 it can be seen that the beginning of the iliac vessel is almost at right angles to the aorta. This is rather an extreme case but a study of other

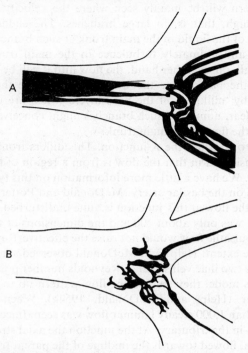

Fig. 4.6. Flow patterns with injected dye at the distal end (the 'bifurcation') of the rabbit aorta These are tracings of single frames of a high-speed film (16 mm) record.
A. during the acceleration phase of systole;
B. during diastole.
There is a marked, but brief, disturbance of flow during systole in the more proximal part of the artery (Fig. 4.1). These drawings, however, serve to show that the presence of a point of branching causes much more marked and prolonged disturbances of flow pattern. The Reynolds number at peak systolic flow in this case was between 800–1,000.

animals indicates that the angle of branching is always greater at the bifurcation than conventional anatomical diagrams suggest.

The difficulties of making direct observations on the interior of intact arteries are severe limitations in surveying this field. As mentioned above, Timm (1942) studied the flow pattern in a glass model which was a faithful reproduction of the anatomical arrangement in the human aorta. Meisner and Rushmer (1963a) made more detailed studies which are described above. From these we can visualize the situation at the origin of the innominate and subclavian branches in these models which will be similar to that of lesser branches leaving a main trunk at right angles. The deflection of the stream causes it to follow a sinuous course, so that the stream entering the branch may first swing over to the far side of the aorta and then curve back into the branch. Presumably the centrifugal force on the curved stream sets up secondary flows at each point where a tributary stream leaves the trunk, and this type of flow pattern will be mainly seen where the velocity of flow in the branch is fairly high, that is, in large branches. The sudden creation of transverse motion of the liquid in the main trunk at such branches would tend to cause vortices and ultimately turbulence in the main trunk. Where the branch is very small, on the other hand, the flow into it will be derived almost exclusively from the blood near the wall, which will be the slow-moving laminae. In fact, by 'milking' off the fluid layers which are undergoing the highest rates of shear, numerous such branches might conceivably contribute to the stability of the flow in the main trunk.

There remains to consider the λ-junction. This differs from the other two types we have considered in that the flow is from a region of lower to higher Reynolds number. We have a little more information on this type of junction because of studies on the basilar artery. McDonald and Potter (1951) showed that in the rabbit the flow at this junction is quite undisturbed. The Reynolds number, however, was only about 100 and the dimensions of this vessel were so small that the pulsatile flow would not raise the effective Reynolds number to any appreciable extent. Helps and McDonald observed similar stability at the junction of the two iliac veins with a Reynolds number possibly as high as 300. Using a glass model they studied the flow pattern up to a much higher Reynolds number (Helps and McDonald, 1954a). When the Reynolds number was less than 1,000 steady laminar flow was seen. Injected dye formed a typical parabola in the tributary. At the junction the axial stream, that is the tip of the parabola, flowed towards the midline of the parent trunk, but owing to the bend between tributary and trunk a circulating movement developed due to secondary flow. The fluid in the axial stream moved towards the midline on either side and then circulated up to, and outwards by, the wall. There were, in fact, two sets of secondary flow set up in each half of the pipe which persisted for some distance down the parent trunk until a new parabola was formed across the single trunk. I have made some high-speed films (1,500 frames/sec) of this phenomenon with Dr. Potter in the basilar artery and the helical course of the streams can be clearly seen.

At a bend the fluid at highest flow rates tends to move to the outer wall and so in a λ-junction it is the faster flowing laminae that meet. Furthermore, where the curve is not smooth, particularly at the inner angle of the λ there is a zone of 'dead water'. As this is contiguous to the confluence of the fast flowing laminae, instability tends to occur at this point.

At rates of flow considerably below the critical Reynolds number (600 in branches, 1,000 in the main trunk) it was observed in the model that vortex rings were formed at this junctional region and were carried down the pipe, and when formed showed no signs of damping out for the length of about thirty diameters that they were followed. This strongly suggests that a λ-junction of this sort lowers the stability of flow across it. The quantitative assessment of this effect is difficult because of the difficulty in making glass junctions without any irregularity of the lumen, and at junctions of blood vessels the smooth tapering of one branch into the other is better managed. It would be interesting to study this problem perfusing an actual venous junction.

The modelling problem has been ingeniously treated by Neumaster and Krovetz (1964) who made models fashioned from the casts of vessel junction. With glass models he (Krovetz, 1965b, Krovetz and Crowe, 1967) found that the presence of a branch origin lowered the critical Reynolds number at which turbulence could occur to a value of between 58 per cent and 89 per cent of the number at which transition occurred in a straight tube (Krovetz, 1965a). Stehbens (1959) studied the break-up of laminar dye patterns in the range (Re) 306–1475 in models of the aortic bifurcation and in curved tubes modelled on the intracranial course of the carotid artery (the 'siphon').

An effect of a side-branch, as in these models, might be caused by the 'milking-off' into a branch of a more stable boundary layer near the wall of the main trunk. In vessels of capillary size this is somewhat analogous to the phenomenon of plasma skimming when no red cells flow into some branches. This has been studied quantitatively in scaled-up models by Bugliarello and Hsiao (1964, 1965). When the branch is smaller than the main trunk the concentration of cell equivalents in the branch is always lower than its parent even when the flow rate through it is 50 per cent higher. Whether this would have any marked effect in vessels which are very large in terms of cell diameter is more doubtful.

VALVES. THE EFFECT OF PROJECTIONS

It is common knowledge that an obstacle projecting into a stream will cause eddies to form, but small ones soon die away. If the disturbance is larger the eddies will grow in size and ultimately will cause a complete breakdown of laminar flow. The size of such an obstacle, as a fraction of the width of the channel, that can be permitted before the laminar flow breaks down depends on the Reynolds number of the flow and to a certain extent the shape of the obstacle. Goldstein (1938, Chapter VII, p. 142) states that for a sharp-edged projection of height ϵ in a pipe of radius r we must have

$$\frac{\epsilon}{r} < \frac{4}{(Re)^{\frac{1}{2}}} (Re = \text{Reynolds number})$$

to maintain laminar flow. For a smooth obstacle of cylindrical cross-section

$$\frac{\epsilon}{r} < 5/(Re)^{\frac{1}{3}}$$

The commonest natural projection is a valve cusp and so the formula for a sharp-edged projection is most valid. At a Reynolds number of 400, for example, the tolerated value of ϵ/r would therefore be $\frac{1}{5}$ and at $(Re) = 1,600$ (ϵ/r) would be $\frac{1}{10}$.

In pathological conditions, such as atheroma, the effect of projecting plaques may be estimated by this formula.

Any breakdown that occurs will be an eddy in the first instance and these will form at the free margin and will break away periodically. The formation of vortices at the free edge of a valve cusp will also have the effect of holding the free edge of the valve away from the wall. This has the important functional effect of presenting a considerable surface to flow in the reverse direction; thus closing the valve immediately there is a tendency for back flow to occur. Equally it means that at every valve there is a projection into the stream. The observation of these eddies at valves can very easily be made (for instance, they are seen in the human axillary vein when it is exposed surgically during a radical mastectomy.) These eddies will cause mixing of blood in the veins. The obstruction due to a sampling catheter will also cause eddies and so increase mixing, an effect that will clearly be greatest in small veins where the catheter will be large relative to the vessel.

At the aortic orifice the presence of valves adds one more factor to those already considered in producing an irregular flow pattern. In addition, the expansion of the aorta, the aortic sinus, immediately beyond the valves will also cause eddy formation. Timm (1942) in the aortic model described above, showed clearly that even in conditions of laminar flow there is a swirling motion of the liquid in this region. The functional significance of eddy formation behind the valve cusps is here not only important for rapid closing, but also prevents the valves from occluding the orifices of the coronary arteries. Bellhouse and Bellhouse (1969) demonstrated, with various models, that the sinuses of Valsalva behind the valve cusps normally trap these eddies completely. If the valve is stenosed, however, they escape into the aortic stream.

The action of the aortic valves in post-mortem hearts was filmed by McMillan (1955); a pump outlet was inserted in the outflow tract of the heart and a ciné camera attached to a tube tied into the aorta while a side-tube conducted the saline away. A graphic view of the triangular opening of the valve cusps and the flittering of the valve margins, which were apparently shedding vortices, was obtained. The action of the aortic valves has been studied in much more detail by Bellhouse and Bellhouse (1968) and Bellhouse, Bellhouse and Reid (1968). In dissections of the origin of the aorta in man, sheep, dogs, pigs, and oxen they have demonstrated that the dilatations of the aorta behind the opened valve cusps (the sinuses of Valsalva) are much deeper than has been assumed; on the average the depth of the sinus is about equal to the radius of the aorta. Externally this is rather obscured by the ventricular muscle. The narrowing of the aorta at the far end of the sinuses is usually marked by a distinct internal ridge. When the valves are fully opened the top of the cusps lie slightly within the sinus below this ridge. They suppose that the necessity of tying a tube into the aorta, as was done by McMillan and others using a similar technique, distorts the exit from the sinuses and makes it appear that the cusps are lying free in the stream. In the configuration they describe the cross-sectional area of the aorta at the sinus ridge is about the same as the somewhat triangular valve orifice. This would account for the apparent absence of a jet effect which was predicted by McDonald (1960). In fact, as noted above, the velocity profile in the ascending aorta recorded by Schultz et al. (1969) was remarkably flat across the ascending aorta as are those of Ling et al. (1968) recorded with a similar technique; earlier recordings by Freis and Heath (1964) had indicated the same lack of a jet. (With stenosed valves, however, Schultz et al. found much higher velocities in midstream than in the regions closer to the wall.) These experimental findings regarding the velocity profile are more fully discussed in Ch. 5.

The stages of valve opening and closing are described by the Bellhouse group in four stages.

(1) *Opening phase*. The cusps present negligible resistance and open widely as the flow accelerates. This is augmented by flow displaced from the sinuses by the opening cusps. This movement of blood close to the wall contributes to the flat velocity profile.

(2) *Vortex generation phase*. The valve is fully open before the aortic flow reaches its peak. A vortex starts in the boundary layer and when it reaches the free margin it rolls up into the sinus. The vortex also bends the streamlines towards the wall so that the sinus ridge becomes a stagnation point (Ch. 2, p. 37). A major vortex thus develops in the sinus, fed by the streamlines on that side of the stagnation point. (These vortices were recorded with the hot-film anemometer that was used by Schultz in the same laboratory, and described above, p. 80). The time available for vortex formation is governed by the duration of systole and the Strouhal number (see p. 81 above in relation to aortic turbulence). The vortex here described quantitatively has previously been noted above in the models of Timm (1942) and Meisner and Rushmer (1963a). They are important functionally in preventing the cusps from being pushed into the sinuses and thus occluding the orifices of the coronary sinus; indeed, they play a part in maintaining a good coronary flow during systole.

(3) *Deceleration phase*. The vortex in the sinus provides a thrust on the valve cusp which grows relatively larger as it is being continually fed during the deceleration of aortic flow. As the ventricular pressure upstream falls relative to the downstream aortic pressure (see Figs. 6.3 and 6.4) the valve bellies out into the stream leading to (4).

(4) *Valve sealing by reverse flow*. The moment aortic flow falls to zero and

starts to reverse, the protruding cusps are snapped shut. They probably seal off flow effectively before they are fully back in the diastolic position and at least part, if not all, of the reverse flow recorded in the ascending aorta is blood movement pushing the valve cusps back rather than regurgitation through them (Schultz, personal communication).

THE AORTA AND LARGE ARTERIES

This account of the vortices necessarily associated with the valve cusps is convincingly documented and accounts for the usual findings of essentially laminar flow in the ascending aorta by Schultz et al. (1969). It was previously assumed (McDonald, 1960) that the vortices of the valves would be shed into the stream and hence cause considerable disturbances in the flow pattern. As noted previously (p. 85) there is some disturbance as seen radiographically. Freis and Heath (1964) also studied this flow with thermal and other methods. Using cool liquid injections directed in different parts of the aortic cross-section and scanning across the aorta with a thermistor they found (a) a flat profile as Schultz and Bellhouse and colleagues subsequently did, and (b) rapid mixing throughout the whole aortic cross-section during systole. This latter finding they attributed to very disturbed or turbulent flow. It was distinctly different from the non-mixing pattern of laminar flow that they found in the descending aorta. The evidence for highly disturbed flow in the ascending aorta was augmented by the recording of sound-frequency (predominantly 100–200 Hz) vibrations with a high-frequency intra-arterial catheter; these faded out in the arch of the aorta. Unfortunately flow velocities could not be derived in these experiments so that they do not necessarily controvert the findings of Schultz et al. for they also found disturbances at high Reynolds numbers.

The conclusion at the present time is that usually flow in the ascending aorta is predominantly laminar, but that radial movement of blood does occur and therefore, there is rapid mixing across the stream. When disturbed flow does occur in the ascending aorta it is unlikely to dissipate much extra energy because we are not only dealing with inlet conditions but with oscillatory flow; both of these will cause largely unsheared flows with a flat velocity profile whether the flow is laminar or turbulent as discussed in Chs. 5 and 6 following.

Blood in the aorta is completely mixed. If it were not then the composition of blood flowing into different branches would vary and withdrawing blood from a peripheral artery would not give a reliable and representative sample of arterial blood. This technique is used so widely in physiology and clinical medicine that the absence of any evidence of variability of samples from different arteries may be taken as proof of this assertion.

We have already seen that passage through the contracting chambers of the heart, together with the motion of the valves, is probably sufficient cause for this mixing. The uniformity of composition does not, therefore, inherently provide any evidence as to whether flow within the arterial system is laminar or turbulent. As this point is of some interest, albeit rather academic, we need more direct evidence.

Cineradiographic investigations by Stauffer *et al.* (1955) showed that radiopaque material injected into the root of the aorta of a dog was very rapidly dispersed throughout the vessel as was discussed above.

In the thoracic aorta several earlier workers had made observations which suggested that aortic flow may be laminar. It was noted above that Freis and Heath (1964) found poor mixing of infused cold saline; they also found a clear streaming pattern with radiopaque injections. The problem of opacity in the aorta of the cat was circumvented by Ralston and Taylor (1945) by inserting a lucite cannula, and watching the flow of injected Indian ink. They reported the presence of streamlines. In a further study, Ralston, Taylor and Elliott (1947) supported these findings by showing that Indian ink injected into the ventricles was not distributed equally to the two renal arteries. This was a similar finding to the classical experiment of Hess (1917) who injected a solution of methylene blue which was of the same viscosity as the blood into the arch of the aorta from a cannula inserted down the cartoid artery, and found that a higher concentration was found in the left iliac artery than in the right. These results show that there is not sustained turbulence in the aorta and that the flow is probably laminar. This is more impressive in the case of Hess' results because he used a large St. Bernard dog, and although data on velocity of flow and size of vessels were not given, it is certainly to be expected that the Reynolds number would be well above 2,000 during part of each cardiac cycle. This would confirm the data discussed above (p. 80) which indicate that transient fluctuations of the Reynolds number above the critical value do not cause turbulence.

Hess also stated that flow in the thoracic aorta was not turbulent because he could hear no murmurs through a stethoscope applied to the surface of the aorta. The statement that murmurs are simply due to the onset of turbulence is made so frequently in physiological and medical textbooks that it was discussed at length by McDonald (1960, pp. 69–77). It was also reviewed by McKuisck (1957, 1958) and by Bruns (1959). All these authors concluded that audible sound was not due to turbulence alone but involved the vibration of solid structures such as the chordae tendinae of the mitral valves or abnormal valve cusps. A good example was given by vibration of the wall of the pulmonary artery during certain stages of the closure of the ductus arteriosus shown as fast oscillations in the pressure record by Dawes, Mott, and Widdicombe (1955). Meisner and Rushmer (1963*b*) showed in models that high degrees of turbulence could cause vibrations in the wall of an elastic tube. This was extended in an elegant and detailed analysis of the Korotkoff sounds produced in an artery during occlusion by the occluding cuff of a sphygmomanometer by Anliker and Raman (1966). They concluded that with reduction of the normal tension in the wall instability developed and the resulting wall movement could result in a large degree of mechanical amplification. This has been studied experimentally by McCutcheon and Rushmer (1967). Thus major disturbances of flow, even though too local to be rigorously classified as turbulence, always appear to be associated with the production of audible sound. The absence of sound cannot, of itself, prove that flow is laminar. Nevertheless, the original contention of Hess (1917) that aortic flow is laminar would appear to be essentially true in the light of the more recent evidence discussed above even though McDonald (1960) regarded it as controversial.

5

The Velocity Profile in Pulsatile Flow

When investigating the stability of pulsatile flow in Ch. 4, the form of the velocity profile was invoked as evidence in some work discussed. It is, therefore, necessary to study the degree to which these findings are in agreement with those predicted by theory. As the flow is not steady, one of the basic assumptions of deriving the Poiseuille equation is violated. Thus, it is to be anticipated that the velocity profile will not be of the same parabolic form that is found in steady laminar flow.

The equation for the motion of a viscous liquid in laminar flow in a tube of circular cross-section, radius R, was derived in Ch. 2 for steady flow (eqn. 2.15). In its general form for an incompressible liquid we can write (Womersley, 1955a, b; 1957a)

$$\frac{\partial^2 w}{\partial r^2} + \frac{1}{r} \cdot \frac{\partial w}{\partial r} + \frac{1}{\mu} \cdot \frac{\partial p}{\partial z} = +\frac{\rho}{\mu} \cdot \frac{\partial w}{\partial t} = \frac{1}{\nu} \cdot \frac{\partial w}{\partial t} \qquad 5.1$$

Following common convention the axis of the tube is taken as the z axis and the velocity in the direction of that axis is w (the velocities in the x and y axes are, respectively, u and v in this convention and for a rigid tube will both be zero).

For steady flow the velocity does not vary with time so that $\partial w/\partial t = 0$; the pressure-gradient $\partial p/\partial z$ can then be measured over a finite distance and written as

$$\frac{P_1 - P_2}{L} = \frac{\partial p}{\partial z}$$

This averaging over a distance L leads to some error with non-steady flow and will be discussed later (p. 136).

The Newtonian coefficient of viscosity is μ (eqn. 2.1) and the density of the liquid is ρ. The kinematic viscosity ν (p. 31) is μ/ρ.

For simplicity the form of the pressure-gradient will be taken as a simple harmonic motion and written in complex form (A* is the complex conjugate of A in Womersley, 1955a)

$$-\frac{\partial p}{\partial z} = A^* e^{i\omega t} \qquad 5.2$$

where $\omega = 2\pi f$ is the angular frequency in radians/sec of the oscillatory motion, with f the frequency in Hz. The solution for this case is especially important because, with the aid of the Fourier series (Ch. 7), any periodic function, such as the arterial pulse, can be represented.

With this substitution we rewrite eqn. 5.1 in the form

$$\frac{\partial^2 w}{\partial r^2} + \frac{1}{r} \cdot \frac{\partial w}{\partial r} - \frac{1}{v} \cdot \frac{\partial w}{\partial t} = -\frac{A^*}{\mu} \cdot e^{i\omega t} \qquad 5.3$$

This may be simplified mathematically by the substitution $w = u e^{i\omega t}$, whence by the cancellation of $e^{i\omega t}$ throughout the equation we obtain

$$\frac{d^2 u}{dr^2} + \frac{1}{r} \cdot \frac{du}{dr} - \frac{i\omega}{v} \cdot u = -\frac{A^*}{\mu} \qquad 5.4$$

This is a form of Bessel's equation (Pipes, 1958) and its solution, appropriate to the boundary conditions, is

$$u = \frac{A^*}{i\omega\rho} \left[1 - \frac{J_0[r\sqrt{(\omega/v)} . i^{\frac{3}{2}}]}{J_0[R\sqrt{(\omega/v)} . i^{\frac{3}{2}}]} \right] \qquad 5.5$$

where an expression of the form $J_0 (xi^{3/2})$ is a Bessel function of the first kind of order zero and complex argument (Pipes, 1958). It is well known and occurs in problems such as the distribution of UHF alternating current in conductors of circular cross-section; in the German literature they are more descriptively called 'cylinder functions' (Jahnke and Emde, 1945). They are also tabulated by Dwight (1961); it is his tables that have been used in the profiles calculated in this chapter.

The quantity $R\sqrt{(\omega/v)}$ is a non-dimensional parameter which characterizes kinematic similarities in the liquid motion. Its relation to Reynolds and Strouhal's numbers has already been noted (p. 82). It is here written as the symbol α

$$\alpha = R(\omega/v)^{1/2}; \qquad 5.6$$

The radius is also made non-dimensional by substituting the fractional radius, $y = r/R$. The solution for the velocity, w, then converts eqn. 5.5. to

$$w = \frac{A^* R^2}{i\mu\alpha^2} \left[1 - \frac{J_0(\alpha y i^{\frac{3}{2}})}{J_0(\alpha i^{\frac{3}{2}})} \right] e^{i\omega t} \qquad 5.7$$

This gives the velocity of motion of the lamina of liquid at a fraction of the radius, y, from the axis of the tube. The corresponding volume flow is derived by integrating across the tube as was done for Poiseuille flow; the oscillatory volume flow is considered in Ch. 6. Although the terminology and derivation of Womersley (1955a, 1957a) is followed here, the same, or essentially similar, solutions have been achieved by other authors previously, notably Witzig (1914), Richardson and Tyler (1929), Sexl (1930), Apéria (1940), Iberall

(1950), Lambossy (1952a) and Morgan and Kiely (1954). Indeed, the solution for the rigid tube case is said to have been set as an examination question. Witzig's work was in a Ph.D. thesis and remained unknown until cited by Lambossy (1952a); it is remarkable in that he actually obtained velocity profiles (at values of α of 4 and 10), like those illustrated in this chapter, in reference to arterial flow. Lambossy also calculated profiles over a range of values of α relevant to the circulation, while Richardson and Tyler (1929) and Morgan and Kiely (1954) were more concerned with the limiting cases; Sexl (1930), Apéria (1940), and Iberall (1950) only dealt with the general mathematical solution.

The numerical solution of equation 5.7 is concerned with complex quantities (Ch. 7) and may be made by separation into real and imaginary parts (the real and imaginary parts of a Bessel function of the first kind are tabulated as Ber and Bei functions)—as Witzig (1914) and later Lambossy (1952a) did. Alternatively they may be expressed as modulus and phase which Womersley regarded as more tractable. This involves the substitutions

$$J_0(\alpha y i^{3/2}) = M_0(y)e^{i\theta_0(y)}$$
$$J_0(\alpha i^{3/2}) = M_0 e^{i\theta_0} \qquad \textbf{5.8}$$

If the real part of the pressure-gradient, $A\overset{*}{e}{}^{i\omega t}$, is also written in modulus and phase form as $M \cos(\omega t - \varphi)$ then

$$w = \frac{M}{\omega\rho}\left[\sin(\omega t - \varphi) - \frac{M_0(y)}{M_0}\sin(\omega t - \varphi - \delta_0)\right] \qquad \textbf{5.9}$$

where

$$\delta_0 = \theta_0 - \theta_0(y)$$

It can be seen that, for the lamina at the wall, $r = R$ and $y = 1$ so that $M_0(y) = M_0$ and $\delta_0 = 0$; the expression in the square brackets is thus zero, i.e. the flow velocity at the wall is zero. This is the same boundary condition that was discussed in relation to Poiseuille's equation (p. 28).

For purposes of calculation, Womersley compressed the equation further by writing

$$h_0 = \frac{M_0(y)}{M_0} \qquad \textbf{5.10}$$

and introduced the terms M'_0 and ε_0 by the following definition,

$$M'_0 = (1 + h_0^2 - 2h_0 \cos \delta_0)^{\frac{1}{2}} \qquad \textbf{5.11}$$

and

$$\tan \varepsilon_0 = \frac{h_0 \sin \delta_0}{1 - h_0 \cos \delta_0} \qquad \textbf{5.12}$$

so that

$$w = \frac{M}{\omega\rho} . M'_0 \sin(\omega t - \varphi + \varepsilon_0) \qquad \textbf{5.13}$$

or since $\alpha^2 = R \cdot \dfrac{\omega\rho}{\mu}$ (eqn. 5.6), eqn. 5.13 may be written as

$$w = \frac{MR^2}{\mu} \cdot \frac{M'_0}{\alpha^2} \cdot \sin{(\omega t - \varphi + \varepsilon_0)} \qquad \textbf{5.14}$$

in this form it can be seen that for steady flow (eqn. 2.5) the term M'_0/α^2 is analogous to $(1 - y^2)/4$, where $y^2 = r^2/R^2$.

(The zero subscript in M'_0 indicates that only Bessel functions of zero order are involved and is modified when functions of a higher order are involved —see Ch. 6).

The forms of the velocity profile created by a pressure-gradient which oscillates sinusoidally were discussed in some detail by Hale *et al.* (1955). Some examples calculated from eqn. 5.14 are shown in Fig. 5.1. The pressure-

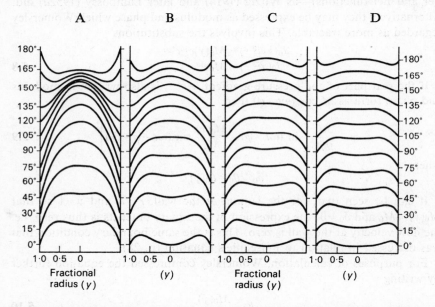

Fig. 5.1A. The velocity profiles, at intervals of 15°, of the flow resulting from a sinusoidal pressure-gradient (cos ωt) in a pipe. In this case, $\alpha = R \cdot \sqrt{\omega/v} = 3.34$, corresponding to the fundamental harmonic of the flow curves illustrated in **Figs. 5.3** and **5.4**. Note that reversal of flow starts in the laminae near the wall. As this is harmonic motion only half a cycle is illustrated as the remainder will be the same in form but opposite in sign, e.g. compare 180° and 0°.

B. A similar set of profiles for harmonic motion of double the frequency of A ($\alpha = 4.72$). The amplitude and phase of the pressure are the same here and in C and D as in A. The effects of the larger α are thus seen to be a flattening of the profile of the central region, a reduction of amplitude of the flow and the rate of reversal of flow increases close to the wall.

C. The third harmonic with $\alpha = 5.78$. The effects of higher frequency noted in B are here further accentuated.

D. The fourth harmonic ($\alpha = 6.67$) shows the same effects again. The rapidly varying part of the flow lies between $y = 0.8$ and $y = 1.0$ and the central mass of the fluid reciprocates almost like a solid core.

gradient was assumed to be of the form $M \cos (\omega t - \varphi)$, the standard expression for one harmonic component of a Fourier series (Ch. 6). In this example, $M = 1 \cdot 0$ and $\varphi = 0$, i.e. the gradient is $\cos \omega t$. The angular frequency ω is respectively in the ratio 1, 2, 3, and 4, which gives α values in the ratios of the square roots, i.e. 1, $\sqrt{2}$, $\sqrt{3}$ and 2. The actual α values used were those taken from an experiment on the femoral artery of a dog in which the pulse rate was $2 \cdot 8$ Hz. Only half a cycle is illustrated (at intervals of 15°) because with simple harmonic motion the second half is the inverted form of the first half—as shown by comparing the profiles at 0° and 180°.

It will be seen from the illustrations that, even at the lowest frequency shown, a true parabolic profile is not formed at any time. There is a phase lag between the applied pressure and the movement of the liquid; being a cosine function, the amplitude of the gradient is a maximum at 0° while the maximum for the total flow integrated across the tube is at about 60° in example A, and at about 77° in example D. The laminae that move first are those nearest the wall and flow successively involves the laminae towards the axis of the tube. At the wall is a lamina of zero velocity; the laminae near the wall always have a low velocity owing to the effect of viscosity. Hence they have a low momentum and reverse easily when the gradient reverses. As we move towards the axis of the tube, the momentum becomes progressively higher relative to the viscous drag so that there is a greater lag between the pressure–gradient and the movement of the liquid in the centre of the tube (see also Fig. 5.4). As the frequency increases there is, as it were, less time in the cycle for the movement to be translated throughout the axial laminae and the velocity profile becomes very flattened, i.e. subject to very low shear. An increase of diameter without change of frequency will, similarly, produce a like alteration in the profile. These changes are shown for higher values of α (such as are found in the low-frequency components of aortic flow) in Fig. 5.2. The liquid in the central part of the tube is virtually unsheared and the significant velocity gradients are only found in the layers near the wall. Thus the liquid begins to behave rather like a solid mass sliding inside a thin layer of viscous liquid surrounding it. For example, in Fig. 5.2c where $\alpha = 20$ the region of high velocity gradient is virtually confined to the outer 5 per cent of the tube radius. In order to visualize the velocity profiles in an artery it is necessary to sum the profiles of the main harmonic components, with their appropriate amplitudes and phases, together with a parabolic profile representing the steady flow component, i.e. the mean forward flow. Such a summation has been done in Fig. 5.3 for a typical cycle for the femoral artery from the four harmonics illustrated in Fig. 5.1. It can be seen that in the fast systolic rush all the harmonics are most nearly in phase and create a profile which approaches the form of a parabola. Then reversal of flow following reversal of the pressure-gradient begins in the peripheral laminae and progressively involves those towards the axis. The oscillations of certain selected laminae throughout

the cycle in relation to the pressure-gradient is shown in Fig. 5.4. Thus, at 135°
of the cycle, the average velocity in the artery is approximately zero; the axial
laminae are still flowing forward when the mural laminae are flowing back-

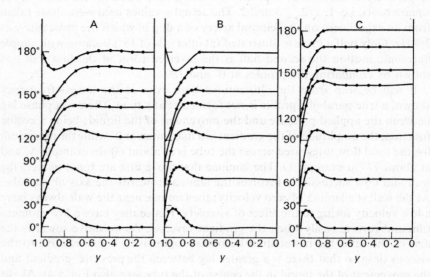

Fig. 5.2. Velocity profiles of a cylindrical tube created by a pressure-gradient of sinusoidal wave-
form. Profiles are given for half the tube at intervals of 30° from 0° to 180° as in Fig. 5.1.
    A. when $\alpha = R(\omega/\nu)^{1/2} = 10$
    B. $\alpha = 15$
and C. $\alpha = 20$.
    The flattening of the profile in the centre of the tube with increasing α that is seen in Fig. 5.1 is
here further accentuated.

ward. During back flow the harmonics are considerably out of phase with one
another and the profile, in contrast to that in forward flow, is very much
flattened. Indeed, the maximum retrograde velocity does not occur at the
axis but in the laminae with a fractional radius of between 0·3 and 0·4. From
Fig. 5.4 it can be seen that even in a vessel as small as the femoral artery the
point of flow reversal in the most peripheral lamina ($y = 0.95$) is about 25°
later than pressure-gradient reversal; in the axial lamina ($y = 0$) reversal
occurs about 40° later still.

Inhomogenous liquid. The viscous behaviour of blood, due to the fact that it
is a suspension of cells in plasma, was discussed in Ch. 3. As the laminae very
close to the wall have a lower concentration of cells, the viscosity in this region
is lower so that the shear is greater than it would be if the viscosity was
uniform throughout. The effect of this on the profile is to make it steeper
at the wall than it would otherwise be. This is illustrated in Fig. 5.5 by some
theoretical examples calculated (in steady flow) by Womersley (cited in

McDonald, 1965). He made the assumption that the mean viscosity was an inverse power function, m, of the radius of a lamina, r,

$$\bar{\mu} = \mu(r/R)^{-m}$$ **5.15**

There is no experimental justification for this equation but it is mathematically tractable and gives a qualitative picture of the effect that will occur to

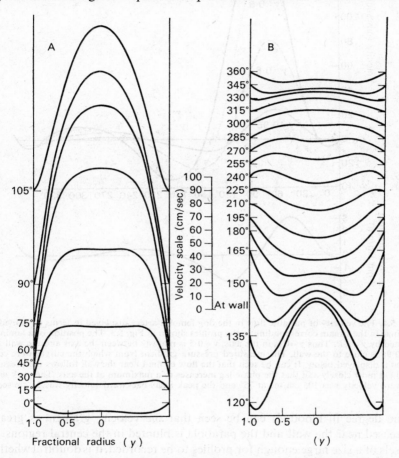

Fig. 5.3. Velocity profiles calculated from the measured pressure-gradient in the femoral artery of the dog. The first four harmonic components with the same values of α as in Fig. 5.1 are summed together with a parabola (axial velocity 30 cm/sec) representing the steady forward flow. The maximum forward velocity occurs in the axis because here the harmonic components are in phase but the maximum backward velocity lies between $y = 0.3$ and 0.4 at $180°$. The reversal of flow beginning near the wall is clearly seen.

The variation in velocity of certain of these laminae is also plotted in Fig. 5.4 in a similar way to that of ordinary average velocity flow curves. *Average* velocity is used for the average of all laminae across the tube at any moment; *mean* velocity is reserved here for the mean value throughout the cycle, i.e. the steady, or constant, term of the Fourier series.

The pulse-frequency in this case was 2.8/sec so that the cycle length was approximately 360. One degree of arc is thus approximately one millisecond.

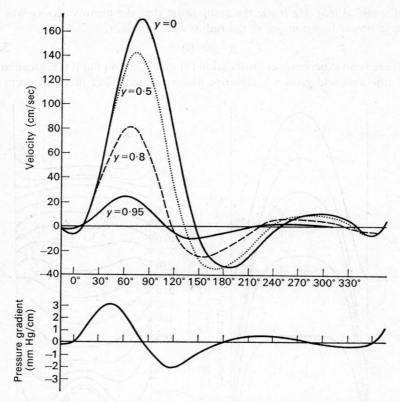

Fig. 5.4. The velocity of pulsatile flow in the dog femoral artery displayed in terms of individual laminae in the stream corresponding to the profiles shown in Fig. 5.3. The position of a lamina is defined by $y=r/R$. Thus $y=0$ is in the axis, $y=0.5$ is midway between the axis and the wall and $y=0.95$ is close to the wall. The measured pressure gradient from which the curves were computed is displayed below. It can be seen that the flow of fluid near the wall follows the pressure-gradient most closely and that the phase lag increases to a maximum at the axis. The peak *mean* forward velocity was 105 cm/sec at 75° and the peak *mean* backward velocity was 25 cm/sec at 165°.

some degree in blood. It can be seen that the velocity gradient is greatly increased near the wall and the parabola is blunted in the central regions. In vessels of a size large enough for profiles to be recorded, it is doubtful whether the magnitude of the effect would be measurable at normal flow rates if the conclusions reached in Ch. 3 about the extent of non-Newtonian viscous behaviour in arteries is correct.

THE INLET LENGTH

In the consideration of the basic assumptions of the Poiseuille equation (pp. 27–30) it was pointed out that, in a pipe leading from a reservoir, the

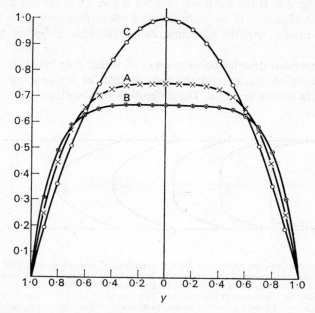

Fig. 5.5. Velocity profiles in steady flow when the viscosity varies as an inverse power of the fractional radius (eqn. 5.15).

A. The power, $m=2$.
B. The power, $m=4$.
C. A parabolic profile for comparison.

It can be seen that this type of inhomogeneity also flattens the profile in the central regions of the tube.

pressure–flow relation was different in the proximal part of the tube. The region between the reservoir and the point where a constant flow regime is 'established' is called the 'inlet' (or sometimes 'entrance') length. When considering the circulation there is a clear analogy with the outflow into the aortic tube from the ventricular reservoir. Strictly speaking, a similar situation occurs when flow is from a larger artery into a smaller branch. The conditions within this region near the entrance may be visualized in this way. At the orifice in the reservoir there is initially the same velocity all the way across. Once inside the pipe the layer of liquid immediately in contact with the wall will become stationary. The laminae close to it begin to slide on it subject to the force of viscosity and form a boundary layer. The bulk of the fluid in the centre of the tube will move as a mass, affected very little by the forces of viscosity, and will have a flat velocity profile. As flow proceeds down the tube, however, the boundary layer will grow in thickness as the viscous drag involves more and more of the liquid. Finally the boundary layer comes to occupy the whole of the tube and steady viscous flow is established. The velocity profile is then parabolic. The stages of development of the profile are shown in Fig. 5.6. If the Reynolds number is above the critical number then the established flow will be turbulent but up to that point, i.e. within the inlet, one cannot, strictly speaking, define the flow as either laminar or turbulent.

This conceptual description of the way in which flow becomes established in the inlet region is essentially the same as that for determining the form of the profile in oscillatory flow. The differences only spring from the fact that

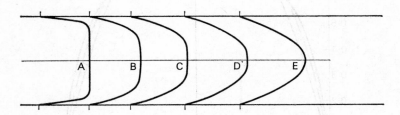

Fig. 5.6. Successive velocity profiles within the 'inlet length' between two parallel walls leading from a reservoir—it is assumed that the pattern in a cylindrical pipe would be similar. Near the inlet (A) the shear in the liquid is confined to a boundary layer near the wall and there is no velocity gradient in the centre of the channel. The boundary layer increases in thickness progressively (B, C and D) with a corresponding diminution of the unsheared region. Finally the parabolic profile (E) of steady laminar flow is established. It is of interest to compare the profile such as A with those of oscillatory flow, e.g. Fig. 5.1D, and of turbulent flow, e.g. Fig. 2.5.

the standard concept in calculating inlet length is an initially flat profile across the tube at the reservoir with only forward flow, whereas with continuously oscillatory flow the profile is never completely flat. From this comparison we can think of the oscillatory flow profile as though it were that of a steady flow which has not had time to become completely established. This analogy is borne out by the flat central regions which are seen in Fig. 5.2 in oscillatory profiles, e.g. the 90° profile in Fig. 5.2A is essentially similar to the profiles within the inlet length, e.g. Fig. 5.7A. We should, therefore, expect the inlet length for oscillatory flow to be shorter than for steady flow; indeed the higher the value of α the shorter one would expect the oscillatory inlet length to be.

The effect of inlet length conditions will be to cause a flattening of the central region of the velocity profile. This may be, in practical applications, of less importance than the change in pressure–flow relations. The pressure-gradient in the inlet length is higher for a given rate of flow than when the same flow is established. This correction has been made somewhat empirically (eqn. 2.17) for the quantitative application of Poiseuille's equation. For the derivation of aortic flow from pressure-gradient measurement, it is necessary to estimate what the magnitude of this effect is.

Formulas for the calculation of the inlet length for steady flow are given in all standard hydrodynamic texts. They are all of the form, for an inlet length L, when the established flow is laminar,

$$L = n \cdot r \cdot (Re)$$

where r is radius, (Re) the Reynolds number and n a numerical factor derived mathematically. It is, therefore, somewhat confusing to find a range of values for n in various sources. Goldstein (1938, cited by McDonald, 1960) gives $n = 0.057$. Prandtl and Tietjens (1934), however, say that this is a lowest limit which is too short and recommend an experimentally determined value of $n = 0.1$; the highest value quoted by Chang and Atabek (1961) is $n = 0.13$. These last authors use $n = 0.08$ and as they are the only authorities to have determined it for oscillatory flow their value is used here. (Values quoted are modified for use of (Re) calculated from diameter and not from radius; the variation in the calculated lengths presumably arises from differing degrees of stringency in defining fully established flow.)

The length of the inlet length for steady flow component in arteries is therefore taken as

$$L = 0.08 \cdot r \cdot (Re) \qquad \qquad 5.16$$

Some numerical examples will indicate what lengths this involves in the arterial tree.

(a) *Dog aorta.* Radius 0.5 cm; mean flow velocity 20 cm/sec; kinematic viscosity 0.04 stokes. The Re is 500 and the inlet length is 20 cm; this is approximately the length of the intra-thoracic aorta.

(b) *Human aorta.* Radius 1.25 cm; flow velocity 20 cm/sec. The (Re) is 1,250 and the inlet length calculated is 180 cm. This greatly exceeds the lengths to which the dimensions used would apply but shows that inlet length conditions should be considered as being operative throughout all major arteries in man.

If the flow of the liquid in the reservoir is turbulent then the inlet length is much shorter. The formula given by Goldstein (1938) is

$$L = 1.386 \cdot r \cdot (Re)^{1/4} \qquad \qquad 5.17$$

Calculating the two examples above with this formula we obtain: (a) dog aorta, $L = 2.6$ cm, or shorter than the ascending aorta; (b) human aorta, $L = $ approx. 10 cm, or within the arch of the aorta.

It is clear from the evidence considered in Ch. 4 that the flow out of the heart is predominantly laminar and that the blood in the heart, although well-stirred perhaps, is not really turbulent. The inlet lengths calculated from eqn. 5.17 are, therefore, manifestly too short. On the other hand, the heart is not the very large still reservoir of hydrodynamic experiments so that we can equally argue that the value calculated from eqn. 5.16 are unrealistically long. From the flow patterns recorded near the valves (p. 95) it appears that the outflow tract of the ventricles should be considered as part of the inlet.

E

The investigation of the inlet length for oscillatory flows was specifically undertaken by Chang and Atabek (1961) to clarify the situation in the circulation. The problem is extremely intractable for a purely oscillatory flow for during half of each cycle reversal of flow would take place, i.e. flow from the tube into the reservoir; in a tube of finite length it would thus be necessary to consider inlet conditions at the far end. The case that was analysed was one in which an oscillatory flow was superimposed on a steady flow component which was large enough to maintain a forward flow into the tube throughout the cycle. The actual equation used was a flow velocity, $u = (1-0.5 \cos \omega t)$. The examples computed are for $\alpha = 4$ and, in an experimental paper (Atabek, Chang, and Fingerson, 1964), for $\alpha = 5$. They are not thus directly applicable to the aortic situation where $\alpha > 10$ and the mean flow velocity is not double the amplitude of the larger, low frequency, components.

Their conclusions are briefly as follows: (a) the inlet length varies with the velocity although its fluctuations lag behind the flow oscillations; (b) this variation of inlet length is smaller in magnitude than the variation of the flow velocity. As the Reynolds number varies directly with the flow velocity this also expresses the relation of inlet length to the instantaneous Reynolds number, also for the laminar flow case. In Chang and Atabek (1961, Fig. 7) the inlet length increases in the ratio 0.222/0.16 when the (Re) increases by 50 per cent of its steady flow value, at an $\alpha = 4$. In the higher α range of the aorta one can assume that the 'foreshortening' of the inlet length will be greater; but as the peak systolic flow velocity will be at least four times the velocity of the steady flow it can be predicted that the inlet length then would be two to three times the length calculated above, if the fundamental assumptions hold. Conversely in diastole it will fall to a very low value; (c) the increase in the pressure-gradient is also calculated by Chang and Atabek (1961, Fig. 6). At a distance of one-eighth of the inlet length from the entrance the gradient is about 10 per cent greater than for fully established flow. The steady flow gradient in the aorta is so small that such a change would be undetectable; at high values of α one presumes that the effect on the oscillatory gradient would be much less than this because the effective viscous boundary layer is so much narrower as discussed in relation to Fig. 5.2 above. Certainly the applications of the Womersley equation—which assumes established flow—to aortic flow has not shown a discrepancy of as much as 10 per cent (Chs. 6 and 13).

The predicted inlet length velocity profiles were shown to fit very well with experimental data by Atabek et al. (1964); the flattening effect on the profile is illustrated from their curve (Fig. 5.7). From the discussion above it can be seen that there is some considerable uncertainty as to the actual length of the effective 'inlet' in various stages of the cardiac cycle. The measurements of the velocity profile that have been made experimentally in the aorta, however, clarify the situation to some degree.

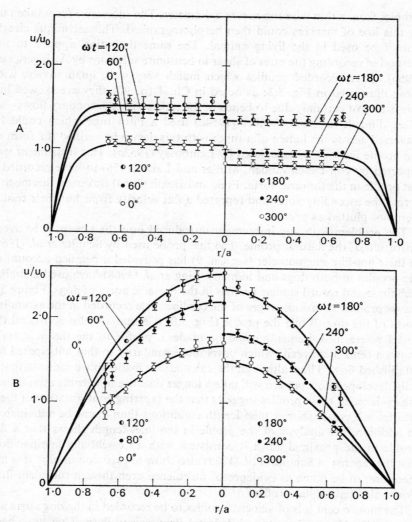

Fig. 5.7. The sets of velocity profiles for sinusoidal flow near the entrance to a tube. In this case there is steady flow present so that there is no reversal of flow at any part of the cycle. The solid lines give the theoretically predicted curve and the circles mark experimentally measured points. Profiles are given at 60° intervals alternately on the left and right half of the figures.

A. The profile very close to the inlet.

B. The profile when flow is almost fully established. (From Atabek, Chang and Fingerson, 1964.)

EXPERIMENTAL MEASUREMENTS OF THE VELOCITY PROFILE

The technique used for recording the velocity profile by Atabek *et al.* (1964) in their models involved the pulsed electrolytic release of a line of minute bubbles from a thin wire run across a diameter. The successive form taken up by this line of markers could then be photographed. This technique clearly cannot be used in the living animal. The same limitation applied to the method of recording the rates of shear in bentonite solutions by Attinger *et al.* (1966). They recorded profiles which match very well, qualitatively, with those illustrated in Fig. 5.2; as noted in Ch. 4 (p. 90) they are skewed but this is almost certainly due to bends in the pipe causing secondary flows—an effect difficult to avoid. Müller (1954a) used a Pitot tube which could be traversed across the lumen of a tube; with this device he verified the form of the profile for $\alpha = 6\cdot43$ calculated by Lambossy (1952a). This instrument was reported by von Deschwanden, Müller and Laszt (1956) to have recorded a flat profile in the thoracic aorta. Freis and Heath (1964) traversed thermistors across the ascending aorta and reported a flat velocity front but their results were not plotted as profiles.

The problem with any instrument introduced into the stream is to avoid distortion of the natural profile. The fine probe used by Schultz *et al.* (1969) in their hot-film anemometer (see Ch. 9) has provided a detailed account of the profiles in both dogs and humans. Ling *et al.* (1968) have used a similar technique and record similar profiles in the thoracic aorta of dogs. Figure 5.8 shows profiles at various stages of the cardiac cycle recorded in the ascending aorta of the dog. While the profile (Fig. 5.8) is essentially flat across all the vessel where measurements could be made, a profile in the thoracic aorta shows a central convexity which bears more similarity to that anticipated for established flow. Thus, although the calculations made above indicate that a fully developed flow pattern will take a longer distance to become established, the evidence of these profiles suggests that the tapering conformation of these arteries will create shorter inlet length conditions than might be anticipated. In addition, the analysis of the profile in the inlet length shows that a flat profile in the proximal aorta is consistent with an essentially laminar flow that the records of Schultz *et al.* (1969) also show to exist commonly. It is not therefore, to be taken as evidence of turbulence even though turbulent flow would also have a flat profile.

The most recent sets of velocity profiles to be recorded in the dog aorta are those of Dr. Hinglais' group at L'Hôpital Broussais in Paris. They have been using the pulsed Doppler flowmeter which is described in Ch. 9 (Peronneau and Leger, 1969; Peronneau *et al.*, 1970). No extensive account of these researches has appeared in English (and the full account in French is in an electrical engineering journal which is difficult to obtain in this country). As with the other profiles one picture is worth a thousand words (Fig. 5.9). With this technique, the profile can be measured in a matter of milliseconds and it thus can make a virtually continous traverse, which gives it an advantage over the heated-film technique where only certain spots in the traverse can be made. The pulsed Doppler also can measure velocity right up to the wall. The

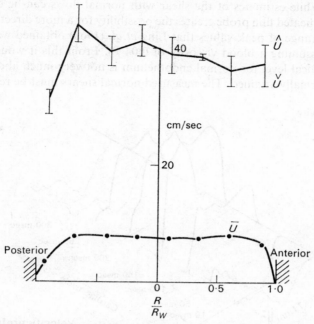

Fig. 5.8. Measurements of velocity across the transverse plane of the arch of the aorta in a dog. Maximum and minimum flow velocity profiles are shown as measured from the points on a traverse of the vessel with a hot-film needle flow probe. The vertical bars on the upper curves represent the standard deviation. (From Schultz *et al.*, 1969.)

sequence of velocity profiles in the descending aorta shown in Fig. 5.9 shows little tendency to convexity in the centre of the vessel. The high velocity-gradient close to the wall is also clearly seen and both these characteristics suggest that this region is, in fact, still in the inlet length region. At the present time while the difficult experimental study of the velocity profile is still in its infancy these questions cannot be settled but the general similarity of this data to those predicted theoretically is very encouraging.

The paper by Ling *et al.* (1968) is of especial interest in that they attempted to measure the actual shear at the wall of the thoracic aorta. In a group of very interesting papers, Fry (1968; 1969*a, b*) has studied the acute yield stress of the vascular endothelium subjected to the shearing stress of the blood flow in the aorta. In order to increase the stress of a localized region of the endothelium, he introduced, into the thoracic aorta of a dog, a plastic plug with a restricted channel machined on one side. The linear velocity of flow would thus be greatly increased in this channel and the adjacent endothelium consequently subjected to an increased shear. Damage to the endothelial cells was assessed histologically from cell configuration and also by the abnormal uptake of dyes. The shear stress was calculated from the relevant hydrodynamic equations. It was estimated that the acute yield was 379 ± 80 (SD) dyn/cm². While estimates of the shear with normal flows can be calculated (Ch. 3), the heated film probe creates the possibility for a more direct measurement. The range of peak values that Ling *et al.* (1968) obtained was 80–160 dyn/cm² (assuming a blood viscosity of 0·04 P). From this it would appear that the critical level for normal endothelium is not very much above shears that are normally attained. The measured normal shears must be regarded as

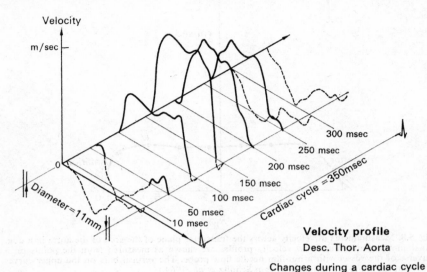

Fig. 5.9. A set of velocity profiles in the descending thoracic aorta of a dog recorded with a pulsed Doppler flowmeter. Profiles are recorded at 50 m/sec intervals and are drawn obliquely to represent the time sequence; reverse flow is shown by a dashed line. (From Peronneau *et al.*, 1970.)

tentative because the heated probe should be precisely flush with the internal surface—a condition very difficult to achieve. Nevertheless, this work provides the first definite relationship between hydrodynamic stresses in the arterial wall and the genesis of arterial disease. (Fry also found that where an intra-arterial catheter made contact with the wall, abnormal staining reactions appeared in the endothelial cells.) Even an increase in the permeability of endothelial cells, without gross structural damage, might well facilitate the accommodation of lipids in the arterial wall which is the dominant feature of arteriosclerosis. It has long been suspected that mechanical and hydro-dynamic factors (notably turbulence) are concerned in the genesis of athero-sclerosis but have hitherto been largely speculative. Duguid and Robertson (1957) discussed the role of the radial stresses in the wall and the whole sub-ject is considered more fully by Mitchell and Schwartz (1965). The advances that have been made in the study of stress factors of the wall in recent years should, in the light of the remarkable findings of Fry in the endothelium, enable us to provide comparable data for the other tissues of the wall.

The role of sheer stress at the wall in relation to the incidence of athero-sclerosis has been restudied by Caro *et al.* (1971). Taking a view quite con-trary to that of Fry, these authors maintain that the optimal sites for the location of arteriosclerosis plaques is at points of minimal shear.

The figures for wall shear are expressed as a mean shear index—Q/d^3 (where d is the diameter of the vessel and Q is the volume flow). A large number of resin casts were made and the area-ratio (see Table 2.2) calculated (β); the ratio of the wall shear stress in the daughter branches to the parent trunk expressed as a value γ; $\gamma_\infty \sqrt{2}\beta^{-3/2}$ so that the wall stress is less in the daughter branches whenever $\beta > 1·26$. Work was done in the arterial system of 24 human subjects. From the arterial cast a hollow model was made of precisely the same form as the anatomical tree. A flow of air through the model was used as an analogy of the flow of blood; the air carried a small concentration of nitrogen dioxide and the wall of the cast was thinly coated with a starch paste containing litmus and sodium hydroxide. Thus where the mass transfer from the flowing fluid was greatest the litmus changed from blue to red. The photographs show that all the red areas are in low shear regions and do, indeed, mimic the main distribution of atheromatous plaques in humans with extraordinary fidelity such as has not been seen in any previous experimental work. Furthermore, the basic concept that the initiat-ing process in atherogenesis is the mass transfer of cholesterol, and possibly calcium, from the blood to the arterial wall is, intuitively, a very plausible one. It is easy to see that this process will be more easily carried out in low shear regions. Biologically this is a more dynamic one and can be tied to the very elegant work on cell membranes and lipid bi-layers that has been done by Urry and Goodall and their colleagues in the past 2 years. The paper by Caro *et al.* (1971) seems destined to be a signpost in changing the direction of our thought away from the purely mechanical one of structural damage to that of metabolic interchange. One reason to doubt the mechanical thesis would be that men leading strenuous lives would damage their endothelia the most and thus be most prone to arterial disease, which is the exact reverse of the epidemiological situation. Indeed, the data above (p. 116) of Ling and Fry would indicate that a man who increased his cardiac output by some 4–5 times might damage his aortic endothelium severely.

6
The Relation between Pulsatile Pressure and Flow

One of the conditions for the application of Poiseuille's equation (2.3) is that the flow be 'steady', i.e. that it does not vary with time (a condition also known as 'stationary flow'). It has long been realized that the equation could not be applied to arterial flow which is highly pulsatile. While flow measurements were confined to determinations of mean flow only with the use of such instruments as Ludwig's *stromuhr* the problem aroused little interest. This probably accounts for the complete neglect of pioneering mathematical analyses such as that of Witzig (1914) which was noted in Ch. 5 (p. 103). A somewhat empirical approach to the problem was made by Shipley, Gregg and Schroeder (1943) as a result of their detailed study of pulsatile flow patterns in a wide range of arteries using an orifice meter (p. 233). They could find no clear relation between the pressure and the flow wave-forms and, with considerable insight, suggested that flow was more closely related to the derivative of the pressure rather than to the pressure itself. They did not pursue the quantitative relationship and their comment seems to have escaped notice for it was generally assumed that an increase in pulsatile pressure would cause an increase in pulsatile flow.

A physiologist getting interested in the problem for the first time in the early 1950s, as I did, had this consensus of opinion to work from. Most haemodynamics of that time were based on simple applications of *Windkessel* theory (Ch. 1, p. 10) which treated the arterial tree as a chamber in which pressure rose as blood was pumped into it. As an approximation for calculating the stroke volume this analysis was quite useful (p. 284), but it was quite inadequate to predict the instantaneous flow rate, as Peterson (1954) showed. When flow velocity can be measured continuously we find a situation like that illustrated in Fig. 6.1. Although the increase in flow starts more or less synchronously with the pressure rise the peak flow velocity precedes the peak pressure. On the basis of previous reasoning this would appear to violate the laws of inertia. The apparent anomaly was resolved when it was realized that it was the pressure-gradient along the artery which determines pulsatile flow (McDonald 1955a) just as it determines steady flow in Poiseuille's equation. This elementary observation can only be described adequately, in the late J. B. S. Haldane's phrase, as a 'blinding glimpse of the obvious'.

118

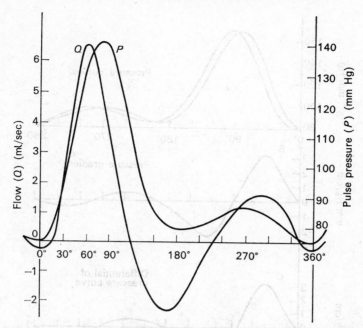

Fig. 6.1. A flow velocity pulse (*Q*) and the arterial pressure pulse (*P*) recorded simultaneously in the femoral artery of a dog. The flow velocity was recorded by high-speed cinematography but the corresponding volume flow has been plotted as the ordinate (left). Although superficially similar in shape when plotted on a comparable scale, the fact that the peak flow occurs before the pressure peak shows that there is no simple relation between these curves. The flow is, in fact, determined by the pressure-gradient (see text).

The pulse-frequency was 2·75 Hz in this experiment. The abscissa representing time in this and all subsequent curves is plotted as fractions of the cycle length, i.e. as degrees of arc. As noted in the legend to Fig. 5.1 with pulse-frequencies of this order one degree of arc is about one millisecond.

The pressure-gradient may be determined by recording the pressure at two points a short distance apart along the artery and subtracting the pressure from the downstream point from that at the upstream point at each moment (the deviation of the gradient over a finite distance from the gradient at a point, dp/dz, is discussed below (p. 136). The record of such a measurement is shown in Fig. 6.2A. Owing to the fact that the pressure-pulse generated in the aorta by the expulsion of blood by the heart travels along the arteries, the crest of the wave reaches the first recording point a short time before it reaches the downstream point. At this time the pressure is higher at the first than at the second point and the pressure-gradient slopes in this direction. The situation rapidly reverses and when the crest has reached the second point the pressure-gradient is in the opposite direction. Any secondary 'bumps' in the wave form will cause similar oscillations. The resultant pressure-gradient, therefore, is one that oscillates about a mean as shown in Fig. 6.2B. As we have a travelling wave in all arteries then all arterial pressure-gradients will be

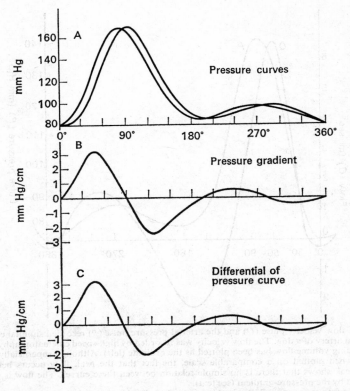

Fig. 6.2. A diagram that shows how a travelling pressure wave creates an oscillatory pressure-gradient.

A. Two waves recorded a short distance apart in the femoral artery of a dog. The downstream wave is here identical with the upstream one.

B. The pressure-gradient (mm Hg/cm) derived by subtracting the pressure at the downstream point from that at the upstream one at 15° intervals and dividing by the distance between recording points. (It should be noted that this gives a gradient opposite in sign to the usual mathematical convention for slopes.)

C. The derivative in respect to time of the upstream pressure wave (dp/dt). The form of this curve and that of pressure-gradient (which in the limiting case of a very small interval is the derivative in respect of distance, dp/dz) is very similar. In this case the only difference is due to the transmission time over the interval necessary to determine the gradient. The vertical lines demonstrate the small phase differences that this creates. In the presence of the usual distortion of the wave as it travels this similarity between time-derivative and space-derivative no longer holds with any precision (see text).

of this form. This gradient is directly related to the flow that is occurring just as the gradient and flow always occur together in Poiseuille flow.

The factors involved in moving a fluid by a pressure that oscillates in this way is clearly much more complex than those required for steady flow. The mass of fluid may be thought of as being at rest at the start of the cycle—as indeed it is, virtually, in the ascending aorta at the end of diastole. When a force, in the form of a pressure, is applied it will first appear to resist movement because of its inertia. As it accelerates it acquires ever increasing momentum; it will continue to accelerate as the pressure-gradient increases. With increasing velocity the viscous drag also increases. If the pressure gradient suddenly fell to zero the momentum of the blood would keep it moving until the opposing viscous forces brought it slowly to rest. In fact, because we are dealing with a travelling wave the gradient reverses when the pressure has passed its peak, as illustrated in Fig. 6.2. This reversal causes a rapid deceleration of the flow; only if the reversal of gradient continues after the forward flow has been brought to a halt does it lead to a reversal of flow. This is commonly seen in the femoral artery and is illustrated in Fig. 6.9.

In the ascending aorta, however, this reversal does not occur to any significant extent (Fig. 6.3) owing to the presence of valves. Noble (1968) has

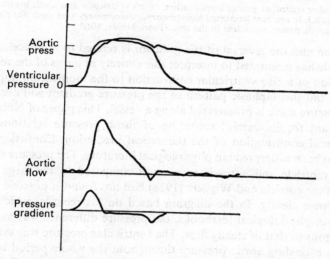

Fig. 6.3. This record shows the relations between the pressure-gradient and the flow at the root of the aorta. With the beginning of ventricular contraction there is a rapid rise in ventricular pressure (from the diastolic pressure which is near atmospheric) until it exceeds the aortic pressure when the valves open. A rapidly accelerating ejection of blood occurs while the pressure-gradient is positive. The rate of muscular shortening then slows and the ventricular pressure falls slightly below the aortic pressure and this reversal of the pressure-gradient decelerates the aortic flow until the aortic valves close (marked by a dip in all the traces). With high-frequency manometers it can be seen that there is no large overshoot of ventricular pressure. (Record from our own laboratory.)

made careful and accurate recordings of the simultaneous pressures in the outflow tract of the left ventricle and the root of the aorta (Fig. 6.4). This shows that initially the ventricular pressure is higher than that in the aorta immediately after the aortic valves open. During the latter part of systole as the ventricular pressure begins to fall, the aortic pressure is higher, i.e. the pressure-gradient has reversed. The point of reversal coincides approximately with the time of peak aortic flow. As the forward pressure-gradient is greatly in excess of that required to maintain a steady flow, there is initially a rapid

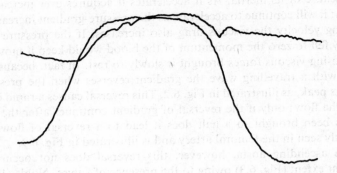

Fig. 6.4. Another record, at greater amplification, of left ventricular and aortic pressure to compare with Fig. 6.3. In this case implanted high-frequency manometers were used. See discussion of the form of aortic pressure-gradient in the text. (From Noble, 1968.)

acceleration and the reversal of the gradient is related to the deceleration of flow. Noble has attempted to interpret this entirely in terms of the relation of the duration of active ventricular contraction to the momentum imparted to the blood but this biphasic pattern of the pressure gradient will occur wherever a pressure wave is propagated along a vessel. This paper of Noble (1968) is important for its careful recording of those pressure relations for the experimental confirmation of the theoretical prediction. Confusion on this matter has been widespread in physiological literature. The pressure difference between ventricle and aorta is very small compared to the large pressure swing in the ventricle and Wiggers (1928) had not found it possible to define the difference clearly. In the diagram based on his records, which became standard in physiological textbooks, the pressure difference was assumed to be analogous to that of steady flow. The ventricular pressure was thus always shown as exceeding aortic pressure throughout the whole period of systolic ejection. Using strain-gauge manometers attached to catheters Spencer and Greiss (1962) reported that the pressure in the ventricle exceeded the aortic pressure during a brief period after the opening of the aortic valves, and thereafter the ventricular pressure was less than the aortic pressure. The brief period was a spike in the pressure recording and due to manometer artifact in a system which was underdamped and of a relatively low resonant frequency. This is exactly analogous to overswing of such a system in response to a step-function of pressure (and the very rapid rise in ventricular pressure is, in effect, such a function) and is succeeded by a train of oscillations which are used to determine the frequency response of manometers (Fig. 8.1). In fact, such after-oscillations can be seen in the Spencer and Greiss recordings. With the introduction of the very high-frequency catheter-tip and disc manometers used by Noble (1968) the true form of the ventricular pressure curve has been established.

We have seen in Ch. 2 that the solution of the factors involved in the laws for steady flow could not be determined without an adequate mathematical theory. In the case of oscillating flow it was essential that we should have a mathematical solution of the problem from the start. Such a solution was made by Womersley (1955b) and has been discussed in relation to the velocity profile in Ch. 5 (eqns. 5.1–5.14). The flow in a tube, in which any dilatation is neglected, was considered when the pressure-gradient varied periodically in the form of a sine-wave. With a Fourier series the flow related to any periodic pressure-gradient could be described.

THE RELATION OF FLOW TO AN OSCILLATORY PRESSURE GRADIENT

The derivation by Womersley (1955b, c) has already been described in Ch. 5 (eqns. 5.1–5.7).

The equation of motion of the liquid if the pressure-gradient varies with time (rearranging eqn. 5.1) is

$$\frac{\partial^2 w}{\partial r^2} + \frac{1}{r} \cdot \frac{\partial w}{\partial r} - \frac{1}{v} \cdot \frac{\partial w}{\partial t} = -\frac{1}{\mu} \cdot \frac{\partial p}{\partial z} \qquad \textbf{6.1}$$

If we take the pressure difference over a distance L as the pressure-gradient (if L is small the approximation is negligible) and represented by a simple harmonic motion then

$$\frac{P_1 - P_2}{L} = \frac{dp}{dz} = A^* e^{i\omega t} \qquad (5.2)$$

and the solution for the velocity, w, of the lamina at a distance $(y = r/R)$ from the axis is

$$w = \frac{A^*}{i\omega\rho} \left\{ 1 - \frac{J_0(\alpha y i^{\frac{3}{2}})}{J_0(\alpha i^{\frac{3}{2}})} \right\} e^{i\omega t} \qquad (5.7)$$

where

$$\alpha = R\sqrt{\frac{\omega}{v}} = \sqrt{\frac{2\pi f \cdot \rho}{\mu}} \qquad (5.6)$$

where f is the frequency in Hz.

To obtain the volume flow it is necessary to integrate the velocity across the lumen of the tube. Integrating eqn. 5.7 gives the volume flow $Q = $ ml/sec as

$$Q = \frac{\pi R^2 \cdot A^*}{i\omega\rho} \left\{ 1 - \frac{2J_1(\alpha i^{\frac{3}{2}})}{\alpha i^{\frac{3}{2}} J_0(\alpha i^{\frac{3}{2}})} \right\} e^{i\omega t} \qquad \textbf{6.2}$$

where J_1 is a Bessel function of the first kind and of order one. The expression in the braces was termed $[1 - F_{10}]$ by Womersley (1955b, c) and was tabulated by him in his monograph of 1957.

When the real part of the gradient is written as $M \cos (\omega t - \varphi)$, eqn. 6.2 can be written

$$Q = \frac{\pi R^2}{\omega \rho} . M . [1 - F_{10}] \sin (\omega t - \varphi) \qquad \textbf{6.3}$$

and may be calculated in this form using the real and imaginary parts of $[1 - F_{10}]$ given in Table B (p. 453). The physical interpretation of the equation is, however, easier if the function $[1 - F_{10}]$ is expressed in modulus and phase form; (modulus M'_{10} and phase ε_{10}). These terms are analogous to M'_0 and ε_0 (eqns. 5.11 and 12) in the equations for velocity discussed in Ch. 5 with the subscripts modified to indicate which Bessel functions are involved.

Equation 6.3 then becomes

$$Q = \frac{\pi R^2}{\omega \rho} . M . M'_{10} \sin (\omega t - \varphi + \varepsilon_{10}) \qquad \textbf{6.4}$$

The analogy with Poiseuille's equation is more easily seen if the term $\alpha^2 = R^2 . \omega / \nu$ is substituted

$$Q = \frac{\pi R^4 . M}{\mu} . \frac{M'_{10}}{\alpha^2} \sin (\omega t - \varphi + \varepsilon_{10}) \qquad \textbf{6.5}$$

because $M'_{10}/\alpha^2 \rightarrow 1/8$ as $\omega \rightarrow 0$ and $\varepsilon_{10} \rightarrow 90°$ so that $M \sin (\omega t - \varphi + 90°)$ becomes $M \cos (\omega t - \varphi)$ which is $\Delta P/$, eqn. 2.6.

The kinematic similarity of oscillatory flows in pipes is characterized by the non-dimensional parameter α which as seen above (eqn. 5.6) is a function of the radius, frequency and kinematic viscosity. Assuming the viscosity to be constant it is clear that the same α may arise from a lower frequency in a wide tube as from a higher frequency in a narrower tube. The velocity profiles will then be identical; the volume flow from a given gradient, however, is also a function of the cross-sectional area and so will only be similar in its phase relations. Although the dimensionless parameter α does not appear explicitly in eqn. 6.4 it must be remembered that both M'_{10} and ε_{10} are determined by it; they should properly be written $M'_{10}(\alpha)$ and $\varepsilon_{10}(\alpha)$ but the form has not been used in order to avoid making the equations more cumbersome than they need be.

The variations of M'_{10} and ε_{10} with α are shown in Fig. 6.5. In order to relate them to the steady flow equation the ratio M'_{10}/α^2 is plotted as a ratio of the Poiseuille constant $1/8$ and ε_{10} is plotted as the phase lag, or $(90 - \varepsilon_{10})°$, for the range of α from 0 to 10. Further details of the numerical values of these functions is given in Table A.

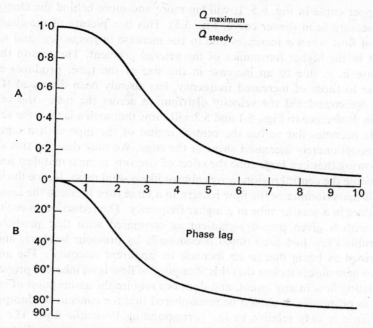

Fig. 6.5. The effect of changes in value of the non-dimensional constant α (eqn. 5.6) on the amplitude and phase of oscillatory flow generated by a pressure-gradient of simple harmonic form.

A. The amplitude as a ratio with the corresponding steady, or Poiseuille, flow. As the Poiseuille formula value is 1/8, the ordinate is, in fact, eight times the value of the term M'_{10}/α^2 tabulated in the appendix. For simplicity M' is usually written in the text for M'_{10} except where direct comparison with Womersley's paper might cause confusion.

B. The phase lag of the flow with respect to the pressure-gradient. The ordinate here is $(90 - \varepsilon_{10})°$ in Womersley's notation.

It will be seen that as α increases the phase lag is tending towards 90° and the amplitude term becomes very small (M' is tending to 1·0 and ε to 0°—see Fig. 7.6). At values of $\alpha < 1·0$, however, there is little deviation from Poiseuille's formula.

To consider the behaviour of the oscillating components of flow in an artery the best physical analogue is that of a pipe connecting two water reservoirs. If these reservoirs are supported on either end of a beam which is rocked about a fulcrum in the centre, the head of water, and so the pressure-gradient, will vary rhythmically. It is clear that as one reservoir rises water will begin to flow out of it along the pipe into the other reservoir. The flow, however, will build up more slowly than the upward movement of the reservoir, i.e. more slowly than the applied pressure, because of its inertia. Hence there is a phase lag, $(90 - \varepsilon)°$, of flow behind pressure. Equally when the movement of the reservoir is reversed the flow will continue in its original direction due to its momentum. As the rate of oscillation increases it is easy to see that the amount of flow generated in the pipe will also become smaller at the same head of water due to the inertial effect, and this is expressed quantitatively by the upper curve in Fig. 6.5. It will lag more and more behind the changes in the pressure head (lower curve, Fig. 6.5). This is a picture of the change in type of flow when α increases due to the increase in frequency, and will be found in the higher harmonics of the arterial gradient. The reason that an increase in α, due to an increase in the size of the tube, produces effects similar to those of increased frequency, has already been discussed (Ch. 5) when we considered the velocity distribution across the tube—the velocity profile. Reference to Figs. 5.1 and 5.2 will show that with a large α the velocity profile becomes flat across the central region of the pipe with a region of disproportionately increased shear at the edge. We may describe this simply as showing that in a large tube the effect of viscosity is most manifest near the wall while the central region moves almost like a solid mass. Hence the inertia of this mass dominates the flow pattern in a large tube in much the same way as it does in a smaller tube at a higher frequency. The reduction in oscillating flow with a given pressure-gradient as compared with that predicted by Poiseuille's law had been noted occasionally by previous workers, and was explained as being due to an increase in 'apparent viscosity'. The analogy drawn here makes it clear that this 'damping' of flow is an inherent property of oscillating flow in any liquid, and does not require the assumption of strange viscous properties. It should be remembered that the concept of 'damping' in this sense is only relative to the corresponding Poiseuille flow. The actual volume flow, Q, does, in fact, increase in a larger pipe with oscillating flow because R^4 increases in magnitude much faster than M'/α^2 decreases.

THE CALCULATION OF FLOW FROM THE PRESSURE-GRADIENT

With a characteristic arterial pressure-gradient such as that shown in Fig. 6.2B, measured in the femoral artery of a dog, the first step necessary is to resolve it into its harmonic components by a Fourier analysis (Ch. 7). The first four harmonic terms of such a curve are shown graphically in Fig. 6.6 together with their resynthesis to form the original curve. Each pressure oscillation has a corresponding flow term which is also of sinusoidal form. The conversion factors depend on the values of α for each harmonic term (for α increases as the frequency increases) and are derived from the tables prepared by Womersley. Figure 6.7 shows the relation between individual pressure and flow components, calculated from eqn. 6.5.

To derive the total flow due to the pressure-gradient as recorded the harmonic components of the flow are added together and the result is shown in Fig. 6.8. The final curve requires some further explanation because a mean flow has been added to it and this is shown by lowering the line representing zero flow. This is necessary from the nature of the analysis. The harmonic terms are all sine waves, that is they have a mean value of zero and so the

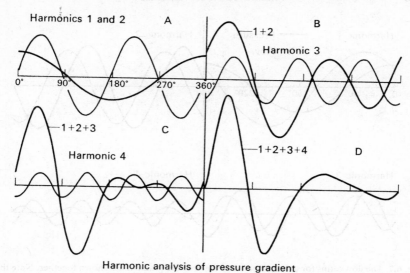

Harmonic analysis of pressure gradient

Fig. 6.6. The first four Fourier components of the pressure gradient of one experiment in the form $M \cos (\omega + \varphi)$.

A. 1 and 2 are the sine waves representing the first, or fundamental, harmonic ($n = 1$) and the second harmonic ($n = 2$). The modulus (M) of the second harmonic is 1·32 and that of the fundamental is 0·78. φ is $+0° \ 39'$ for the first harmonic and $-82° \ 45'$ for the second.

B. 1 and 2 represent the sum of the first two harmonics represented in A and the third harmonic (3) is superimposed ($M = -0.74$ and $\varphi = +26° \ 30'$).

C. $1+2+3$ is the sum of the first three harmonics and the fourth is superimposed ($M = -0.41$, $\varphi = -16° \ 39'$).

D. $1+2+3+4$ is the sum of four harmonics.

This figure is slightly modified from Fig. 4 of McDonald (1955a) because there is a small error in the calculated third harmonic. Curve D now represents the correct resynthesis but the other curves have not been withdrawn. The discrepancy between the resynthesized curve and the recorded gradient are now mainly, as always with a Fourier series taken to only a few terms, at the points of sharp inflection.

summation of a series of sine waves also can only sum to zero over a complete cycle. Where the mean value is not zero, it is represented in the Fourier series (eqn. 7.3) by the constant term A_0. The flow through an artery must have a positive mean value of this sort because after all its function is to convey blood from the heart to the tissues of the body. The simplest way of representing this has been to take the mean value of the pressure-gradient over the whole cycle and assume that this generates a steady flow of Poiseuille type which is added to the oscillating term. This method has two defects, one practical and one theoretical. The *practical* difficulty is that the mean positive pressure-gradient is of very small dimensions—in the case illustrated the mean flow is only 1 ml/sec which corresponds to a mean gradient of only 0·13 mm Hg/cm of artery. It is, therefore, at the mercy of manometric errors for, even measuring over an 8 cm length of femoral artery, this only amounts to a pressure drop of about 1 mm Hg. This accuracy can only be attained by using

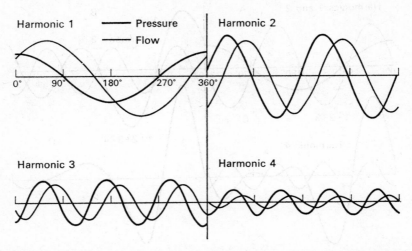

Fig. 6.7. The flow terms for each harmonic of the pressure gradient are shown together. Note that there is a phase shift (φ) due to the inertia of the fluid. 1 is the fundamental, 2, 3 and 4 the next three harmonics. φ is 31° 14′ in 1, 19° 57′ in 2, 15° 50′ in 3 and 13° 99′ in 4. The composite modulus is 2·4 in 1, 2·33 in 2, 1·12 in 3 and 0·34 in 4 and the curves show how the resultant flow is progressively damped in the higher harmonics. The ordinates are on an arbitrary scale.

a good differential manometer. In the illustrations the mean flow has been checked by direct observation. The *theoretical* objection is that the system is non-linear so that there is an interaction between the oscillating flow and the steady flow and so they cannot truly be treated as separate terms. This is discussed in Ch. 11. At the peak of the systolic flow in one case Womersley (1955c) calculated that the alteration in steady flow would be of the order of 15 per cent. In terms of the shape of the pulsatile flow curve this is negligible because the steady flow is itself small compared with the oscillating components of the flow. As regards the steady flow itself the correction cannot be disregarded. As the complexity of the calculation of the correction is coupled with the inherent inaccuracies of the measurement of the mean pressure-gradient we can see that this method is of no practical application in the prediction of mean flow in an artery. The work surveyed later, however, shows that important physiological data may be derived from the phasic variations in the pattern of flow and these are well predicted by the calculated curves.

Figure 6.9 shows the comparison between an observed flow curve and one calculated from the 'pressure-gradient' measured at the same time, and it can be seen that the correlation, allowing for experimental error, is fairly good. Mathematically the convincing aspect of these two curves is that the phase relations are accurately predicted. Discrepancies in amplitude may easily arise from experimental error in view of the very precise manometry required. The points of reversal of flow are much less subject to error in the observed

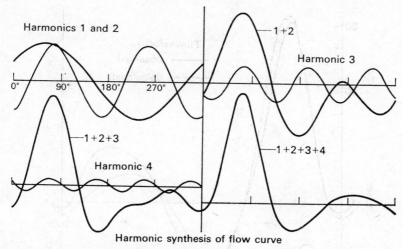

Harmonics 1 and 2

1+2

Harmonic 3

0° 90° 180° 270°

1+2+3

1+2+3+4

Harmonic 4

Harmonic synthesis of flow curve

Fig. 6.8. The flow components shown in Fig. 6.7 are here shown singly and then summed successively as the pressure components were in Fig. 6.6. In the final summation $1+2+3+4$ the zero line has been moved to represent the addition of the mean flow, as the sine waves only represent the oscillating part of the flow. Because of the damping of the flow in the higher harmonics the flow due to the fifth and sixth harmonics is too small to show on this graph.

There is here a correction of Fig. 6 in McDonald (1955a), necessary because of the error in the analysis of the gradient noted in the legend to Fig. 6.6. As these figures are only shown to illustrate the method of calculation only the final curve has been redrawn—this time correctly.

curves than in the calculated. Nevertheless the prediction of the diastolic part of the curve is not satisfactory and the explanation of this is discussed below (p. 442). Another comparison, under conditions of vasodilatation, is shown in Fig. 6.10.

THE EFFECT OF THE SIZE OF THE ARTERY ON THE FLOW PATTERN

A return to the formula (6.5) for the oscillating flow shows that it differs from the formula for Poiseuille's law. For oscillating flow

$$Q = \frac{\pi R^4}{\mu} \cdot \frac{M'_{10}}{\alpha^2} \cdot M \sin(\omega t - \varphi + \varepsilon_{10})$$

where the pressure-gradient $\dfrac{P_1 - P_2}{L} = M \cos(\omega t - \varphi)$

whereas for steady flow $\quad Q = \dfrac{\pi R^4}{\mu} \cdot \dfrac{1}{8} \cdot \dfrac{(P_1 - P_2)}{L}$ **6.6**

With an oscillating pressure the amplitude of the flow no longer varies linearly with the pressure-gradient but is modified by the term M'/α^2. Furthermore the flow lags behind the pressure by an angle $(90 - \varepsilon)°$. When α is small

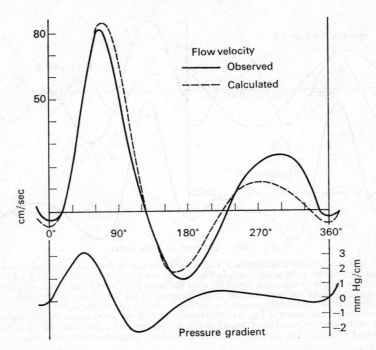

Fig. 6.9. The flow velocity in the dog femoral artery recorded by high-speed cinematography compared with that calculated from a derived 'pressure-gradient' (lower curve). The so-called gradient was calculated from the time-derivative of the pressure and the value for the 'peak-to-peak' wave velocity recorded in a series of animals by Hale *et al.* (1955). As discussed in Ch. 13 where the arterial input impedances of this experiment are shown (Fig. 13.7), the amplitude of the calculated flow is almost certainly too great. There are, however, reasons to believe that this method of recording flow also tends to give values that are too high (Ch. 6). The correspondence between the two curves, which is reasonably good, suggests, therefore, that even these approximations, the equations on which the calculation is based are satisfactory.

The pulse-frequency in this experiment was 2·85/Hz. The abscissa is expressed as degrees of arc of a cycle (360°) because of the method of calculation (see Fig. 6.1).

M'/α^2 approximates to the value 1/8 which is the constant in Poiseuille's law. At the same time the value of ε tends to 90° so that the term $M \sin(\omega t - \varphi + \varepsilon_{10})$ becomes $M \sin(\omega t - \varphi + 90°)$ or $M \cos(\omega t - \varphi)$, i.e. $(P_1 - P_2)/L$. The formula for the flow thus approximates to Poiseuille's law in small vessels. Where α is 0·5 or less for the fundamental harmonic the difference between the two formulae is negligible. The approximation is quite good in a vessel such as the saphenous artery ($\alpha = 0·8$) so that in small vessels even if the pressure-gradient varies the flow will vary, approximately linearly, with it.

With large vessels the oscillating flow deviates very greatly from the Poiseuille formula. When α is 10 it can be seen from Fig. 6.5. that the amplitude of the flow is about 1/15 of that predicted by Poiseuille's formula and furthermore is more than 80° out of phase. The limiting condition as α gets very large is that the flow excursion decreases to a very small value and is 90°

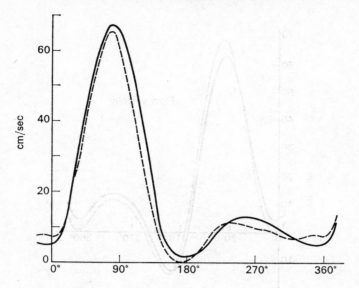

Fig. 6.10. The observed (whole line) and calculated (broken line) flow velocity curves in the dog femoral artery after an intra-arterial injection of 100 μg of acetylcholine, i.e. with marked peripheral vasodilatation. Observed and calculated curves were obtained in the same way as those in Fig. 6.9. The improved correspondence of the curves compared with that figure is attributed to the reduction of reflections (see text). The pulse frequency was 2·1 Hz.

out of phase. The phase relation is then analogous to the relation of an alternating voltage to the current it produces in an inductance. Such a situation will be reached in the aorta where the α of the fundamental will be between 10–15 so that the fourth harmonic can reach 30. A calculated flow curve for aortic flow in a dog is shown in Fig. 6.11 and it can be seen that there is an increased lag between flow and pressure-gradient.

THE VALUES OF α FOUND IN THE CIRCULATION

From values calculated for dogs we have seen above that α at the pulse-frequency was less than 1 in the saphenous artery, about 3 in the femoral artery and about 10 or higher in the aorta. These values were for particular individuals and they will show variation in the same individual with changes of pulse-frequency and between individuals because of differences in calibre. It is interesting to compare the range of values found in different species. Because small animals, which have small arteries, tend to have fast heart rates, and vice versa, the value of α tends to vary over a surprisingly small range at comparable anatomical sites. Some estimated values are given in Table 6.1.

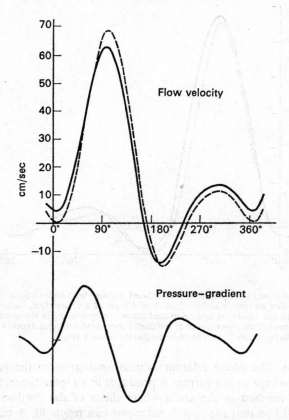

Fig. 6.11. Flow velocity curves calculated from a pressure-gradient measured in the proximal aorta—the recording points were estimated to lie 2 and 7 cm from the aortic valves. The pulse frequency was 2·85/Hz.

The *unbroken line* represents the curve calculated from full eqn. 6.5—for the fundamental frequency, $\alpha = 10·7$; the *broken line* shows the calculated curve when the effects of viscosity were neglected and the asymptotic values for M' (1·0) and for ε (0°) were used. The discrepancies between the two curves show that the effect of the blood viscosity is to reduce both the amplitude and the phase lag with respect to the pressure-gradient. In vessels of this size, however, this effect is very small and neglecting it is of little practical importance. The motion of the blood in large arteries is mainly determined by its inertia.

Only four harmonics were used to calculate these curves; this is quite insufficient to represent accurately a pulse form such as that in Fig. 6.3 so that comparisons of shape are of little value. The mean flow is also arbitrary in this case and was largely determined by setting end-diastolic flow at, or near, zero as in the method of Fry *et al.* (1956).

Although the larger species tend to have somewhat larger values there is quite a remarkable correspondence of values. This suggests that the circulation in various mammals has a dynamic or kinematical similarity and lends comforting theoretical support to the application of results derived from lower animals to the interpretation of observations made in human beings.

TABLE 6.1. Some values of α in different mammalian species

A: *Site*—Root of aorta (from data in Clark, 1927, relating to heart rates and aortic cross-sectional area)

Species	Pulse rate/min	Radius (cm)	α (fundamental)
Mouse	600–730	0·03–0·04	1·19–1·74
Rat	360–520	0·045–0·095	1·38–3·5
Rabbit	205–220	0·17	3·92–4·07
Cat	180	0·2	4·4
Dog	72–125	0·55–0·6	8·27–10·68
Man	55–72	1·08–1·11	13·5–16·7
Ox	43	2·0	21·1
Elephant	40–50	4·47	48–51

The range of average body-weights of the same species ranges from 35 g (mouse) to $2 \cdot 0 - 2 \cdot 5 \times 10^6$ g (elephant) (Clark, 1927).

B: *Site*—Femoral artery

Species	Pulse rate/min	Radius (cm)	α (fundamental)
Rabbit	210–360	0·06	1·4–1·8
Dog	72–180	0·12–0·15	1·65–3·25
Man	60–72	0·2–0·25	2·5–3·5

The higher range of pulse rates allowed here in the rabbit and dog are based on personal observations in animals anaesthetized with pentobarbitone (nembutal).

THE RELATIONSHIP OF THE PRESSURE-GRADIENT TO THE TIME–DERIVATIVE OF THE PRESSURE

The pressure-gradient we have considered up to this point is one measured directly by the difference in pressure measured at two points in an artery. It was pointed out earlier in this chapter that it is this gradient that must be considered as the force related to the flow and not the pressure curve itself. Nevertheless the form of the gradient is clearly related to the form of the pressure pulse. In Fig. 6.2 the pressure-gradient is drawn as the difference in pressure between the two points divided by the distance separating these two points. If the distance is Δz then we may write the gradient as $\Delta p/\Delta z$. If the distance between the recording points is very small the expression for the gradient becomes, in the terms of the calculus, dp/dz—that is, the derivative of the pressure in respect of distance. The pressure curve may be differentiated by putting the output from an electrical manometer through a suitable circuit or by differentiating the Fourier series of the curve. Figure 6.2c shows that the time-derivative of the arterial pressure obtained in this way is, in fact, of the same form as the pressure-gradient. By differentiating the pressure we are deriving the coefficient in respect of time, dp/dt. It is, however, clear that the relation between dp/dz and dp/dt is simply

$$\frac{dp}{dz} = \frac{dp}{dt} \cdot \frac{dt}{dz}$$

and dz/dt, or the coefficient of space in respect to time, is the velocity, c, of propagation of the pulse-wave. The sign convention for slopes of curves also requires that the actual gradient is $-dp/dz$ (representing a 'downhill' slope) so that the relation is written

$$\frac{-dp}{dz} = \frac{1}{c} \cdot \frac{dp}{dt} \qquad \qquad 6.7$$

The rate of flow which is dependent on the pressure-gradient is, therefore, also seen to be dependent on the rate of change of the pulse-pressure although not on its absolute value. As noted above a qualitative relationship of flow and the rate of change in pressure was noted by Shipley, Gregg and Schroeder (1943) although they did not determine a quantitative relationship. Indeed it is difficult to see how one could ever be found without a fundamental theoretical analysis, such as has been made by Womersley.

The relationship between the pressure-gradient and the time derivative of the pressure-wave looks seductively simple but its implications need examining more closely. As it stands it is true for a pressure-wave of sinusoidal form and the value, c, is then called its phase velocity. In a linear system it will also be true of a compound wave in which all its harmonic components are travelling at the same phase velocity. The phase velocity is, however, only independent of the frequency in a perfectly elastic tube filled with inviscid fluid which is so long that no reflection of the wave occurs. The wave will then travel without distortion. When eqn. 6.7 was originally used by McDonald (1955a) and Womersley (1955b) this condition, that it was only valid if the wave travelled without distortion, was stated although the implications of this condition were not discussed. Nevertheless, the time-derivative was used for calculating flows. This was not because we imagined that the blood had no viscosity or that the arterial wall was perfectly elastic but because the magnitude of these two effects was known to be small, especially in comparison with the errors inherent in measuring the pressure-gradient by differencing two manometers. Further work has shown that major errors may be introduced by this method due to the presence of reflection of waves in the arterial tree. The detailed discussion of these factors in general is deferred to Chs. 12 and 14 and here we are only noting the conclusions presented there.

In spite of these serious reservations raised by McDonald (1960) the gradient derived from the time-derivative of the pressure from eqn. 6.6, but using a constant value of c taken as the foot-to-foot wave velocity, has been used by several authors, e.g. Jones et al. (1959). Greenfield et al. (1962) and Boyett et al. (1966). As in all these cases the application was in the ascending aorta where the effect of reflected waves is relatively small (Ch. 11) the approximation was not particularly severe, especially when only the stroke volume was measured. Nevertheless Greenfield and Fry (1965b) criticized it severely while using the substitution themselves; their criticisms are more aptly discussed below with a consideration of the equation used by Fry to calculate flow.

The effect of the viscosity of the fluid on the transmission of a wave is to damp it in amplitude and also to reduce its velocity. These effects are described mathematically by expressing the wave velocity as a complex number. If the complex value of c is used in eqn. 6.7 the effect of viscosity is, therefore, allowed for. The wave velocity under these circumstances increases with its frequency and in a free elastic tube its limiting value is the velocity that the wave would have in an ideal, non-viscous liquid (see Fig. 11.3). The damping also increases with frequency. From the figure, however, it can be seen that at values of α above 3 the change in velocity is small and for this reason it was considered that the difference in phase-velocity of the components of the pulse wave over the range of α that we have considered in the femoral artery could be neglected. They would only be of the order of 2–3 per cent at most and this is smaller than the errors involved in measuring the velocity of the pulse. The non-linear elastic behaviour of the arterial wall would also cause an increase in wave-velocity with frequency (Ch. 12) and, although we do not have such quantitative data for this effect, it also may be regarded as small over the frequency range with which we are concerned.

The possible effect of reflections on the phase velocity was suggested by the fact that predictions of flow curves from the time-derivative of the pressure were, in early experiments in 1955 and 1956, very much in error when there was marked vasoconstriction produced by intra-arterial injections of adrenaline. It was realized that this was a condition likely to produce reflections—which until then had been assumed to be negligible. This conclusion was supported by the finding that with increasing vasodilatation, and so reduced reflections, the fit became very good (Fig. 6.10). Here there is a good correspondence even in the diastolic portion of the curve, a region where there is a discrepancy in the 'normal' curve (Fig. 6.9). The effect of wave reflection is discussed in Ch. 12 and the effect on arterial impedance in Chs. 13 and 14. Here, it is sufficient to note that one effect is to cause large alterations in the apparent rate of travel of the various harmonic components with frequency for a change in frequency alters the distance, in terms of wave-length, of any point from the reflecting site.

In the presence of reflected waves it is, therefore, necessary to measure the apparent phase velocity, c', of each harmonic component and use this velocity as the value of c in eqn. 6.7 because the use of a single wave velocity for all the components in the pressure-wave is invalid. Even this will lead to some errors in predicting the wave form because it neglects the fact that, as noted above, the wave-velocity is complex (which is further discussed in Ch. 11). The substitution of a wholly real value for the wave velocity fails to predict the phase relations between the components of flow accurately which leads to a distortion of the shape of the wave after resynthesis. The nature of this distortion is more easily considered in terms of the phase of the input impedance and is discussed in Ch. 15. The use of the apparent phase-velocity with the time-derivative of the pressure, however, predicts the amplitude of the harmonic components accurately.

The use of the time-derivative has the technical attraction that it is easier to measure it accurately than to measure the pressure-gradient, but it can be seen that, in the arterial system, it has pitfalls associated with the factors that distort the shape of the pressure wave as it travels. Nevertheless, the simple form of the equation has, as noted above, been used by several workers; this led Greenfield and Fry (1965a) to compare critically this method with the pressure-gradient approach of Fry, Mallos and Casper (1956) which is discussed in a subsequent section (pp. 139–142). An elementary demonstration of this can be appreciated if, in eqn. 6.7, we replace dp/dz by the flow equivalent given by eqn. 6.4, given the assumption that the liquid is inviscid (as is essentially the Fry approach). The values of M'_{10} and ε_{10} will then be, respectively, 1·0 and 0·0° for all frequencies. Taking a single constant value for the wave velocity, c', thus allows a simple integration of pressure and flow in respect to time and the form of the flow wave will be identical to that of the pressure wave. This will always be so with a liquid of negligible viscosity where there are no reflected waves (an assumption made in assuming c to be independent of frequency). This is discussed further in Ch. 12. Greenfield and Fry (1965b) also demonstrate this experimentally. In fact, it is well known (e.g. Figs. 6.1 and 12.2) that the flow and pressure waves are very different in form which, of itself, shows that the simple interpretation of eqn. 6.7 is not adequate. Greenfield and Fry actually interpret the discrepancies in terms of the electrical components in their analogue computer but it seems easier to interpret in terms of the effects of wave-reflection and, as noted, the discussion is deferred to later chapters.

The pressure-gradient, by contrast, is directly related to flow that is occurring and is also modified by such factors as wave reflections that modify the flow. It must be realized, however, that in the mathematical analysis we are considering the rate of change of pressure in respect to distance, the space-derivative, at a point. In measuring the gradient over a finite interval we are only obtaining an approximation to this. The effect due to wave-travel between the two points of measurement can be seen by comparing the gradient (Fig. 6.2B) with the time-derivative (Fig. 6.2C). In this diagram the wave is represented as travelling without distortion and the forms of the gradient and the time-derivative are identical but it can be seen that the gradient is displaced in time. The error due to measuring over a finite interval has been analysed by Taylor (1959c) and also, in more detail, by Gessner (personal communication). The magnitude of the error in measuring both amplitude is given approximately by

$$\varepsilon = \frac{\Delta z}{2\lambda} = \frac{\Delta z \cdot f}{2c} \qquad \qquad 6.8$$

that is, the ratio of half the interval to the wave length, λ, of the oscillation. While for the lower frequency components this is very small it becomes appreciable, for any precise work, in the higher frequency components especially in the large vessels where the wave-velocity is relatively small. For example, if a 4 cm interval is used in the ascending aorta where the wave velocity is c. 4 m/sec, the error at 1·0 Hz will only be 0·5 per cent or 1·8° (Nichols and McDonald, 1972). As the gradient must be measured over a finite interval, the error in measurement is unavoidable, but can be allowed for in subsequent calculations.

THE VALIDITY OF THE WOMERSLEY EQUATIONS WHEN APPLIED TO ARTERIES

As with the derivation of the Poiseuille equation for steady flow, it is necessary to review the basic assumptions on which the mathematical analysis of Womersley was based. The two derivations share many of these assumptions although they need to be stated in a somewhat different form:

(1) *That the flow is laminar.* The evidence of the distribution of laminar flow in arteries has been discussed in Ch. 4 where it was seen that in peripheral vessels such as the femoral artery this is almost certainly the case. McDonald (1960) suggested that, because of the high Reynolds numbers attained during systole, the laminar pattern almost certainly broke down in large arteries near the heart during part of the cycle. The evidence of Schultz *et al.* (1969) (Ch. 4, p. 80) indicates that even in the human ascending aorta any appearance of turbulence, if detected, is very brief in normal circumstances. Only in diseased conditions, notably with stenosis of the aortic valve, is any large-scale disturbance seen. As, with the high values of α found in these large vessels, the resistive component is small compared to the inertial components, one would expect that deviations from laminar flow would only make a small difference in the predicted flow.

(2) *That the length of the tube is long compared to the region being studied.* This is the 'inlet length' problem which was considered in Ch. 4. While the length of the 'inlet' for the oscillatory flow in the systemic and pulmonary arterial trees has not been determined, clearly the ascending aorta and pulmonary artery (the regions of especial interest) will be fully within it. The theoretical and experimental work of Chang and Atabek (1961) shows that this will introduce an error but it is small compared to the probable error in pressure measurement and may be neglected.

(3) *That the fluid is homogenous and does not have anomalous viscous properties.* While this assumption, as stated, is untrue, it was seen in Ch. 3 that the effects of anomalous (non-Newtonian) viscosity in blood at high shear rates only became important in very small vessels of arteriolar dimensions. In oscillatory flow, however, there are periods in every cardiac cycle

when the shear rate becomes very low. While no experimental work has been done to test the effects of this, a detailed theoretical investigation by Taylor (1959a) showed that the error would not be more than 1–2 per cent.

(4) *That the flow is through a cylindrical tube whose diameter remains constant.* While superficially this assumption would appear to involve a large approximation the experimental evidence shows that the actual radial dilatation of arteries during the cardiac cycle is in fact small; at the largest in the proximal aorta it is usually c. ±2·5 per cent around the mean diameter. The error due to this approximation is discussed in Ch. 11 and again is small compared to the probable error of measurement of flow.

(5) *That the flow may be expressed as a sum of harmonic components calculated from the individual harmonic terms of the pressure-gradient.* This is discussed in terms of non-linearity in relation to hydrodynamic equations in Ch. 11 and to the non-linear elastic behaviour of the arterial wall in Ch. 12. In terms of pressure and flow it is generally agreed that non-linear terms are very small.

(6) *That no 'slip' occurs at the wall.* The justification for this was discussed with the assumptions underlying Poiseuille's equation in Ch. 2, and it is clear that this assumption is always true for liquid flow.

The Womersley equations have been tested experimentally in rigid tubes by Linford and Ryan (1965) over a wide range of values for α. They found a very close agreement between the theoretical and measured flows; they further showed that, as anticipated, only very small differences occurred when turbulent flow was present at high values of α ($\alpha > 10$). The comparison made by Kunz and Coulter (1967), using blood in tubes, has been discussed in Ch. 3. Again, over the great part of the range, the agreement between theory and experiment was very close but, at very low frequencies, discrepancies appeared attributable to the anomalous viscous properties of the blood. Greenfield and Fry (1965a) made a detailed comparison between flow measured in the thoracic aorta with an electromagnetic flowmeter and the flow predicted by both the full Womersley equation and the simpler approach introduced by Fry, Mallos, and Casper (1965)—which is discussed in the next section. The predicted flow showed close agreement between the two methods; while the comparison of predicted and measured values was good, there was found to be a small, random, difference of between 2–10 per cent. This, however, is most likely to be attributable to the experimental error in measuring the pressure-gradient. The experimental situation in a living animal will always make a precise testing of the basic equations used extremely difficult.

In summary, the simple Womersley equation cannot be rigorously applied to arteries but, nevertheless, it is almost certainly as close, or closer, a practical approximation as Poiseuille's equation is for steady flow in arteries.

FRY'S SOLUTION FOR PRESSURE–FLOW RELATIONS IN THE AORTA

Fry (Fry, Mallos, and Casper, 1956) made an analysis of the pressure–flow relationship in a large artery that is of a simpler form than that of Womersley and has been widely used for deriving the flow in the aorta. His derivation was based directly on the Navier–Stokes equations. These equations are extensions of the Euler equations of motion for a three-dimensional entity of inviscid fluid; they were extended to include viscous fluids by Navier (1827) and Poisson (1831) and later derived more rigorously by St. Venant (1843) and Stokes (1845). The derivation of these equations is given in standard textbooks (e.g. Prandtl and Tietjens, 1934, Newman and Searle, 1957; they are discussed in a particularly lucid way in the reviews of Fry, 1959a, b, and again, with especial reference to the Womersley equation, by Fry and Greenfield, 1964, and Attinger, 1964, also gives a general account of those aspects of hydro-dynamics relevant to haemodynamics). For an incompressible fluid, i.e. liquids, the motion in the x-axis is given by

$$\frac{\partial u}{\partial t} + u\frac{\partial u}{\partial x} + v\frac{\partial u}{\partial y} + w\frac{\partial u}{\partial z} = X - \frac{1}{\rho}\cdot\frac{\partial p}{\partial x} + v\left[\frac{\partial^2 u}{\partial x^2} + \frac{\partial^2 u}{\partial y^2} + \frac{\partial^2 u}{\partial z^2}\right] \qquad \textbf{6.9}$$

The motions in the y-axis and the z-axis have flow components of, respectively, v and w and the two corresponding equations for these axes are written with the appropriate substitutions for x and u in eqn. 6.9. Fry took the x-axis as the axis of the artery and he made the assumption (as did Womersley) that there were no flow components at right angles to the axis of the tube, i.e. that the radius was invariant (the 'rigid' tube), so that these other equations reduce to zero on both sides because v and w are zero.

The term X on the RHS is the force component in the x-axis and, assuming irrotational flow over the whole cycle, will be zero. By rearranging and multi-plying both sides by ρdx the following equation may be written

$$\frac{-\partial p}{\partial x}\cdot dx = \rho\cdot\mathbf{q}\,\nabla u\cdot dx + \rho\frac{\partial u}{\partial t}\cdot dx - \mu\nabla^2 u\cdot dx \qquad \textbf{6.10}$$

where $\mathbf{q}\nabla u$ is the sum of the rates of change of u in the three axes on the LHS of eqn. 6.9 using the vector $\mathbf{q}$ and $\nabla^2 u$ is the sum of the second order derivatives in the brackets on the RHS of eqn. 6.9 (LHS and RHS are abbreviations for left- and right-hand side). This was further simplified by making further approximations. The third term on the RHS defines the viscous drag which, because it would be relatively small, was approximated by a linear frictional term a and written $a.u(t)$. Further, arguing from a more generalized form of the relationship between dp/dz and dp/dt given in eqn. 6.7 it was assumed that the rate of change of u in the x-axis would be very small (by virtue of the factor $1/c$) compared to the rate of change of u in respect of time. It could, therefore, be regarded as negligible. The term involving $(\mathbf{q}.\nabla u)$ therefore also disappeared. The equation was thus finally reduced to

$$p(t) = \rho \Delta x . \frac{du}{dt} + au(t) \qquad \qquad \textbf{6.11}$$

where $p(t)$ is the pressure difference, as a function of time, over the interval Δx.

The solution of eqn. 6.11 is

$$u(t) = \frac{\exp\left(\dfrac{at}{\rho \Delta x}\right)}{\rho \Delta x} \int_0^t p(t).\exp\left(\frac{at}{\rho \Delta x}\right).dt + C_1.\exp\left(\frac{at}{\rho \Delta x}\right) \qquad \textbf{6.12}$$

The second term on the RHS is the transient solution which, for steady-state conditions, may be ignored.

The equation also assumes that there is no frequency dependence of any terms; this is analogous to the limit of the inviscid case in the Womersley equation. Such flow would have a flat velocity profile and is, in fact, a not unreasonable approximation for flow in the inlet length of a large tube with the Womersley parameter $\alpha > 10$ (see Ch. 5). A comparison of a synthesis of the first four harmonics of flow in the thoracic aorta between the curve computed with the actual values of α used in the Womersley equation and with α taken as infinitely large (i.e. with zero viscosity) is illustrated in Fig. 6.11. The discrepancy between the two curves is not large. Linford and Ryan (1965) also demonstrated that for $\alpha > 7$ the approximation introduced by Fry makes only a small difference.

As no account is taken of this frequency of the oscillation there is no necessity to perform a Fourier analysis and the solution of the equation can be made with a simple electrical analogue. The equation for electrical components analogous to eqn. 6.9 is

$$I = \frac{CdE}{dt} + \frac{E}{R}. \qquad \qquad \textbf{6.13}$$

where the voltage drop E was taken as the analogue of the velocity u, the current I as analogous with the pressure drop p, R as the fluid resistance and the capacitance C as equalling $\rho \Delta x$. Fry, Noble and Mallos (1957) built an electric circuit to solve this equation and this has been used by all subsequent workers using this approach.

The mean flow is not given by the above equations and this was approximated on the assumption that the flow in the latter part of diastole is zero and the curve of the analogue solution was displayed and the components were adjusted until the diastolic flow was zero.

At the time when it was introduced, digital computers were rarely available in physiological laboratories and the practical advantages of this method were great; indeed as flowmeters were also both relatively rare and unreliable it was important as a method for deriving the flow velocity in the ascending aorta. Later, comparison with flow curves measured with flowmeters showed that the somewhat sweeping assumptions made in the derivation were, indeed, justified in vessels such as the ascending or thoracic aorta. A comparison of a derived curve and one measured with a flowmeter is shown in Fig. 6.12.

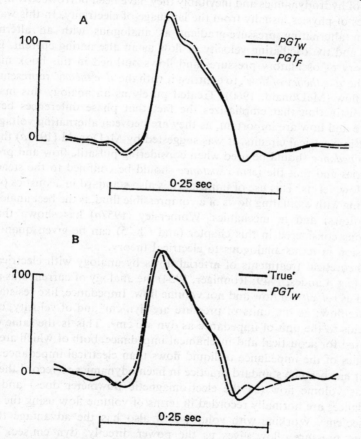

Fig. 6.12A. A comparison of the pulsatile flow curve in the thoracic aorta as calculated from the pressure-gradient using the Womersley equations (solid line———PGT_W) and the Fry equation (broken line - - - - - - -PGT_F).

B. A comparison between the same flow curve calculated from the gradient as in A by the Womersley equations (broken line - - - - - - - PGT_W) and an electromagnetic flowmeter (solid line———'True').

It can be seen that the Fry equation gives a result very close to the Womersley equations when applied to a large artery; and that both are not significantly different from the flowmeter recording. (From Greenfield and Fry, 1965a.)

As the method has been often used in estimating ventricular output a more detailed consideration of the results obtained with this method is deferred to Ch. 15.

The approximations made, however, render the equation inadequate for deriving flows in smaller and more peripheral arteries and in those situations the full Womersley equation should be used.*

The concept of impedance. Because the behaviour of oscillating liquid flow is not generally familiar we do not have a set of technical terms peculiar to this branch of hydrodynamics and inevitably they have been borrowed from other branches of physics, usually from the language of electricity. In this way, we treat an alternating pressure-gradient as analogous with an alternating voltage and the oscillating velocity of flow as an alternating current. Hence the theory of oscillatory pressures and flows outlined in this book may be called the '*a–c theory of flow*', to contrast it with the '*d–c theory*' represented by steady flow (McDonald, 1960). Treated purely as an analogy this makes a useful distinction that emphasizes the fact that phase differences between pressure and flow are important, as they are between alternating voltage and current in electrical circuits. It was suggested by McDonald (1955a) that the term *impedance* should be used when considering pulsatile flow and pressure in arteries and that the term *resistance* should be confined to the steady, or mean flow, terms. This use of impedance is also standard in acoustics (which, in dealing with oscillating flows of a compressible fluid, is the best analogy for liquid flows) and in mechanics. Womersley (1957a) has shown that the equations considered in this chapter (and Ch. 5) can be given quantitative expression in terms analogous to electrical theory.

In theoretical treatments of arterial flows by analogy with electrical networks (e.g. Landes, 1949; Ronniger, 1954) the analogy of current was always treated as *velocity* of flow and not volume flow. Impedance, like resistance, is pressure/flow; as the units of pressure are dyn/cm^2 and of velocity, cm/sec, this leads to the unit of impedance as $dyn\ sec\ cm^3$. This is the same unit as that used for acoustical and mechanical impedance, both of which are closer analogies of the impedance to liquid flows than electrical impedance. However, it has become standard practice in haemodynamics to record the blood flow as volume flow (as the electromagnetic flowmeter does) and hence impedances are normally recorded in terms of volume flow using the unit of $dyn\ sec/cm^5$. Working with volume flow also has the advantage that the product pressure × flow gives us the power directly, dyn cm/sec. This is analogous with the derivation of electrical power as voltage × current. The conversion from one to the other is, of course, simple in that the conversion

---

* A much improved analogue computer which is based on the Womersley equations has been built by Gabe (1965a, b). It has been used successfully for recording blood flows in human arteries (Gabe, 1965a, b) and has been shown to be as accurate as a digital computer used for the same purpose.

factor only involves the cross-sectional area. In later chapters the impedance is usually expressed in terms of volume flow. Where generalizations about the whole vascular bed are being made, however, there is an advantage in using the linear velocity of flow in calculating the impedance because, as was seen in Ch. 2 (p. 38), the changes in velocity of flow are determined by changes in the total cross-sectional area of the branches at any level; the impedance calculated from volume flow only expresses the impedance of a single vessel out of an array of vessels in parallel.

Writing the pressure-gradient in exponential form we have

$$\frac{P_1 - P_2}{L} = A\overset{*}{e}^{i\omega t} \qquad\qquad 6.14$$

and the corresponding term for the average velocity across the pipe is

$$\overline{V} = \frac{Q}{\pi R^2} = \frac{A^* . R^2}{i\mu} . \frac{M'_{10}}{\alpha^2} e^{i\epsilon}{}_{10} . e^{i\omega t} \qquad\qquad 6.15$$

The *longitudinal impedance*, Z, is defined as the impedance per unit length of the pipe and is thus given by

$$Z_L = \frac{A\overset{*}{e}^{i\omega t}}{\overline{V}} = \frac{i\mu}{R^2} . \frac{\alpha^2}{M'_{10}} . e^{-i\epsilon}{}_{10} \qquad\qquad 6.16$$

$$= \frac{\mu\alpha^2}{R^2 . M'_{10}} \sin \epsilon_{10} + \frac{i\mu\alpha^2}{R^2 M'_{10}} . \cos \epsilon_{10} \qquad\qquad 6.17$$

(or, where volume flow is used, the R^2 is replaced by πR^4).

The electrical complex impedance analogous to flow in a rigid pipe is written

$$Z = R + i\omega L \qquad\qquad 6.18$$

where R is resistance and L is the inductance, and hence the real part of eqn. 6.17 may be called the fluid resistance and the imaginary part the inductive term or reactance. Thus

$$\text{Fluid resistance} = \frac{\mu\alpha^2}{R^2 . M'_{10}} . \sin \epsilon_{10} \qquad\qquad 6.19$$

and

$$\text{Fluid reactance} = \frac{\mu\alpha^2}{R^2 . M'_{10}} . \cos \epsilon_{10} \qquad\qquad 6.20$$

Expanding the term α^2 ($= R^2 . \omega\rho/\mu$) we can also write

$$\text{Resistance} = \frac{\omega\rho}{M'_{10}} . \sin \epsilon_{10} \qquad\qquad 6.21$$

and

$$\text{Reactance} = \frac{\omega\rho}{M'_{10}} . \cos \epsilon_{10} \qquad\qquad 6\cdot22$$

so that

$$\text{Inductance} = \frac{\rho}{M'_{10}} . \cos \epsilon_{10} \qquad\qquad 6.23$$

F

Normalized values for the inductance and the resistance with changing α are shown in Fig. 6.13. It can be seen that the inductance falls slowly with

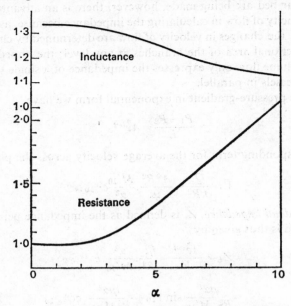

Fig. 6.13. Fluid inductance (eqn. 6.23) and resistance for oscillatory flow in a rigid pipe plotted as a function of α. The values for resistance are given relative to the steady-flow, or Poiseuille, resistance and are 1/8 times that given by eqn. 6.19. As α is a function of the square root of the frequency it can be seen that both these components of the fluid impedance are frequency-dependent in contrast to the analogous electrical quantities. The application of the fluid resistance in oscillatory flow to the manometer equations is discussed in Ch. 8.

increasing α and tends, in the limit, to $1 \cdot 0$. The limiting value of the reactance is, therefore, ω. The fluid resistance, on the other hand, remains close to the Poiseuille resistance up to $\alpha = 3$ and then rises steadily with α (i.e. with $\omega^{1/2}$); with $\alpha > 4$ the relationship is almost exactly linear. Fry, Griggs, and Greenfield (1964) found that, in the proximal aorta, they could substitute a weighted mean value of $1 \cdot 1$ for the inductance and $1 \cdot 6 \times$ the Poiseuille resistance for the resistance term over the frequency range represented in the pressure-gradient. These are approximately the values at $\alpha = 7$.

When considering a conducting system along which the wave of oscillatory flow is propagated we define the *characteristic impedance*, Z_0, and the velocity of propagation, c, so that

$$Z_0 = Z \cdot c/i\omega \qquad\qquad 6.24$$

so that from eqn. 6.16, after expanding α^2, we obtain

$$Z_0 = \frac{\rho c}{M'_{10}} \cdot e^{-i\varepsilon}{}_{10} \qquad\qquad 6.25$$

Applying the relation between the complex wave velocity c (see Ch. 11) and the real part of the velocity, in a longitudinally restrained elastic tube, derived by Womersley (1957a, b) we have

$$Z_0 = \frac{\rho c_0}{\sqrt{(1-\sigma^2)}} \cdot \frac{1}{(M'_{10})^{\frac{1}{2}}} e^{-i\epsilon_{10}/2} \qquad 6.26$$

where c_0 is the velocity derived from the Moens–Korteweg equation (10.56) for an elastic tube filled with an inviscid liquid.

The characteristic impedance is defined as the ratio of oscillatory pressure to flow at the input of a pipe in which no reflected waves return to the origin, i.e. that the tube ends in a matched impedance, or is so long that any reflected waves arising from the termination are completely attenuated before they reach the origin.

The term *input impedance* is used to express the ratio of oscillatory pressure to flow at the input to any region of the circulation and is modified by reflection. The frequency dependence of the input impedance due to the interaction with reflected waves is discussed in Ch. 12 and the experimental work on the subject is reviewed in Ch. 13. The input impedance in rubber tubes was analysed by Hardung (1958) and the components of the characteristic impedance investigated in detail by Taylor (1959b). An excellent review of the topic in visco-elastic tubes by Hardung (1962) goes into greater detail than is considered in this work. When the measured phase-velocity is used to derive a value for the pressure-gradient from the time-derivative of the pressure (eqn. 6.7) then the modulus of the impedance can be expressed in terms of the wave-velocity. This relation is explored in Ch. 14 (p. 398) (and its application to measuring cardiac output in Ch. 15) and provides a valuable cross-check on the accuracy of the measurements made. The concept of impedance has proved a fertile extension of the concept of peripheral resistance (Ch. 2) which is widely used in physiology; indeed it can be seen that the resistance is the impedance at zero frequency.

7

The Numerical Analysis of Circulatory Wave-forms

In Chs. 5 and 6, the problems of pulsatile flow have all been dealt with in the case of an oscillation in simple harmonic motion, i.e. of sinusoidal form. The conversion of repeating, or periodic, wave records, such as pressure and flow pulsations, to numerical form is done by Fourier, or harmonic, analysis. Although this type of analysis was little used in physiology until introduced by Womersley (1955b) and McDonald (1955) it had been used theoretically by Frank (1927) in addition to the emphasis on transient phenomena in the *Windkessel* analysis. As this type of analysis is unfamiliar to many physiologists a general account of the nature and application of the Fourier series is given here, without any attempt at mathematical rigour, especially in relation to the type of curves that we are concerned with, which cannot be defined as a function of an algebraic variable on which the processes of integration can be performed but have to be dealt with as a finite sum of measured values.

A periodic function is defined as one which repeats itself after a time, T, the period. This may be expressed thus: if

$$y = F(t) \quad \text{then} \quad F(t+T) = F(t)$$

This is familiar in the definition of a sinusoidal wave which repeats after 2π radians so that

$$\sin x = \sin (x + n2\pi)$$

as the frequency f is $1/T$ then the angular frequency, in radians/sec, ω, is given by

$$\omega = \frac{2\pi}{T} \text{ or } T = \frac{2\pi}{\omega} \qquad \textbf{7.1}$$

The Fourier theorem may be stated: if $y = F(t)$ is any continuous function of the variable, t, which repeats with a period, T, then

$$F(t) = A_0 + A_1 \cos \frac{2\pi t}{T} + A_2 \cos \frac{4\pi t}{T} + \ldots + A_n \cos \frac{2n\pi t}{T} +$$

146

$$B_1 \sin \frac{2\pi t}{T} + B_2 \sin \frac{4\pi t}{T} + \ldots + B_n \sin \frac{2n\pi t}{T} \qquad \textbf{7.2}$$

or, as $\omega = 2\pi/T$,

$$F(t) = A_0 + A_1 \cos \omega t + A_2 \cos 2\omega t + A_3 \cos 3\omega t + \ldots + A_n \cos n\omega t$$

$$+ B_1 \sin \omega t + B_2 \sin 2\omega t + B_3 \sin 3\omega t + \ldots + B_n \sin n\omega t \qquad \textbf{7.3}$$

where n has an integral value.

The successive values of A and B are called the Fourier coefficients.

To evaluate the coefficients both sides of eqn. 7.3 are first multiplied by dt and integrated between the limits 0 and 2π. Thus,

$$\int_0^{2\pi} F(t)dt = A_0 \int_0^{2\pi} dt + A_1 \int_0^{2\pi} \cos \omega t . dt + \ldots + A_n \int_0^{2\pi} \cos n\omega t . dt$$

$$+ B_1 \int_0^{2\pi} \sin \omega t . dt + \ldots + B_n \int_0^{2\pi} \sin n\omega t . dt \qquad \textbf{7.4}$$

and every term except the first disappears, giving

$$\int_0^{2\pi} F(t)dt = 2\pi A_0 \quad \text{or} \quad A_0 = \frac{1}{2\pi} \int_0^{2\pi} F(t)dt$$

To evaluate A_n both sides of eqn. 7.3 are multiplied by $\cos n\omega t . dt$ and integrated so that we obtain

$$\int_0^{2\pi} F(t).\cos n\omega t . dt = A_0 \int_0^{2\pi} \cos n\omega t . dt + A_1 \int_0^{2\pi} \cos \omega t . \cos n\omega t . dt + \ldots +$$

$$A_n \int_0^{2\pi} \cos^2 n\omega t . dt + B_1 \int_0^{2\pi} \sin \omega t . \cos n\omega t . dt + \ldots +$$

$$B_n \int_0^{2\pi} \sin n\omega t . \cos n\omega t . dt$$

and the only term on the right-hand side (RHS) that is not zero is

$$A_n \int_0^{2\pi} \cos^2 n\omega t . dt = \frac{1}{2} A_n \int_0^{2\pi} (1 + \cos 2n\omega t)dt = \pi . A_n$$

so that

$$A_n = \frac{1}{\pi} \int_0^{2\pi} F(t) \cos n\omega t . dt$$

and, similarly,

$$B_n = \frac{1}{\pi} \int_0^{2\pi} F(t) \sin n\omega t . dt.$$

We can also see that A_0 is the mean value of the function over the period, T, or from 0 to 2π.

This is the mathematical method for determining the Fourier series of an algebraic function. As an example, let us take the saw-tooth function (Fig. 7.1) which repeats with a period of 2π and has the form

$$y = x, \ (0 < x < 2\pi)$$

Thus,

$$A_0 = \frac{1}{2\pi} \int_0^{2\pi} \tau \,.\, d\tau = \pi$$

and,

$$A_n = \frac{1}{\pi} \int_0^{2\pi} x \,.\, \cos nx \,.\, dx = \frac{1}{n\pi} \int_0^{2\pi} x \,.\, d \,(\sin x)$$

Integrating by parts

$$A_n = \frac{1}{n\pi} \left[(x \sin nx) \Big|_0^{2\pi} - \int_0^{2\pi} \sin nx \,.\, dx \right]$$

and both these terms disappear so that there are no cosine terms in the expansion. Analogously, we write

$$B_n = \frac{1}{\pi} \int_0^{2\pi} x \,.\, \sin nx \,.\, dx = -\frac{1}{n\pi} \left[(x \,.\, \cos nx) \Big|_0^{2\pi} - \int_0^{2\pi} \cos nx \,.\, dx \right] = \frac{-2}{n} \cos 2n\pi$$

and so we have

$$y = x = \pi - 2 \left(\sin x + \frac{1}{2} \sin 2x + \frac{1}{3} \sin 3x + \ldots + \frac{1}{n} \sin nx \right) \qquad \textbf{7.5}$$

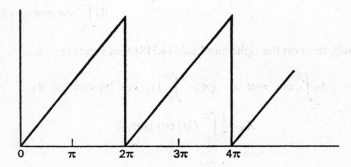

Fig. 7.1. A simple repetitive 'saw-tooth' function where $y=x$ between 0 and 2π. There is a sharp discontinuity at the end of each cycle when y has the value of both 0 and 2π.

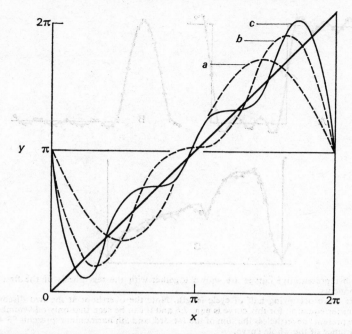

Fig. 7.2. The partial Fourier resynthesis of the function shown in Fig. 7.1. The Fourier series of this function is given as eqn. 7.5. Curve (a) represents the mean plus the first harmonic, i.e. $\pi - 2 \sin x$; (b) with the second harmonic added, i.e. $\pi - 2 \sin x + \sin 2x$; (c) with the third harmonic added, i.e. $\pi - 2 \sin x + \sin 2x + 2/3 \sin 3x$. The series in this case (and for Fig. 7.3A) converges slowly.

The progressive summation of the first three terms is shown in Fig. 7.2 which demonstrates how a straight line may be approximated by a small number of terms of a Fourier series.

In a similar way, a square wave which, for example, has a value of 1 in the interval 0 to π and of zero in the interval π to 2π will be analysed as the sum of the respective intervals. This expansion gives

$$y = \frac{1}{2} + \frac{2}{\pi}\left[\sin x + \frac{1}{3}\sin 3x + \frac{1}{5}\sin 5x + \ldots\right] \qquad 7.6$$

and the resynthesis of these terms is shown in Fig. 7.3A. In both this case, and that illustrated in Fig. 7.2, it will be observed that there are discontinuities in the function. Thus, the square wave has both the values of zero and one when $x = 0$ and $x = \pi$. The Fourier resynthesis will then always have a value that is a mean of these two values at these points; this is a general property of the series. The rule concerning discontinuities is generalized as the 'Dirichlet condition' which states that 'a function with a finite number of finite discontinuities may be represented by a Fourier series'. The illustration in

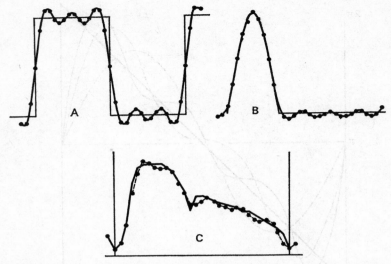

Fig. 7.3. These representative curves are shown together with the resynthesis of the first five Fourier components.

A. A square wave occupying half of cycle length. Note the overshoot at the two discontinuities. The Fourier equation for this curve is eqn. 7.6 and it can be seen that only odd-numbered harmonics are present; nevertheless the sum of the 1st, 3rd, and 5th harmonics represents 93·4 per cent of the variance of the whole curve.

B. A half-rectified sine-wave, one-third of the duration of the cycle. The fit of the resynthesized curve is much better than in A; the 5 harmonics here represent 98·7 per cent of the variance of the curve.

C. A central aortic pulse; the resynthesis with 5 harmonics here should be compared with the resynthesis with 10 harmonics in Fig. 7.7. Here 97·6 per cent of the variance is represented (see Fig. 7.8 which shows typical values of the variance with varying numbers of harmonics). (Thirty ordinates per cycle were used in each case.)

Fig. 7.3A also shows that at the jump of the discontinuity the graph of the series overshoots at both extremes; this is known as the Gibbs phenomenon.

For further pursuit of the properties of the Fourier series, mathematical and physical texts should be consulted, such as Newman and Searle (1957), Franklin (1958) or Pipes (1958).

The analysis of a curve which cannot be described by an algebraic function is performed by drawing a number, $2r$, of equally-spaced ordinates that will each have the value y_r. Then we may write,

$$A_0 = \frac{1}{2r} \sum_{r=0}^{(2r-1)} y_r$$

and

$$A_n = \frac{1}{r} \sum_{r=0}^{(2r-1)} y_r \cos \frac{n\pi}{r}$$

7.7

$$B_n = \frac{1}{r} \sum_{r=0}^{(2r-1)} y_r . \sin \frac{n\pi}{r}$$

Thus, if we take $r = 12$, then each interval is $\pi/12$ or $15°$ and for the value of A_1 we take the sum $1/12 \, (y_0 \cos 0° + y_1 \cos 15° + y_2 \cos 30° + \ldots + y_{23} \cos 345°)$ and for A_2 the sum $1/12 \, (y_0 \cos 0° + y_1 \cos 30° + y_2 \cos 60° + \ldots + y_{23} \cos 330°)$ and so on.

It will be recalled that a function of the form of a sine or cosine constitutes a Simple Harmonic Motion (SHM) which is also defined as the function of the movement, with respect to time, of the foot of a perpendicular drawn from the radius vector of a circle, on to the x-axis, as the vector rotates counterclockwise around the circle. Each pair of terms $A_n \cos n\omega t$ and $B_n \sin n\omega t$ in eqn. 7.3 may thus be represented graphically in Fig. 7.4A as two such rotations represented simultaneously. The sum of these two functions represents the SHM of a single vector of length M starting its rotation at an angle φ below the x-axis (Fig. 7.4B). From Pythagoras' theorem we can see that

$$M = \sqrt{(A^2 + B^2)}$$

and $\qquad \tan \varphi = B/A \text{ or } \varphi = \tan^{-1} B/A.$ $\qquad$ **7.8**

Thus, we may write

$$A \cos \omega t + B \sin \omega t = M \cos (\omega t - \varphi) \qquad \textbf{7.9}$$

where M is called the modulus, or amplitude, of the oscillation and φ its phase, or argument.

From Fig. 7.4 we also see that

$$A = M \cos \varphi \text{ and } B = M \sin \varphi \qquad \textbf{7.10}$$

To demonstrate the equivalence we expand the RHS of eqn. 7.9

$$M \cos (\omega t - \varphi) = M \cos \varphi \cos \omega t + M \sin \varphi \sin \omega t = A \cos \omega t + B \sin \omega t \qquad \textbf{7.11}$$

which is the simplest proof that the angle φ in this equivalence must be written as $-\varphi$. If, as is often done, eqn. 7.9 is written as $\cos (\omega t + \varphi)$ then $\tan \varphi = -B/A$.

In Chs. 5 and 6 the harmonic motion is often written in complex numbers. By use of the operator, $i = \sqrt{-1}$ the point, P, can be defined as $(A - iB)$. Here A is a length measured along the x, or real, axis and is the *real* part of the number; B is measured along the y, or imaginary, axis and is called the *imaginary* part of the number. The manipulation of complex numbers is described in mathematical texts (e.g. Franklin, 1958; Pipes, 1958) and may be summarized by saying that this is identical to that of more familiar algebraic symbols but the real and imaginary parts must always be kept separate. All complex numbers have, as it were, a 'mirror image' in the x-axis and this is

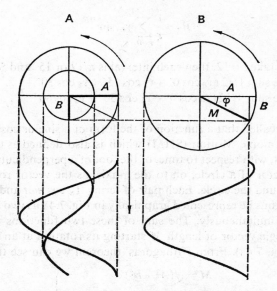

Fig. 7.4. Diagrammatic representation of a simple harmonic motion in terms of its Fourier coefficients.

A. A pair of Fourier terms $A \cos \omega t + B \sin \omega t$; for convenience the sine term is drawn as if it were a cosine projection 90° behind the true cosine component. Thus at $\omega t = 0°$, $\cos \omega t = A$ and $\sin \omega t = 0$; when $\omega t = 90°$ the two vectors A and B have rotated anticlockwise through that angle and $\cos \omega t = 0$ and $\sin \omega t = B$; with $\omega t = 180°$, the cosine is $-A$ and the sine zero. The waves traced out by the points moving around the circles are shown below—the direction of the vertical arrow indicates the values of the two terms as the points move around the circles (curved arrow). The sum of these two curves is shown in the oscillation in the lower part of (B).

B. The circular diagram shows how the resultant single oscillation described in A can be described as a single wave; its initial point is at $-\varphi$ and the amplitude is M. It is thus the curve of $M \cos (\omega t - \varphi)$. It can be seen that $M = \sqrt{(A^2 + B^2)}$ and that $\tan \varphi = B/A$ (eqn. 7.8).

called the complex conjugate, e.g. the complex conjugate of $(A - iB)$ is $(A + iB)$. The algebraic manipulation of complex numbers needs to bear in mind the properties of i; i.e. $i^2 = -1$, $i^3 = -i$, and $i^4 = +1$, etc., thus the product of $(A - iB)$ with its complex conjugate $(A + iB) = A^2 + B^2$, a real number. This equivalence is used when dividing by a complex number; both numerator and denominator are multiplied by the conjugate of the latter so that the denominator becomes real.

The use of i in exponents may be explained by referring to the series expansion of e^x.

$$e^x = 1 + x + \frac{x^2}{2!} + \frac{x^3}{3!} + \frac{x^4}{4!} + \dots \qquad 7.12$$

so that

$$e^{ix} = 1 + ix - \frac{x^2}{2!} - \frac{ix^3}{3!} + \frac{x^4}{4!} + \dots \qquad 7.13$$

and
$$e^{-ix} = 1 - ix - \frac{x^2}{2!} + \frac{ix^3}{3!} + \frac{x^4}{4!} - \ldots$$
                                                      7.14

so that
$$e^{ix} + e^{-ix} = 2\left(1 - \frac{x^2}{2!} + \frac{x^4}{4!} - \ldots\right) = 2\cos x$$
                                                      7.15

and
$$e^{ix} - e^{-ix} = 2i\left(x - \frac{x^3}{3!} + \frac{x^5}{5!} - \ldots\right) = 2i\sin x$$
                                                      7.16

Hence,
$$\cos x = \frac{e^{ix} + e^{-ix}}{2} \quad \text{and} \quad \sin x = \frac{e^{ix} - e^{-ix}}{2i}$$
                                                      7.17

Thus
$$e^{ix} = \cos x + i\sin x$$
                                                      7.18

and a Fourier term such as in eqn. 7.9 may be written as the real part of

$$Me^{i(\omega t - \phi)}, \text{ i.e. } A\cos \omega t + B\sin \omega t$$
                                                      7.19

while its complex number equivalent will be $A - iB$.

This relationship leads to a condensed way of writing a Fourier series in exponential form. The eqn. 7.3 above is the equivalent of

$$F(t) = \frac{A_0}{2} + \sum_{n=1}^{n=\infty} (A_n \cos n\omega t + B_n \sin n\omega t)$$
                                                      7.20

where ω is the angular frequency of the pulse frequency (the fundamental). From eqns. 7.17 and 7.18 we may rewrite eqn. 7.20 as

$$F(t) = \frac{A_0}{2} + \frac{1}{2} \cdot \sum_{n=1}^{n=\infty} (A_n - iB_n)e^{in\omega t} + \frac{1}{2}\sum_{n=1}^{n=\infty} (A_n + iB_n)e^{-in\omega t}$$
                                                      7.21

This can be simplified by introducing negative values of n; since $\cos(-\theta) = \cos\theta$ and $\sin(-\theta) = -\sin\theta$ then also $A_{-n} = -A_n$ and $B_{-n} = -B_n$. The last term of eqn. 7.21 can then be changed, thus

$$\frac{1}{2}\sum_{n=1}^{n=\infty} (A_n + iB_n)e^{-in\omega t} + \frac{1}{2}\sum_{n=-1}^{n=-\infty} (A_n - iB_n)e^{in\omega t}$$
                                                      7.22

and eqn. 7.21 simplifies to

$$F(t) = \sum_{n=-\infty}^{n=+\infty} F(n)e^{in\omega t}$$
                                                      7.23

where $$F(n) = \frac{1}{2}(A_n - iB_n)$$ **7.24**

for $n = 0, \pm 1, \pm 2, \pm 3$, etc.

By a similar process, writing the function in terms of the period T (eqn. 7.2) we find that

$$F(n) = \frac{1}{T}\int_{-T/2}^{+T/2} F(t)e^{-in\omega t}.dt$$ **7.25**

Equations 7.23 and 7.25 are defined as the Fourier transforms of each other. In amplitude and phase form

$$F(n) = \sqrt{(A_n^2 + B_n^2)}.\exp\left[i\tan^{-1}\left(\frac{-B}{A}\right)\right]$$ **7.26**

Travelling waves. The exponential form is also a useful way of compactly designating a travelling wave. Thus, an undamped wave travelling at velocity c in the direction of the z-axis (conventionally denoting the axis of a tube) then at any distance z_1 from the origin it is defined (for $n = 1$) as

$$Me^{i\omega(t-z_1/c)}$$

and later at z_2 as $Me^{i\omega(t-z_2/c)}$ or, in terms of eqn. 7.19, as $Me^{i(\omega t - \phi_1)}$ and $Me^{i(\omega t - \phi_2)}$. The interval $(\varphi_2 - \varphi_1)$ is called the phase shift so that

$$(\varphi_2 - \varphi_1) = \frac{\omega}{c}(z_2 - z_1)$$

or

$$c = \frac{\omega(z_2 - z_1)}{(\varphi_2 - \varphi_1)} = w\frac{\Delta z}{\Delta\varphi}$$ **7.27**

The velocity c is termed the phase velocity.

PROCEDURES FOR CALCULATING A FLOW CURVE

In Fig. 7.5 there is illustrated a femoral artery pressure pulse and the pressure difference measured over a distance of 5 cm.

The values of the harmonic components are given in Table 7.1.

TABLE 7.1. Fourier analysis of the pressure-gradient (mm Hg/cm)

Harmonic	A (cosine)	B (sine)	Modulus (M)	φ
1	+1·024	+0·240	1·052	13·2°
2	−0·126	+1·346	1·352	95·23°
3	−0·819	+0·477	0·948	149·79°
4	−0·305	+0·002	0·305	179·62°
5	−0·260	−0·144	0·380	209·33°

Mean value = +0·335 mm Hg/cm

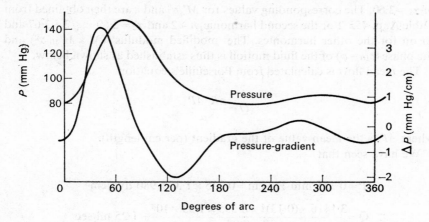

Fig. 7.5. Simultaneous recordings of a femoral artery pressure pulse and the pressure-gradient measured between two points 5 cm apart. The gradient curve is subjected to a Fourier analysis and the corresponding flow terms calculated in the text (pp. 154–56).

Note that the angle determined by eqn. 7.8 must be placed in the correct quadrant according to signs of the cosine and sine terms, i.e. from 0° to 90° both are positive, from 90° to 180° the cosine is negative and the sine is positive, etc. When there is a marked peak to the curve as in this case, it will be found that there is a progressive increase in the angle φ with increase of harmonic order; this is because the 'peak' is the sum of maxima of the components. In terms of the whole cycle, i.e. of the fundamental, the peak occurs at about 45°, which will be equivalent to 90° of the cycle of the 2nd harmonic, 135° in the 3rd harmonic, etc. This progression of the phase angle is a useful practical guide to detecting errors that may have occurred in computation.

CALCULATION OF FLOW COMPONENTS

Method 1

There are alternative methods of calculating the flow according to which form of the equation is used. The simplest one would appear to be that using eqn. 6.6.

$$Q = \frac{\pi R^4}{\mu} . M . \frac{M'_{10}}{\alpha^2} \sin (\omega t - \varphi + \varepsilon_{10})$$

First, the values of α for each harmonic have to be calculated. In the present example $R = 0.13$ cm, the pulse-frequency, $f = 2.4$ Hz, we take $\mu = 0.04$ Poise and $\rho = 1.055$ g/ml.

As $a = R_n \sqrt{(2\pi n f \rho / \mu)}$, then, for the first harmonic (i.e. $n = 1$) this gives a value of $\alpha_1 = 2\cdot60$. The corresponding values for M'/α^2 and ε are then obtained from Table A, p. 452. For the second harmonic, $n = 2$ and $\alpha_2 = 2\cdot60 \times \sqrt{2} = 3\cdot67$ and so on for the other harmonics. The 'modified modulus' $(M \times M'_{10}/\alpha^2)$ and the phase $(\varepsilon_{10} - \varphi)$ of the fluid motion is thus established as shown below.

The mean flow is calculated from Poiseuille's equation

$$Q = \frac{\pi R^4 \Delta P}{8\mu}$$

where ΔP is the mean value of the gradient (per cm length).

We have seen that

$$\Delta P = 0\cdot335 \text{ mm Hg/cm} = 0\cdot335 \times 1\cdot36 \times 980 \text{ dyn/cm}^3$$

$$\therefore \quad Q = \frac{3\cdot1416 \times (0\cdot13)^4 \times 0\cdot335 \times 1\cdot33 \times 10^3}{8 \times 0\cdot04} = 1\cdot25 \text{ ml/sec}$$

TABLE 7.2

Harmonic	α	M'/α^2	ε°	$M \times M'/\alpha^2$	$(\varepsilon - \varphi)^\circ$
1	2·60	0·0819	42·86	0·0862	+29·66
2	3·67	0·0508	27·31	0·0687	−67·92
3	4·49	0·0363	21·17	0·0344	−128·62
4	5·20	0·0282	17·83	0·0086	−151·79
5	6·80	0·0233	15·76	0·0089	+166·43

The factor $\pi R^4/\mu$ is common to all terms and is calculated separately (with the conversion of mm Hg into dyn/cm^2, i.e. $1\cdot36 \times 980$); here its value is $29\cdot83$ so that the total flow (including the mean flow) is given by the equation

$$Q = 1\cdot25 + 2\cdot57 \sin (x + 29\cdot66^\circ) + 2\cdot05 \sin (2x - 67\cdot92^\circ) +$$
$$1\cdot03 \sin (3x - 128\cdot62^\circ) + 0\cdot23 \sin (4x - 151\cdot79^\circ) +$$
$$0\cdot27 \sin (5x + 166\cdot43^\circ)$$

where x (or ωt) is, as before, successively 0°, 12°, 24°, etc. Care has to be taken with regard to the sign of the sine. As the sine is positive from 0° to 180° and thereafter negative, angles between 180° and 360° have been written as negative angles.

This method has the great disadvantage that the sines of every individual term of each harmonic has to be looked up in tables of trigonometrical functions.

Method 2
When it is recalled that, in the harmonic terms of the pressure-gradient,

$$A = M \cos \varphi \text{ and } B = M \sin \varphi \text{ (reference Fig. 7.4)}$$

we can expand eqn. 6.6 into this form, where Q_n is the oscillatory flow of the nth harmonic

$$Q_n = \frac{\pi R^4}{\mu} \cdot \frac{M'_{10n}}{\alpha_n{}^2} (A_n \sin \varepsilon_n - B_n \cos \varepsilon_n) \cos nx +$$

$$\frac{\pi R^4}{\mu} \frac{M'_{10n}}{\alpha_n{}^2} (A_n \cos \varepsilon_n + B_n \sin \varepsilon_n) \sin nx \quad \textbf{7.28}$$

This only necessitates looking up the sine and cosine of each value of ε and so, provided a desk calculator is available to do the greatest number of multi-plications, is much less tedious than the previous method. Not only does it minimize reference to standard tables but it obviates the need to calculate the modulus and phase of the pressure component.

When $\alpha > 10$ the tables do not apply but simple asymptotic expansions are available to compute M' and ε. Thus

$$M'_{10} = 1 - \frac{\sqrt{2}}{\alpha} + \frac{1}{\alpha^2} \qquad \textbf{7.29}$$

and

$$\varepsilon \text{ (radians)} = \frac{\sqrt{2}}{\alpha} + \frac{1}{\alpha^2} + \frac{19}{24(\sqrt{2})\alpha^3} \qquad \textbf{7.30}$$

These values are plotted graphically for $10 < \alpha < 20$ in Fig. 7.6. When $\alpha > 20$ eqns. 7.29 and 7.30 may be used (e.g. for vessels the size of the aorta). Even then, when $\alpha = 20$, M'_{10} is less than 7 per cent from its limiting value of $1 \cdot 0$ and ε is only $4 \cdot 2°$, so that relatively little error will be introduced by taking $M'_{10} = 1 \cdot 0$ and $\varepsilon_{10} = 0°$ (cf. Fig. 6.10), but with a computer this calculation is normally done routinely.

Method 3

A further method of calculation is that using the form of the equation for flow given by eqn. 6.2. This may be written as

$$Q = \frac{\pi R^4}{i\mu} \cdot \frac{M}{\alpha^2} [1 - F_{10}]e^{i\omega t} \qquad \textbf{7.31}$$

and expanding α^2 this becomes

$$Q = \frac{\pi R^2 \cdot M}{i\omega\rho} [1 - F_{10}]e^{i\omega t} \qquad \textbf{7.32}$$

where the pressure-gradient is the real part of $Me^{i(\omega t - \phi)}$, that is

$$Re[Me^{i(\omega t - \phi)}] = A \cos \omega t + B \sin \omega t$$

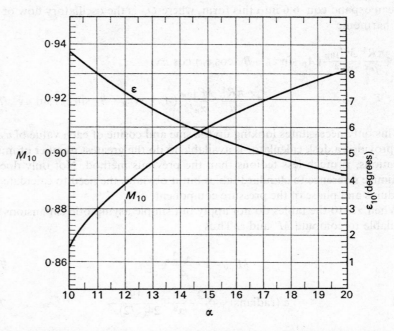

Fig. 7.6. M'_{10} and ε_{10} for values of α from 10 to 20 to supplement Table A. More accurate estimates may be derived from the asymptotic expansions given in eqns. 7.29 and 7.30. Note that it is M'_{10} which is being plotted rather than M'_{10}/α^2 as the latter becomes very small and changes slowly over this range.

Once again A and B are the Fourier coefficients and the gradient may be written as the complex number $(A - iB)$.

The value of $(1 - F_{10})$ in real and imaginary parts is given in Table B, p. 453, as a function of α and may be written $(C + iD)$.

Therefore to compute eqn. 7.32, we write

$$Q = \frac{\pi R^2}{i\omega\rho} \cdot (A - iB)(C + iD)e^{i\omega t} \qquad \textbf{7.33}$$

As dividing by i is equivalent to multiplying by $-i$ we get

$$Q = \frac{\pi R^2}{\omega\rho}(-B - iA)(C + iD)e^{i\omega t} \qquad \textbf{7.34}$$

and following the normal rules of multiplying complex numbers we obtain

$$Q = \frac{\pi R^2}{\omega\rho}[(AD - BC) - i(AC + BD)]e^{i\omega t} \qquad \textbf{7.35}$$

of which the real part is to be taken, as we are using the real part of the pressure-gradient. Therefore, for each harmonic the oscillatory flow is

$$Q = \frac{\pi R^2}{\omega \rho} (AD - BC) \cos \omega t + (AC + BD) \sin \omega t \qquad \textbf{7.36}$$

In the example worked above these terms have been tabulated below (the values for A and B are set out on p. 154).

TABLE 7.3

Harmonic	α	$(1 - F_{10})$ C (Real)	$(1 - F_{10})$ D (Imag.)	Flow terms $(AD - BC)$	Flow terms $(AC + BD)$
1	2·60	0·4061	0·3738	+0·2884	+0·5063
2	3·67	0·6075	0·3137	−0·8572	+0·3457
3	4·49	0·6835	0·2647	−0·5428	−0·4335
4	5·20	0·7269	0·2337	−0·0727	−0·2212
5	6·80	0·7436	0·2195	−0·2256	+0·0504

Thus, the flow is calculated, as in other methods, by substituting the appropriate value of $(AD - BC)$ and multiplying, successively, by the cosine of the interval used and of $(AC + BD)$ multiplied by the corresponding sine of the interval for each harmonic. The mean flow is also added.

This last method appears more elaborate than the previous ones but is in practice faster because the values of the cosine and sine of the 30 intervals once tabulated for the initial analysis are used throughout. The only additional reference to a table required (which is always the most time-consuming procedure in a computation of this sort) is to read off the value of $(1 - F_{10})$. The similarity of eqn. 7.36 to eqn. 7.28 will be seen to be dependent on the fact that the Real part of $(1 - F_{10})$ is $M'_{10} \cos \varepsilon_{10}$ and the Imaginary part is $M'_{10} \sin \varepsilon_{10}$.

The steps of the procedure have been written out in full but relatively simple apparatus can be made to carry out much of the work. The model developed by Taylor (1958a)—an improved version of that described by Rymer and Butler (1944)—will perform both Fourier analysis and synthesis. All that is required is the setting of the values of the co-ordinates read from the curve. With adequate computer support that can operate in complex arithmetic the procedure is simple.

For some purposes the resynthesis of the flow curve is unnecessary, for example, in the calculation of the input impedance. In this case it is necessary to divide the pressure components for each harmonic by the corresponding flow terms. If the calculation is in modulus and phase form then the modulus of the impedance is given by

$$|Z_0| = M(\text{Press.})/M(\text{Flow})$$

and the phase by the difference

$$Ph(Z_0) = \varphi(\text{Press.}) - \varphi(\text{Flow})$$

If the calculation is kept in real and imaginary parts it is necessary to follow the procedure of dividing complex numbers. If the arterial pressure has each harmonic term, $P = (A' - iB')e^{i\omega t}$ and for the flow velocity (following the usage of Ch. 6 in calculating impedance from the average velocity) we set $\overline{V} = (E - iF)e^{i\omega t}$; E and F are $(AD - BC)$ and $(AC + BD)$ in the table above when flow has been calculated from the pressure-gradient.

$$\therefore Z_0 = P/\overline{V} = \frac{A' - iB'}{E - iF} \quad \text{or} \quad Z_0 = \frac{P}{Q} = \frac{A' - iB'}{\pi R^2(E - iF)}$$

($1/\omega\rho$ appears when eqn. 7.33 is converted to $\overline{V}$ from Q, i.e. dividing by πR^2.)

As noted above, to divide by a complex number it is necessary to make the denominator real; in this case, we multiply the top and bottom of the fraction by $E + iF$ so that

$$Z_0 = \omega\rho \frac{(A' - iB')(E + iF)}{(E - iF)(E + iF)} = \omega\rho \left[\frac{(A'E + B'F) + i(A'F - B'E)}{(E^2 + F^2)} \right] \qquad \textbf{7.37}$$

To take an example from Fig. 7.5, the Fourier coefficients of the fundamental component of the pressure curve was computed (A', B') and the results were as follows:

A'	B'	E	F	$(A'E + B'F)$	$(A'F - B'E)$
$+6.65$	$+23.96$	$+0.2884$	$+0.5063$	$+15.486$	-3.144

then multiplying by $\omega\rho/((E^2 + F^2)$

$Z_0 = +610.0 - i123.8$ 　　　Modulus, $|Z_0| = 6.2 \times 10^2$ dyn.sec/cm^3
　　　　　　　　　　　　　　　　Phase $= -11.5°$

This is the method for calculating the arterial input impedance from the arterial pressure and the pressure-gradient used by Bergel *et al.* (1958).

While the above was written for those who wish to perform the analysis with a manually-operated machine, in most laboratories today it will be performed with a digital computer. Nevertheless, the steps in the procedure will be essentially similar to one of those set out. The procedure varies with the capacity of the computer but with a reasonably sized one the sampling rate is set without regard to the length of the cycle; this requires that each value of the cosine and sine terms has to be calculated using the series expansions in eqns. 7.15 and 7.16 (with x as radians). In my laboratory a sampling rate of 100/sec is a common rate using the QRS complex of the ECG to trigger the beginning and end of sampling over one cycle. Working in the aorta where the value of α is greater than 8.0 for the fundamental the series expansions (eqns. 7.29 and 7.30) for M'_{10} and ε_{10} are used. A provision is made in the programme to allow a computer write-out of the resynthesis of each curve analysed, superimposed on the original curve to check the accuracy of the analysis.

REQUIREMENTS AND LIMITATIONS OF A FOURIER ANALYSIS

Number of sample intervals

The number of samples that need to be taken is determined by (a) the frequencies present in the record and (b) the number of harmonics that it is desired to determine. The limiting rule under (b) is simple; if N intervals are taken in one cycle then the number of harmonics that can be determined are $N/2$. All higher harmonics are indeterminate. Thus if twelve points are taken (a manual method given in Franklin, 1958), six harmonics would be valid. When the sampling rate is set per second the same rule applies to the maximum frequencies that are analysable, i.e. 100 samples/sec allows up to 50 Hz to be analysed. The number of harmonics this represents depends on the heart-rate; e.g. if this is 2·0 Hz it is twenty-four harmonics whereas with a rate of 3·0 Hz it is only sixteen harmonics. If there are frequencies present beyond the limit set by the sampling rate (the 'folding' frequency) then they will introduce errors into the components analysed. This phenomenon is known as 'aliasing' and is discussed by Blackman and Tukey (1959) and by Attinger, Anné and McDonald (1966). In general, it may be said that if the folding frequency is F then a frequency of $(F+f)$ will be analysed with the component at a frequency $(F-f)$, i.e. with our folding frequency of 50 Hz the main contamination will be with 60 Hz noise (the commonest intruder) which will distort the computed value for a component at 38 Hz. As we do not, in practice, ever use any frequency term above 30 Hz in our analysis, we regard our sampling rate as sufficiently high. This has been verified by comparing analyses at 200 and 100 samples/sec; the higher frequency will eliminate aliasing at 60 Hz but no significant difference is found. Increasing the number of samples carries a considerable penalty in the time taken for computation of the series, even on a computer, so that a compromise has to be reached. It is preferable to insert a filter in each of the lines to be computed to cut off frequencies above those required for analysis but this requires care in matching the filters on each channel and in ensuring that no phase-distortion occurs in channels that are analysed. Active, rather than passive, filters are to be preferred.

The accuracy of measurement of the ordinates of the samples taken is a limiting factor for the possible accuracy of the analysis. With an Analogue–Digital converter the limit would appear to be set by the number of 'bits' available in the conversion. Thus a 6-bit convertor samples to an accuracy of one part in 2^6 (64), approximately 1·5 per cent of the width of the channel, and accuracy would apparently be increased by changing to 8- or 10-bit conversion. This may be illusory for with FM recording on magnetic tape the accuracy of retrieval is often no better than 1 per cent although some manufacturers claim to be accurate to 0·5 per cent. While this appears to be a trivial error in biological recording, it becomes of significance in measuring the phase angle of the higher harmonics, for, to derive tan φ, the ratio of 2 small numbers is required. Even at 1 Hz a 1 per cent error in 360° is 3·6° so that discrimination of very small phase shifts is impossible, and leads to a considerable standard deviation in the measurement of the phase velocities of those components.

THE SIGNIFICANT HARMONIC TERMS IN THE FLOW AND PULSE WAVES

The variance of a curve

The reproduction of the original wave from a given number of harmonic terms can, by inspection, give a qualitative check on the adequacy of the analysis. Examples of the resynthesis of a flow and a pressure wave with 10 harmonics is shown in Fig. 7.7.

For a more quantitative measure the *variance* of the wave and of the Fourier series is compared. The variance of a curve is familiar as a statistical procedure for it is the square of the standard deviation. Thus, for a curve delineated by m ordinates with a mean value of $\bar{y}$ we have

$$\text{Variance} = \frac{1}{m} \sum_{i=1}^{i=m} (y_i - \bar{y})^2 \qquad 7.38$$

or, more usually, calculated as

$$= \frac{1}{m} \sum_{i=1}^{i=m} y_i^2 - \left(\frac{1}{m} \sum_{i=1}^{i=m} y_i \right)^2 \qquad 7.39$$

The variance of a Fourier series is given from the following equation resulting from Parseval's theorem

$$\text{Variance (series)} = \frac{1}{2} \sum_{n=1}^{n=n} M_n^2 \qquad 7.40$$

i.e. half the sum of the squares of the moduli of the harmonic terms used.* The graphs shown in Fig. 7.8 give the progressive sum of the variance of

* As a corollary to this we note a valuable property of the Fourier series: the representation by n-terms is the best approximation possible for this number of terms, and increasing the number of terms will increase the accuracy without any necessity for recalculating the lower terms. This is in marked contrast to other series such as the exponential series, where adding an extra term requires a recalculation of the whole set.

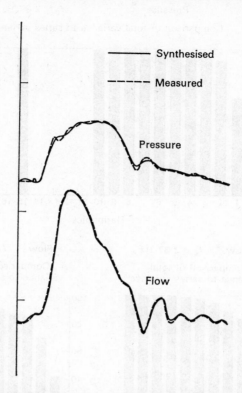

Fig. 7.7. The resynthesis by 10 Fourier harmonic components of a pressure and flow curve in the ascending aorta. The sampling frequency was 100 samples/sec; cycle length 0·48 sec. The fit of the curves is very good even at points of sharp inflection and appreciably better than that shown for 5 harmonics in Fig. 7.3c. A resynthesis of this type is a quick check on a computer to ensure that there are no calculating errors; these examples are taken from one of our routine checks during an experiment.

series representing a typical aortic pressure and flow curve as a percentage of the variance of the original curves. It can be seen that better than 99·5 per cent of the variance is included, a point often reached by the 7th or 8th harmonic. No appreciable improvement is achieved by going to 20 harmonics and the residual loss appears to consist entirely of noise in the recording systems and the low energy content of cardiovascular sounds. It is on such evidence that we state that no significant propagated waves in relation to blood flow exist above 30 Hz and those above 20 Hz are small. The original curves and their resynthesis from ten harmonics is shown in Fig. 7.7 and demonstrates the degree of accuracy that this number of harmonics gives. As the pulse-frequency was only a little over 2 Hz (2·37) in this case this shows that there are only very small components detectable in the arterial system at frequencies above 20 Hz.

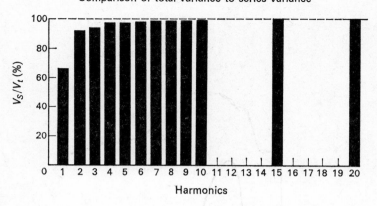

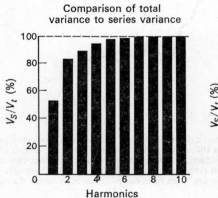

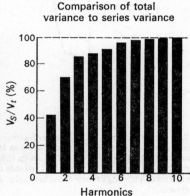

Fig. 7.8A. The columns represent the cumulative variance of the Fourier series (V_s) to the total variance of an aortic pressure curve (V_t). This example was specially taken to 20 harmonics for demonstration purposes.

B. The variance represented by 10 harmonics of the flow curve simultaneously measured in the ascending aorta as the pressure curve analysed in A. Although the first and second harmonics contribute a smaller proportion of the total variance than in the pressure curve, a 99 per cent total is actually achieved in the flow at a lower frequency than in the pressure.

C. The variance of a flow curve at a lower heart rate than in **B.** Ten harmonics are still more than adequate even though the 10th harmonic is only at 12·8 Hz. (From Nichols, 1970.)

THE VALIDITY OF FOURIER ANALYSIS IN THE CIRCULATION

Any series of which all the terms are sine and cosine functions must be periodic. The heart beat is normally periodic but doubts have been raised as to whether the variations in cycle length that do occur make the analysis invalid. Although, mathematically, the phrase can only be used for a function that has repeated itself from minus infinity and will continue for an infinitely long time in the future, in physical analysis it is applied to systems said to be in *steady-state oscillation*. When a train of pulses is first started in a quiescent system the initial excitation will produce changes that will decay exponentially with time due to the damping of the system and which will be superimposed on the periodic excitation. Once the initial excitation has died away and has become undetectably small, the system is said to be in steady-state oscillation. In other words, there is no way of detecting how long the oscillation has been in progress. The length of time required to achieve this is not known exactly but we do know that the viscous damping is high (Ch. 14). From studies of the after-effect of a transient imposed on the arterial system there is strong evidence that, in the dog, the steady-state is a period of about 0·5 sec (Fig. 7.9) or within the duration of one heart-beat.

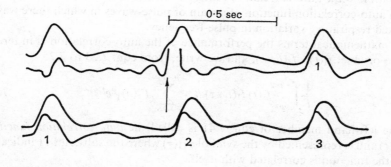

Fig. 7.9. A record of the femoral artery pressure (upper trace) and the pressure-gradient over a 4 cm interval (lower trace) during and after occlusion of the artery. The artery was clamped 3 cm beyond the distal pressure site and released at the point marked by the arrow. The cardiac cycles following the release are shown in the second row (part of cycle 1 is repeated for ease of continuity). Analysis of successive pressure and gradient curves showed no significant variation after one complete cycle following release. Thus, the system was again in steady-state oscillation in little more than 0·5 sec and must be highly damped (see discussion in text).

Therefore, following a sharp discontinuity in periodicity, as with an ectopic heart-beat followed by a pause, a steady-state will have been reached again by the end of the next normal beat. Transient irregularities of the heart-beat are thus of little moment for analysis of later curves.

There are also periodic fluctuations of heart-rate, especially due to the slower respiratory rhythm (sinus arrhythmia). The inaccuracies due to such causes may be checked by analysing a long train of pulses and determining its periodogram or its *power spectrum*.

POWER SPECTRUM

The technique of performing statistical analyses such as this was introduced into circulatory physiology by Randall (1958) and a fuller account is given in standard texts such as Blackman and Tukey (1959) or Lee (1960). The first step in analysing a time-series such as a train of pulse waves is to perform an *auto-correlation*. This is, in essence, a correlation of points in the curve with points occurring later delayed by a variable time-lag, τ. When the delay lag $\tau = 0$ then the correlation of each point is with itself and the correlation is $1 \cdot 0$. If the function is, for example, a sine wave then the correlation will become $1 \cdot 0$ again when the delay $\tau = T$, where T is the period of the sine-wave and the auto-correlation function is itself a sine wave. If the period varies slightly the auto-correlation function will approximate to a sine wave but with $\tau > 0$ the correlation will never be $1 \cdot 0$. When the function is compounded of harmonic components, as is the pulse-wave, then, equally, we get a corresponding oscillation in the auto-correlation function. An example is shown in Fig. 7.10 of an auto-correlation function of a train of pulse-waves in which there was a marked respiratory variation in pulse-frequency.

In mathematical terms the performance of the auto-correlation is in terms of the product $f_1(t) \times f_1(t + \tau)$, and we write, from eqn. 7.23 to 7.25

$$\frac{1}{T} \int_{-T/2}^{+T/2} f_1(t) f_1(t + \tau) dt = \sum_{n=-\infty}^{n=+\infty} |F_1(n)|^2 e^{in\omega\tau} \qquad \textbf{7.41}$$

The left-hand member of eqn. 7.41 is called the *auto-correlation function* of $f_1(t)$ and is represented by the symbol $\varphi_{11}(\tau)$ where the subscript 11 indicates that the function is correlated with itself.

The power spectrum is represented by the symbol $\Phi_{11}(n)$ so that

$$\Phi_{11}(n) = F_1(n)^2 \qquad \textbf{7.42}$$

In terms of these symbols

$$\varphi_{11}(\tau) = \sum_{n=-\infty}^{n=+\infty} \Phi_{11}(n) e^{in\omega\tau} \qquad \textbf{7.43}$$

and, inversely,

$$\varphi_{11}(n) = \frac{1}{T} \int_{-T/2}^{+T/2} \Phi_{11}(\tau) e^{-in\omega\tau} d\tau \qquad \textbf{7.44}$$

From eqns. 7.43 and 7.44 we can say that the auto-correlation function and the power spectrum are Fourier transforms of each other.

The power spectrum of the auto-correlation function shown in Fig. 7.10A is illustrated in Fig. 7.10B. It can be seen that there is a peak at a little over

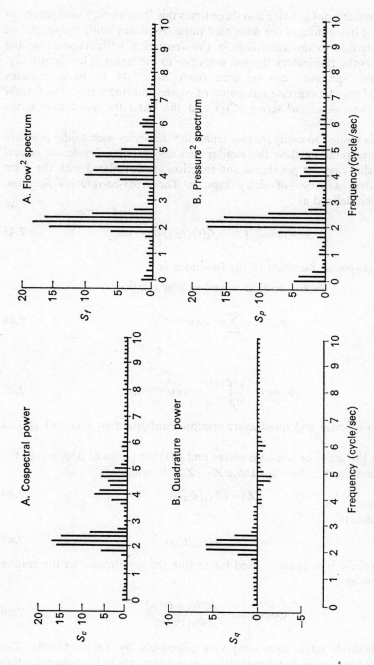

Fig. 7.10. Left: Each ordinate of these curves represents the amount of pulsatile power in a frequency band of 0·167 Hz. Units are in mm Hg × ml/min. A. Spectral distribution of pulsatile power from pressure and flow components in phase with one another. B. Spectral distribution of pulsatile power resulting from pressure and flow components 90° out of phase with one another.

Right: Each ordinate represents the amount of activity in a frequency band of 0·167 Hz. A. Spectral distribution of statistical variance of flow about its mean. Units—(ml/min)²; B. Spectral distribution of statistical variance of pressure about its mean. Units—(mm Hg)². (From Randall, 1958.)

2 Hz and smaller ones at twice and three times this frequency. These represent the first three harmonics of the dominant pulse frequency while the spread on either side is due to the variations in this frequency with respiration; the fluctuation at the respiratory rhythm gives rise to the terms at low frequency.

The power spectrum can be seen from eqn. 7.44 to be a complex quantity and may be expressed as a sum of cosine and sine terms. The former are called the *co-spectral* terms (C_{11}) and the latter the *quadrature* terms (Q_{11}).

When it is wished to compare two separate time-series such as the pressure and the corresponding flow the similar process of *cross-correlation* is employed. In this case the points on one function are correlated with those on the other over a series of delay lags, τ. The *cross-correlation function*, $\varphi_{12}(\tau)$, is then defined as

$$\varphi_{12}(\tau) = \frac{1}{T}\int_{-T/2}^{+T/2} f_1(t).f_2(t)\,(t+\tau)dt \qquad \textbf{7.45}$$

and the *cross-power spectrum* of the functions is

$\Phi_{12}(n)$, so that we get similar relations

$$\varphi_{12}(\tau) = \sum_{n=-\infty}^{\infty}\Phi_{12}(n)e^{in\omega\tau} \qquad \textbf{7.46}$$

and

$$\Phi_{12}(n) = \frac{1}{T}\int_{-T/2}^{+T/2}\varphi_{12}(\tau)e^{-in\omega\tau}d\tau \qquad \textbf{7.47}$$

with the co-spectral and quadrature spectra symbolized by C_{12} and Q_{12} as above.

If $f_1(t)$ is the series of pressure waves and $f_2(t)$ the series of flow waves the ratio between them is the impedance $Z = |Z|e^{-i\phi}$ where

$$|Z| = (\Phi_{11}/\Phi_{22})^{\frac{1}{2}} \qquad \textbf{7.48}$$

and the phase is

$$\varphi = \tan^{-1}(Q_{12}/C_{12}) \qquad \textbf{7.49}$$

The *coherence* is a quantity used for testing the significance of the results and is given by

$$\text{Coherence} = \frac{(C^2_{12} + Q^2_{12})}{(\Phi_{11}.\Phi_{12})^{\frac{1}{2}}} \qquad \textbf{7.50}$$

These methods have been used very effectively by Taylor (1966). The spectrum of frequencies in a long train of pressure waves in the femoral artery when the heart was of a normal regularity is shown in Fig. 7.11A. He then stimulated the pacemaker in a random fashion so that the heart-rate was very irregular, as it may be with atrial fibrillation. The spectrum then appeared as illustrated in Fig. 7.11 and now represents more nearly a continuous series of frequencies. In particular, components can be seen down to very low frequencies which are much below those that can be obtained by pacing the heart regularly or by imposing a heart block. As a result he has been able to explore the impedance of various vascular beds (Ch. 13) into this interesting range of frequencies which cannot be measured by single pulse analysis. Equally by comparing these results with those of the harmonic analysis of a single pulse it can be seen that, under normal conditions, slight variations of pulse-frequency introduce little error into the results.

LINEARITY

The use of simple harmonic analysis in defining the physical relations also assumes the *linearity* of the system. Some confusion regarding the limits of its applicability in a non-linear system tends to arise in discussion of this point so that it is as well to redefine them. For numerical description of a periodic phenomenon such as the pulse-wave the Fourier series is perfectly valid whether the system is linear or not. A resynthesis of the harmonic components will recreate the original wave to whatever accuracy is defined by the number of terms taken. In this sense it is valid as a means of describing a single wave even if it is solitary. If, however, the Fourier series is taken term by term and related causally to the corresponding terms of the flow wave then this presupposes a linear system. In a non-linear system there will be interaction between the harmonic components and addition and difference frequency components will be created.

The arterial system is clearly non-linear in the precise sense of the term. The equation of motion between the pressure-gradient and the flow contain the second-order terms of the Navier–Stokes equations (Ch. 6, p. 139). The relation of pressure to flow in an elastic tube contains further non-linear terms due to the changes in radius with pressure (Ch. 11). Finally, the elastic properties of the arterial wall (Ch. 10) are markedly non-linear in that the wall gets stiffer with increasing strain. The assumption of linearity in the system is, therefore, of necessity an approximation. If the predicted non-linearities are not greater than the order of accuracy of our measuring devices they are virtually impossible to detect and therefore, in an experimental situation, may be deemed not to exist. This assumption has, however, to be re-examined from time to time as improvements in instrumentation occur.

The experimental evidence relating to the detection of non-linear behaviour is discussed at various places throughout this book where it is relevant to the various aspects of the system being considered. The methods used have fallen

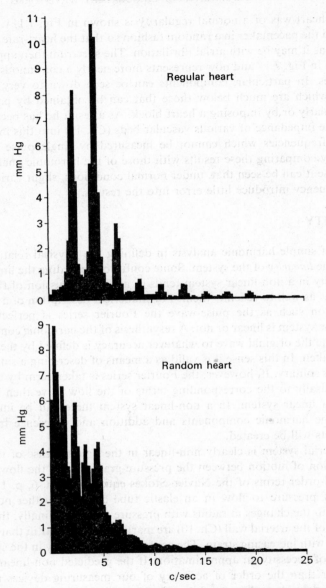

Fig. 7.11A. The frequency spectrum of a long sequence of pressure pulses with a 'regular' heart rate. The peaks are seen to fall at integral multiples of the lowest frequency—c. 2 Hz, i.e. represent the harmonic components. The fact that a heart rate is never exactly regular is shown by the low level between the main peaks.

B. The frequency spectrum of a train of pulses while the heart is being excited at a randomly varying rate. A much more continuous band of frequency components has been created; in particular a large number of these fall below the normal pulse frequency; this frequency region is especially useful in studying the arterial impedance (Ch. 13). (From Taylor, M. G., 1966.)

under three general headings. (1) The system is excited by a single harmonic frequency and the creation of higher harmonic frequencies has been studied. In a simple system this is an elegant method and was used effectively by Taylor (1959c) in a long single rubber tube in relation to the creation of a second harmonic (Ch. 11). He found that the second harmonic term grew in amplitude with distance from the origin and reached a maximum at one to one-and-a-half wave-lengths along the tube and diminished thereafter. In the arterial system, a similar study is difficult because the whole system is short and only attains a length of a wave-length at the frequency of the fourth, or higher, harmonics which are small in amplitude. Attinger, Anné and McDonald (1966) did attempt this type of analysis in a perfused isolated aorta attached to a sinusoidal pump and could not regularly detect any higher frequencies. They concluded, therefore, that the non-linear terms did not amount to more than 5 per cent which they considered to be the limit of accuracy of their studies. (2) The system *in situ* is studied when driven by the heart at different frequencies without changing the properties of the peripheral bed. The argument underlying this approach is that the behaviour of the bed, e.g. the input impedance at 3 Hz should be constant independent of the heart-rate. If the heart is driven successively at 1·0, 1·5, and 3·0 Hz, the component at 3 Hz will be successively the third, the second, and the fundamental harmonics. If there is no consistent change in the impedance at 3 Hz in these cases, then the system may be considered as functioning linearly. Data summarized in Ch. 13 show that this is the case. (3) A more precise and explicit method as an extension of (1) and aimed solely at detecting non-linearity is to excite the system simultaneously with two frequencies that are not integral multiples of each other, and look for the appearance of addition and difference frequencies. This was done by Dick *et al.* (1968) who replaced the flow input of the heart with two sinusoidal pumps; these were run at 2 and 3 Hz and the power spectrum of the pressure was analysed. The only 'stray' frequency of appreciable magnitude that they could detect was the addition frequency of 5 Hz, but that was only 1–2 per cent of the input amplitude in the abdominal aorta. They therefore concluded that the arterial system, for all practical purposes, behaved as a linear system at least in regard to pressure and flow relations.

While to biologists bred with the legend of the 'exactness' of the physical sciences this may appear as a crude approximation, it should be emphasized that such approximation is universal in physics for, strictly speaking, no precisely linear system exists in the real world. The transmission of sound is, for example, non-linear but this has not hampered the widespread application of harmonic analysis to it; where sound transmission becomes markedly non-linear, as in loudspeaker output (McLachlan, 1941) the cross-terms in the Fourier series can be defined and analysed. With digital computers available, a similar analysis could be made but the pursuance of such a goal would have to be tempered by the decision as to whether, in terms of the available accuracy of our raw data, the extra precision would have any significant meaning or be worth the far greater computation time necessary.

ERRORS IN RESYNTHESIS

There is a tendency in a number of abbreviated methods for obtaining the Fourier components of a wave-form to concentrate on the amplitude of the components and neglect their phase relations. For a lot of purposes such as in electrical transmission line studies where one is often concerned with detecting a small signal in the presence of noise this is sufficient. Errors in determining the phase-relations can, however, cause large changes in the form of the resynthesized curve even though the representation in terms of its variance (eqns. 7.38 to 7.40) will be unchanged. A simple example is given in Fig. 7.12

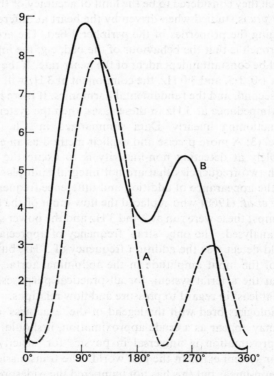

Fig. 7.12. A simple example to show that errors in measuring the phase of harmonic terms can produce a great distortion in resynthesizing a curve. Curves A (- - - -) and B (———) are a combination of a first and second harmonic of equal magnitude; however, in curve B the second harmonic has been shifted by 45° as compared to A. (See also discussion in text of Ch. 15.)

in which a first and second harmonic are added together in two ways, in one of which the second harmonic is shifted by 90°. It will be seen that in one case the total oscillation appears to be markedly greater than in the other. A more complex example is given in Fig. 15.6, where an ascending aortic flow curve is first resynthesized with the correct phase relations of the harmonic components and then with the phase relations of the corresponding pressure wave. This illustrates the errors that will arise in methods of comparing flow curves from pressure measurements without measuring these phase shifts (which constitute the phase of the complex input impedance discussed in Ch. 13). This error is referred to again in relation to measuring output in Ch. 15. In spite of the marked distortion in the shape of the curve the area under it (the stroke volume) remains the same. Thus, stroke volume is predicted accurately but the peak flow velocity is markedly inaccurate.

8
The Design of Manometers

The study of pulsatile pressure in the circulation anticipated that of pulsatile flow by many decades because the technical development of manometers was simpler than that of flowmeters. The theory of manometer design capable of producing adequate instruments was initiated by Otto Frank (1903) and remains essentially the same today. Frank's manometers used short, wide cannulas and rubber membranes and were used extensively in Wiggers' exhaustive studies of pressure-wave forms such as those reported in his classic monograph of 1928 *The Pressure Pulses of the Cardiovascular System*. In the 1930s a substantial improvement was made by Hamilton who replaced the membrane with thin beryllium–copper, and increased the sensitivity of the optical recording system (Hamilton, Brewer and Brotman, 1934). This improved the frequency characteristics considerably. The technical advances in electronics due to World War II, when applied to manometry, made dramatic changes in design with respect to miniaturization and frequency response. This allowed them to be used with long, fine catheters so that pressure measurements over a large part of the arterial tree could be made from a single insertion in a peripheral artery; this immediately opened the way to the extensive clinical use in human beings with which we are familiar. However, it is still often not appreciated fully that optimal performance can only be achieved by exercising great care in the setting-up procedure. As the quantitative analysis of arterial pressure waves requires a detailed knowledge of the accuracy of the measurements made with regard to the manometer response in terms of frequency, it is necessary first to survey the theory of manometer design (Gabe, 1972). (A fuller account is given in Appendix 1.)

THE THEORY OF MANOMETER BEHAVIOUR

Free vibrations

A manometer may, in the first instance, be regarded as analogous to a simple oscillating system consisting of a weight suspended from a spring. If this is displaced and released it will oscillate in simple harmonic motion and, if the system is ideal, these oscillations will continue unchanged at a constant

174

frequency. This frequency is termed its natural frequency, ω_0 (radians/sec). This is given by the equation

$$\omega_0 = \sqrt{\frac{S}{M}}$$

8.1

where S is the stiffness, or elastance, of the spring and M is the mass attached to it.

If there is a resistance to the movement which is proportional to the velocity of movement of the mass this is termed viscous damping, R. The damping of the system, β_0, is denoted by

$$\beta_0 = \frac{R}{2M}$$

8.2

The behaviour of the system on displacement and release of the mass will depend on relative magnitudes of the damping and the undamped natural frequency and can fall into one of three categories.

(1) If the damping factor is equal to the natural frequency, i.e. $\beta_0 = \omega_0$, the mass will not oscillate after release but will return exponentially to its equilibrium position. This is called the condition of *critical* damping.

(2) If $\beta_0 > \omega_0$ then the rate of return to equilibrium is also non-oscillatory but is slower and the system is said to be *over-damped*.

(3) If $\beta_0 < \omega_0$ the mass will oscillate but the amplitude of the oscillations will decay exponentially until it comes to rest. The frequency of these oscillations, ω_D, is also lower than the undamped natural frequency although the difference in these frequencies may be very small. The system is thus said to be *under-damped*. All manometers that we are considering are used in this condition and the derivations below apply only to the under-damped situation as defined in this way. When applying these concepts to a manometer system the term S represents the 'stiffness' of the transducer; this will be, in essence, a water-filled chamber with a deformable membrane at the wall. The volume elasticity, E, of the system (transducer plus attached catheter) $(E = \Delta P / \Delta V)$ replaces the spring constant, S. Hence, increasing the stiffness of the membrane increases the natural frequency of the manometer. The mass M is now the mass of the liquid that moves. As the cross-sectional area of the transducer is usually very large in relation to the cross-sectional area of the catheter it may normally be defined solely in relation to the kinetic mass of the liquid in the catheter, i.e. its velocity is inversely proportional to the cross-sectional area. Hence M is given by

$$M = \frac{L \cdot \rho}{\pi r^2}$$

8.3

G

where L and r are the length and internal radius of the catheter and ρ is the density of the liquid (which, being water, will be taken as $1\cdot0$ in further derivations).

Rewriting eqn. 8.1 we then obtain

$$\omega_0 = \sqrt{\frac{\pi r^2 E}{\rho L}} \quad \text{or} \quad r\sqrt{\frac{\pi E}{\rho L}} \qquad \textbf{8.4}$$

The true frequency observed, ω_0, on applying a brief transient change of pressure and allowing the system to vibrate freely is given by

$$\omega_D = (\omega_0{}^2 - \beta_0{}^2)^{\frac{1}{2}} \qquad \textbf{8.5}$$

It can be seen that ω_D is very close to ω_0 when β_0 is relatively small and unless it is small there are insufficient values, in practice, to measure the frequency accurately.

Thus the natural frequency varies as the radius of the catheter and inversely as the square root of its length with any given transducer—provided that the stiffness of the catheter wall is sufficiently great to maintain the elastance of the whole system. The natural frequency of the transducer itself can be increased by making the membrane stiffer though this increase will only be proportional to the square root of the increase in the value of E. The smaller deflection of the stiffer membrane will lead to a decrease in sensitivity and must be compensated.

The damping term, β_0, can similarly be written in a form applicable to a liquid-filled system. The value for the resistance R was taken by Hansen (1949) as the Poiseuille resistance (eqn. 2.31).

$$R = \frac{8\mu L}{\pi r^4} \qquad \textbf{8.6}$$

Hence, taking M again as given by eqn. 8.3 we get (assuming $\rho = 1\cdot0 = M$)

$$\beta_0 = \frac{R}{2M} = \frac{4\mu}{r^2} \qquad \textbf{8.7}$$

This value is only significant in relation to the natural frequency of the manometer and is usually described as a fraction, or percentage of critical damping, the condition where $\beta_0 = \omega_0$. The relative damping, β, can be simply derived from eqns. 8.4 and 8.7.

$$\beta = \frac{\beta_0}{\omega_0} = \frac{4\mu}{r^2}\sqrt{\frac{\rho L}{\pi r^2 E}} = \frac{4\mu}{r^3}\sqrt{\frac{\rho L}{\pi E}} \qquad \textbf{8.8}$$

Hence, in respect to the choice of catheter, it can be seen that the damping varies only as the square root of the length but inversely as the cube of the radius. This sensitivity of the damping to changes in the internal radius of the catheter must be borne in mind when considering the possible effects of fibrinogen deposition on the inside of the catheter. The fact that the term E appears in the equation also emphasizes that if the effective elastance is decreased, as by even a minute air-bubble in the system, not only will the resonant frequency be reduced but the damping will be increased.

The derivation of eqn. 8.8 is not, however, strictly accurate, for the value of the Poiseuille resistance (eqn. 8.6) is only valid for steady flow. The correct solution for oscillatory flow was first obtained by Lambossy (1952a). The resistance he used was mathematically the same as that derived by Womersley and discussed in Ch. 5. From eqn. 6.19 and Fig. 6.13 it can be seen that the resistance rises with frequency; if plotted against the parameter, α, the resistance rises linearly, relative to the Poiseuille resistance, for values of α above 3.

From the expression derived for the oscillatory resistance (eqn. 6.19) we may write it in a different form

$$\beta_0 = \frac{\mu}{2\rho r^2} \frac{\alpha^2}{M'_{10}} \cdot \sin \varepsilon_{10} = \frac{\omega \sin \varepsilon_{10}}{2M'_{10}} \qquad \textbf{8.9}$$

The values of M'_{10}/α^2 and ε_{10} are given in Table A and the second form has the expression for α cancelled out and values of M'_{10} and ε_{10} for the appropriate value of α may be taken from Fig. 7.6. A simpler, but more approximate, method that is adequate uses the values for the ratio of the oscillatory value of R to the Poiseuille resistance that are plotted in Fig. 8.3. If the values of β_0 or β calculated from the Poiseuille resistance (eqns. 8.7 and 8.8) are then multiplied by the factor read from the graph for the appropriate value of α the true damping at that frequency may be obtained. This refinement is only necessary if the damping needs to be calculated accurately in the low-frequency working range of the manometer–catheter system, where, because of the narrow bore of catheters normally used, the value of α is low. It only applies when the damping is calculated at the resonant frequency as in the common free-vibration method. This technique and numerical examples of this correction are given below (p. 197).

This discussion describes the behaviour of a manometer when it vibrates freely after a single deflection. It is important to appreciate that critical damping and hence, from common usage, all damping coefficients are derived by analysis of behaviour under such conditions. The behaviour of a manometer in practice, however, is determined by the fact that it is being continually driven by the force of the arterial pressure. This is the condition of forced oscillation, or forced vibration.

Forced vibrations

A manometer system that is being driven will respond only to the applied frequency. In an under-damped system the amplitude of the manometer response will increase as the applied frequency increases until it reaches a peak, when it is said to resonate. The resonant frequency will be close to, but rather less than, the natural undamped frequency. Thereafter the amplitude of response falls off rapidly with frequency (Fig. 8.1). In addition to the ampli-

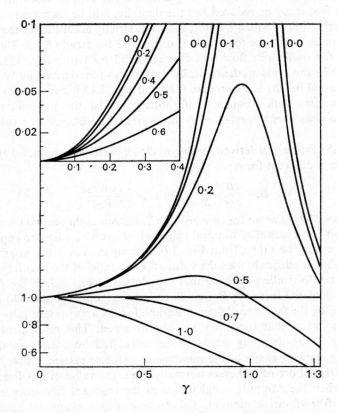

Fig. 8.1. The amplitude response of a manometer, under different conditions of damping, when driven by an oscillatory force of unit amplitude and varying frequency. Abscissa—the ratio of driving frequency (ω) to the undamped natural frequency (ω_0), denoted by γ, as in the text. Ordinate—amplitude of response. Inset square (top left) is a more detailed display of the behaviour at relatively low driving frequencies. Figures by each curve indicate damping as a fraction of critical damping. The corresponding phase changes are shown in Fig. 8.2. To make recordings that are reasonably accurate with regard to both amplitude and phase it can be seen that one needs a manometer with a natural frequency of the order of ten times the highest frequencies it is wished to record.

tude response there is also a phase lag in the response. This increases with frequency but the rate of increase varies with the damping (Fig. 8.2). In all cases, however, the phase lag is 90° when the driving frequency equals the resonant frequency and increases to 80° at frequencies above that.

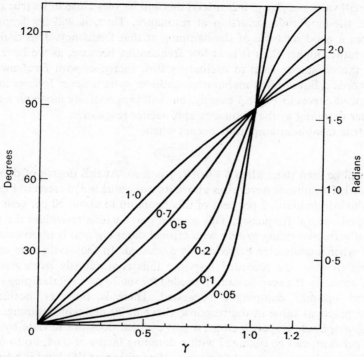

Fig. 8.2. The phase-lag in a manometer driven by an oscillatory force of constant amplitude. With zero damping there is no phase-lag up to the point of resonance and then a sudden change to 180°. Abscissa—ratio of driving frequency to natural frequency (cp. Fig. 8.1); ordinate—phase-lag in degrees (left scale) and radians (right). It will be noted that phase distortion is marked unless the damping is kept very low (e.g. less than 0·1 of critical damping).

If we call the manometer response x and express it as a ratio of its true value and denote the driving frequency as a fraction, γ, of the natural frequency, ω_0, so that the applied pressure is of the form $\sin \gamma t$ we find that

$$x = \frac{1}{[(1-\gamma^2)+4\beta^2\gamma^2]^{\frac{1}{2}}} \sin \left(\gamma t - \tan^{-1} \frac{2\beta\gamma}{1-\gamma^2} \right) \qquad \textbf{8.10}$$

so that the amplitude, A, relative to its true value, is determined by the term

$$A = \frac{1}{[(1-\gamma^2)^2+4\beta^2\gamma^2]^{\frac{1}{2}}} \qquad \textbf{8.11}$$

It is this function that is shown graphically in Fig. 8.1 for various values of β.

From eqn. 8.11 it can be seen that when the manometer is driven at its natural undamped frequency, i.e. $\gamma = 1.0$, then

$$A = \frac{1}{2\beta} \qquad \textbf{8.12}$$

With small values of β (e.g. 0·2 or less) this will be very close to its true maximum at the amplitude excursion at resonance. Thus, it will be, from this equation, a good measure of the damping at that frequency. This damping will be rather higher than it is at low frequencies because, as we have seen above, the resistance term in oscillatory flow increases with frequency. In other words a liquid-filled manometer–catheter system never follows any of the graphed curves in Fig. 8.1 exactly, but will progressively move on a curve of higher damping as the frequency approaches resonance.

The true maximum amplitude occurs when

$$\gamma = \sqrt{(1 - 2\beta^2)} \qquad\qquad \textbf{8.13}$$

and it will be seen that, when $\beta = 0.707$, γ is zero. At this degree of damping the recorded amplitude never rises above its true value but, as seen in Fig. 8.1, it remains within about 2 per cent of this figure up to about 50 per cent of its undamped natural frequency. This gives a curve which resembles the behaviour of a free-vibrating system with critical damping and is often confused with it when manometer behaviour is discussed. In fact, with true critical damping ($\beta = 1.0$) the recorded response falls continuously from zero frequency upwards. If a specific name is needed for the 70 per cent damping curve, the term 'optimal' damping is suggested. There is, however, nothing of especial practical value in the response curve at 70 per cent damping. Considering amplitude response alone, a curve which does not deviate by more than 2 per cent, can be obtained with a damping factor of 0·64, up to 67 per cent of the undamped natural frequency. If precision of this kind is required, then these values have to be modified by including the changes in oscillatory resistance and Lambossy (1952b) has calculated values for curves which would be optimal under these conditions.

The phase lag, φ, of the manometer response in relation to the driving pressure is shown in eqn. 8.10 to be given by

$$\varphi = \tan^{-1} \frac{2\beta\gamma}{1 - \gamma^2} \qquad\qquad \textbf{8.14}$$

and is shown graphically in Fig. 8.2 for various degrees of damping. It can be seen that only with low damping is the phase lag small over any part of the frequency range, and, indeed, if accurate phase recording is required, then the damping should be less than 0·1. At this value, for example, the phase lag is some 2·3° at 0·1 of the natural frequency. With modern catheter-tip manometers with resonant frequencies from 5 to 15 kHz the problem does not arise. With an increase in damping the phase error at this relative frequency increases approximately linearly as the damping.

The errors in phase introduced by a manometer were not regarded as very important until the measurement of such complex quantities as impedance became of interest within the last decade. Here both the amplitude and phase must be measured to define the parameter and the phase distortion inherent in recording must be known. This was in spite of the fact that they had been calculated and displayed by Hansen and Warburg (1950). Even when only the form of the pressure wave is of interest distortion of shape will result from shifts of phase of the harmonic components relative to each other. An extreme example is shown in Fig. 7.12 where there are two curves composed of a fundamental and a second harmonic component; in one curve, the second harmonic is shifted 90° in relation to the other and it can be seen that the combined wave form is drastically altered. On the other hand, the total excursion is not much changed. Phase distortion will be progressively more marked at the higher frequencies but, as we have seen (Ch. 7) the harmonics above the fifth are relatively small so that if the larger distortions are confined to these components neither the form nor the amplitude of the wave will be altered appreciably.

Ideally, one would wish to have no phase errors at all. The nearest approach to this is achieved with catheter-tip manometers which commonly have their resonant frequencies in the kilocycle range; the relevant frequencies in the pulse-wave are then only 1 or 2 per cent of the resonant frequency and the phase lag can hardly be discriminated from zero. Where fine catheters have to be used it was recommended by Hansen (1949) that a damping coefficient of around 0·7 be used. It can be seen from Fig. 8.2 that, in this case, the phase lag varies virtually linearly with frequency from zero to resonance. In a recording with such a manometer all the harmonics will be recorded with the same delay in actual *time* (for the phase angle is referred to the cycle length at each frequency). This will be equivalent to recording the composite wave undistorted but delayed in time. If the precise time relations of the wave are not important this is a satisfactory solution; if, however, the transmission time were being related, for example, to the ECG, it would introduce an error. It is this lack of relative phase distortion, coupled with the relatively flat response that led Hansen (1949) to recommend damping coefficients of 0·6–0·8 as optimal. However, unless special manometers are built which allow for adjustable damping, as Hansen did with his oil-damped capacitance manometer, this situation is very difficult to achieve; and once achieved is difficult to maintain with any assurance throughout an experiment.

In situations where a manometer and catheter system cannot achieve a satisfactorily high resonance frequency some workers have corrected their pressure curves by calculating the true amplitude response from the equations governing the theoretical curves shown in Figs. 8.1 and 8.2. This is quite easily done when a digital computer is available; the pressure curve is first subjected to an harmonic analysis and the amplitude and phase correction applied to each frequency component. It is in this situation that errors will be introduced unless the oscillatory resistance derived from Womersley's equation (6.10) and incorporated into the term β_0 as shown in eqn. 8.9. Two examples are shown in Figs. 8.4 and 8.5. In each figure the curve marked Obs. is the amplitude response when the manometer–catheter system is driven by a pump (see section on calibration by forced vibration, p. 200). The curves marked W are the amplitude calculated using the oscillatory or Womersley resistance and they can be seen to be reasonably close to the observed curve. The curves marked H use the steady-flow or Hansen resistance and it can be seen that the discrepancy from the true curves is large; in Fig. 8.4 for example the predicted amplitude at resonance is more than double the true value. Clearly if such a curve is used to 'correct' a pressure curve an error of over 100 per cent can be introduced. If such corrections are deemed necessary the value of α of each frequency component is first calculated. The value of the required oscillatory damping is then derived by increasing it by the factor of the relative resistance in relation to α which is shown in Fig. 8.3.

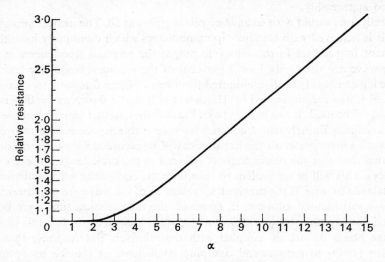

Fig. 8.3. A graph of the resistance component of the impedance in oscillatory flow (see eqns. 6.19 through 6.23). The ordinate is plotted as the Relative Resistance, i.e. the ratio of the oscillatory resistance to the Poiseuille resistance for the same tube. The parameter α is plotted as the abscissa. As discussed in the text the true damping in a manometer–catheter system will exceed that calculated from Hansen's equation (eqn. 8.8) by a factor which is that of the relative resistance plotted here in terms of the appropriate value of α. Examples of this correction are shown in Figs. 8.4 and 8.5.

THE PRACTICAL PROBLEMS OF MANOMETER DESIGN

It is apparent that it is impossible to construct a manometer that does not distort the amplitude and/or phase if it is necessary to measure a wide band of frequencies. The best approach to simultaneous accuracy for both these characteristics is to have a manometer with a high resonant frequency and very small damping. The highest frequencies that we normally need to record

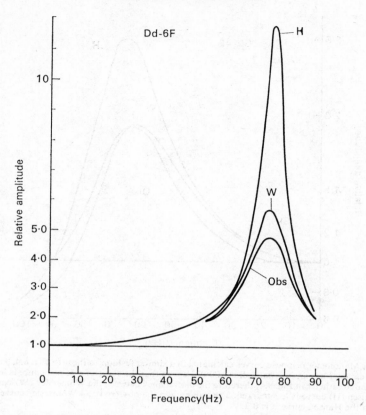

Fig. 8.4. The curve marked Obs. is the amplitude response (cp. Fig. 8.1) of a Statham P23Dd transducer attached to a standard no. 6 French catheter and tested with a pump running to 90 Hz (Yanof *et al.*, 1963). The curves marked H and W are the theoretical curves calculated with the catheter radius, 0·046 cm, given by the manufacturers. The elastance of the whole system is calculated from the observed resonant frequency. In curve H, the standard Hansen equation, using the Poiseuille resistance, is used as it is in Fig. 8.1. In curve W the oscillatory resistance, as derived by Womersley and plotted in Fig. 8.3, is used to calculate the damping. Thus the relative damping measured by the observed curve is 0·1, and that predicted by the curve W is close to this at 0·09; by contrast the curve H predicts a damping of only 0·04 so that the use of the Hansen equation could lead to a large error. It will be noted that the discrepancies of all three curves are small up to a frequency about 70 per cent of the resonant frequency. The use of this correction is discussed in the text.

accurately in arteries are 25–30 Hz in dogs and probably considerably less than this in man. The most striking technical advance in recent years has been in the construction of miniature transducers which can be placed on the tip of a catheter and thus eliminate the hydraulic damping consequent on having a fluid-filled catheter between the transducer and the point in the artery where the pressure is measured. One of the first to be introduced (c. 1962) was the Statham SF-1 (see description below (pp. 188–89)). Its external diameter was c. 2 mm and its resonant frequency c. 2,000 Hz with an effective damping

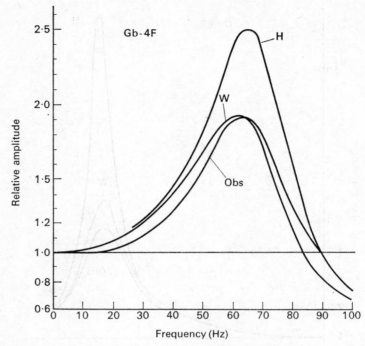

Fig. 8.5. Manometer response curves calculated in a similar fashion to those in Fig. 8.4. The no. 4 French catheter has an internal radius of 0·023 cm so that the value of α at resonance is less than for the no. 6 catheter in Fig. 8.4; therefore the discrepancy between the Womersley (W) curve and the Hansen (H) curve is less marked. The damping in the observed and Womersley curve is 0·27 while in the Hansen curve it is 0·2.

<1·0 per cent of critical (Yanof *et al.*, 1963). They were, however, rather fragile, and thus rather expensive to use routinely. They were nevertheless in very widespread use by the late 1960s. About this time they were withdrawn from production by Statham who replaced them by their model P866 catheter-tip manometer. This is smaller with an OD c. 1·5 mm (and also a good deal more expensive). The Telco (inductance) manometer—which was introduced in France in 1959 (p. 190 below)—is also still in use in some laboratories. The use of semiconductor transducers has, however, revolutionized the development of catheter-tip manometers, which have also been made in the form of small discs which can be chronically implanted in the larger arteries or the chambers of the heart (see p. 189 below). These are constantly being improved and made more rugged and any detailed account is apt to be out of date by the time it appears in print.

Nevertheless, there is still a large usage of transducers with a catheter attached for routine clinical work and in animal experiments where small vessels are involved. In these cases, the recording characteristics discussed above must be considered carefully, and frequency calibration must be carried out on each occasion they are used.

TYPES OF MANOMETER IN USE

The great technical developments in manometer manufacture of the past few years make it impossible to give detailed information on all makes available. A brief survey of the principal techniques that have been applied is given here, followed by a more detailed discussion of the types in most frequent use on which reliable performance data are available. Additional information is given in reviews by Piemme (1963) and Yanof (1965) which illustrate and discuss constructional details and the principles of operation in a fairly elementary way; Franke (1966) has provided a more technical review which is useful, and has been used as a source for some of the data reported here.

Optical manometers

The simplest inertia-free method of recording the bending of a membrane is by the deflection of a beam of light reflected from a mirror mounted on it. Membranes made out of beryllium–copper which can be made as stiff as required, were introduced by Hamilton (Hamilton, Brewer and Brotman, 1934). The practical limitation of this type is that, with membranes of a stiffness needed to give a good frequency response, a beam of light several meters long is necessary to obtain a reasonable deflection on photographic paper. As a result, they have largely been superseded by methods using electrical methods of recording. One such optical manometer of which I have personal experience (made by the Cambridge Scientific Instrument Company, England) was based on the design of Müller and Shillingford (1954). In this model a rectangular beam of light is reflected on to two photo-electric cells arranged side by side so that a deflection of the beam causes a change in balance of the output of the two cells. This is amplified and recorded. An advantage of this design is that the light beam can operate through water so that a differential manometer can be easily made by applying a different pressure simultaneously on either side of the membrane. The sensitive membranes required for measuring arterial pressure-gradients, however, had a rather low frequency response; even with wide-bore catheters we were only able to record a flat amplitude response up to about 8 Hz.

Recently, refinements in techniques of fibre-optics has revived interest in optical techniques. Franke (1966) has described a manometer in which light conducted down a 'light-guide' made of glass fibre is reflected from a membrane that is deformed by pressure. The reflected light is passed through a narrow gap, one side of which is formed by the membrane; hence the flux of light through it varies as the size of the slit is changed. The light passing through the gap is picked up by another light-guide and channelled to a photo-multiplier. This device can be made as small as an intravascular catheter and is reported to have an amplitude response which is flat to 200 Hz but the design has problems in achieving a satisfactory signal-to-noise ratio.

Another design which is in the experimental stage uses a light-guide which is divided longitudinally into two parts. Light passing down one side is reflected from the back of a diaphragm in a terminal capsule and is reflected back. Movements of the membrane will cause variable interference between the reflected and incident beams which can be detected and amplified as a signal. As the movements of the membrane need to be restricted to less than the wave-length of light, high resonant frequencies can be obtained. With modern fibre-optic technology it is forecast that the overall diameter can be reduced to less than 1 mm. (Without the terminal membrane and using the arterial wall as a reflecting surface the technique is also being developed as a means of measuring the radial dilatation of small arteries.)

Capacitance manometers

The capacitance manometer was introduced into physiology by Lilly (1942) in America and developed by Hansen (1949) who used it in the detailed studies on manometer performance reported in that important monograph. In the following decade, it was the most widely used high-frequency manometer in England. Among electronic methods of recording it can combine high sensitivity with high-frequency characteristics and with relative simplicity of manufacture of the transducer.

The principle is that the membrane which is moved by the applied pressure forms one side of a condenser. Deflection of the membrane, therefore, alters its capacity. To detect this, the capacitance is made part of an oscillator circuit. Change in this capacitance alters the oscillatory frequency and thus is measured by a frequency modulation technique.

The main problem in its practical application is that, in a high-frequency manometer, the capacitance of the transducer must be very small. Other capacitances in the circuit, notably the capacitance of the cable, will be large; furthermore, the effective cable capacitance may be altered by changes in cable position. Good circuit design can virtually eliminate the problem and, in practice, it never troubled us with the English (Southern Instrument Co.) capacitance manometers we used for many years. Franke (1966) discussed the electronic problem briefly and points out that in this type of manometer there is a problem in getting a satisfactory response in the *low*-frequency range. The audio-frequency range is relatively simple to deal with and the technique is widely used in condenser microphones.

Nevertheless, in spite of the pioneer work in high-frequency response manometers using this method, they have virtually dropped out of use. This is probably due to the relative complexities of the electronic circuits compared to those using strain-gauges. However, a new application has been reported by Coon and Sandler (1967). This is a catheter-tip manometer in a range of sizes of which the smallest is a little over 1 mm in diameter. This is considerably smaller than has been achieved so far with other techniques, and would greatly enhance their usefulness in clinical work. The resonant frequency is reported to be 6–8,000 Hz. These manometers were designed and built at the Ames (NASA) Research Center in California and, at the time of writing, it is not clear if they will become commercially available.

Strain–gauge manometers

The change in ohmic resistance which occurs in a wire when it is strained has been widely used in a large variety of gauges. The change in resistance is measured by setting the gauge as the arm of a Wheatstone bridge; straining the wire by an applied pressure unbalances the bridge and the voltage produced is a measure of the pressure. This method has the advantages of stability and simplicity in its electrical circuits. The voltage applied to the bridge has usually been energized by an a.c. source to avoid problems, such as zero drift, in d.c. amplifiers. In this case, a phase-sensitive demodulation circuit needs to be included and, of course, the carrier frequency needs to be filtered out. The technical aspects of the circuity are discussed by Franke (1966), Stacy (1960) and Yanof (1965). The carrier frequency used limits the frequency range that can be recorded accurately; this is always ample for the frequencies recorded in the arterial pulse but often limits calibration procedures which depend on determining the resonance-frequency of a manometer system, especially with the advent of catheter-tip transducers. For example, the widely used Sanborn carrier amplifier has an activation frequency of 2,400 Hz. I have taken, empirically, that one can work up to a quarter of the activation frequency (i.e. 600 Hz in this example). Franke (1966), on the other hand, states that the carrier frequency should be 10 times that of the highest frequency recorded. Reference to Table 8.1 will show that the less stringent

Table 8.1. Resonant frequencies of various manometer–catheter systems

	Catheter (internal radius, cm)			
	4F 0·023	5F 0·033	6F 0·046	7F 0·058
Transducer				
Db	49	65	74	83
Dd	60	78	86	110
Gb	75	90	114	130

All catheters were standard cardiac catheters manufactured by United States Catheter and Instrument Corporation (USCI) and were 112 cm long.

All resonant frequencies in Hz. Values given are arranged from Yanof et al. (1963), Nichols (1970), and McDonald and Navarro (unpublished data, 1965).

criterion will easily cover all available external transducers, with the exception of the Statham SF-4. As filling, with its consequent problems with trapped air-bubbles, is no difficulty with catheter-tip manometers, they do not often require frequency-calibration so that this limitation is not serious. Nevertheless, good d.c. amplifiers are now available and d.c. excitation of the strain-gauge is feasible and satisfactory. It is now used in my laboratory (Honeywell amplifiers).

The manometers of this type that are by far the most widely used are the P23 series made by Statham Physiological Transducers. The performance characteristics of the current models are given in Table 8.1 and it can be seen from the very small volume displacement that the design has been highly perfected. These all are unbonded wire strain-gauges, in which the wire is wound around pegs on a sliding element and on a fixed frame. The sliding element moves when the flexible diaphragm is deformed by the applied pressure. The strain-wire resistance is balanced against a similar wire which is not strained to compensate for temperature effects. Wire can only be subjected to tensile strains; under a compressive stress they will buckle. Hence, the wire is prestretched to allow for recording below atmospheric pressure. With a volume of water in it of approximately 1·0 ml the volume elasticity of the P23G transducer is $1·3 \times 10^{10}$ dyn/cm^5 while that of water at 20°C is about $2·3 \times 10^{10}$ dyn/cm^5. It is clear that very little increase in frequency response can be made by making the membrane stiffer; it was calculated by Yanof et al. (1963) that about 60 per cent of the reported volume displacement was taken up by compression of the water and only 40 per cent by displacement of the membrane. It was also estimated from this calculation that the membrane displacement for an applied pressure of 100 mm Hg was of the order of 260 mμ (or nanometers, nm).

This compares well with the estimate of 300 nm based on electrical measurements by the manufacturers. The fact that this is about half the wave-length of green light gives a vivid idea of the technical refinement involved in modern manometers.

Increase in frequency response involves an increase in volume elasticity (p. 176); the effect of the compressibility of water can be minimized by reducing the volume of the transducer. This has been done in the Statham SF-1 catheter-tip manometer developed from an original design by Warnick and Drake (1958). This transducer is essentially a fluted cylinder with the wire wound around the outer surface; pressure applied to the inside of the cylinder expands it and strains the wire. This cylinder is enclosed in an outer brass cylinder, with an OD of c. 2 mm, which is seen at the catheter-tip. The wire connections pass back in the walls of the cardiac catheter to which it is attached. These walls are a little thicker than the normal catheter; the lumen is that of a size-6 French catheter and the OD is that of 6·5 French size (see Table 8·1 for catheter dimensions). The initial report by Warnick and Drake

(1958) stated that the resonant frequency filled with water was 2,000 Hz and I have recorded a similar value; Franke (1966), however, lists a value of 800 Hz. (The description of its construction given here is based on information received from Statham Inc. in 1962 and also appears, with illustration, in Yanof (1965); Franke (1966), however, incorrectly states that it used a silicon element and classifies it as a piezo-resistive instrument.)

The main disadvantage of this manometer is its fragility. The transducer element itself is probably sturdy but the wiring in the flexible catheter appears to break. The transducers are also very temperature sensitive. This may appear to contradict the statement above that strain-gauge transducers are compensated for temperature changes; in this case it arises from a different cause. Between the inner sensing cylinder and the protective outer cylinder there is a trapped air space. Thermal expansion on this air creates, as it were, a back pressure. As the outer cylinder is of brass it responds very quickly to changes in temperature and a static calibration in the laboratory may be difficult if it is not protected from air-current or careless handling. This gives the impression that it is very unstable. In fact, it causes only a base-line shift. The actual calibration in terms of applied pressure has been performed in my laboratory by W. W. Nichols and is found not to vary between 20°C and 38°C. When in use inside the body, the blood stream acts as a thermostat and I have found this manometer very stable in physiological use. To keep a control on this, I normally connect a P23 type manometer to the lumen of the catheter and check the mean pressure continuously and check the calibration at intervals with it. The same transducer has been adapted for use outside the body attached to a needle or catheter. It is then given the code name of SF-4. It is potentially of value in situations where a fine catheter is essential because it has a much higher frequency-response with any given catheter than the P23 series; this is due to the higher volume-elasticity noted above. The volume displacement given by the manufacturers is only 0·001 mm³/100 mm Hg pressure, so that the requirements for ensuring that the system is free from gas bubbles is even more stringent than for the larger transducers (see p. 195).

Semiconductor transducers

Under this heading we note a variety of solid-state elements and resistance is altered where they are strained and this is arranged to cause an imbalance in a Wheatstone bridge as with the strain-gauge manometers discussed above. One of the first to be used was introduced by Anliker and his group (developed at the Ames (NASA) Research Center, California, and later marketed by the Bytrex Corporation), which had a good sensitivity and a high natural frequency of c. 6 kHz. Disc transducers of similar design performance were also developed and, as noted above (p. 184), were found to be highly satisfactory for chronic implantation for long-term studies in dogs. The earlier models tended to be very temperature-sensitive but, although the relative constancy of blood temperature minimizes this problem, improved design has virtually eliminated this defect. Silicon chips appear to be favoured material and catheter-tip transducers with resonant frequencies of 10–15 MHz are made by a variety of manufacturers, e.g. Kulite, Inc., Whittaker Corp., etc. The ones routinely used in my laboratory are those made by Millar Instruments, Houston, Texas, and these are very sensitive and, so far, have proved to be very free of breakdowns. These manometers have an external diameter of slightly less than 2 mm and a resonant frequency of 14 kHz. Any frequency that we require to measure is usually below 30 Hz so that, in terms of the curves in Figs. 8.1 and 8.2, this is about 1/500 of the resonant frequency; the maximum value of α in these graphs will be c. 0·002. Thus, there will be no measurable distortion of amplitude or phase.

Inductance manometers

The variation in electrical current induced in a coil when an iron core, or its equivalent, is moved in it have been applied in various ways to manometer design. Where such a core is actually moved its mass needs to be very small to achieve suitably high natural frequencies. In other designs, a membrane has been made to alter the width of an air-gap in a magnetic circuit and, as a result, alters the amount and distribution of flux in the circuit.

The inductance principle has not, however, been very effectively used with transducers to be used with fluid-filled catheters. It is important because the first very small manometers that could be used intravascularly used this technique. Wetterer (1944) was the first to build one on a straight metal sound; this was later improved by Wetterer and Pieper (1952). The device had a small iron core which was displaced within a differential transformer; the core was attached at one end to a metallic membrane which was displaced by the applied pressure. A similar principle was used by Gauer and Genapp (1950) and its experimental use was described by Ellis, Gauer and Wood (1952). A commercial manometer apparently similar to the Gauer manometer was developed commercially in France as the Telco manometer which was attached to a No. 8 French catheter—about 3 mm in diameter. A detailed report of its performance in clinical application was made by Laurens *et al.* (1959) and it has been widely used in cardiology units since that time, particularly for recording intraventricular pressure. Laurens *et al.* (1959) reported a natural frequency of 800 Hz.

Other types of manometer

The present-day requirements of fidelity over the range of frequencies of significant amplitude in the arterial pulse have rendered a lot of manometers, using other physical principles, obsolete. (Where only the mean pressure is required, however, adequate recording can be made quite simply. There is still quite a lot to be said for the directness of the mercury manometer although it is not very easy to convey the reading to an electrical signal for display on a recorder.) Some of these techniques should be noted for use in special applications.

(a) *Piezo-electric transducers*. Certain materials such as quartz develop an electrical potential when they are mechanically stressed. The group of sintered ceramics such as barium titanate are now used more often than quartz. They have the advantages that they can be used at high frequency (e.g. up to 4 kHz) and for this reason have been used as microphones in the study of cardio-vascular sound. Their main disadvantage is that the potential developed during static deformation is very small and, even with good insulation, leaks away. Thus, only the oscillatory terms are recorded and they cannot measure mean pressure. They have been used for measurement of arterial pressure by extravascular application through the intact skin. This is a highly desirable objective but here the calibration is also dependent, in part, on the force with which the gauge is applied to the artery and so may be affected by such things as slight lateral movements of the vessel. Okino (personal communication) has reviewed these problems critically. Where wave-form, rather than the precise amplitude, is the required measure, they can be valuable. A good example is the use of them made by Porjé (1946) in studying the apparent phase velocities of the harmonic components of the human arterial pulse. Spencer (1964) developed a device in which a titanate crystal was incorporated in a cuff which was implanted around an artery in an animal which was free-ranging subsequently (in particular for use in giraffes).

They have also been incorporated in catheter-tips for use intravascularly but the important contributions they have made are pre-eminently to the study of sound generation (Wallace *et al.*, 1957, 1959; Lewis *et al.*, 1959).

(b). *Servo micropipette manometer*. This device is really basically different from all others discussed. Instead of recording the deformation produced by a change of pressure, in this technique a counter-pressure is produced to nullify the effects of the applied pressure. It was specifically designed to measure pressures in the microcirculation, mainly vessels with a diameter of less than 100 μm. This is very difficult with conventional methods. A saline-filled micropipette (tip from 0·5 to 5 μm diameter) is used as the transducer which is introduced into the small vessel. The pressure will displace blood into the tip, which alters its electrical impedance. This change in impedance is sensed and made to activate a hydraulic system which applies a counter-pressure until the original null-point is reached. The pressure in the hydraulic system is measured by a conventional transducer. Developed in Seattle by Wiederhielm and colleagues, they reported an assessment of its use in the vessels of the frog's mesentery (Wiederhielm *et al.*, 1964) and a detailed description of the technique has also been given by Wiederhielm (1966). As reported here it has a flat frequency response to c. 10 Hz. With the marked attenuation of the higher frequency pulse-wave components that will occur by the time the wave reaches the arterioles this is probably adequate; with further refinement of the servo-mechanism this frequency might well be increased if it is deemed to be necessary. This is a remarkable example of the application of a special technique to a difficult situation.

(c). *Conductance manometer*. There will be a conductance change of a solution in the space between two plates when pressure is applied to them. This was made the basis of a differential manometer by Pappenheimer (1954). This was capable of high sensitivity although at the expense of frequency response. It does not appear to have come into general use.

(d). *Mechano-electric transducer*. Green (1954) used the transducer tube, RCA 5734, which has a probe attached to the anode, as a basis for a mano-meter. This is the same tube which has been used as the sensing unit for the bristle flow-meter (Ch. 9). In this case, a metal plate was attached to the probe. Doubts were raised as to its zero stability and this particular design does not appear to have been used elsewhere. It is suggestive of similar techniques that might be applied.

AMPLIFIERS AND RECORDERS

All the discussion of the behaviour and design of manometers tacitly assumes that there is no subsequent distortion of the recorded pressure. The enormous variety of amplifier circuits and recording devices that have been used makes it impossible to make more than a few general observations. For precise quantitative work it is necessary that the response of the recording system in respect of amplitude and phase should be known over the frequency range to be analysed. This is especially true of phase where variable electrical damping is used in an additional circuit or where mirror galvanometers are used with electrical or hydraulic damping. If frequency-response calibration can be performed with the recording apparatus used for experimental work, then separate calibration of the recorder is less important. In practice, calibration of the resonant frequency of the system may be too high to register satisfac-torily on a recorder that is suitable for the experimental range. It is then necessary to use a higher frequency recording device such as a cathode-ray oscilloscope which has very different characteristics to the normal recorder.

With these general observations in mind, the choice of recording device is a matter of personal preference (and availability).

(a) *Cathode-ray oscilloscope*. In terms of accuracy of recording over a wide frequency range this is undoubtedly the first choice. Its only disadvantage in terms of making permanent records is that the scope face needs to be photo-graphed and the film subsequently processed, although rapid-development techniques can minimize this inconvenience.

(b) *Magnetic tape-recorder*. For subsequent analysis by computer this is rapidly becoming the standard method of recording for haemodynamic data to be analysed quantitatively. In any reputable tape-recorder designed for scientific work again the frequency response far exceeds the range required in studies of the arterial pressure pulse.

(c) *Pen-writers.* The present-day pen-writers have a remarkably good frequency response. Yanof *et al.* (1963) reported that an Offner RS recorder (now Beckman), tested with a beat-frequency oscillator, recorded within the accuracy of measurement (estimated as $\pm 1\cdot 5$ per cent up to 125 Hz; it was only down 14 per cent at 150 Hz. This is achieved by compensating circuits and there was a slight tendency to over-read in the 60–70 Hz range. A Sanborn instrument tested in 1964 had a very similar response with an ink-writing pen. The heated stylus used for rectilinear recordings is heavier and the 'flat' response is to 80 Hz but was only down 3 per cent at 100 Hz. The distortion due to the fact that the tip of the pen describes an arc was also considered. This is often quoted as a limitation but if the deviation from the midline constitutes an angle θ radians the percentage distortion of amplitude only amounts to $100 (1 - \sin \theta/\theta)$. With a 10 cm pen a deviation from the mid-line of ± 1 cm gives a θ of $0\cdot 1$ radian and the error is $0\cdot 2$ per cent; a deviation of ± 2 cm has an error of $0\cdot 7$ per cent and a deviation of ± 4 cm (which is more than most recorders are calibrated for), the error is only $3\cdot 4$ per cent. Using the heated stylus which gives a rectilinear trace the corresponding error is $100 (1 - \tan \theta/\theta)$ and is approximately twice that of the pen-writer. A blind trial, with three observers, suggested that no measurement on the curves could be made with a greater accuracy than $0\cdot 5$ mm. As the excursion of a pen-writer has to be quite severely limited this emphasizes the difficulty of doing accurate wave-analysis and it is doubtful if they are ever used for this purpose. They are valuable, however, for making visual records of all variables recorded, in fact as a monitor, to act as a reference to recording on a tape-recorder for computer analysis.

(d) *Direct-writing optical recorders.* With the introduction of self-developing reversal paper activated by u.v. light has resulted in a popular type of recorder; these are dominated by the Visicorder introduced by Honeywell Inc. and although it is a trade-name, all this group tend to be called by that name in the laboratory. The use of mirror galvanometers eliminates the inertial of the lever and can be used the whole width of the recording paper. Higher paper traverse speeds are also usually available so that curves can be recorded on a much longer scale than on a pen-writer. This lessens the errors in reading the traces if this is necessary (i.e. when a tape-recorder and analogue–digital conversion are not available). In my own laboratory a large number of analyses have been done on such traces with a Gerber digitizer which punches out cards for use in an IBM computer. Mirror galvanometers are available with high natural frequencies (e.g. up to 350 Hz). High frequency is attained at the expense of sensitivity. To minimize the preamplification required, recorders sold for physiological purposes usually have galvanometers which are of relatively low natural frequency and which are damped so as to be flat only out to 25–35 Hz. As remarked in the general comments above this is apt to introduce a phase shift which needs to be checked.

THE PERFORMANCE OF STRAIN-GAUGE MANOMETERS

The strain-gauge tranducers manufactured by Statham Physiological Trans-ducers Inc., Puerto Rico, have very extensive use in present-day laboratories. They have been carefully tested with a variety of catheters and the results are tabulated below. The calibration methods are described in the next section. It will be noted that some internal inconsistencies apper, such as a failure to obtain a higher frequency with a catheter of larger bore. Also, the natural frequencies recorded with the free-vibration method tend to be lower than those recorded with the forced oscillation technique. While this discrepancy may be inherent in the methods or due to individual differences in transducers of the same series, it is more likely that it is due to incomplete elimination of air from the system. The values given, therefore, are only to be regarded as what can be achieved with reasonable care. As catheter-lengths were not the same in all cases, a more direct comparison can be made if the effective volume-elasticity of the transducer–catheter system is calculated. This calculation is from an inversion of eqn. 8.4.

$$\omega_0 = 2\pi f_0 = r \sqrt{\frac{\pi E}{\rho L}} \qquad\qquad \textbf{8.4}$$

Thus

$$E = \frac{\omega_0^2 \rho L}{\pi r^2} = \frac{4\pi f_0^2 . \rho L}{r^2} \qquad\qquad \textbf{8.15}$$

Comparison of this value with that of the transducer alone (calculated from the manufacturer's data) also indicates how much compliance is contributed by the catheter. It will be seen that the small no. 4 catheter gives volume elasticity values nearest to that of the transducer alone and hence is the stiffest catheter. This is largely due to the fact that the ratio of wall-thickness to radius is greatest in the small sizes. For this reason the relation between catheter dimensions and natural frequency cannot be exactly transferred from one size to the other. Nevertheless, in terms of their length these cardiac catheters have an extremely small compliance (all were standard Cournand type cardiac catheters manufactured by USCI Inc., Glen Falls, N.Y.). By comparison, the responses of two 120 cm lengths of polyethylene tubing are included. In this case, the high compliance of the catheter completely domin-ates the frequency response of the system which was undistinguishable whether a P23Dd or the higher-frequency Gb was used.

Values for damping given are all calculated at the resonant frequency of the system. They are thus higher than they will be in effect at the frequency range used in recording the arterial pressure pulse. This effect is discussed in the theoretical outline given above (p. 174) and in more detail in a subsequent section. The correction for this is not usually important.

THE CALIBRATION OF MANOMETERS

Manometers that are used with catheters fall into a special class of recording instruments in that their frequency-response needs to be checked every time they are used. The reason for this can be seen from the theoretical analysis given above (pp. 174–85) because their behaviour depends on the effective volume-elasticity of the transducer–catheter system. Any air that is trapped in the system on filling will obviously change the volume-elasticity and hence the resonant frequency and the damping. Furthermore, during its use in the blood-stream the effective lumen of the catheter may alter due to the deposition of fibrin, so that the damping will increase and the resonant frequency will decrease from their initial values. To obviate this, flushing of the system at intervals is usually undertaken; this in turn creates the risk of introducing air bubbles if the dramatic effect of even minute amounts of air in the system are not appreciated.

Human nature being what it is, we want to have methods of testing frequency response that are as simple as possible while still giving adequate information. A brief discussion of magnitude of the gas bubble effect will help to emphasize the vital importance of this artifact. The volume displacements of some modern transducers have already been quoted and, in the Statham series for example, may vary from 0·04 mm^3 in the P23Dd to 0·001 mm^3/100 mm Hg applied pressure in the SF-4. It would seem intuitively obvious that a bubble of gas of minute size size will drastically reduce the effective volume-elasticity of the system. Even if it was in one of the transparent parts of the transducer it would be difficult to detect. In fact, it is much more likely to be trapped at a metal connection or in a stopcock. Inspection of the system will, therefore, be of no value.

Assuming the volume of liquid in a P23 type manometer with catheter is 1 ml then the effective bulk modulus k for the liquid-filled transducer, from the values given in Table 8.1, will range from 0·5 to 1·1 $\times 10^{10}$ dyn/cm^2. The *bulk modulus, k,* or modulus of volume elasticity (see Ch. 10) is defined as $k = -V.dP/dV$; its reciprocal is called the compressibility. The bulk modulus of water at body temperature is close to 2·2 $\times 10^{10}$ dyn/cm^2. That of a gas may easily be derived from the gas laws; as temperature is held constant we may simply use Boyle's law for an ideal gas:

$$PV = \text{Constant} \qquad\qquad \textbf{8.16}$$

hence
$$\frac{dP}{dV} = -\frac{C}{V^2}$$

So
$$k = -\frac{V.dP}{dV} = \frac{C}{V} = P \qquad\qquad \textbf{8.17}$$

Under the oscillatory conditions in a manometer the actual relation will more closely approximate to an adiabatic compression where

$$PV^{\gamma} = C \qquad\qquad \textbf{8.18}$$

$$\text{and then } k = \gamma P \qquad\qquad \textbf{8.19}$$

For air, the value of $\gamma = 1.41$. The value of P is that of atmospheric pressure or about 10^6 dyn/cm^2 so that we may take the bulk modulus of air as approximately 1.5×10^6 dyn/cm^2; that is, smaller than that of the transducer by a factor of at least 3×10^3. In other words, a bubble of air which is this fraction of the volume of the transducer system will undergo the same volume change and would double the volume displacement. For the system of 1 ml capacity we have been considering this would represent a bubble of 0.3 mm^3 volume (for the smaller SF-4 transducer the bubble would be correspondingly smaller). Doubling the volume displacement reduces the volume elasticity, E, to half its previous value and from eqn. 8.4 would reduce the resonant frequency to approximately 70 per cent of its previous value. This analysis is simplified to illustrate magnitudes; in practice, the application of the manometer equations does not apply very well when gas and liquid are both present. For example, the presence of an air-bubble increases the damping more than would be predicted from these equations by the change in frequency response.

In practice it would seem that bubbles of this order of size are normally the smallest that we have to cope with. This is deduced from the fact that with successive flushing, etc., to improve a frequency-response, progress is usually made by a series of jumps of at least 10–20 Hz and is therefore obvious on quite a cursory inspection of the record after a little experience.

The use of the tables of characteristic performances of commonly used manometers and catheters will make this procedure quicker. A knowledge of the expected frequency-response makes it possible to avoid the otherwise tedious task of numerous tests, after reflushing, to determine when the best possible response has been achieved. The somewhat different values given in the tables using forced oscillations or free vibrations illustrates how difficult it is to determine whether a slight difference in response is due to small variations between individual transducers, or catheters, or is merely to get an optimal response in any one case. Where a catheter size not listed here is used an approximate prediction of the likely frequency response can be derived from one of the listed catheters by substituting the new values for radius and length in eqn. 8.4. If transducers are used other than those numerated in the Table a lot of time can ultimately be saved if a series of preliminary tests of this kind are performed.

The methods used are either (a) the *free-vibration* methods using a step-function of pressure (in lab. slang often called the 'pop' technique) or (b) the *forced-oscillation* method using some form of a pump with a wide range of frequencies. There is no very simple or quick way to eliminate gas-bubbles. The most important step is to use water or saline from which all, or most, of the dissolved air has been removed by boiling (the use of sterilized saline will normally achieve this in any case). Desaturation of the liquid has the result that small bubbles will then tend to dissolve spontaneously. It is not, in my opinion, to prevent separation of air-bubbles from the water; normally all pressures recorded are above the atmospheric pressure at which solution occurred. The spontaneous solution of air may be rather slow and filling the transducer–catheter system overnight will usually save time at the start of an experimental day. Carbon dioxide is more soluble than air and for testing procedures where catheters need to be changed at intervals, the displacement of all air with CO_2 before filling with liquid is recommended. In the completely liquid-filled pump system it was an invaluable technique.

The use of preliminary cleansing with alcohol or detergent has been recommended by some workers. It only appears to be important where new plastic catheters are used for the first time to get their inner surface thoroughly wet. Very small amounts of detergent also seem to minimize the trapping of small bubbles at connecting joints; exuberant use of wetting agents, however, may create foam which is very difficult to remove.

Free-vibration method

This method requires that a sudden change in pressure be imposed at the end of the manometer–catheter system. I have found that the simplest and most reliable way to do this is by rupturing a rubber membrane closing one end of a chamber that is inflated with air. The design of such an apparatus can be very varied. The one I use simply consists of a section of a sturdy lucite cylinder of ID about 4 cm and some 10–12 cm in length. This is clamped in a vertical position; the lower end is filled with a rubber bung, with two tubes piercing it. One tube passes at least halfway up the chamber and has an inflation bulb attached (a bulb from a sphygmomanometer is usually used). The end of the catheter to be tested passes through the other; for catheters we currently use a small glass chamber with a rubber seal at the lower end between two metal discs which screw together. Formerly, a catheter was held in the glass tube with artists 'modelling clay' (in England 'Plasticine' works very well). This only protrudes through the bung as the tip of the catheter must be kept under water. As flushing the system with boiled distilled water is carried out the necessary liquid level in the chamber is achieved.

The rubber membrane used is commonly cut from discarded surgical gloves but is better purchased in flat sheets. This needs to be stretched lightly, without an air-leak, over the end of the chamber. We commonly hold it in place by a rubber band wound around the top of the chamber under tension and held by a haemostat; a thicker piece of rubber with a circular hole cut in it and pulled over the membrane is quick and convenient (D. H. Bergel— personal communication). With a chamber such as described inflation produces a pressure of 40–50 mm Hg when the rubber is distended. A chamber such as described here is illustrated by Yanof (1965).

The most rapid and reliable method of rupturing the membrane appears to be burning (a lighted match or cigarette is very effective). This breaks the membrane explosively and causes an audible 'pop' (hence the nickname for the technique). The time for the pressure to drop to atmospheric is less than 1 msec judged by a high-frequency manometer such as the Statham SF-1. The pressure is displayed on an oscilloscope triggered to sweep when the pressure begins to drop and the sweep photographed. To save time (and rubber) an approximate idea of the resonant frequency can be obtained by giving a sharp tap to the catheter; if the same sweep speed is used (we standardize at 10 msec/cm) a little practice soon enables one to estimate the time between peaks. Thus, if an end-result of 80–100 Hz is expected it is easy to spot when the oscillations are markedly lower than this in the early stages of setting-up. A photograph is necessary for any accurate measurement of resonant frequency and for measuring the damping.

The main artifact in this technique is due to vibration of the cylinder support and this needs to be made extremely rigid so that its natural frequency is far higher than that of the manometer system. Even vibration of the chamber may introduce errors into the measurement of damping and is discussed below when considering analysis.

The problem of adequate support and after-vibrations is the reason why I have not adopted the attractively quick technique of Hansen (1949). This uses a syringe with a hole through the plunger and stem; an aperture is arranged on the stem so that it can be closed by a thumb, or finger, while withdrawing the plunger. The negative pressure thus produced can be suddenly released by lifting the thumb. A device of this kind can be easily made from a glass syringe with a hollow plunger; large holes can be blown in the end of the plunger and in the side of the neck. In my experience, it needs to be operated with a quick-withdrawal and release and I have found it difficult to do this without vibrating the whole system.

Analysis of results. A typical record made with a manometer system of low damping is shown in Fig. 8.5 which has the characteristic overshoot with oscillations dying away exponentially. The frequency is derived directly from the period between points of like phase in successive oscillations (time from peak-to-peak is normally measured). In Hansen's nomenclature, this frequency, in the presence of damping, is f_D (and the period correspondingly is designated T_D). In cases where the damping is as low as in the examples given in Table 8.1 the difference between the value of f_D and f_0 (the frequency if there were no damping) is not usually significant experimentally and the subscripts are only used when it is necessary to distinguish them.

The damping is calculated from the logarithmic decrement, Λ, from cycle to cycle. Hansen (1949) measured the deviation from the equilibrium position; I find it easier to measure the total excursion every half-cycle, i.e. from maximum deviation in one direction to maximum deviation in the other as shown in Fig. 8.6. The logarithmic decrement is then given by

$$\Lambda = 2 \, (\ln \theta_1 - \ln \theta_2) \qquad\qquad \textbf{8.20}$$

(where ln signifies the logarithm to base e).

This method has the practical advantage that (a) it is not necessary to

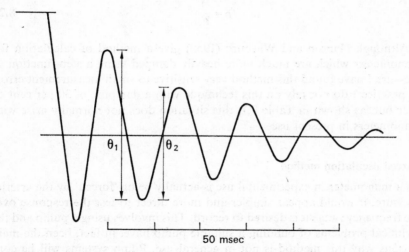

50 msec

Fig. 8.6. A sample trace enlarged from an oscillograph photograph of the vibrations created by a sudden pressure drop in a transducer–catheter system. The horizontal line at the start is the initial pressure before rupturing the membrane; the long horizontal line is the equilibrium position. The sweep velocity of the oscilloscope trace is marked along the bottom so that the resonant frequency is calculated from the period of each completed cycle.

The measures of θ_1 and θ_2 in successive half-cycles are used to measure the logarithmic decrement (eqn. 8.20) and thus the damping (eqn. 8.21) as described in the text.

record a base line separately and (b) if there is vibration of the apparatus distorting the apparent zero it is largely compensated by measuring deviations to either side. Nevertheless, there may be appreciable variation between the logarithmic decrement of each cycle and an average value of as many cycles as possible should be measured.

Figure 8.6 both illustrates the method of calculations and the cycle-to-cycle variation. Although Fig. 8.6 appears to be free of ectopic variations there is considerable variation in decrements that may be found. Plotting the measured pressure swings on semilogarithmic graph paper and drawing a mean slope is in many ways simpler.

The relative damping, β, is then given by

$$\beta = \frac{\Lambda}{\sqrt{(4\pi^2 + \Lambda^2)}} \qquad\qquad 8.21$$

The undamped natural frequency, f_0, if required, is given by

$$f_0 = \frac{\sqrt{(4\pi^2 + \Lambda^2)}}{2\pi T_D} \qquad\qquad 8.22$$

and it can be seen that when Λ is small compared to 2π then f_0 is close to

$$f_D = \frac{1}{T_D} \qquad\qquad 8.23$$

Although Hansen and Warburg (1950) give a method of calculation for manometers which are much more heavily damped using a step-function of pressure I have found this method very sensitive to small measurement error. In practice I do not rely on this technique with a damping of 30 per cent or over but, as shown in Table 8.1, this situation does not normally arise with manometers in present use.

Forced oscillation method

As a manometer in experimental use is actually being 'forced' by the arterial pressure, it would appear simpler and more direct to test the response over the frequency range it is desired to record. This involves using a pump and the technical problems of building a suitable pump have, in fact, been the main reasons why this method is not in general use. Pump systems will be considered in two categories; (i) completely water-filled, and (ii) with an air chamber above the liquid.

It is preferable to use a pump which develops a pressure oscillation which is known to be of constant amplitude over its whole frequency range. In a water-filled system, this requires a considerable amount of power and such constancy is most easily obtained with a mechanically-driven pump. As the pressure is created by compressing the water in the system, the volume displaced by the pump must be very small if the pressure oscillation is kept to a reasonable size. Yanof, Rosen, McDonald and McDonald (1963) used a sinusoidal pump with a frequency range of c. 0·5–90 Hz; the results in Table

8·1 (b) were from this paper. The eccentricity of the pump was of the order of $3-6 \times 10^{-4}$ cm and the stroke volume with a small plunger was about 0·23 mm³. The pressure oscillation this produced was about 60 mm Hg with a pump-chamber some 60 ml capacity. Figures 8.7 and 8.8 show records made

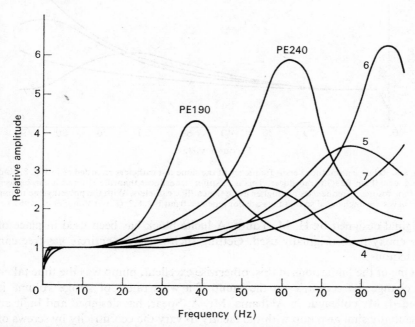

Fig. 8.7. Graphs made of records of relative pressure amplitude using a mechanical pump attached to a system comprising a Statham P23Dd transducer attached to a variety of catheters. Abscissa—pump frequency in Hz. Ordinate—relative pressure amplitude. Single numbers on curves refer to French sizes of USCI cardiac catheters; the two PE numbers refer to polyethylene tubing—ID. PE-190 was 0·06 cm, ID of PE-240 was 0·084 cm—which were larger in bore than any of the cardiac catheters. The low resonant frequency in these cases is due to the large distensibility of the polyethylene tubing compared to the transducer. This is emphasized by the fact that Fig. 8.8 shows how the resonance frequency in all the cardiac catheters systems is increased by using a stiffer transducer but the amplitude curves of the polyethylene tubing is not changed (and hence not repeated in that figure). (From Yanof *et al.*, 1963.)

with this pump. Such an eccentric would be hard to duplicate although a larger one would be tolerable if a larger pump chamber was used. The essential features of the design are given by Yanof *et al.* (1963) but my present pump is modified in certain small details. The gears in the drive-shaft are eliminated; the maximum frequency is thereby limited to 60 Hz but the direct drive would make it possible to drive an harmonic resolver from the main shaft. The use of glass syringes has also been eliminated. Stroke volume is varied by using interchangeable brass plungers with a Teflon cuff in the orifice of the pump block. The sloping top of the pump chamber with the location of a bleed-tap at the apex to facilitate removal of all air has been retained as in the

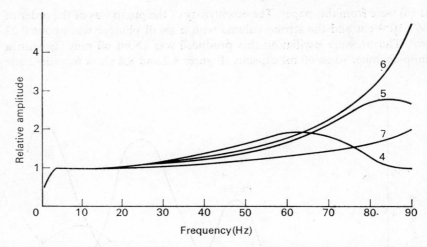

Fig. 8.8. Relative amplitude versus frequency of the same test catheters recorded as in Fig. 8.7 but using a Statham P23Gb transducer. This is a 'stiffer' transducer than the Dd and it can be seen that the resonant frequencies are higher using the cardiac catheters. With the polyethylene tubing the curves are unchanged so that they are not repeated from Fig. 8.7. (From Yanof *et al.*, 1963.)

original designed by H. M. Yanof. A lucite block has been used in place of the epoxy resin originally used. Getting such a system entirely gas-free can be tedious.

One of the limitations in this, otherwise excellent, pump was the time taken to change the eccentric on the pump if a wide range of stroke volume is needed. My colleague in Alabama, Mr. A. Spear, has designed and built an essentially similar pump with the facility to vary the eccentricity by screws of fine pitch; this has avoided the usual difficulties with designs using Scotch yokes in that they commonly have an intolerable amount of backlash.

A much wider frequency range can be more easily achieved with a diaphragm which is electrically driven. A neat little apparatus of this kind was designed by Linden (1958) in which a brass diaphragm was driven by a barium titanate crystal made to oscillate by an applied sinusoidal voltage. The behaviour of the titanate unit he originally recommended was, however, dubious below 20 Hz—an important part of the range for physiological purposes—and needed a sinusoidal voltage of some ±200 V to produce a reasonable pressure which we found difficult to achieve. The principle seems both simple and effective and modern piezo-electric ceramics may eliminate some of the difficulties we found ten years ago. Vierhout and Vendrick (1961) have also described an electrically driven pump with circuits designed to maintain a constant displacement in spite of variations in load which is reported to give good results. Hansen and Warburg (1950) described five different devices and Hansen (1949) designed and used a magnetic pump.

Some of the problems relating to a completely liquid filled system can be avoided by using an air-chamber over the liquid. Such a system may be driven mechanically (e.g. Ball and Gabe, 1963) or electrically driven (e.g. Fry, Noble and Mallos, 1957a). In this case, however, the pressure generated by a pump of constant stroke varies with frequency in the lower frequency range owing to adiabatic compression effect. Thus, the pressure oscillation increases with frequency until it reaches a steady value as given by eqn. 8.18 for an adiabatic change. This was measured specifically by Ball and Gabe (1963) and means that the pressure generated by the pump must be monitored by a second manometer, known to be accurate over the range being tested, attached to the pump chamber. Such a system was used by Fry et al. (1957a) in their thorough, and pioneer, investigation of a wide range of manometers available at that time. A monitor was also deemed necessary in this case to ensure that the pressure created by the electrically driven diaphragm was accurately known. These authors incorporated the membrane of a Lilly capacitance manometer into the wall of the compression chamber; they state that this device had a flat response to 1,000 Hz.

ARTIFACTS IN PRESSURE RECORDING

(1) End-pressure artifact

Pressure is defined as the force exerted per unit area on the walls enclosing a fluid. A flowing liquid also has a kinetic energy by virtue of its motion; this is discussed more fully in Ch. 9 in relation to flow-meters. On arresting the flow this energy will appear as a pressure. Thus, if the tip of a catheter points upstream it will record the sum of the lateral pressure and the converted kinetic energy. The kinetic energy per cm³ of blood (KE) in these circumstances is given by

$$KE = \frac{\rho V^2}{2} \text{ dyn cm}$$

where V is the velocity in the streamlines impacting on the catheter tip and ρ is the density of the liquid. The pressure equivalent of this energy is relatively small. If V is 100 cm/sec and the density of blood is taken as 1·0 the equivalent pressure is given by

$$P = \frac{(100)^2}{2} \text{ dyn/cm}^2 = \frac{10^4}{2(1333)} \text{ mm Hg} = 3\cdot76 \text{ mm Hg}$$

Similarly for a velocity of 50 cm/sec it will be one-fourth this (i.e. less than 1 mm Hg) but for a flow velocity of 200 cm/sec it would be 15·0 mm Hg. Flow velocities of the order of 100 cm/sec or higher are only found as peak velocities (Ch. 6) in the large vessels close to the heart. In more peripheral vessels the kinetic energy will be very small in terms of absolute magnitude. However, the peak velocity of flow, e.g. Fig. 6.1, commonly precedes the pressure peak and hence an end-pressure artifact will show as a hump on the rising phase of the pressure limb. Undoubtedly a lot of the discussion on the 'anacrotic wave' of the pulse wave in the older literature was, in fact, concerned with such an artifact.

The actual magnitude of the kinetic energy artifact will be more unpredictable than the simple exposition above suggests. Unless the velocity profile is known the velocity of the flow impacting on the catheter end will not be known. In all flow patterns—even in the very 'flat profiles' (Ch. 3) which almost certainly occur in the large vessels close to the heart—the velocity falls rapidly close to the wall. Therefore, if the catheter tip lies against the wall the kinetic energy there will be small. Usually, a long moderately stiff catheter introduced from a peripheral artery will be held against the wall by its springiness on passing around any bend, such as the junction of the iliac artery and the aorta. It is not, however, at all certain. As it is difficult to allow for an artifact of unpredictable amplitude, it is best avoided. This is achieved by closing the tip and having lateral holes. When using a catheter-tip manometer such as the SF-1 this can be achieved by fitting a small cap, suitably perforated over the brass tip. I have found good tips made of a short length of polyethylene tube satisfactory.

Even so, it is possible, when recording in the ascending aorta, that a catheter passing around the arch of the aorta may lie obliquely across the lumen so that a 'lateral' hole may be subject to some flow impact. Very precise measurements in this area, as for the determination of pressure-gradients, is thus subject to some uncertainty.

To summarize, the end-pressure artifact is usually small but should be guarded against as a source of distortion of the shape of a pressure-curve; for accurate quantitative analysis, it clearly needs to be eliminated.

(2) Catheter impact artifact

Whenever the liquid-filled catheter is hit a transient pressure is created by the acceleration; any frequency component of this transient which coincides with the resonant frequency of the manometer system will create a pressure oscillation imposed on the recorded wave-form. When intracardiac catheters are used every heart-beat creates such a transient. The frequencies that cause this effect rarely exceed 50 Hz; the higher the resonant frequency of the system above 50 Hz the less intrusive this distortion is. In addition, very rapid changes of pressure such as in the rising phase of intraventricular pressure, or the 'incisura' caused by the closure of the aortic valves, can also cause free vibration of this kind. Inspection of a record by looking for such transient vibrations will give a very good estimate of the resonant frequency of the system in use.

It is not always appreciated how much the superimposition of such transients may distort measurements made from such a pulse-curve. An example is shown in Fig. 8.9 in which the pressure in a human left ventricle is recorded

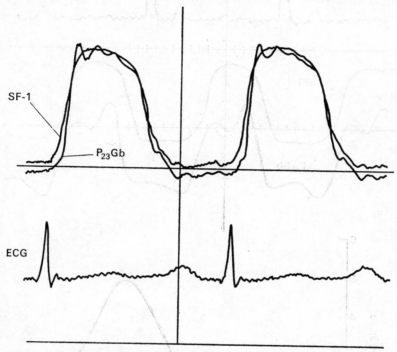

Fig. 8.9. Two simultaneous tracings of the left ventricular pressure in a human subject. A Statham SF-1 catheter-tip manometer was introduced into the ventricle; the transducer in the catheter-tip has a very high resonant frequency of 2,000 Hz. The pressure recorded with this transducer is marked SF-1. Simultaneously a Statham P23Gb recorder was attached to the lumen of the catheter via approximately 6 ft of wide-bore polyethylene tubing so that the transducer could be kept well away from the patient. In spite of very careful flushing to remove all air bubbles the resonant frequency of this system was only about 25 Hz.

Comparing the two pressure traces it can be seen that the high-frequency trace of the SF-1 shows a smooth-rounded top to the ventricular pressure. By contrast the low-frequency P23 trace overshoots in a 'spike' with after-vibrations—for many years this spike was taken as a normal component of the ventricular pressure. Furthermore, the rate of rise of the pressure in the low-frequency curve is much steeper than the high-fidelity recording; in fact, the maximum value of dp/dt is artificially increased some 40 per cent in the low-fidelity recording.

simultaneously with a catheter-tip (SF-1) manometer and with a P23G gauge attached to the lumen through a considerable length of polythene tubing.* From the small oscillations seen throughout the cycle it can be deduced that the resonant frequency of this system was about 25 Hz while the resonant frequency of the SF-1 was c. 2,000 Hz.

* This record was made on a patient with a congenital heart defect by the late Dr. Weizmann and Dr. Honey in the Department of Cardiology, St. Bartholomew's Hospital, London, in 1962. The system was well flushed and the low resonant frequency was almost certainly due to the polyethylene tubing which had been used routinely up to that time.

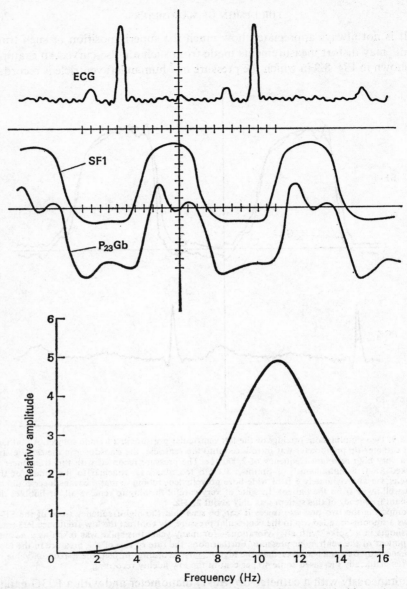

Fig. 8.10A. Two recordings of ventricular pressure, made in the dog, recorded with a catheter-tip SF-1 manometer. The lower trace was made through the lumen of the catheter to which a P23Gb transducer was directly connected. When thoroughly free of air bubbles the tracings from both channels were indistinguishable. The frequency response was then deliberately degraded by introducing a small air-bubble and when this was done the overshoot and secondary hump appeared on the top of the pressure tracing. The frequency response of the upper trace is c. 2,000 Hz; by the analysis shown in Fig. 8.10B below the resonant frequency of the lower trace is only c. 11 Hz.

B. A Fourier analysis of both curves was performed and the amplitude of the lower frequency trace relative to that of the SF-1 was plotted as a graph which shows a typical resonance curve similar to those shown in Fig. 8.1. This illustrates how the use of a low-frequency manometer system can introduce distortions into a pressure curve.

In spite of the general belief that high rates of pressure change are only recorded by high-frequency manometers it can be seen that the apparent rate of rise is higher in the P23G recording. Coupled with the spike at the top of the rise, it is clear that superimposition of a transient oscillation has given a spuriously high value to the rate of pressure rise which is recorded correctly by the SF-1. In fact, the maximum dp/dt is approximately 40 per cent too high in the low-frequency recording.

In my experience, the presence of this initial spike on a ventricular pressure record is always an artifact of this kind (if the record is made in the outflow tract a kinetic energy artifact may also occur). With an even lower frequency system appearances may be even more deceptive. Fig. 8.10A shows two records made in a similar way in a dog ventricle; in this case, the P23 system response had been deliberately degraded by introducing a small bubble. The resonant frequency of the P23 system was 11 Hz but it produces a wave which many physiologists would regard as normal. Figure 8.10B compares the amplitudes of the harmonic components of the two curves (normalizing to the amplitudes of the SF-1 record). They form a classic resonance curve of the type shown in Fig. 8.1.

The example of the high-frequency record made with the SF-1 shows that impact and resonance artifacts can be eliminated with a high enough resonant frequency. If a catheter-tipped manometer is not available the values given in Table 8.1 show that, with care in setting up, resonant frequencies of the order of 100 Hz and above can be achieved with straingauge manometers and cardiac catheters.

The use of increased damping

In so far as these artifacts are due to resonance, an attractive way of eliminating them appears to be by increasing the damping. In the initial theoretical section above, it was pointed out that a damping coefficient of 0·7 can give an accurate curve. To this end, electrical damping circuits are often incorporated in commercial amplifiers for blood-pressure recording; methods of hydraulic damping are also variously used. The practical difficulties that this introduces, if precise analysis is to be made, are not, however, often appreciated. (i) An 'optimally' damped response is only 'flat' (within 5 per cent of true value) to about 60 per cent of the undamped resonant frequency. Thus, the trace in Fig. 8.6 with a resonant frequency of 25 Hz could only be made good in terms of amplitude to 15 Hz; (ii) As discussed in Methods of Calibration, a measure of the damping in such a case is only possible if a good pump system is available. (iii) The phase shift is only linear with frequency (Fig. 8.2) if the damping is very close to 0·7. The damping coefficient is very sensitive to catheter diameter; eqn. 8.8 shows that it varies inversely as the cube of the radius. Thus, if a layer of fibrin is deposited in the catheter it may change markedly during the course of an experiment, or in a long series of clinical

H

observations. To take an example, if a film of fibrin only 20 μm thick were deposited in a no. 4 French size catheter (int. radius 0·23 mm) the damping would be increased such that an initial measured damping of 0·7 would be increased to 0·94. Reference to Fig. 8.1 shows that the recorded amplitude would then fall continuously with increasing frequency and the phase lag (Fig. 8.2) would also increase markedly if the initial damping was 0·2, how-ever, the increase would be to 0·27 and would produce little amplitude change over the working frequency range (but would increase the phase lag by about 30 per cent in this range). Teflon catheters of approximately this bore are commonly left *in situ* for long periods in clinical investigations. In such a catheter a film of 50 μm thickness would more than double the damping and if the initial situation was with 0·7 damping the effect would be disastrous but would be tolerable at least in terms of amplitude. With a larger catheter the effect would naturally be smaller. In a no. 7 French catheter (int. radius 0·56 mm) a 50 μm film would produce a result similar to that of a 20 μm film in a no. 4 F catheter.

Thin layers of fibrin are very difficult to prevent by the use of anticoagu-lants, if blood is allowed to enter the catheter at any time. Use of continuous flushing with a slow flow of saline can be used; such a flow in a long, narrow catheter requires an appreciable head of pressure which will distort the measured mean pressure unless it is very carefully controlled.

To summarize: Modern pressure transducers used with standard cardiac catheters have a high resonant frequency with low damping when scrupu-lously filled with liquid. This allows accurate amplitude measurement with very small phase shift up to rather more than 20 per cent of the resonant frequency. This usually covers the physiologically significant frequency range. The resonant frequency and damping in these circumstances are easily measured.

A flat amplitude response up to 50 per cent of the undamped natural frequency can be obtained by increasing the damping to 0·7; the phase lag is then linear with frequency and is thus predictable. Damping of this order is more difficult to measure yet must be known fairly accurately because the characteristic response curves change rapidly with deviations from this damping. Either condition is capable of producing accurate results if the system is well-calibrated. The danger with arbitrarily increasing the damping is that it may be used as a short-cut that avoids the tedium of obtaining the maximal response from the manometer–catheter system in the first place; a heavily damped system with an initially low resonant frequency will have very poor performance characteristics.

9
Flowmeters for Pulsatile Flow

Until relatively recently techniques for measuring the pulsatile flow in arteries lagged a long way behind pressure measurement techniques. This was a severe limitation on the analysis of the hydrodynamics of the circulation. The advances that have been made in the present decade may be appreciated by quoting my own assessment of the situation in 1959 (McDonald, 1960): 'the development of an accurate flowmeter is, in my opinion, the principal problem in fundamental work on the circulation today. The variety of meters that have been used is, of itself, sufficient comment on their generally unsatisfactory nature.'

Today, a flowmeter of at least tolerable accuracy is virtually standard laboratory equipment. In the majority of cases, this is an electromagnetic flowmeter, with ultrasonic meters as an alternative choice. In 1960 the electromagnetic flowmeter was regarded as the most likely to be effective but results from different models varied widely and no calibration data were available. At that time, the ultrasonic flowmeter was only briefly noted under 'Other Methods'. This illustrates how rapidly a technical account can become overtaken by events; this is now apparent in the rapid development of miniature intravascular probes. The present chapter will, therefore, only survey the principles involved and the performance characteristics where they are well-established. Brief notice is also taken of other methods which may be regarded as obsolete at present, but may yet come into use again. More detailed reviews have been made by Wetterer (1963) and Mills (1972). In the section edited by Fry (1966, in Vol. 11 of *Methods in Medical Research*) a wide range of flow measurement techniques is surveyed both for mean and pulsatile flows with especially recommended chapters on the electromagnetic flowmeter (Bergel and Gessner, 1966) and the pulsed ultrasonic flowmeter (Baker, 1966). A whole symposium devoted to flowmeters has appeared and comprises a wide survey (Cappelen, 1968).

THE ELECTROMAGNETIC FLOWMETER

This meter uses the principle of magnetic induction. When an electrical conductor moves across the lines of force of a magnetic field a potential difference is created. Michael Faraday himself, in 1832, attempted to measure such an induced voltage created by the flow of the river Thames in the earth's magnetic field. He failed to detect it but, as Sharcliff (1962) points out, he lived to hear of Woolaston's success, in 1851, in measuring voltages induced by tidal currents in the English Channel. In 1917 a device for measuring the speed of ships was patented; it measured the voltage induced between two electrodes on the hull with a magnetic field created by the ship. But not until 1930 was the possibility investigated of using the technique as a flowmeter (by E. J. Williams, cited by Sharcliff, 1962).

As blood is a conductor of electricity its velocity of movement may be measured by aligning a blood-vessel across a magnetic field and recording the induced e.m.f. Provided that (1) the field is uniform, (2) the conductor moves in a plane at right angles to the field, and (3) the length of the conductor extends at right angles to both field and direction of motion, then the potential difference is given by the following equation (Jochim, 1948):

$$E = H . L . \overline{V} . 10^{-8} \hspace{3cm} \textbf{9.1}$$

where E is the potential difference in volts, H the strength of the magnetic field in gauss, L the length of conductor within the field in cm, i.e. the internal diameter of the vessel, and $\overline{V}$ the velocity of the conductor in cm/sec. As a typical example, if the field density is 300 gauss, the diameter of the vessel is 0·5 cm and a velocity of 100 cm/sec (a diameter and a peak velocity likely in a dog aorta) the voltage predicted will be 300 μV; in fact, it will be rather less. The discrimination of such small signals was the problem in the delayed development of the technique for so long. If H and L are kept constant it can be seen that the potential difference recorded varies linearly with the velocity of flow and, in fact, the velocity recorded is the average velocity across the pipe (Kolin, 1945; Shercliff, 1962). The calibration curve is thus a straight line passing through the origin.

After a preliminary model made by Fabre (1932) which attracted little attention, the instrument was introduced into physiology independently by Kolin (1936, 1937) in the United States and Wetterer (1937) in Germany. Its advantages are the linear calibration noted above and that it can be applied to an unopened vessel. It also records backflows as well as forward flows.

The problem of creating a uniform magnetic field forms a practical obstacle in applying the meter to some arteries, but, with improvement of design, small electromagnets have been developed which can be applied to any reasonably accessible vessel. Interference due to the electrical potentials created by the heart which was earlier thought to limit its use, was soon overcome, for Wetterer and Deppe (1940) used it successfully on the ascending aorta (Fig. 9.1) and its use there is now commonplace.

The simplest form has a constant magnetic field (the d.c. type) and the recording system has to use a direct-coupled amplifier. Surface potentials

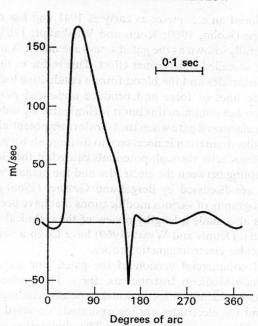

Fig. 9.1. A flow curve recorded in the ascending aorta of a dog (Wetterer and Deppe, 1940) with an electromagnetic flowmeter (redrawn from Wetterer, 1954).

Forward flow is virtually confined to the period of systolic ejection, the end of which is marked by a sharp but brief backflow.

formed at the electrodes are relatively large compared with those induced in the flowing blood and it is difficult to discriminate between them in a d.c. system. The d.c. meter also suffers a lot from zero drift due to the polarization caused by the small current generated. Jochim (1948) attempted to minimize the electrode potentials by embedding them in Perspex blocks which fitted closely around the artery. A similar apparatus was used by Richards and Williams (1953). Inouye, Kuga and Usui (1955) and Inouye and Kosaka (1959) have also used this type of meter, as have Feder and Bay (1959). They find it satisfactory for intermittent short runs which do not allow significant polarization.

It is interesting to find that the electromagnetic flowmeter has an important application in measuring the flow of liquid metals such as sodium, which are used as heat-exchange materials in nuclear reactors. The very detailed theoretical analysis by Shercliff (1962) arose from this application. As polarization due to electrolysis is no problem here these meters are usually of this d.c. type.

To avoid polarization effects some form of alternation of the current generating the magnetic field is now virtually always used in meters for physiological use. This alternation may be sinusoidal, the a.c. meter, or use a specific wave-form as in the square-wave and trapezoidal-wave flowmeters.

Kolin had introduced an a.c. meter as early as 1941 and has developed and improved this type (Kolin, 1960; Kolin and Wisshaupt, 1963) to the satisfactory form generally known as the gated sine-wave meter. A major difficulty has been with the so-called transformer effect. This is due to the fact that the electrode leads, electrodes and the blood form a conductive loop which is cut by some magnetic lines of force and produce undesired potentials. Good design of the probe can minimize this but it is eliminated by only sampling the signal through an electronic gate when the transformer potential is zero. In the a.c. meter phase-discrimination is necessary to distinguish forward from back flow. Other problems arise through potentials caused at the electrode–artery interface and coupling between the electrodes and the magnet winding. These technical aspects are discussed by Bergel and Gessner (1966) (they also give an extensive bibliography of various modifications that have been introduced); Wyatt (1961) has also made a lengthy review of the technical problems, and sources of artifacts. Dennis and Wyatt (1969) have taken a very critical look at some intravascular electromagnetic probes.

A widely used commercial version of the gated sine-wave meter is the 'Medicon' (Statham-Medicon Instruments, Inc.). The probes are made of plastic of the order of 2 mm thick in which coreless windings to create the magnetic field and the electrodes are incorporated; standard sizes available range from 2 to 22 mm internal diameter. The elimination of an iron core removes errors due to hysteresis but greatly reduces the strength of the magnetic field created (to increase sensitivity they are retained in the small sizes) and the signal-to-noise ratio, of a signal of only a few microvolts, is very small. The development of a meter and probes for use on the coronary arteries and small vessels generally has been specially studied by Khouri and Gregg (1963), Khouri et al. (1968). Understandably, care in grounding the animal is necessary and metal in the vicinity of the probe needs to be reduced to a minimum. A metal operating-table, for example, makes it virtually impossible to achieve a noise-free record.

The introduction of the square-wave electromagnetic flowmeter was due to Denison, Spencer, and Green (1955) as a way to avoid the problems they had found with an a.c. meter (Richardson, Denison, and Green, 1952). The magnet's current is pulsed in a square-wave form in which the polarity is reversed and the signal is sampled by a gate during the stable part of the field at the top of the square-wave. As this model uses iron-cores in the probes there is considerable oscillation of the field each time the current is reversed. The time available for sampling the flow signal is thus very short (the Carolina Medical Electronics, Inc., model uses 240 Hz; the Avionics Research Products Corporation model used 330 Hz). To improve the possibility of accurate gating Yanof (1961) developed a trapezoidal-wave model and this problem of design is discussed in this paper and also in Yanof (1965). The metal cores of the square-wave model also tend to heat up considerably. Nevertheless, it is in wide use although its calibration characteristics are far worse than the gated sine-wave meter (Bergel and Gessner, 1966).

Another electromagnetic flowmeter that is presently in common use is that made by Biotronex, Inc. The system is described as a pulsed logic system and appears to incorporate some features of both the gated sine-wave and square system. Like the Medicon it uses air coils in the probes with a metal core (in fact, the Medicon and Biotronex probes can be used interchangeably).

Performance characteristics

The simplicity of eqn. 9.1 would suggest that calibration of the electromagnetic flowmeter is simply a matter of knowing the field strength and the diameter of the vessel. In fact, the measured signal is less than that predicted by the equation; (i) the use of short probes inevitably causes a non-uniformity of the magnetic field with the result that the effective strength is less than that calculated for a given coil winding; (ii) some of the signal is shunted around the outer surface of the arterial wall and the fluid on its surface both of which are electrically conductive (Gessner, 1961).

In addition, the validity of the assumption of linearity needs to be considered. Shercliff (1962) has shown theoretically that eqn. 9.1 is valid for $\bar{V}$ as a representation of the average velocity of flow across the tube, whatever the velocity profile, provided that it is symmetrical about the axis. This result, which Shercliff attributes originally to Thürlemann in 1941, is intuitively surprising and he refers to it as a mathematical fluke. Thus, it is immaterial whether the flow is laminar or turbulent and disturbances produced by valves will not produce a distortion unless the effect is asymmetrical, which is unlikely with a normal valve. As a result, this factor has, in general, been ignored. The secondary flows produced by bends (Ch. 4) will, however, produce asymmetry of flow profile; the most prominent example is the arch of the aorta and thus recordings made in the upper thoracic aorta are particularly likely to be distorted from this cause. This factor has been investigated by Goldman, Marple, and Scolnick (1963).

These various factors underline the necessity for calibration. Each probe needs to be tested for its output signal in terms of flow; this can be regarded as a calibration factor and will include any theoretical error under (i) above. If it is calibrated using a length of artery with blood in it then the error under (ii) will be mostly included. The magnitude of this effect will, in part, depend on the contact between the electrode and the wall. This will change with variations in the distension of the artery with changes of arterial pressure. In practice, considerable change in artery size seems to be able to occur without any measurable change in effective contact. Some workers deliberately choose a probe that will produce a marked constriction of the artery to minimize this effect. Such a constriction, however, produces distortions both of pressure and flow patterns. I always aim to produce as good a fit as possible without visible constriction of the artery. If experiments are planned in which large drops in mean pressure are anticipated for any length of time, as in studying the effects of haemorrhage, it is better to change to a smaller probe when the artery becomes visibly too small for the larger probe.

Testing the effects of non-symmetrical profiles is more difficult and should be done with the probe *in situ* with a known flow imposed with a pump. The velocities created should be equivalent to those in the living animal if equivalent effects on the profile are to be achieved.

The dynamic response of the main types of electromagnetic flowmeters have been tested by Gessner and Bergel (1964) and Bergel and Gessner (1966). They tested them both hydraulically with a sinusoidal pump and electrically by imposing an electrical signal on the electrodes. They found no significant difference between the two methods indicating that the dynamic characteristics were determined by the electrical circuitry. Once this has been measured, therefore, it is not necessary to repeat it except at long intervals. Their results for the Medicon K-2000 model and the Carolina square wave model are shown in Fig. 9.2. The gated sine-wave meter has an amplitude response which is virtually constant to 10 Hz and then falls off almost linearly to about 81 per cent at 40 Hz. The phase lag is also virtually linear and amounts to about 3·6° per Hz and is thus easily corrected for. With colleagues in Philadelphia I obtained very similar results in the later Medicon M-4000 model using only a hydraulic model and a sinusoidal pump (described under pressure calibration in Ch. 8, p. 200). However, we found the amplitude response virtually flat to 20 Hz with a slight tendency to over-read above that. However, the records above 20 Hz tended to be noisy because the excised arterial segment vibrated and there is uncertainty about these higher frequency results. The phase lag was found to be linear and of approximately the same amplitude. It is much larger than one would desire but, because of its linearity, is easy to correct in individual harmonic components for the time-lag is the same. For a dog with a pulse-frequency of 2 Hz the amplitude response is good to 5 harmonics and within 5 per cent appreciably beyond this. Thus, it would cover all harmonics of any significant size (Ch. 7).

The response of the square-wave meter was far less satisfactory. It is 'flat' only to about 5 Hz and then falls rapidly to about 80 per cent at 10 Hz and is only 30 per cent at 40 Hz. Equally, the phase lag increases approximately linearly to 45° at 10 Hz and then more slowly to reach 100° by 30 Hz. Calibration data have also been reported by O'Rourke (1965).

If harmonic analysis is being performed and detailed curves of response characteristics are available then correction for any flowmeter can be made. Furthermore, except in special circumstances referred to above, once the characteristics of probe and meter have been determined, they will remain sufficiently constant for only a periodic check to be necessary.

The discussion above had assumed throughout that a probe applied to the outside of the artery has been used. The ability to measure flow in an un-opened artery is one of the major advantages of the electromagnetic flow-meter. In addition, its linearity and the relative indifference to the form of the velocity profile which is theoretically calculated and experimentally confirmed give it formidable advantage.

For reasons of stability and increased sensitivity, cannulatory probes are still used on occasions. These are usually only for small vessels (e.g. c. 2 mm diameter) where low sensitivities, and obtaining a good fit with an external probe, are problems. The distortions introduced by the introduction of a rigid cannula were discussed at considerable length by McDonald (1960). For cannulae the length of a present-day probe they were found to be negligible. Lengths of tubing of the order of 15 cm which had been used by some workers to take the flow to an externally placed meter were found to introduce

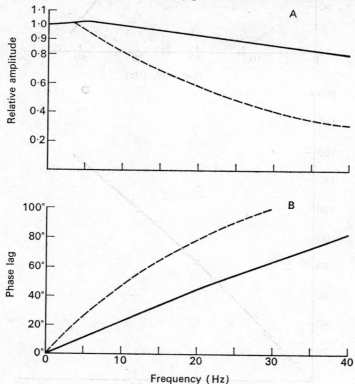

Fig. 9.2A and B. Frequency responses of two electromagnetic flowmeters—A shows amplitude response; B—shows phase lag. The solid line (——) gated sine-wave flowmeter (Medicon Model 2000). The broken line shows response of square-wave flowmeter (Carolina Medical Electronics). Calibrations were done both electrically and hydraulically with no significant difference between the two (data derived from Bergel and Gessner, 1966).

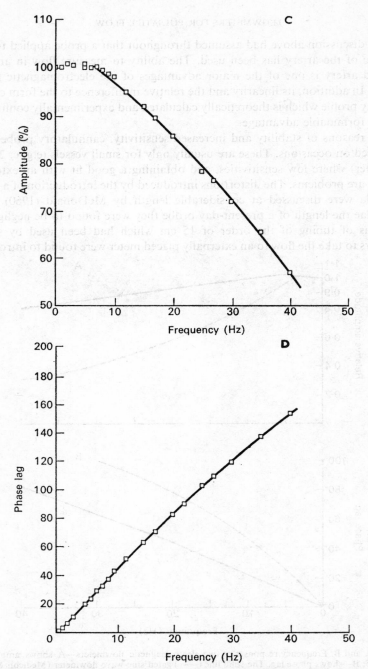

Fig. 9.2C and **D.** Corresponding amplitude and phase components of one of our current Statham Medical Model 4001 flowmeters (electrical calibration) which is in current use in my laboratory. This differs considerably from the calibration reported in the text for another flowmeter of the same model number in 1965. (Record made by Dr. Michel Gerin.)

very marked damping. As no such meter is now in use, the calculations will not be repeated here.

The main weakness of the electromagnetic flowmeter is in the precise determination of its zero. Meter zero obtained by switching off the magnet current is fallacious. The most reliable way is to arrest flow by occluding the vessel; to prevent the wall falling away from the probe the occlusion should be downstream of the probe but with no intervening branch. With the large vessels this puts a big strain on the heart; also some pulsatile flow remains because the occluded stump is distensible. Gated sine-wave meters commonly have a device which allows a 90° shift in the position of the gate when a flow signal should be zero. In practice, one sets this to the position of minimum oscillation but again a very flat zero line is not usually obtained, and in an aortic flow curve the uncertainty of the zero reading may be as much as 5–10 ml/sec. The problem of precise measurement of the zero or the integrated mean flow is inherent in the fact that in major arteries the peak flow is commonly at least six times as great as the mean flow so that flow curves should be recorded on as big a vertical scale as possible.

Measurement of flow in small vessels is also not very reliable with an electromagnetic flowmeter but this is common to nearly all meters; in fact, many of the types described below can only be used on large vessels.

An electromagnetic flowmeter that is built on to the end of a catheter and can be used intravascularly has been described (Mills 1966; Mills and Shillingford, 1967; Bond and Barefoot, 1967). It is discussed below (p. 226) in relation to other flowmeters which may be used intravascularly; this important technical development is advancing very rapidly at the present time.

ULTRASONIC FLOWMETERS

The velocity of sound in a flowing fluid is the algebraic sum of the characteristic velocity of sound in the fluid and the stream velocity. For flow of a liquid in an elastic tube the sound frequency has to be high to ensure that the elastically determined wave-velocity (Ch. 10) does not interfere and that the velocity of transmission is determined exclusively by the properties of the liquid. Frequencies in the range 1–8 MHz are now routinely used. The principle has been used for the measurement of the velocity of fast-flowing liquids but it was originally felt that the velocities of flow found in the bloodstream were so small relative to that of sound as to make it technically impossible to build an apparatus that was sufficiently accurate. The impossible has, however, been achieved by four different methods. When one remembers that the velocity of sound in water is about 1,500 m/sec and the peak velocities reached in the ascending aorta are about 150 cm/sec or 1/1,000 the velocity of sound, it will be appreciated that a precision of 1 in 10^5 is necessary to detect flow velocities within 1–2 cm/sec.

The methods used have been (a) phase-shift detection; (b) pulse transit time; (c) Doppler frequency shift, and (d) the recently introduced pulsed Doppler technique.

(a) *Phase-shift detection* has priority from the historical point of view for a meter of this type was described by Haugen, Farrell, Herrick and Baldes (1955). They used crystals with a frequency of 300–400 kHz, and a flow velocity of 100 cm/sec only represented a phase shift of about 3°, so that an ability to discriminate phases down to 1/100 of this was required. This needed extremely elaborate phase-stabilizing circuits and was very expensive to build. Little has been published on its physiological use apart from a report by Marshall and Shepherd (1959). It does not appear to have been developed further although the technique becomes more feasible with the higher frequency crystals that became available a few years later.

(b) *Pulse transit time* is measured in the type of meter that has come to be known as the pulsed ultrasonic flowmeter. First reported by Franklin, Ellis and Rushmer (1959), later versions have been described in more detail by Franklin, Baker, and Rushmer (1962) and Baker (1966). The principle is very simple. A cuff is placed around a length of artery which incorporates two crystals diagonally placed at the ends. Both crystals can act as transmitter and receiver. A short tone-burst of 5 MHz is first emitted at the upstream end and the time of transmission to the far end recorded; the next burst is sent in the reverse direction. Transit time is measured by starting a ramp voltage rising with each pulse emitted and which is stopped by the reception of the pulse; the voltage is than a measure of the time t. As the line of transmission is oblique the expression for the average velocity is given by

$$t = \overline{V}(2d/c^2) \cos \theta \qquad \qquad \textbf{9.2}$$

where $\overline{V}$ is the average velocity in the line of the sound beam, d is the diagonal distance between the two crystals, c is the velocity of sound in the liquid and θ is the angle between the line of the sound beam and the axis of the tube.

The angle θ is made quite large in the later probes to keep the length of the cuff down to 1–3 cm according to the size of the vessel it is designed for. In Rushmer's group they have been used extensively as chronically implanted probes on vessels ranging in size from the hepatic and renal arteries to the ascending aorta and superior vena cava.

Baker (1966) reports that the response is linear for steady flows from 0 to 180 ml/sec and that the electrical circuitry has a uniform frequency response from 0 to 50 Hz. Hydraulically it is found to have a flat response up to 10 Hz, which was the limit of the pump available. Comparison with an electromagnetic flowmeter shows a close matching.

The rate of sampling can be varied and appears to be normally done a few hundred times per second. Baker (1966) states that the cycle from pulse emission to reception and recording takes only 120 μsec so that several meters on various arteries can be used simultaneously on a 'time-sharing' basis with a single electronic unit.

The theoretical relation between the velocity measured and the velocity profile has not been investigated with the thoroughness with which it has been done for the electromagnetic flowmeter. Baker (1966) discussed the 'averaging' facility in terms of the beam width of the emitted sound. As the crystal is commonly $\frac{1}{4}$–$\frac{1}{2}$ of the ID of the vessel considerable averaging would occur. He concludes, reasonably, that the only precise value would be obtained with a flat velocity profile. Errors from this source are unlikely to be great provided the profile is symmetrical.

Zero calibration can theoretically be checked when flow has been stopped by reversing the sequence of pulse emissions; this would cause a reversal of flow pattern but will cause no shift if there is no flow. The problem of creating zero flow in large vessels is the same as with the electromagnetic flowmeter.

The fact that a rigid cuff has to be placed on the artery makes the general limitations to its use much the same as for electromagnetic probes. Indeed, the ultrasonic cuffs are usually longer and rather more difficult to place without interference from branches. The only superiority claimed for the pulsed ultrasonic flowmeter is its greater stability but it has so far been less widely used than the Doppler effect model or than the electromagnetic flowmeter.

(c) *The Doppler effect* is the cause of the familiar experience of hearing a rise in pitch (i.e. of frequency) of the sound of a train whistle that is approaching and the fall in pitch that occurs when the train passes and begins to recede. The alteration of frequency of an emitted wave when the source is moving relative to the observer is, of course, not limited to audible sound. The Doppler flowmeter uses this effect when the effective source is the origin of a wave from a stationary source reflected from a moving object. In the case of blood the reflection arises from the flowing erythrocytes and is usually referred to as 'back-scatter' to distinguish it from reflection from moving solid surfaces such as the arterial wall.

The use of ultrasonic waves and the Doppler effect in its present form was first reported by Franklin, Schlegel and Rushmer (1961); later reports came from Baker *et al.* (1964), and Baker (1965). It was originally demonstrated to a Biomedical Engineering Conference in 1964 (where especial interest was aroused, in an evening session, when Rushmer showed that it would monitor the flow of beer down the oesophagus—apparently due to the gas-bubbles in it, as water flow could not be measured). The design of the probe is simple in that an angled titanate crystal used for emission is mounted next to another crystal used for receiving the back-scattered waves. The reflected wave is used to modulate the emitter frequency and the resultant frequency due to the Doppler shift is in the audio-range, so that for qualitative monitoring the signal may be used to drive a loud-speaker.

The angle at which the crystal is set depends on the location in which it is to be used. As with the pulsed ultrasonic meter it is advantageous to have the beam directed as near the line of flow as possible. The probe can be used directly applied to a vessel wall and may also be mounted on an intravascular catheter (p. 229). The early main development of the meter has, however, been for measuring flows in arteries within the body from a probe applied to the intact skin (Stegall, Rushmer, and Baker, 1966).

With a flow velocity of V with the emitting crystal at an angle α to the axis of the artery and the receiving crystal β the frequency shift Δf is given by

$$\Delta f = f - [f.(c - V \cos \alpha)/(c + V \cos \beta)] \qquad 9.3$$

where c is the velocity of sound in blood and V is in the direction away from the crystal. If flow is towards the crystal then $(-V)$ should be substituted for (V).

As V is very small compared to c the equation may be approximated by (Stegall *et al.*, 1966)

$$\Delta f = [(0·2f. \cos \gamma)/c]V \qquad 9.4$$

where

$$\gamma = (\alpha + \beta)/2$$

Using a crystal with a resonant frequency of 5 MHz, taking c as 1,500 m/sec and with crystals at 50 and 70 degrees respectively, then a flow velocity of 100 cm/sec produces a frequency shift of 3,300 Hz.

In most versions in use the algebraic sign of the frequency shift is unknown so that the meter is unable to discriminate between forward and backward flow which is quite a serious limitation, as all fluctuations are recorded as forward flow. Further elaboration of the circuitry will doubtless allow this defect to be eliminated. The pulsatile movement of the arterial wall causes a small frequency-shift which is removed from the flow record by filtering out frequencies below 200 Hz. As a result, it is not possible to discriminate flows below about 6 cm/sec. Equally, care has to be taken with spurious signals from such moving structure as the heart valves.

Calibration for steady flows in a Lucite flow channel and in a perfused femoral artery are reported to be linear (Stegall, Rushmer, and Baker, 1966) but does not appear to have been done with oscillatory flows. Thus, there is no information, or analysis, of the effect of varying velocity profiles during the cardiac cycle (Ch. 5). An initial analysis of recording of a reflected beam directed obliquely through the complex oscillatory profile has been made by Gessner (1961) which will lead to a much better understanding of this problem. Current developments in the use of the pulsed Doppler meter (in the next section) are aimed specifically at the problem created by the velocity profile which will, we anticipate, lead to an improvement in the accuracy of the Doppler flowmeter.

As a meter which can be used transcutaneously, it has great potentiality for qualitative clinical use. Such applications as detecting fetal blood flow, detecting regions of occlusion in diseased peripheral arteries, and making records from human arteries, ranging from the aorta to digital arteries in the hand, have been discussed by Rushmer *et al.* (1967), Fronek (1972), and Tunstall-Pedoe (1972). No absolute calibration has been attempted in these cases and indeed would be very difficult, but present devices incorporate an electrical calibration based on a standard frequency shift—assuming a stated angle of reflection.

Built into a cuff which is implanted on an artery where the relation between the crystals and the arterial wall can be kept constant, it can be used as a quantitative instrument. The back-scattered frequency band is, however, quite wide and it would seem to have less inherent accuracy than the pulsed ultrasonic meter. Nevertheless, it is being used with chronic implantation by several laboratories, possibly because a modulated frequency signal is easier to telemeter than other types (telemetry has been used dramatically on free-ranging wild animals). Not enough published data is available at the present time to evaluate the Doppler flowmeter in comparison to other meters which can be used in this way.

The severe limitation that all these Doppler shift meters have is that they are unable to discriminate between the frequency shift due to forward or backward flow and both are recorded as forward flow. In arteries where the normal flow pattern is known it is relatively easy to guess which peak represents backflow, but as the main advantage of the transcutaneous type is its use in clinical diagnosis this limitation can be a major disadvantage where unknown backflows occur in such conditions as incompetence of the aortic valve. A Doppler flowmeter in which there is good discrimination of the direction of flow was reported by MacLeod (1967) and has been further developed (McLeod, 1970). This necessitates some elaboration of the circuitry but, nevertheless, in spite of its manifest advantages it has not been adopted in America. Kalmanson and his colleagues in Paris have also developed an instrument which enables discrimination of the direction of flow to be made and have put it to extensive clinical use (Kalmanson *et al.*, 1968; Chiche *et al.*, 1968*a, b*; Kalmanson *et al.*, 1970, 1972) in recording arterial and venous flows outside the thorax. They have also made some records of the flow in the output tract of the right ventricle. While calibration in terms of volume flow remains difficult they have shown what a valuable addition to cardiological diagnosis this instrument can be, in studying valvular incompetence. This has been made possible by mounting it as a catheter-tip instrument.

(*d*) *The pulsed Doppler shift instrument* by Peronneau and Leger (1969) combines the features of both (*b*) and (*c*) above. Whereas the Doppler device uses a continuous emission of ultrasonic frequency in this modification the tone emission is divided in short bursts (μsec) at rapidly repeated intervals.

The emitting and receiving crystal is applied to the vessel and angled into the blood-stream. The pulses of reflected waves will vary in their time of arrival back at the wall according to the distance the wave travelled into the lumen before being reflected back to the source. The distance from the wall at which flow is being recorded can be determined from the velocity of sound in blood; by varying the timing of the receiving gate a complete scan of the interior of the blood vessel can be obtained. The velocity of flow at each point is determined by the Doppler frequency shift of each pulse; in spite of the short pulse duration when emitting frequencies of 3–8 MHz are used it will be seen that each pulse contains a long series of waves and may be treated as being in steady-state oscillation. The ability to scan the flow velocities within the blood vessel has led to its use for recording the velocity profiles which were discussed in Ch. 5. In 1970 the Paris group was the only one that had experience with it but its potentialities have stimulated laboratories in America who have the necessary sophistication in electronics so that rapid development may be expected in the future. A cather-tip model has been developed in Paris to increase its application in the living animal. The technical problem here is that it must be held against one wall so that the position of the crystal within the vessel is precisely known. It is not clear how this can be done without wall damage so that its application in human beings will depend on future modifications.

THERMAL METHODS

The *Thermostromuhr* was introduced by Rein some forty years ago and, although designed to record only mean flow, it is of interest because it was the first meter that could be applied to an intact artery. The principle is simple in that liquid flowing through a heated region will show a rise in temperature; the rise in temperature is inversely proportional to the rate of flow. In practice, the temperature of the blood flowing into the meter needs to be monitored by a second temperature measurement upstream of the heating coil. Its stability and performance were improved by Baldes and Herrick (1937) who worked with it for many years. When compared to an orifice meter by Gregg, Pritchard and Shipley (1948) it was observed that when used on arteries with a backflow during the cycle it could give erroneous results. For example, they showed that occluding the femoral vein the mean flow in the limb was decreased when recorded by an orifice meter; this was largely caused by a marked increase in the backflow phase. The *thermostromuhr* on the contrary recorded an increase of flow. It is clear that a reversal of flow past the heating coil will heat the upstream control point and by reducing the temperature difference will record an increase of flow. Later improvements (Aschoff and Wever, 1956; Wever and Aschoff, 1956) were said to have made the instruments sufficiently rapid in response to follow pulsating flow. It does not appear to have been used for this purpose; it has, however, been tested critically for measuring mean flows by comparing it with the bubble flow-meter and the rotameter (Janssen *et al.*, 1957). Thermal flowmeters have been reviewed by Galle (1966).

Methods using thermistors

To obtain response fast enough to follow pulsatile flow at all accurately miniaturization has been necessary. The introduction of thermistors (a term derived from Thermally Sensitive Resistors) in which the resistance element is a semi-conductor and which characteristically show a decrease of resistance with a rise in temperature meets this need. Thermistors can be made extremely small and very sensitive (some can detect a temperature change of 10^{-4} degrees C). Their sensitivity has found an application as sensors in the thermal-dilution flow method; this is a version of the indicator-dilution technique in which saline at a temperature different from the blood (usually colder) is used as the indicator (Wilson *et al.*, 1972). Small thermistors have a rapid response time and so can respond to rapid changes of flow.

Their first use in this manner appears to have been by Mellander and Rushmer (1960) in an instrument called the 'isothermal flowmeter'. It was inserted intravascularly. A small thermistor and heating element were built on the tip which was maintained at 1°C above the blood-stream. As the flow tended to cool the thermistor, a servo-loop increased the current in the heating element to keep its temperature constant. The fluctuations in current necessary provided a measure of the flow. It was reported to have a uniform amplitude response from 0 to 5 Hz. A similar technique has been used by Kuether, Higgs, and Richards (1966) who used a platinum ribbon in place of the thermistor in order to improve the frequency response. A response time of 0·003 sec in the sensor and a valid calibration up to 500 cm/sec and a frequency of 50 Hz has been reported.

Another possible technique using thermistors applies the *thermostromuhr* principle of measuring the rise in temperature of the blood after flowing past a heated element or various combinations of the two techniques (Grahn, Paul, and Wessel, 1969; Kinnen, 1966). This has been built with a catheter-tip flow probe and consequently is noted below in the discussion of intravascular flowmeters.

The hot-wire anemometer

This, as its name suggests, is mainly an instrument for measuring air-flow but has been adapted to measure blood-flow. In principle, it depends on a wire heated above the surrounding temperature; flow past the wire cools it proportionately to its velocity. The change in temperature is followed by recording the resistance change. It is capable of a high-frequency response.

Machella (1936) used such an instrument to record the pulsatile flow in the carotid artery. The flow records appeared to have a marked phase lag in them but the technique was not pursued at the time.

Recently, the principle has been used in the form of hot-film anemometry in which the wire is replaced by a thin metal film on a probe which is inserted into the artery through the wall (Ling *et al.*, 1968; Schultz *et al.*, 1969). They were introduced for the study of velocity profiles (Ch. 5) although Ling and Atabek (1966) published some aortic flow curves recorded with this device; Schultz *et al.* have used it extensively for recording flow in dogs and in man. The thin metal film on the tip of a needle probe is heated to maintain it some 5°C above the blood temperature. Flowing blood would thus cool it in proportion to its velocity. By arranging a sensitive feed-back loop the heating current is varied so that the film is maintained at a constant temperature. Variations in this current are thus a measure of the flow velocity. Because the heat capacity is low this instrument can record flow variations at frequencies up to 10 MHz. The effect of the deposition of a thin film of fibrin would appear likely to alter its performance and so may limit its use for any length of time without withdrawal and cleaning. This may limit its use as a standard recording device but it has undoubtedly been a valuable tool for studying velocity profiles in blood vessels and the flow patterns around the aortic valve and the mitral valve (Ch. 4). Its high-frequency response enables it to record turbulence and eddies in the flow so that it is to be hoped that it will be developed for application by more laboratories. A catheter-tip version holds promise in this respect.

INTRAVASCULAR FLOWMETERS

There is no doubt that a reliable method of measuring blood-flow in the human being, with no more trauma than the introduction of an intravascular catheter, would be extremely valuable in the diagnosis and treatment of heart disease. It is for this reason that so much attention has been paid to methods of deriving the stroke output of the heart from pressure measurements made close to the heart. These methods are discussed separately (Ch. 15). As noted there, the information derived may give (a) the integrated stroke volume from the ventricle only, or (b) the actual form of the flow pulse. The flow pulse can be integrated to give the stroke volume, but can, if the pressure is measured too, also give additional information regarding the power output of the ventricle and the input impedance of the arterial tree and the peripheral resistance. For haemodynamic studies the ability to measure flow and pressure at the same site is a necessity.

All the methods described here have not been widely used yet but their potentialities will be discussed with these criteria in mind. Furthermore, it must be borne in mind that all these meters primarily record linear velocity of flow and not volume flow. This latter requires, in addition, a knowledge of the internal radius of the artery at the point of measurement; this is not peculiar to these meters, but the implantation of a rigid probe on the outside of an artery at least determines the outside diameter at that time. All the evidence in animals with chronically implanted external probes indicates that they soon become firmly attached to the vessel wall so that the diameter becomes fixed by fibrin and the wall may be thickened. The internal diameter thus requires to be determined radiographically. If we assume, from the data presented in Ch. 10, that the pulsatile dilatation with each cardiac ejection is about $\pm 2 \cdot 5$–3 per cent of the radius, even the best radiograph cannot give an accuracy greater than this. Thus, the cross-sectional area will be indeterminate to at least ± 5 per cent; any flow derived from velocity measurement cannot expect to be more accurate than this. The second problem involves our knowledge of the distribution of the velocity across the artery and, in particular, the relation of the velocity measured by the meter to mean velocity across the pipe. From the evidence surveyed in Ch. 5, it is highly probable that the velocity profile will be fairly 'flat' in large vessels, i.e. uniform across most of the artery with the region of shear limited to a narrow region at the wall. Nevertheless, without fairly precise knowledge of the width of the region of shear, the relation of the velocity of the central region to the mean velocity is uncertain. As the unrestrained tip of a catheter will usually rest against, or close to, the inner wall of a systemic artery when introduced towards the heart, the velocity near the wall becomes important. The smallest size of probe so far reported is about 2 mm and it may be reasonable to assume that by acting as a 'baffle' it will produce an averaging effect. Further miniaturization is desirable to minimize arterial trauma and by causing less disturbance in the velocity distribution this problem will, paradoxically, become more acute. In the pulmonary artery, on the other hand, an intravascular flowmeter will pass through the pulmonary valves and so tend to remain in the more central part of the stream. An unsupported central position will tend to show catheter whip which may cause artifacts of itself.

The problem of stable catheter position in the lumen was solved by Mellander and Rushmer (1960) and by Pieper (1958, 1963), who attached an expanding wire cage which held the catheter tip in the centre of the vessel. The device could be operated from the proximal end of the catheter. While excellent, in principle, the effect of this cage on the endothelium of the artery, if left in position for any length of time, would seem likely to be damaging. A simpler device, in an intravascular meter used for rather a different purpose by Kolin et al. (1967), used a single wire. When it was tensed it bowed the catheter so that it was held firm against the opposite walls of the artery; some modification of this method might be conceived which held the sensing element in a known position without damaging the wall. The flow meter described by Kolin (1969*a*) has radial rubber vanes which place it centrally but are much less damaging to the endothelium.

The types of meter that have been adapted for intravascular use are (a) electromagnetic, (b) ultrasonic, (c) viscous drag, and (d) thermal, in principle.

(a) Electromagnetic

A meter which is built on the end of a catheter has been designed by Mills (1966). The physical analysis of such a system was made by Kolin (1944). Further design modifications and detailed calibration characteristics have been reported by Mills and Shillingford (1967). This probe uses the same principle as the electromagnetic flowmeter with the probe external to the artery. In the intravascular version, the magnetic field is external to the probe and the blood flows around, and not through, it. The magnetic field is created by a sinusoidal current through longitudinal coils in the tip. Therefore, the signal will be generated by the velocity of flow in the region around the probe —it is estimated that the velocity is an average across the annulus which is one probe radius wide, i.e. a little more than 1 mm in the smaller models. There is a hollow core through which pressure may be measured simultaneously.

The calibration characteristics were reported in some detail and compare favourably with more conventional electromagnetic flowmeters. Calibration was carried out electrically and hydraulically; the latter with steady and oscillatory flows in both laminar and turbulent regimes. Tests were made with the probe at various angles to the tube axis because in experimental conditions it is difficult to control their orientation; it was interesting to note that sensitivity was decreased much less than theory predicted which suggests that local flow tended to run parallel to the probe. Records made in the pulmonary artery of a dog with a cuff probe as well as an intravascular one showed close agreement between the two. A simultaneous record of pressure and flow in the human pulmonary artery was also shown. A comparison of the flow recorded with the intravascular probe and an external flow probe in the thoracic aorta of the dog is shown in Fig. 9.3. This instrument has been extensively used in my laboratory and found to be very satisfactory. Occasionally, on moving the probe, a sudden diminution of signal occurs; this is apparently due to the contact of one of the pick-up electrodes with the arterial wall for the full signal is restored by manipulating the catheter into a new position. With modification of design in later models this is reported to be only a minor problem.

This model has been used in the study of humans. An investigation of venous flow velocities was made by Wexler *et al.* (1968); a study of arterial flows and pressures was made in a series of patients by Gabe *et al.* (1969) and used to measure cardiac output (see also Ch. 15). This led to a wide survey of arterial impedance studies by Mills *et al.* (1970) which is the most complete

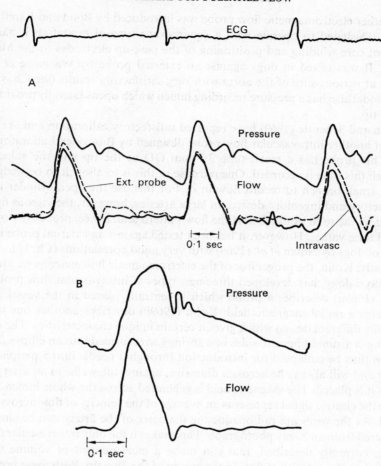

Fig. 9.3A. Comparison between the flow curve in the thoracic aortic of the dog recorded with two different probes.

The solid line is the tracing made with the Mills (1968) intravascular flow probe. The broken line is the tracing from an external flow probe (Statham-Medicon) placed at the same level. It can be seen that the two traces are virtually identical but the intravascular probe trace tends to drift back and forth a little in the period of the respiratory cycle.

(The pressure trace is recorded through the lumen of the Mills probe and is a poor one because the channel was not adequately flushed free of air bubbles.)

B. A pressure and flow recording made in the ascending aorta with the same probe as used in A. The pressure recording here is the optimal one that can be done through the narrow lumen of this early model. A larger lumen is available in the present model. The flow trace may be compared with that in Fig. 9.1. (Nichols, unpublished.)

report on the human arterial system to date (Ch. 14). A further report has been made by Mason *et al.* (1970) on findings in humans. The probe can thus be regarded of established value in clinical studies and constitutes a major advance in both clinical diagnosis and in the relatively unexplored field of clinical haemodynamics.

Another electromagnetic flow probe was introduced by Bond and Barefoot (1967). Designed to operate with a square-wave type of excitation it has a different core winding and positioning of the pick-up electrodes to the Mills probe. It was tested in dogs against an external probe by Warbasse *et al.* (1969) at various sites of the aorta with very satisfactory results (see Ch. 15). This model also has a pressure recording lumen which opens laterally proximal to the tip.

Stein and Scheutte (1969) have reported satisfactory calibration and *in vivo* tests of another intravascular flow probe designed by Biotronex Laboratories Inc. This probe has a small tube 3·7 mm OD at the tip and the velocity through this tube is recorded. One purpose of this is to allow it to be wedged into a small branch to record flow in it. For this use the open cylinder is a satisfactory and ingenious device. In large arteries, however, the viscous drag caused by the tube would distort the flow pattern and, hence, probably would record false values. However, it has been tested against an external probe in a series of dogs by Nolan *et al.* (1969) with very good correlations (Ch. 15).

Finally, Kolin, the progenitor of the electromagnetic flowmeter as we know it in physiology, has developed three new types of intravascular flow probes. Kolin (1969a) describes a probe which is centrally placed in the vessel and generates a radial magnetic field. Kolin (1969b) describes another one of a radically different design which gives it certain unique characteristics. The coil winding is around opposite sides of a springy wire formed into an ellipse. The tip can thus be collapsed for introduction through a needle into a peripheral artery and will always lie across a diameter, against the walls, in an artery in which it is placed. The magnetic field is generated across the whole lumen and hence the electric signal represents an average of the velocity of flow across the vessel. As the wires are radiopaque the diameter of the artery can be simply measured from an X-ray photograph. This makes it the only intravascular flow probe, currently described, that can make a measurement of volume flow rather than the velocity of flow in the region of the flow tip. Both these probes were demonstrated on a hydraulic model by Dr. Kolin in my laboratory in 1969 and compared with a Mills probe on which we had done extensive tests. Their performance was excellent and the second model (Kolin, 1969b) had considerably greater sensitivity than the others. Another modification of this probe (Kolin, 1970) uses it only to carry the pick-up electrodes and the magnetic field is generated external to the animal. A different type of intravascular probe was described by Kolin, Archer, and Ross (1967). This is specifically designed to measure flow through aortic branches. A small flow probe with an orifice at right angles to the axis of the aorta is carried by the catheter which introduces it. The probe is positioned, under radiographic control, with the orifice over the mouth of a branch. A wire-tensing device then bows the catheter so that the orifice of the probe is held firmly over the origin of the branch. Illustrative records of flow in the renal and superior mesenteric arteries were shown. All these models appear to be excellent instruments and the only limitation is that, at present, there is no provision for the simultaneous measurement of pressure, but doubtless this can be overcome.

The difficulty of making a magnetic field that is strong enough to create a detectable induced current in the flowing blood makes it tempting to increase the current through the field coil. The possibility of leakage of this current needs to be carefully assessed in considering the use of these instruments especially when close to, or within, the heart in human beings because such leakage could cause ventricular fibrillation. In addition, high current densities will increase heating of the tip. Jones and Wyatt (1970) have done a detailed survey of some electromagnetic catheter-tip flow probes with these points in mind. They conclude that the Mills type probe is acceptable for human use. The square-wave type probe that they tested, however, carried a much larger current load and the heat dissipation was so high that it was able to boil stationary liquid. This has been disputed by Buchanan and Shabetai (1972). Prior testing of all such instruments and continuous careful monitoring of insulation is, therefore, necessary before using such devices in patients.

Specific reports on ultrasonic catheter-tip devices have not yet been made. In view of the fact that they require much smaller electrical currents to activate them it is anticipated that these problems will not arise.

(b) Ultrasonic

Two piezo crystals have been mounted on the tip of a Dallon–Telco manometer (see Ch. 8) by Stegall, Stone, Bishop, and Laenger (1967). This instrument was slightly less than 3 mm in diameter, but has been reduced in later models. With two such crystals the meter is normally operated on the Doppler shift principle and, because it is directed along the axis of the vessel, it can be made relatively more sensitive than the type for external application. The flow record was found to agree within 10 per cent of an externally applied Doppler probe and its frequency response was good up to 50 Hz. The region from which the back scatter of sound was occurring was estimated to be from 0·5 to 4 cm ahead of the tip of the probe. The accuracy of the device has yet to be established as with all Doppler flowmeters. The linking of the flow probe with a high-frequency manometer is an excellent feature of this instrument although it should be appreciated that the points at which pressure and flow are measured are separated by an appreciable distance. This flow probe has been used to measure pulsatile flow in the thoracic aorta in patients with cardiac arrhythmias by Benchimol et al. (1969). A disadvantage of the first model was that large echoes from the aortic valves prevented its satisfactory use in the ascending aorta. By slight angling of the two crystals the point of focus has been brought closer and this limitation has been overcome (Stegall, personal communication).

Another limitation of this probe was that it was unable to discriminate between forward and backward flow. Directional discrimination as used by MacLeod (1967) and in the instrument used by Kalmanson (see above) avoids this difficulty. The Kalmanson device has been successfully mounted in a catheter-tip and he uses it routinely, by intravenous insertion, to record the velocity flow patterns due to the action of the right atrio-ventricular (tricuspid) valve in the heart. This is the most direct way of detecting incompetence of the tricuspid valve. In dogs it is also being used to study the flow through the mitral valve. Such studies of the pulsatile patterns of the velocity of blood flow show that the development of the intravascular flow probe can greatly extend the application of flowmeters beyond the field of measuring vascular flow. A catheter-tip probe which measures the changes in ultrasonic pulse transit-time has also been used by Pardue, Hedrich, Rose, and Kot (1967) and also appears a promising instrument.

Another type developed by a group at the Eidgenossiche Technische Hochschule (ETH), Zürich, utilized the phase discrepancy caused by the velocity of flow between 7 MHz pulses of $5 \mu sec$ duration transmitted in opposite directions by two lead zirconate crystals. Originally described by Plass (1964) it was rather large for routine use and it could not discriminate the direction of flow; it has been reduced in size and in the latest version described by Borgnis and Fruiger (1969) the tip is only 1·5 mm in diameter while the housing for the crystals is 2·3 mm in diameter. In this model also the flow is directed through a tube at the tip and so may have problems due to this cause.

(c) Viscous drag

Pieper (1963, 1964) has developed a miniature version of the concentric cylinder type of meter originally described by Pieper and Weterer (1953a, b). In this a central, hollow cylinder sliding on a core is moved against a spring by the drag of the flow. The movement is detected by a differential transformer. Records made with the instrument appear satisfactory and the position of the probe in the centre of the artery is elegantly arranged. It is not easy to arrange for simultaneous pressure measurements to be made at the flow measuring site. It is probably smaller in size than any other intravascular probe so far reported.

The wire ribs that are used to centre the instrument in the vessel can also be arranged to move a differential transformer and thus record changes in diameter of a vessel or a heart-chamber (Pieper, 1966). The two instruments have been combined in one (Pieper and Paul, 1968) which makes it a versatile experimental tool, although there is still some doubt about the phase-lag of the flow recording (see p. 236).

(d) Thermal

The catheter-tip devices with electrically-heated metallic or thermistor elements of Kuether et al. (1966), Grahn et al. (1969) and Kinnen (1966) have already been discussed (p. 223). Of the few flow curves published so far, the best seem nevertheless to show low peak flows compared to those normally recorded with electromagnetic flow-meters. Also, no provision so far has been made for simultaneous pressure measurements. The technique is ingenious and appears potentially valuable. Its inherent weaknesses would seem to be that as the rate of heat transfer across the surface is crucial it might well be especially vulnerable to fibrin deposition on the surface and also to stream distortion patterns caused by the catheter itself. Thus, it is particularly desirable that their behaviour in detailed performance tests should be known.

All the types discussed above have concerned themselves with following the pulsatile flow changes accurately. The application of thermal-dilution techniques to measure mean flow locally seems a distinct possibility, with the sensitivities now possible with thermistors. A promising technique of this type was described by Fronek and Ganz (1960) in which a catheter was used to make small repeated injections of saline in a vein and the temperature a few centimetres downstream was recorded. Ganz et al. (1964) used it successfully in the femoral artery; Ganz (personal communication) has also used it with success in the coronary sinus. As with all indicator-dilution methods in which the distance between injection and sampling is small, a major problem is to be sure that thorough mixing of indicator and blood is achieved. Another application of this type of approach has been made by Alfonso (1966).

The hot-film probe described above (p. 224) requires insertion through the arterial wall into the blood-stream and hence is an intravascular probe by definition. The usual meaning that workers have in mind, however, is an instrument that can be threaded along a vessel fron a single point of insertion. It is possible to mount the heated film into the tip of a catheter and thus introduce it into the proximal aorta from a peripheral artery. Such models have been built in Schultz's laboratory in Oxford and have been tested *in vitro*. No reports are currently available on their use in living animals where it is necessary to prevent the tip from resting against the arterial wall. The special advantage of this probe in studying flow patterns that are not parallel to the wall makes it desirable that its range should be extended as much as possible.

BERNOULLI METERS

The types of meters that come into this category most commonly used in physiology are the *Pitot tube* and the *orifice meter*. Both use applications of Bernouilli's theorem (Ch. 2, p. 35) which states that

$$P_1 + \tfrac{1}{2}\rho V_1^2 = P_2 + \tfrac{1}{2}\rho V_2^2 = C \qquad \textbf{9.5}$$

In the *Pitot meter* there is a tube in which the tip is bent at right angles so that it points in the direction of the flow. The flow of fluid is dammed up immediately in front of the tip and divides the flow round it, but in the centre of the dammed-up region there is a 'stagnation point' where the fluid comes entirely to rest. The pressure, P_1, at this point is called the 'total pressure' and

$$P_1 = P_0 + \tfrac{1}{2}\rho V_0^2 \qquad\qquad \textbf{9.6}$$

where V_0 is the velocity of flow and where P_0 is the 'static', or lateral, pressure in the vessel. The term $\tfrac{1}{2}\rho V_0^2$ or $(P_1 - P_0)$ is called the 'kinetic', or dynamic pressure (Prandtl, 1952). The term P_0 is measured by a second tube directed perpendicular to the flow. The difference of pressure between the two tubes is therefore proportional to the square of the velocity of flow. Sometimes, the second tube is bent at the tip so that it points directly downstream and so it should, theoretically, record a pressure P_2 where

$$P_2 = P_0 - \tfrac{1}{2}\rho V_0^2 \qquad\qquad \textbf{9.7}$$

so that the differential pressure, $P_1 - P_2$, will be ρV_0^2 and the sensitivity doubled.

One technical difficulty in making a Pitot tube accurate is that the upstream tube causes eddies and so distorts the measurement of P_0 and the problem of design is largely concerned with minimizing this effect (Prandtl, 1952). Green (1948) makes the comment that the Cleveland group abandoned its use for measuring arterial flows on account of the oscillations that developed in their pressure records, and these were probably due to this cause. For the same reason, the reduction of pressure at a tip pointing downstream is not equal in magnitude to the rise at the upstream point and separate calibration curves must be made. Hardung (1957) has discussed the problems connected with the use of Pitot tubes for measuring pulsatile flows.

A second problem is that the velocity, V_0, measured, is that of the laminae in the line of the tip and so it is necessary to know the form of the velocity profile and the exact position of the tip within the vessel. This is usually done by centring it in a cannula and inserting the cannula in the vessel. Müller (1954a) has designed a very small Pitot tube that can be advanced across the lumen of the tube in which it is inserted and so establish the shape of the velocity profile before using it for flow determinations. Results obtained in arteries remain to be published although a preliminary report stated that the velocity profile in the dog aorta is very flat (p. 114). Baxter and Pearce (1951) also designed a Pitot tube meter which they used in the pulmonary trunk of the cat. It had the elegant addition of a 'square-rooting' device so that a linear calibration was achieved. It was, however, not calibrated with oscillatory flow. In a further paper, Baxter, Cunningham, and Pearce (1952) compared its mean flow recording with the cardiac output measured by the direct Fick method and found that it averaged some 15 per cent too high, but it seemed a promising instrument.

The *orifice meter* depends, as its name suggests, on placing a cannula containing a narrowed orifice in the lumen of the tube. Technical details are given by Green (1948). This increases the linear velocity of the flow. In eqn. 9.5 above, V_2^2 is then greater than V_1^2 so that P_2 is less than P_1. If the lateral pressure is measured on either side of the orifice and the pressure difference $(P_1 - P_2)$ measured on a manometer (Shipley, Gregg, and Schroeder, 1943) then

$$P_1 - P_2 = \tfrac{1}{2}(V_2^2 - V_1^2) \qquad\qquad \textbf{9.8}$$

This principle was used by Broemser (1928) in his 'differential sphymograph' which ingeniously avoided the necessity for cannulation by applying an external constriction to an intact artery.

If the radius of the orifice is R_2 and that of the cannula in which it is mounted is R_1 then

$$V_2 = \left(\frac{R_1}{R_2}\right)^2 . V_1 \qquad\qquad \textbf{9.9}$$

and

$$P_1 - P_2 = \tfrac{1}{2}V_1^2 \left[\left(\frac{R_1}{R_2}\right)^4 - 1 \right] \qquad\qquad \textbf{9.10}$$

so that it can be seen that a reduction of the size of the orifice greatly increases the sensitivity of the meter; however, it also greatly increases resistance and this is its greatest disadvantage.

In pulsatile flow the pressure difference across the meter, if there were no orifice, would be the oscillating pressure-gradient that is normally present in an artery. As was seen in Ch. 6, this is different in form from the flow curve. The orifice must, therefore, cause sufficient change in velocity for the Bernoulli term to be very large in comparison with the pressure-gradient so that the latter may be neglected. This sets a limit to the extent in which the orifice may be enlarged to reduce the impedance of the meter.

It is not easy to forecast precisely the changes in the flow pattern due to the obstruction of the meter. Gregg and Green (1939) stated that 'at flows of 60–80 ml per minute the net loss of the pressure head in the stream is not more than 3 to 4 mm Hg'. The 'resistance' of meters is often defined in this way and in terms of the drop in mean pressure from the large arteries to the capillaries a fall in the pressure head of 3–4 mm Hg may seem very small. Looked at another way, however, we saw from the consideration of pressure-gradient in the femoral artery that at a mean flow of this magnitude the mean gradient is only of the order of 0·1–0·15 mm Hg/cm, so that even expressed in terms of steady flow it is, as it were, equivalent to introducing an extra length of some 20–30 cm of artery. The effect of a rigid cannula on the oscillating components of the flow was considered with the description of the electromagnetic flowmeter as this is a problem common to both. The 'resistance' of a meter, used for pulsating flow, defined in terms of a steady flow is not very helpful, for we need to know its impedance in terms of oscillatory flow.

A further point regarding the use of meters in arteries concerns the role of alternative channels. There are two femoral arteries, for example, and the introduction of a meter of appreciable impedance will tend to enhance the flow in the contralateral leg at the expense of the observed leg. With phasic recording this will alter the pattern of the flow curve. Reactive hyperaemia in one leg, for instance, can markedly enhance the backflow phase in the contralateral one. It would be of considerable interest to see if the insertion of orifice meters symmetrically into both femoral arteries altered the flow patterns as compared with those recorded from a single one.

To summarize, the orifice meter is sound in principle and has advantages in relative ease of application. With it, Shipley et al. (1943) and Pritchard et al. (1943) have recorded phasic patterns in a greater variety of arteries than any other workers. Its main disadvantage appears to lie in its relatively high impedance which will cause damping. This damping will not only modify the amplitude of the recorded phasic variations in flow but will also cause a distortion of the shape of the flow curve due to the accompanying shift in phase. Furthermore, a meter with a marked impedance probably causes significant alteration in the flow pattern by causing a redistribution of flow into other vascular beds.

A well-designed Pitot tube may be preferable for detailed investigation if its use is restricted to very large arteries such as the aorta so that its impedance can be kept small. The accuracy of the Pitot tube is greatest where the velocity gradient across the pipe is very small and, as we have seen above (p. 113), we appear to have this condition in the aorta.

All types of differential pressure flowmeters require accurate differential pressure manometers. The membranes must be sensitive to very small pressure changes and so of a lower 'stiffness' than conventional manometers. This lowers their frequency response (Ch. 8) and the compromise this requires in their design raises special problems. Thus, it is likely that the amplitude of pressure, and hence of derived flow, in the meter used by Shipley et al. (1943) is somewhat too large. The Sanborn differential electro-manometer has been used by Fry et al. (1956, 1957a) and has satisfactory characteristics. Betticher, Maillard, and Müller (1954) have gone to considerable trouble to design and build their own differential manometer for use with the Pitot tube used by Müller (1954a). The optical manometer with photo-electric recording designed by Müller and Shillingford (1955) has been used for recording pulsatile venous flow. The Statham differential manometer (P23H) has the same frequency response as the P23Db (Table 8.1) and has been used by O'Rourke and Milnor (1967), and McDonald (unpublished) to measure pressure-gradients.

THE HYDRODYNAMIC PENDULUM OF CASTELLI. 'BRISTLE' FLOWMETERS

If a pendulum is suspended so that it is free and lies in liquid then flow in that liquid will cause the pendulum to move. The movement can be used to measure the rate of flow and a device of this sort was first used by Castelli (1577–1644), a pupil of Galileo, to measure the flow velocity of mountain streams. Under the name of 'haemodrometer' an instrument of this sort was used by Chauveau and associates in 1860 (Hill, 1900) and extensively by Marey (1881). It must, therefore, have seniority as a phasic flow recorder. In its simplest form, inertia and hence slowness of response are obviously its main technical problem. Bergmann (1937) improved it greatly by using a flexible bristle in an instrument known as the *Stromborste*. The introduction of thermionic valves that can function as mechano-electronic transducers have made the construction of a very refined version of this type of meter possible. Similar models were introduced independently and almost simultaneously by Scher, Weigert and Young (1953); Pieper and Wetterer (1953b); Brecher (1954); and Müller (1954b). Brecher has used the instrument extensively in studying venous flow and has named it the bristle flowmeter, presumably to acknowledge its relationship to Bergmann's *Stromborste*. Müller (1954b) gives an account of the problems connected with this type of meter, and a technical account is given by Brecher (1960); it is briefly discussed by Bergel in Cappelen (1968).

In order to maintain a rigid support for the sensing probe it is necessary to mount the device into a cannula but this can be kept very short. The valve movements of the external probe move the grid and so cause changes in the anode current. It is thus possible to keep the probe very rigid as very little movement is required, hence the orientation of the probe remains virtually constant. It is, however, very difficult to calculate the forces that a pulsating liquid stream will exert on a structure thrust across a diameter of the tube without precise knowledge of the extent to which the flow is deformed by the obstruction. Scher et al. (1953) considered two types. With a streamlined rod the force is in the nature of viscous drag and the deflection varied approximately linearly with the mean flow in their model—more precisely, deflection $= K(V)^{\frac{1}{2}}$. In order to increase sensitivity a second type was made with a paddle on one end; with this the deflection is roughly proportional to $(\overline{V})^2$. Increasing the size of the obstruction will also obviously increase the impedance of the meter. Brecher (1956) appears to use the latter type exclusively in recording venous flow (in fact he used a piece of watchspring—personal communication). He has also used it in the pulmonary artery (Brecher and Hubay, 1954) and Müller and Laszt (personal communication) have used it in the aorta, but the only results published to date are in the coronary artery

(Laszt and Müller, 1957). One cannot, therefore, compare the results with this meter with others on systemic arterial flow at present. In view of its relative simplicity and the fact that, with the available sensitivity in the tube, a thin probe can be used with approximately linear behaviour, this type of meter deserves much more attention as a phasic meter for use in the larger arteries. Laszt and Müller, however, found that the deposition of fibrin was so fast that it needed to be withdrawn and cleaned after 30 sec.

Pieper and Wetterer (1953a) also introduced a flowmeter which has a cylinder held in the axis of the steam in a cannula. The displacement of the cylinder is detected by a differential transformer outside the cannula.

Taylor (1958b) has made a theoretical analysis of the behaviour of flow-meters of the bristle and pendulum type. This will clearly be dependent on the distribution of flow velocity across the tube which, as was seen in Ch. 5, changes greatly in oscillatory, compared with steady, flow. From Taylor's results it appears that the true 'bristle' meter with a fine probe gives the most satisfactory results. In fact, the distortions introduced remarkably little changes. The use of a pendulum or 'paddle' on the probe greatly increases the distortion; the meter with the axial cylinder (Pieper and Wetterer, 1953a) is shown to introduce very large phase lags in the recorded flow although the amplitude is quite faithfully recorded.

HIGH-SPEED CINEMATOGRAPHY

In the 1950s, in the absence of any reliable flowmeter, the tracking of markers such as injected O_2 bubbles, was found to be a reasonably accurate—if rather tedious—method of recording pulsatile arterial flow velocity. Although that use may be regarded as obsolete it still has potential value for recording flow velocity or velocity distributions in situations where meters cannot be used. As the only detailed technical description (McDonald, 1960) is now out of print and enquiries are still occasionally made, the method is reported again (Appendix 2).

CALCULATION OF PHASIC FLOW FROM THE PRESSURE-GRADIENT

In a rigid tube steady flow is commonly measured by recording the pressure-gradient and using Poiseuille's law to calculate the flow. As was shown in Ch. 6, it is now possible to calculate pulsatile flows in a similar way. This is not considered at length in the present chapter as an independent experimental method (but see Ch. 15) because the calculations involved are somewhat lengthy, although, with increased use of computers, this may soon be a small objection. Also, the estimates of mean flow are subject to error. The oscillatory terms may be predicted with fair accuracy but the steady flow is dependent on such a small pressure-gradient that manometers at present available are not able to measure it precisely. All the calculated curves presented have had the mean flow checked by direct observation. For the measurement of arterial impedance, the measurement of the gradient has been used by Bergel *et al.* (1958). The method of Fry *et al.* (1956) for computing flow curves in the root of the aorta from the pressure-gradient has already been discussed and it is a very promising application of the method to a special region. The assumptions on which it is based make it equally applicable to recording flow in the pulmonary artery.

10
The Elastic Properties of the Arterial Wall

In consideration of the pressure–flow relationships of oscillatory flow in Chs. 5 and 6, the vessel was treated as a cylindrical tube of unvarying diameter. In reality, an artery is an elastic tube whose diameter will vary with a pulsating pressure; in addition, it will propagate pressure and flow waves, created by the ejection of blood by the heart, at a certain velocity which is largely determined by the elastic properties of the wall. It was also shown that this wave-velocity in part determined the relation of the pressure-gradient to the pressure wave (eqn. 6.7). The model considered, therefore, was inconsistent in that it was treated partly as a rigid tube in that its diameter was invariant and partly as an elastic tube, in that the velocity of the pulse wave was given its real value in the body. For, in a rigid tube filled with an incompressible liquid, the wave-velocity would be infinitely high, and filled with a real liquid it would be the velocity of sound in blood—about 1,500 m/sec.

Analyses of the behaviour of pulsatile flows in various kinds of elastic tube have been made and are considered in Ch. 11. There it will be seen that many of the physical conditions we are concerned with, such as the viscosity of the blood, the damping of the propagated waves and the presence of reflected waves change the velocity of propagation of the pulse-wave. The degree of this change can only be measured experimentally if the 'natural' velocity, that is, the wave-velocity of the vessels being studied due to the properties of the wall alone, are known. To study the hydrodynamics of the arterial system a knowledge of the elastic constants of the arterial wall, from which one can predict the 'natural' velocity, is of fundamental importance. In many cases, in the living animal, these constants can best be derived from the wave-velocity. In order to ensure that we are relating the one to the other correctly, it is necessary first to consider briefly the physical definitions in which studies of elasticity should be based to allow such quantitative studies to be made; in few fields of physiology has such a proportion of the experimental data that has been collected been useless to other workers because essential measurements have not been recorded.

THE PHYSICAL CONSTANTS OF AN ELASTIC BODY

No solid body is completely rigid. When forces act on it without displacing it, they will deform it; that is, cause a movement of the various parts of the body relative to one another. If the body regains its original form exactly when the force is removed it is said to be *perfectly elastic*. If the body retains the deformation then it is said to be *plastic*.

The theory of elasticity deals with the relations between the forces applied to a body and its consequent deformation. The force per unit area is called the *stress*; the deformation described as the ratio of the deformation to its original form is called the *strain*. Because it is a ratio, strain is dimensionless. The ability to withstand a stress is a property that distinguishes a solid from a fluid, for a fluid when stressed will undergo a viscous flow (Ch. 2). Nevertheless, a large number of substances exhibit properties appropriate to both an elastic solid and a viscous liquid, and the deformation suffered by such a material will depend on both the magnitude of the stress and on the rate at which it is applied. Such substances are called *visco-elastic* and it is to this large class that the arterial wall belongs. When deforming stresses are applied slowly, however, the viscous behaviour may be neglected so we will first outline the purely elastic properties.

No substance is perfectly elastic when very large forces are applied to it but for the small deformations that are considered in such materials as steel wire, which are the main study of elastic theory, the deformation is proportional to the force applied. This proportionality was first described by Robert Hooke in 1676 in the famous phrase *Ut tensio sic vis* (as the (ex)tension so the force) and is known as Hooke's Law. The point at which Hooke's Law ceases to apply is known as the *elastic limit* and when the solid has been deformed beyond this point it cannot regain its original form and acquires a *permanent set*. With larger loads still, the *yield point* is reached when the deformation continues to increase without further load and usually leads rapidly to breakage. The classical theory of elasticity stems from behaviour below the elastic limit and throughout bases itself on two assumptions—that the deformations are infinitesimally small and that the structure of the material is continuous and uniform, or homogeneous. (For a full theoretical development the reader is referred to Love (1944) or Southwell (1941) or the briefer treatment by Newman and Searle (1957). The brief treatment below follows the excellent summary by Bergel (1960) very closely.) It will be seen that neither of these two assumptions apply well to the arterial wall. In the first place, it is easily extensible and is more analogous to substances such as rubber which are often classed as *elastomers* and undergo large deformations. (The detailed consideration of such properties is dealt with in texts such as Treloar (1958), Green and Zerna (1960), and Green and Adkins (1960).) In the second phase

I

the main elastic components of arterial wall are *collagen* and *elastin* which are fibrous in nature and are supported in a fluid, or semifluid, matrix of water and mucoproteins. It is, therefore, far from homogeneous. Nevertheless, the majority of analyses of arterial elasticity is based on classical theory so that it is necessary to consider its main elements.

Strain

When a body of length L_0 is extended to a length L_1, then the relative increase in length $(L_1 - L_0)/L_0$ is the *longitudinal* strain. An increase in length is a positive, a decrease a negative, strain. When there is a change in volume there is a *compressive* strain; when there is an angular deformation, that is, a displacement of two points in parallel planes in a direction parallel to those planes, we refer to a *shear* strain. Considering only longitudinal strain we know from common experience that a substance that is stretched simultaneously gets thinner in the transverse direction. Expressed mathematically, we have the tensile, or longitudinal, strain e, where

$$e_1 = \frac{L_1 - L_0}{L_0} \qquad\qquad \textbf{10.1}$$

While in the width and breadth, or a and b directions we have

$$e_2 = \frac{a_1 - a_0}{a_0} = -\sigma_2 e_1 \qquad\qquad \textbf{10.2}$$

and

$$e_3 = \frac{b_1 - b_0}{b_0} = -\sigma_3 e_1 \qquad\qquad \textbf{10.3}$$

The symbol σ, the ratio of transverse to longitudinal strain, is called the *Poisson ratio*. This ratio is a characteristic property of the material and for small strains it is constant but we cannot necessarily assume that $\sigma_2 = \sigma_3$. Similarly with primary extensions in the a and b directions we obtain four more Poisson ratios making six in all; these may, or may not, be of the same value, depending on the nature of the material.

If we consider an infinitesimally small cube within the substance of an object that has faces parallel to the axes x, y and z, then the strain at any face can be resolved into three components in directions at right angles to each other. These will be one tensile and two shearing strains which may be written e_{xx}, e_{xy} and e_{xz}, where e_{xx} indicates a strain separating two points on the x-axis in the direction of the x-axis and e_{xy} a strain separating these points on the y-axis, etc. We thus have nine components of strain at a point:

$$e_{xx}, \ e_{xy}, \ e_{xz}, \ e_{yx}, \ e_{yy}, \ e_{yz}, \ e_{zx}, \ e_{zy}, \ e_{zz}$$

It may be shown (Love, 1944) that the strains of the form e_{xy} and e_{yx} are identical so that three may be eliminated and we are left with six independent components of strain:

$$e_{xx}, e_{xy}, e_{yy}, e_{yz}, e_{zz}, e_{zx}$$

and the corresponding six independent Poisson ratios

$$\sigma_{yz} \ \sigma_{zx}, \ \sigma_{xy}, \ \sigma_{zy}, \ \sigma_{xz}, \ \sigma_{yz}$$

and the value of σ can be shown to fall in the range $-1 < \sigma < 0.5$ but, although theoretically possible, no isotropic material is known to possess a negative Poisson ratio, so that the effective range is 0–0.5. For small extension, with a ratio of 0.5, the volume of the solid remains the same when it is stretched—an *isovolumetric* deformation. The value for rubber, and rubber-like substances, is usually close to this (rubber, 0.48, Newman and Searle, 1957). For most metals it lies in the range 0.25–0.4 so that they undergo an increase of volume in stretching; when $\sigma = 0$, the increase in volume will be proportionate to the change in length. The value of σ for arterial wall is almost certainly close to 0.5; the evidence is considered below (p. 266).

Reconsidering the cube of dimensions x_0, y_0 and z_0 subjected to a tensile strain e_{xx}, after deformation the dimensions are

$$x_1 = x_0 (1 + e_{xx})$$
$$y_1 = y_0 (1 - \sigma_{yx} \, e_{xx}) \qquad \textbf{10.4}$$
$$z_1 = z_0 (1 - \sigma_{zx} \, e_{xx})$$

The new volume V_1 is $x_1 y_1 z_1$ compared to the original volume V_0 which was $x_0 y_0 z_0$. The change ΔV is

$$\Delta V = V_1 - V_0 = x_0(1 + e_{xx}) y_0 (1 - \sigma_{yz} e_{xx}) z_0 (1 - \sigma_{zx} e_{xx}) - x_0 y_0 z_0 \qquad \textbf{10.5}$$

and if e_{xx} is small so that its powers may be neglected

$$\Delta V = e_{xx} + e_{xy} + e_{xz} = e_{xx}(1 - \sigma_{yz} - \sigma_{zx}) \qquad \textbf{10.6}$$

If the material has the same elastic properties in all these axes it is said to be *isotropic* and all the values of σ will be the same so that we may rewrite eqn. 10.6 as

$$\Delta V = e_{xx}(1 - 2\sigma) \qquad \textbf{10.7}$$

which demonstrates that, for small strains, a value of σ of 0.5 leads to no change in volume. Furthermore, even if the elastic properties in each direction are not the same, but is isovolumetric under strain, then the average values of σ must be equal to 0.5. This is because the average overall value of σ must be 0.5; thus if some are less than 0.5 then others will need to be greater than 0.5 or negative. These considerations need to be borne in mind when assessing experimental work which has studied the arterial wall as an *anisotropic* material—a difficult procedure with biological tissues—and which is discussed below (p. 276).

Stress

Stress is the intensity of force acting across a given plane in a body and, if it is evenly distributed over the area A, the stress is F/A. The units of stress are thus force per unit area (FL^{-2}) or, in fundamental units, (mass) $\times$ (length)$^{-1}$ $\times$ (time)$^{-2}$ or $ML^{-1}T^{-2}$.

The stress on a point in a plane may be resolved into those normal along the axis (tensile or compressive) and tangential to the axis (shearing stresses). The components along the three axes are designated by subscripts thus, X_x, X_y, X_z, Y_x, etc., where the capital letter indicates the direction of the stress component and the subscript the plane across which it acts. It can also be seen that pairs of components such as X_y and Y_x must be equal or a rotational resultant of force would exist. We are therefore left with six independent components of stress:

$$X_x,\ X_y,\ Y_y,\ Y_z,\ Z_z,\ Z_x \qquad \textbf{10.8}$$

The relationship between stress and strain

Hooke's Law states that, within certain limits, strain is proportional to stress. This may be expanded into a generalized statement of Hooke's Law: 'Each of the six independent components of strain may be expressed as a linear function of the six components of stress, and vice versa.' With six stress components and six strain components it can be seen that this will lead to thirty-six constants of proportionality; of these, fifteen can be shown to be interrelated leaving some twenty-one constants to be considered when the material is anisotropic.

If, however, the material is isotropic and has the same elastic behaviour in each of the three axes then the number of constants of proportionality is reduced to two. For a material that is macroscopically inhomogeneous, as the arterial wall is, this is an uncertain assumption although much experimental evidence indicates that under *in vivo* conditions this is approximately true. It can be seen that the advantages, in simplicity, for making such an assumption, if possible, are very great.

The relation between stress and strain is expressed as an *elastic* modulus. As strain is a ratio, and therefore dimensionless, all these moduli will have the dimensions of stress, force per unit area, i.e. dyn/cm^2.

The modulus in the longitudinal direction is called the *Young's modulus* in honour of the pioneer work of Thomas Young (1808, 1809) and is designated by E or Y (in this text E is used). Thus:

$$E = \frac{\text{Longitudinal force per unit area}}{\text{Extension per unit length}} = \frac{X_x}{e_{xx}} \qquad \textbf{10.9}$$

The *shear modulus*, or modulus of rigidity, μ (written as n in McDonald, 1960, and also sometimes as C) is the ratio of shear stress to angular strain

$$\mu = \frac{X_y}{e_{xy}}$$ 10.10

(μ is the common conventional symbol for shear modulus in the standard texts, so is used here in spite of the fact it has also been used for viscosity of a liquid.)

The bulk modulus, K, is the ratio of compressive stress to strain, that is, to the relative change in volume. Taking a cube under compression the mean stress is

$$-(X_x + Y_y + Z_z)/3$$ 10.11

This is commonly considered as a pressure, P, which will exert the same force in all directions (Pascal's law) so that

$$P = X_x = Y_y = Z_z$$ 10.12

The change in volume ΔV is given by

$$\Delta V = e_{xx} + e_{yy} + e_{zz}$$ 10.13

and the volumetric strain is $-\Delta V/V_0$
so that

$$K = \frac{P \cdot V_0}{\Delta V} = \frac{(X_x + Y_y + Z_z)V_0}{3(e_{xx} + e_{yy} + e_{zz})}$$ 10.14

In addition, a generalized longitudinal modulus (λ or χ) is defined as

$$\frac{\text{Longitudinal load per unit area}}{\text{Longitudinal strain}}$$

so that, with the Poisson ratio, we have five elastic constants that are defined. In an isotropic material only two need to be evaluated independently and all five may be expressed in terms of any two of them, thus:

$$E = 2(1+\sigma)\mu = \frac{9K\mu}{(3K+\mu)}$$ 10.15

$$\mu = \frac{E}{2(1+\sigma)}$$ 10.16

$$K = \frac{E}{3(1-2\sigma)} = \frac{2(1+\sigma)\mu}{3(1-2\sigma)}$$ 10.17

$$\sigma = \frac{3K-2\mu}{2(3K+\mu)}$$ 10.18

$$\lambda = \chi = \frac{E\sigma}{(1+\sigma)(1-2\sigma)} \qquad \textbf{10.19}$$

In the treatment that follows in Ch. 11, the two elastic constants that have been used to characterize the wall are the Young's modulus, E, and the Poisson ratio, σ.

From these, we derive certain approximations when $\sigma \doteqdot 0.5$ which are often quoted without stating this condition e.g.

$$E = 3\mu$$

and it will be seen from eqn. 10.17 that as σ approximates to 0·5 the bulk modulus must become very large. The bulk modulus for arterial wall has not been determined but as it contains some 70 per cent of water its bulk modulus will be of the same order of magnitude. This modulus for water is $2.2 - 2.3 \times 10^{10}$ dyn/cm² (Bridgman, cited in Newman and Searle, 1957) while the Young's modulus for arterial wall is in the range $2 - 8 \times 10^{6}$ dyn/cm²; so we see that this condition is satisfied.

THE BEHAVIOUR OF AN ELASTIC TUBE UNDER A DISTENDING PRESSURE

We have seen that within its elastic limits the increase in length of an elastic material is proportional to the tension applied to it. In the case of a tube of cylindrical cross-section this will be the circumferential tension in the wall due to the lengthening caused by a distending pressure. For a very thin wall, as for example a cylindrical soap bubble, this tension is simply given by

$$T = P.R \qquad \textbf{10.20}$$

and the dimensions of T will be dyn/cm and is often called the longitudinal tension. (This relation is commonly called the law of Laplace since Burton (1954) introduced this term, but its derivation is very simple and appears to date back to at least the early eighteenth century long before Laplace.)

If the wall has a thickness h then the circumferential stress τ is given by

$$\tau = \frac{P.R.}{h} \qquad \textbf{10.21}$$

(often known as Lamé's equation).

It will be seen from eqns. 10.20 and 10.21 that the tension or stress will not vary linearly with the distending pressure so that even though the elastic properties of the wall are Hookean the pressure–volume (so often used in physiology) will not be a straight line. To avoid this confusion tension–volume or tension–circumference plots should be made to study non-Hookean properties of the wall.

Some interesting properties of this relationship were pointed out by Burton (1954). If

$$T = P.R$$

then a small increase in P, δP, will cause an increase in tension, δT, so that we obtain

$$(T + \delta T) = (P + \delta P)(R + \delta R) = PR + R\delta P + P\delta R + \delta R\delta P$$

and if δR and δP are small then

$$\delta T = R.\delta P + P.\delta R \qquad\qquad \textbf{10.22}$$

The strain in the circumferential length of the wall is $2\pi\delta R/2\pi R$ so that from eqn. 10.9 we can write

$$\delta T = E.A. \frac{2\pi\delta R}{2\pi R} = E.A. \frac{\delta R}{R} \qquad\qquad \textbf{10.23}$$

If the length of the tube is L and the tube is isotropic this length will remain constant (eqn. 10.33) and the cross-section of wall, A, may be written $A = h.L$ so that from eqns. 10.22 and 10.23 we have

$$R\delta P + P\delta R = E.h.L. \frac{\delta R}{R} \qquad\qquad \textbf{10.24}$$

so that at the limiting value we have

$$\frac{dR}{dP} = R \bigg/ \left(\frac{Eh.L}{R} - P\right) \qquad\qquad \textbf{10.25}$$

In terms of volume we have

$$\frac{dV}{dP} = \frac{dV}{dR} \cdot \frac{dR}{dP} = 2\pi R \frac{dR}{dP} \qquad\qquad \textbf{10.26}$$

so that

$$\frac{dV}{dP} = \frac{2\pi R^2}{\left(\frac{Eh.L}{R} - P\right)} = \frac{2\pi R^3}{(Eh.L. - P.R.)} \qquad\qquad \textbf{10.27}$$

From this it is clear that if the elastic modulus remains constant the rate of increase of volume with pressure will increase until, at the point where $Eh.L/R = P$, it will become infinite and the tube will burst as tyre tubes do. As will be seen below, however, the elastic modulus of blood vessels increases as the circumferential strain increases and this enables arteries and veins to remain stable over a wide range of pressures. The shape of the resultant curve is more complex than these relations suggest, because with increasing disten-sion, the wall gets thinner and the ratio h/R becomes smaller. Furthermore, although the length, L, remains constant with a vessel in situ, this is not true for an isolated segment over the whole pressure range unless the vessel is held at a constant length. If the tension–circumference graph is a straight line then the elastic behaviour obeys Hooke's law and the Young's modulus is the slope of the curve. If the curve is concave towards the tension axis this indicates an increase in Young's modulus with tension and this is characteristic of the arterial wall and is discussed below (p. 260).

The ratio of the wall-thickness to the radius of an artery is considered below (p. 258) but under physiological pressures lies in the range 0·15–0·20. While this may be approximated quite well by the 'thin-wall' relations above, for accurate measurements we need to derive a better relationship. Each element in the wall of a pressurized tube is subject to stresses in the longitudinal, radial, and circumferential (tangential) directions. The strains can be considered additive if the first strain does not alter the second stress and so on. If the strains are small and the tube is isotropic Love (1944) has shown that they may be resolved as follows when the internal radius is R_i with a distending pressure P_i and the outer radius R_0 with a distending pressure P_0; the stresses are

$$\hat{\theta} = \left(\frac{P_i R_i^2 - P_0 R_0^2}{R_0^2 - R_i^2} \right) + \left(\frac{P_i - P_0}{R_0^2 - R_i^2} \cdot \frac{R_0^2 R_i^2}{R^2} \right) \qquad \textbf{10.28}$$

$$\hat{r} = \left(\frac{P_i R_i^2 - P_0 R_0^2}{R_0^2 - R_i^2} \right) - \left(\frac{P_i - P_0}{R_0^2 - R_i^2} \cdot \frac{R_0^2 \cdot R_i^2}{R^2} \right) \qquad \textbf{10.29}$$

$$\hat{z} = \left(\frac{\lambda}{\lambda + \mu} \cdot \frac{P_i R_i^2 - P_0 R_0^2}{R_0^2 - R_i^2} \right) + \left(\frac{e(3\lambda + 2\mu)\mu}{\lambda + \mu} \right) \qquad \textbf{10.30}$$

where
$\hat{\theta} =$ circumferential stress
$\hat{r} =$ radial stress
$\hat{z} =$ longitudinal stress
$e =$ longitudinal extension
$R =$ any chosen radius between R_i and R_0. If the tube is closed at each end by a flat plate so that the forces of the plates will be balanced by the longitudinal tension then

$$\pi(R_0^2 - R_i^2)\hat{z} = \pi(R_i^2 P_i - R_0^2 P_0) \qquad \textbf{10.31}$$

which gives for the longitudinal extension, e,

$$e = \frac{1}{3\lambda + 2\mu} \cdot \left(\frac{P_i R_i^2 - P_0 R_0^2}{R_0^2 - R_i^2} \right) \qquad \textbf{10.32}$$

and substituting for the values of $\lambda + \mu$ in eqns. 10.16 and 10.19 we obtain

$$e = \frac{(1 - 2\sigma)}{2E} \cdot \left(\frac{P_i R_i^2 - P_0^2 \cdot R_0^2}{R_0^2 - R_i^2} \right) \qquad \textbf{10.33}$$

whence it can be seen that for moderately small distensions of a closed isotropic tube the longitudinal extension will be zero if Poisson's ratio σ is 0·5.

Considering distension, if the radial displacement of a shell of radius R is δR then

$$\delta R = AR + \frac{B}{R} \qquad \text{10.34}$$

where

$$A = \left(\frac{P_i R_i^2 - P_0 R_0^2}{2(\lambda + \mu)(R_0^2 - R_i^2)}\right) - \left(\frac{\lambda e}{2(\lambda + \mu)}\right)$$

and

$$B = \left(\frac{(P_i - P_0) \cdot R_0^2 \cdot R_i^2}{2\mu(R_0^2 - R_i^2)}\right) \qquad \Bigg\} \qquad \text{10.35}$$

and from eqns. 10.16 and 10.19 we have

$$2(\lambda + \mu) = 2\left\{\frac{E\sigma}{(1 + \sigma)(1 - 2\sigma)} + \frac{E}{2(1 + \sigma)}\right\} = \frac{E}{(1 + \sigma)(1 - 2\sigma)} \qquad \text{10.36}$$

Substituting the following terms

$P_i = P$
$P_0 = 0$
$e = 0$
$R = R_0$, i.e. taking the displacement at the outer wall.

$$\delta R = \left(\frac{P R_i^2 R_0 (1 + \sigma)(1 - 2\sigma)}{E(R_0^2 - R_i^2)}\right) + \left(\frac{P R_0^2 \cdot R_i^2 \cdot 2(1 + \sigma)}{2E(R_0^2 - R_i^2)}\right) \cdot \frac{1}{R_0}$$

$$= \frac{P R_i^2 2(1 - \sigma^2) R_0}{E(R_0^2 - R_i^2)} \qquad \text{10.37}$$

and

$$E = \frac{P \cdot R_i^2 2(1 - \sigma^2)}{R_0^2 - R_i^2} \cdot \frac{R_0}{\delta R} \qquad \text{10.38}$$

or when $\sigma = 0·5$

$$E = \frac{1·5 \cdot P R_i^2 \cdot R_0}{(R_0^2 - R_i^2)\delta R} \qquad \text{10.39}$$

DYNAMIC BEHAVIOUR OF ELASTIC MATERIALS

The properties of a 'perfectly' elastic body take no account of the rate at which a stress is applied. In many materials, and this includes all living tissues, the time factor is important in that when they are extended rapidly they are stiffer than when they are extended slowly. The analogy for a perfectly elastic solid is that of a spring and its extension is proportional to the force that is applied and remains constant as long as the force is maintained. On the other hand, the force applied to a liquid causes flow, the rate of which is proportional to the force and which is constant while the force is constant. Living tissues show both of these properties and are classed as *visco-elastic*.

While the elastic behaviour is characterized by a spring, with an elastic modulus, E, the viscous flow behaviour is characterized by a 'dashpot'. This is a cylinder containing a liquid of viscosity, η, in which there is a movable vane connected to the spring (Fig. 10.1). The response of the spring to a tension, T, is given by

$$\frac{\Delta L}{L} = \frac{T}{E} \qquad\qquad \textbf{10.40}$$

while that of a dashpot is

$$\frac{dL}{dt} = \frac{T}{\eta} \qquad\qquad \textbf{10.41}$$

If a spring and a dashpot are connected in series we have what is known as a Maxwell element (Fig. 10.1). On suddenly extending such an element only the spring will stretch and the initial tension T_0 will be $(\Delta L/L) . E$; the dashpot

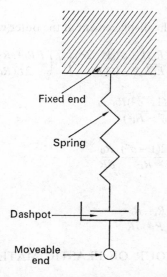

Fixed end

Spring

Dashpot

Moveable end

Fig. 10.1. Model visco-elastic element with one spring and one viscous dashpot in series. This is known as a Maxwell element. As the dashpot contains a viscous liquid which by definition is incapable of sustaining a stress a Maxwell body on its own is, in reality, an elastic liquid.

will, however, begin to move and the tension will begin to decay exponentially to zero according to the formula

$$T = T_0 e^{-Et/\eta} \qquad\qquad \textbf{10.42}$$

This phenomenon is known as stress-relaxation (Fig. 10.3A) and if the analogy with a Maxwell element is adequate the material cannot maintain a stress and is to be classified as an elastic liquid.

At a time $t = \eta/E$ the tension has fallen to $1/e$ of its original value and this is referred to as the relaxation time. If a second spring (modulus E_2) is placed in parallel with the dashpot (Fig. 10.2B) the tension will not decay to zero but its final value will be

$$T = \frac{\Delta L}{L} \cdot \frac{E_1 E_2}{E_1 + E_2} \qquad\qquad \textbf{10.43}$$

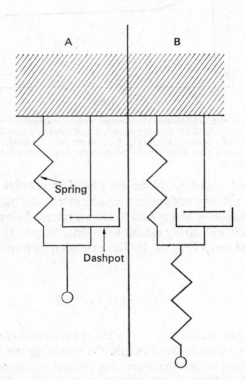

Fig. 10.2A. Simple visco-elastic element with a spring and dashpot in parallel. This is known as a Voigt element. On its own, the arrangement is incapable of a sudden lengthening because of the position of the viscous element.

B. This is a Voigt element with a series spring added and is then commonly known as a St. Venant body.

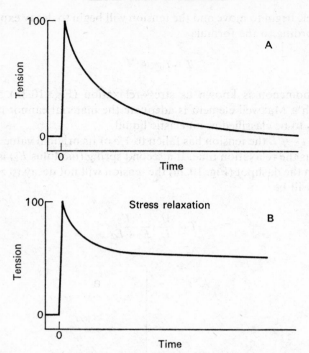

Fig. 10.3. Two types of stresss relaxation; this occurs when a visco-elastic body is suddenly pulled out to a new length and held there. Initially there is a high tension which decays exponentially.
    A. Stress relaxation of a Maxwell body (Fig. 10.1) where the final tension will be zero.
    B. Stress relaxation of a body as in Fig. 10.2B where the final tension is that in the series spring unguarded by a dashpot.

If a spring and a dashpot alone are placed in parallel, it is known as a *Voigt* element. Each unit undergoes the same extension; but the whole cannot respond instantaneously and is said to have a retarded elastic response to an applied force as it will slowly extend to its final length. This phenomenon is commonly called *creep* (Fig. 10.4). The extension in response to an applied force is given by

$$\frac{\Delta L}{L} = \frac{T}{E} (1 - e^{-Et/\eta}) \qquad\qquad \textbf{10.44}$$

and in this case the quantity η/E is called the retardation time, i.e. the time taken to achieve $1/e$ of its final length. On removing the load the converse phenomenon occurs so that the shortening returns on a different curve to that of the lengthening. The two curves thus form a curve which is known as a *hysteresis* loop; the area within the loop represents the energy which has been dissipated by the viscous element.

A combination of a Voigt and a Maxwell element (Fig. 10.2B) is the

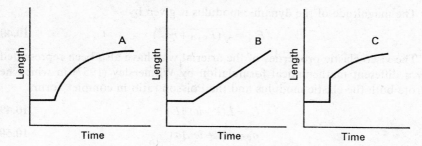

Fig. 10.4. Diagrams to illustrate *creep*. This is the complementary behaviour to stress relaxation in a visco-elastic body. A constant load (or tension) is applied and the element slowly attains (or creeps) to its final length.

A. The type of creep one will get with a Voigt body—see Fig. 10.2A.

B. Linear creep without a final length with a solitary Maxwell body (Fig. 10.1).

C. Creep with a St. Venant body (Fig. 10.2B); the series spring lengthens immediately and lengthening then proceeds as with a Voigt body.

simplest one that has been used to analyse the visco-elastic behaviour of living materials. This type of response has been pursued in considerable detail by Apter and her colleagues (1966, 1967, 1968). The decay in force in stress relaxation is, however, never a simple exponential and it is necessary to postulate a spectrum of such elements.

As the dynamic behaviour of the arterial wall that we are concerned with is the periodic strain imposed by the pulse-wave most workers have preferred to analyse the response of the wall to a stress in the form of a simple harmonic motion. In this case the viscous elements will cause a lag of angle φ, between the applied stress and the resultant strain. The viscosity of the viscous element is symbolized by η.

The first formulation to analyse this in physiology was by Hardung (1952a, 1953, 1962) who expressed the elastic modulus, E', in complex form

$$E' = E_{\text{dyn}} + i\eta\omega \qquad \textbf{10.45}$$

where the real part E_{dyn} is given by

$$E_{\text{dyn}} = \frac{\Delta P}{\Delta l} \cdot \frac{lm}{qm} \cdot \cos \varphi \qquad \textbf{10.46}$$

and

$$\eta\omega = \frac{\Delta P}{\Delta l} \cdot \frac{lm}{qm} \cdot \sin \varphi \qquad \textbf{10.47}$$

where lm and qm are the average length and cross-section of the specimen (Hardung used strips while Bergel (1961b) used segments of cylindrical artery where l would represent circumference); ΔP is the amplitude of the applied stress and $\Delta l/lm$ the strain; ω is the angular frequency; φ, and η, the phase lag and viscosity as stated above.

The magnitude of the dynamic modulus is given by

$$|E'| = \sqrt{(E_{dyn} + \eta\omega^2)} \qquad\qquad \textbf{10.48}$$

The visco-elastic properties of the arterial wall have also been represented by a different mathematical formulation by Womersley (1957) in which he wrote both the elastic modulus and the Poisson ratio in complex form

$$E_c = E(1 + i\omega\Delta E) \qquad\qquad \textbf{10.49}$$

$$\sigma_c = \sigma(1 + i\omega\Delta\sigma) \qquad\qquad \textbf{10.50}$$

This formulation is easier to handle in the wave equations but is more difficult to visualize in a simple physical setting. Its relationship with the formulation of eqn. 10.45 was discussed by Taylor (1959b) and McDonald and Gessner (1968) (Ch. 14); we find that

$$E = E_c = E_{dyn}(1 + i\eta\omega/E_{dyn}) = E_{dyn}(1 + i\omega\Delta E) \qquad\qquad \textbf{10.51}$$

and

$$\frac{\eta\omega}{E_{dyn}} = \tan\ \varphi = \omega\ \left(\Delta E + \frac{2}{3}\Delta\sigma\right) \qquad\qquad \textbf{10.52}$$

when $\sigma = 0\cdot5$. Data derived by the two methods were compared by McDonald and Gessner (1968) and discussed in Ch. 14.

The experimental results are discussed below but it can be noted here that the value of the dynamic modulus which would be expected to rise continuously with frequency (and does with most visco-elastic substances such as plastic tubing), in arterial wall only increases markedly up to a frequency below 2 Hz and thereafter remains virtually constant. Equally, the viscous term η is highly frequency dependent so that the term $\eta\omega$ remains virtually constant with increasing frequency; therefore the 'viscosity' must be regarded as something of a mathematical abstraction and no arrangement of springs and viscous dashpots has yet been found which mimmicks the dynamic elastic behaviour of the arterial wall.

Another way of analysing the behaviour of the wall has been to treat it as an *elastomer*, a class of substances that covers the long-molecular chain polymers. Elastomers are grouped (Stacy et al., 1955) by the properties they have in common. (1) They have a low Young's modulus, of the order of 10^7 dyn/cm^2 compared with most solids which have moduli of the order of 10^{10}–10^{11} dyn/cm^2. They thus include all highly extensible rubber-like substances. (2) They can be stretched to great lengths before their breaking point is reached. (3) Their stress–strain curve is usually sigmoid, or S-shaped. The theory of large deformations in elastomers in terms of the coiling and uncurling of their long-molecular chains using thermodynamic postulates has been quite successful in studying rubber elasticity; on the assumption that these properties are shared by soft body tissues elastomeric theory has been applied in physiology by Guth (1947) and King (1947, 1950) and King and Lawton (1950). A review of their analysis is given by Stacy *et al.* (1955). The mathematical forms, however, are rather intractable and involve inverse Langevin functions which are rarely tabulated so that this approach has not been followed here.

THE VELOCITY OF PROPAGATION IN AN ELASTIC TUBE

The elastic behaviour of the wall of a tube plays an important part in determining the velocity of propagation of a pressure-wave. The study of this problem is closely related to that of the analysis of the velocity of sound in air which was first studied by Isaac Newton. His equation was

$$c_0 = \sqrt{\frac{K}{\rho}} \qquad \qquad 10.53$$

where K was the volume elasticity and ρ the density. The analogy between the velocity of wave-propagation in a compressible fluid (e.g. air) and that in an incompressible fluid (i.e. a liquid) in an elastic tube is very close. Writing eqn. 10.53 out more fully by expanding the volume elasticity, K, we obtain

$$c_0 = \sqrt{\frac{\delta P}{\rho.\delta V/V}} = \sqrt{\frac{\delta P.V}{\rho.\delta V}} \qquad \qquad 10.54$$

which is the form of the equation derived by Hill from the Moens-Korteweg equation (eqn. 10.56) in the classic paper by Bramwell and Hill (1922). The above derivation from Newton's equation was, however, first made by Thomas Young in his Croonian lecture of 1809. Further analyses in the problem were done by E. H. Weber (1850) and later in detail by Résal and Korteweg to whom the final form of eqn. 10.56 was attributed. A stimulating historical review of this subject has been written by Lambossy (1950).

A simple derivation linking Young's treatment with the later work may be made from eqn. 10.54 when expanding $\delta V/\delta P$ as in eqn. 10.26. We may write, with L constant,

$$c_0 = \sqrt{\frac{\pi R^2.\delta P}{\rho 2\pi R.\delta R}} = \sqrt{\frac{R.\delta P}{\rho.2\delta R}} \qquad \qquad 10.55$$

and this form is very useful in calculating the equivalent wave-velocity from measurements of the radial dilatation of arteries *in situ* as by Patel *et al.* (1963) and Greenfield and Patel (1962).

Taking eqn. 10.54 a step further and substituting the derived value for $\delta V/\delta P$ of eqn. 10.27 for a unit length of the circumference, L, and taking the mean value of P as an arbitrary zero we obtain, with E as the Young's modulus in the circumferential direction, and h the wall thickness,

$$c_0 = \sqrt{\frac{E.h}{2R\rho}} \qquad\qquad \textbf{10.56}$$

This is known as the Moens–Korteweg equation. This equation was used with the addition of a constant K in front of the square-root term by Moens (1878) in his experimental studies of the velocity of a pressure-wave in a rubber-tube filled with water. He set the value of his arbitrary constant at 0·9. From the analyses of Womersley (1955c, 1957) which are discussed in Ch. 11 the effect of the viscosity of water in a tube such as that used by Moens would be to reduce the velocity of the wave slightly from that given by eqn. 10.56 and would be equivalent to a value of K of 0·9–0·95, and it is this effect, probably, that made it necessary for him to introduce this constant.

The assumptions underlying the Moens–Korteweg equation (10.56) are that the tube is thin-walled, i.e. $h/2R$ is small; that it is filled with an 'ideal' liquid that is incompressible and has no viscosity. The first two assumptions are quite reasonable; the value of $h/2R$ is normally less than 0·1 and, as was seen on p. 244, the bulk modulus of water is between 10^3 to 10^4 times greater than the elastic modulus of the wall. In the larger arteries the effect of viscosity is also small but will retard the velocity greatly in the smaller vessels—a topic that is discussed at greater length in Ch. 11.

The errors due to assuming that the wall is 'thin' have been explored by Bergel (1960). In the Moens–Korteweg equation (10.56) the wall is assumed to be so thin that there is no appreciable change in wall-thickness. In a wall of finite thickness this is not the case so that the Poisson's ratio has to be incorporated. The full correction equation by Bergel (1960) is given as

$$\left(\frac{c'}{c_0}\right)^2 = \frac{(2-\gamma)}{(2-2\gamma(1-\sigma-2\sigma^2)+\gamma^2(1-\sigma-2\sigma^2)-2\sigma^2)} \qquad \textbf{10.57}$$

where c' is the 'true' derived velocity and c_0 is the velocity calculated from eqn. 10.56; γ is the ratio h/R_{outer}. Taking a Poisson ratio of 0·5 this results in the conclusion that the true derived velocity is higher than c_0 by a factor of $\sqrt{(4/3)}$ even if the wall is very thin. Only when the Poisson ratio is put at zero does the discrepancy disappear. In practice, an effective simplification of eqn. 10.57 in terms of eqn. 10.56 is

$$c' = \sqrt{\frac{Eh}{2\rho R(1-\sigma^2)}} \qquad\qquad \textbf{10.58}$$

The difference between Moens–Korteweg and 'corrected' wave velocities was found by Bergel (1961b) to lie between 16–24 per cent; this discrepancy at that time was not taken to be of great account because the measurement error of the pulse-wave velocity was considerable. Using the technique of measuring wave-front velocities with a delay line (McDonald, 1968a) however, Nichols and McDonald (1972) have been able to reduce the standard error of their measurements to ±3 per cent so that these refinements of relating the elastic constants to the wave-velocity have now become relevant. Careful experiments in wave-velocity and wall-elasticity measured in the same animal still need to be done.

Bergel (1960) also discussed other sources of error; he concluded that the inertial effect due to the movement of the wall would be very small as the radial movement of the wall is small (see p. 271 below). The effects of longitudinal restraint due to the surrounding connective tissue attachments ('tethering'), anistropy, and the effect of the blood viscosity and flow velocity were also discussed but are considered at greater length in Ch. 11.

In general, the calculation of the wave-velocity from the elastic modulus has utilized the Moens–Korteweg equation, 10.56 or eqn. 10.58; the latter is more accurate when visco-elastic effects are allowed for. Various other modifications have been used but have not been proved to be more accurate. Opatowski (1967) has made a theoretical analysis which he considers shows that the definitions for the elastic modulus over-estimate the true value.

OTHER MODES OF WAVE-PROPAGATION

The propagated wave that is considered above is that of the pressure-wave accompanied by a radial dilatation. This is, however, only one of the types of wave that can be transmitted in the elastic substance of the wall. These waves are classified here in so far as there has been some study of them in relation to the elastic constants of the artery. They will be further discussed in Chs. 11 and 14.

(1) *The distension mode or pressure-wave.* Also referred to as Young's mode (Klip, Van Loon and Klip, 1967; Klip, 1969). As the transmission of pressure throughout the arterial system is a major concern in physiological studies it is the only one considered in detail here.

A second mode of wave of this type has been predicted theoretically by Atabek and Lew (1966) but has not been detected experimentally.

(2) *The longitudinal or axial mode.* First described by Lamb (1898) and called the Lamb mode this is a compression wave in the wall of the tube. It propagates at a much higher velocity than the distension wave and is detected by longitudinal movements of the wall. This has been studied in arteries by Anliker, Moritz and Ogden (1968).

(3) *Torsional mode.* A wave form originating in a twisting strain. This has been studied in particular by Klip and Klip (1964), Klip, Van Loon and Klip (1967).

(4) *Flexural mode.* A wave in which the whole tube is displaced laterally; it is analogous to the wave created in a rope that is tethered at one end while the other is shaken up and down.

EXPERIMENTAL INVESTIGATIONS

For technical reasons, it is much easier to measure stress–strain relationships in an excised artery than it is to measure them in the living animal, and a large amount of data has been obtained in this way. It is, therefore, necessary to consider the validity of observations made in this way when applying them to an artery *in situ* in the living animal.

From general principles the obvious reason for doubting their value is that a post-mortem change, such as is usually seen in biological tissues, will have occurred. However, the truly elastic constituents of the wall are the collagen and elastin fibres that form a closely-meshed matrix. These are chemically very stable, in fact, two of the most stable proteins known. There is little evidence that they change their elastic properties until the vessel wall putrefies. There is also a smooth muscle component and, in the absence of an adequate oxygen supply, this will not maintain a contraction; in other circumstances, it may undergo rigor mortis and go into spasm. While in both cases the tension in the wall will alter and thus change the apparent elastic modulus it can be, and has been, argued that as a contractile tissue, like muscle, is not essentially elastic the tissue may be properly studied without the added variations in muscle tension. The effect of smooth muscle on the wall is discussed separately below.

The important confusion in applying measurements on isolated segments to their function under physiological conditions arises from the dimensional changes that occur when they are removed. These will be considered under the headings: (1) the lengths of the segment; (2) the thickness of the wall, and (3) the initial dimensions before applying stress.

(1) The length of an arterial segment

Arteries in the body are naturally under a condition of longitudinal tension. This is demonstrated by the fact that if any artery is severed the cut ends retract a little from each other; when it is dissected free from the surrounding tissues it further shortens by a much greater amount. Although this retraction of excised arteries was studied by Fuchs (1900) at the beginning of the century, the significance of this phenomenon to the study of elastic measurements in excised vessels does not seem to have been appreciated until the work of McDonald (1960) and Bergel (1960). The amount of the retraction varies between animals and it has been shown to decrease with increasing age. Hesse (1926) found that, in the aorta, there was a retraction of 40 per cent at age 12, reducing to 12 per cent at age 65 and nil at 67. The average values for the per cent shortening in terms of *in vivo* length in various arteries found by Fuchs and Bergel were:

TABLE 10.1. Retraction of vessels *in vitro*

	Fuchs	Bergel	(S.E.M.)	(N)
Thoracic aorta	21·0%	31·9%	±0·62	22
Abdominal aorta	33·3%	34·0%	±0·63	17
Carotid artery	33·6%	42·0%	±0·89	22
Femoral artery	37·6%	35·2%	±0·53	29
Iliac artery	—	39·5%	±0·74	9

A contraction of 40 per cent means, of course, that a 5 cm length in the body will shorten by 2 cm. Before the tissue connections are removed the corresponding shortening is found to be only about 0·3–0·5 cm. This observation together with the finding that there is very little, if any, longitudinal movement of the artery during passage of the pulse-wave, led to the concept called *tethering* of arteries. This longitudinal restraint has been studied quantitatively by Patel and Fry (1966); their data and the implications of tethering in the analysis of wave-propagation is discussed more fully in Ch. 11. It does, however, raise the conceptual problem as to the limits of the functional arterial wall when considering excised vessels. Clearly, the effective longitudinal elasticity, at least, will be altered markedly by removing this longitudinal restraint from the outside of the artery. Its implications in measuring the thickness and the composition of the 'true' wall are discussed below.

When the ends of an excised and retracted vessel are blocked and the segment subjected to an internal pressure it will lengthen. This was studied by Fenn (1957). As an isotropic tube of Poisson ratio 0·5 will remain at a constant length when inflated (eqn. 10.33), Fenn concluded that the arterial wall was either markedly anisotropic, with an elastic modulus that was much less in the longitudinal than circumferential direction, or that the Poisson ratio was much less than 0·5. As the evidence discussed below indicates that the Poisson ratio is indeed very close to 0·5, then the vessel must be anisotropic. There is, in fact, no question that the excised retracted artery is markedly anisotropic. For example, McDonald (1960) found that the longitudinal modulus of elasticity of the excised dog femoral artery was c. $2·0 \times 10^6$ cyn/cm^2 up to 90 per cent of its *in vivo* length, while at a distending pressure of 100 mm Hg the circumferential modulus was c. $10·0 \times 10^6$ dyn/cm^2.

The lengthening that accompanies distension is not, however, sufficient to account for all natural lengths of an artery in the body. At a distending pressure of 100 mm Hg Bergel (1960) found that the length of the excised segment was about 90 per cent of its *in vivo* length and that further increases in pressure produced little extra extension and they never reached their natural length. There is some variability between arteries. The thoracic aorta, in my experience, will often regain its *in vivo* length and, at high pressures (e.g. 200 mm Hg) may even exceed it; in the abdominal aorta I have found, with Bergel (1960), that the natural length is never reached and a considerable additional force is needed to pull it out to its *in vivo* length. Arteries in their natural position must, therefore, be always subject to a longitudinal stress. The reason for this is a matter for speculation, and it is postulated that it is due to different growth rates between the artery and the surrounding tissues.

In order to study the circumferential modulus of an excised vessel, it is necessary to measure its length in the body and then extend and hold it at this length during distension; these measurements will then be relevant to the physiological situation. Similarly, measurements of the longitudinal modulus should be made for small extensions around the natural length. Values derived from the force–length curve at initial lengths markedly different from the *in vivo* length will be very different from those at the natural length. Only experimental values obtained by other workers under these conditions will be considered in this chapter. Where the modulus or distensibility has been measured by the change in volume on distension of the unrestrained segment, the inaccuracy is very marked.

Another type of arterial sample that has often been used is the arterial strip. If these are cut in the longitudinal direction then the same considerations apply as for the whole segment. It is more usual, however, to cut the strip in a closely pitched helix as the majority of the muscle cells are orientated in this direction. In this case, it is virtually impossible to estimate the natural length, and data from such preparations must be treated with caution. With arterial rings also there can be no control of the width of the strip. The free edges in all strips also lead to minor distortions (called 'edge-effects' in the elasticity literature).

Before 1960 there was little study of the elasticity of the artery *in situ* although Alexander (1954) had shown that this was feasible. Since the paper of Peterson *et al.* (1960) in which a gauge was used to measure the radial dilatation caused by the pulse wave there have been several studies of this nature with improved gauges. Isolated segments maintained *in situ* have also been used by Patel in a series of papers and this method also has the advantage of maintaining the initial length and the tissue attachments.

(2) The thickness of the arterial wall

Nowhere are the difficulties of applying precise elastic theory to the arterial wall more apparent than in the problem of determining the thickness of the wall. Yet, in ordinary physical studies this would be regarded as very elementary. The imprecision with which one can define the limits of the outer wall in relation to the surrounding tissues has already been mentioned. In addition, the retraction of the segment will cause the wall to thicken. The radial collapse due to removal of the distending pressure will also create wall-thickening. A combination of these factors plus fixation artifacts makes estimates of wall thickness from ordinary histological sections also useless. The estimation of the *in vivo* thickness is then calculated from the assumption that the volume of the wall does not change on extension. This was shown to be the case by Lawton (1954) on arterial strips and, with more confidence, by Carew, Vishnaiv and Patel (1968) on arteries *in situ*.

The method of measurement originally used by McDonald (1960) was to determine the volume (V) of the specimen from weight, (W), and density, (Δ), i.e. from the weight in air and in water. The dimensions of the *in vivo* external radius R_0 and the length (L) allow one to calculate the internal radius R_i, and thus the wall-thickness, h.

$$V = \frac{W}{\Delta} = L\pi(R_0{}^2 - R_i{}^2) \qquad\qquad \textbf{10.59}$$

This method has been used since by the majority of workers. The density, Δ, of the wall is close to 1·06, i.e. very close to that of blood which is 1·05–1·055. McDonald (1960) found no significant difference in the ratio h/R in any artery from the carotid to saphenous. Later values for various arteries are:

TABLE 10.2. Thickness of arterial wall

	Bergel (1960)	Gow & Taylor (1968)	
Thoracic aorta	0·105±0·0046 (15)	0·14	(13)
Abdominal aorta	0·105±0·0061 (9)	0·12	(10)
Femoral artery	0·112±0·0096 (11)	0·13	(16)
Carotid artery	0·132±0·0075 (13)		
	(at 100 mm Hg pressure)	(mean pressure, 105–124 mm Hg)	

Peterson *et al.* (1960) obtained a mean value of 0·15 as did Hürthle (1920), while Patel *et al.* (1969) recorded mean values from 0·123 to 0·10 according to longitudinal extension in the thoracic aorta. Hürthle measured wall thickness in histological sections of arteries fixed *in situ* at a normal distending pressure; Attinger (1968) used the same technique in the femoral artery. Peterson also made a direct measurement. The discrepancies between these estimates can obviously lead to discrepancies in the calculated elastic modulus; however, they probably stem from individual variations in the assessment of outer limit of the arterial wall. That is the decision in answer to the question 'What is artery and what is surrounding connective tissue?'

(3) The 'initial' dimensions of the artery. The incremental modulus

In defining the Young's modulus (eqn. 10.9) as the ratio of stress to strain the length of the initial condition was symbolized by L_0 (eqn. 10.1). In a tube this length is the circumference or $2\pi R_0$. In classical elastic theory R_0 would be the dimension where there is no stress. This would indicate the analogy with the artery when there is zero distending pressure; the length of a segment, L_0, *in situ* we have already seen to be subjected to longitudinal stress. Similarly, an artery that is cut open longitudinally will open up, indicating that there is a residual circumferential stress, even though it is small. Furthermore, it can be seen from Figs. 10.5 and 10.6 that the stress–strain is markedly concave towards

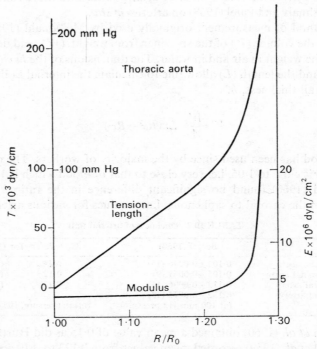

Fig. 10.5. The tension–length relation (elastic diagram) of a segment of the thoracic aorta of a dog subjected to various distending pressures Ordinate—tension in dynes $\times 10^3$/cm (from eqn. 10.20), Abscissa—relative increase of radius (and hence of circumference).

The curve for the Young's modulus is plotted from the slope of the elastic diagram (tangent modulus). If the modulus were calculated with reference to the resting length at zero tension the value at 200 mm Hg pressure would be about 4.2×10^6 dynes/cm². This discrepancy between the two methods only becomes noticeable when there is a marked departure from linearity—for pressures up to 100 mm Hg the elastic behaviour, in this case, is remarkably linear.

the stress axis. If, therefore, the value of R_0 is always taken as that at zero pressure the slope of this line deviates greatly from that of the curve and we are dealing with large strains greatly in excess of the very small strains postulated in Hooke's Law. If, however, the stress is increasing by a series of small steps then the strain at each step can be regarded as the ratio of the increment of extension expressed as a ratio to the length pertaining before the last increment of stress was added. This is the measure commonly used when large extensions are possible in rubber-like material; it is called the *incremental modulus*. Because the limit as the increments get very small is the slope of the

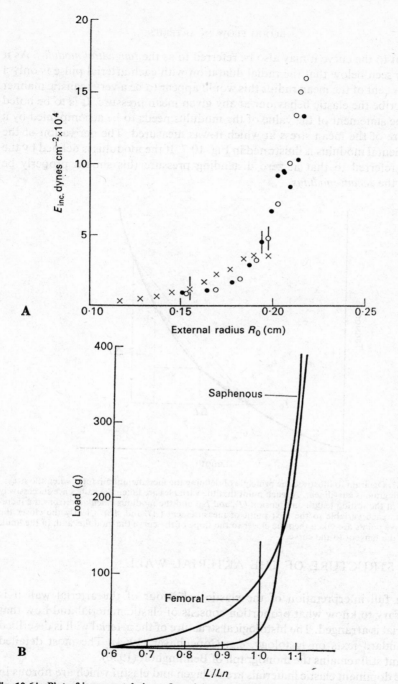

Fig. 10.6A. Plot of incremental circumferential elastic modulus against the radius for a femoral artery in the dog. Three successive runs are superimposed; a different symbol is used for the points on each run. (From Bergel, 1960.)

B. Elastic diagrams for longitudinal extension of specimens of femoral and saphenous arteries of the dog. Ordinate—load in grams; Abscissa—ratio of length to that of the specimen *in the body*. It will be observed that at this length the extensibility of the artery is rapidly increasing.

tangent to the curve it may also be referred to as the *tangential modulus*. As it will be seen below that the radial dilatation with each arterial pulse is only a few per cent of the mean radius this would appear to be a very realistic manner to describe the elastic behaviour at any given mean pressure. It is to be noted that the statement of the value of the modulus needs to be accompanied by a measure of the mean stress at which it was measured. The derivation of the incremental modulus is illustrated in Fig. 10.7. If the modulus is defined by the strain referred to that at zero distending pressure this should properly be called the *secant modulus*.

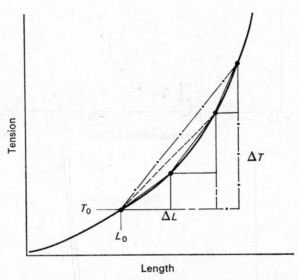

Fig. 10.7. Diagram to illustrate the principle of defining the incremental modulus when the stress–strain diagram is curvilinear. At each point that the variables are taken the values are successively treated at the resting length and tension (T_0 and L_0) and the modulus calculated from the increments in each variable to the next point of measurement (ΔT and ΔL). Clearly the closer the successive points are taken then the closer to the slope of the curve the modulus and, in the limit, will be the tangent to the curve.

THE STRUCTURE OF THE ARTERIAL WALL

For a full interpretation of the elastic behaviour of the arterial wall it is necessary to know what proportion consists of elastic material and how that material is arranged. The histological structure of the arterial wall is described in standard texts on histology, e.g. Copenhaver (1964). The most detailed account still remains the monograph of Benninghoff (1930).

The dominant elastic materials are collagen and elastin which are fibrous in nature although the latter tends to be formed into more or less continuous sheets. The third major constituent is smooth muscle which, while contributing to the tension in the wall, cannot properly be regarded as a true elastic material. The collagen and elastin are complexed with an amorphous substance formed of mucoprotein which, while not itself elastic, contributes greatly to the tensile properties of the collagen, at least. For example, Wood (1954) demonstrated that chemical treatment, e.g. a change in pH, that causes no change in histological structure, even when studied with the electron-microscope, can virtually destroy the tensile strength of collagen.

The blood vessel wall is divided into three zones; the tunicas intima, media and adventitia. The demarcation between the tunica intima and media is by the internal elastic lamina. This is a complex structure which consists of a fenestrated membrane of elastin lined on the intimal side by a coarse fibrous network. The intima consists of the vascular endothelium which is a single layer of cells together with a thin layer of elastin and collagen fibres by which it is anchored to the internal elastic lamina. Fry (1968, 1969a, b) has shown that the endothelium may be damaged quite easily by shearing stresses not greatly in excess of those normally encountered in the circulation due to viscous drag. It may be relatively easily detached from the internal lamina but has considerable powers of regeneration (Poole, 1964; Poole et al., 1958, 1959).

The outer elastic lamina demarks the media from the adventitia. This latter is a region of collagen and some elastin tissue which merges with the surrounding connective tissue and contains the vasa vasorum—the small vessels which run into and supply the wall of the large arteries with blood, nerves and lymphatics.

The tunica media forms the large part of the wall. The intermediate layers have a fibrous structure, the fibres running circularly or in a tight helix. Between these layers lie smooth muscle cells mostly parallel to the elastin though some are oriented longitudinally.

The structure of the tunica media has been subjected to detailed study by Wolinsky and Glagov (1964) who describe it as being made up of an orderly array of lamellar units. At physiological distending pressures elastin and collagen fibres and smooth muscle cells are precisely orientated and form well-defined layers. Relatively thick elastin bands are seen as concentric plates while finer elastin fibres form networks between them. Collagen fibres are dispersed in the interstices and are arranged circumferentially. Although the finer elastin fibres connect with the elastin lamellae no attachments between collagen and elastin fibres can be demonstrated. The smooth muscle cells extend circumferentially between adjacent lamellas among the fine elastin and collagen fibres.

ELASTIC PROPERTIES OF THE COMPONENTS

When studying the elastic behaviour of a material which has such a complex structure as arterial wall it is natural that attempts should be made to interpret the results in terms of the various components. Collagen may be studied in a relatively pure form in tendons; elastin has not been isolated in such a pure form but certain ligaments have a high concentration, e.g. the ligamentum nuchae of the ox is formed of elastin with some 9 per cent collagen. The elastic modulus of collagen is much higher than that of elastin. Values from Krafka (1939) and Bergel (1960) indicate values for the Young's modulus as: collagen, $0\cdot5-1\cdot0 \times 10^8$ dyn/cm^2; elastin, $0\cdot4-1\cdot0 \times 10^7$ dyn/cm^2. Relaxed muscle develops virtually no tension until it is stretched to great lengths and may be regarded as contributing solely viscous properties to the wall. At maximal contraction Somlyo and Somlyo (1968) estimate that vascular smooth muscle can exert a force of $1-3 \times 10^6$ dyn/cm^2 or possibly higher; this is of the same order of magnitude as the values of $3\cdot5-8 \times 10^6$ dyn/cm^2 found by Abbott and Lowy (1958) for molluscan smooth muscle (adductor muscle). The differences in stiffness between elastin and collagen have been used to explain the length–tension diagram of the arterial wall. It may be postulated that at short extensions it is only the elastin which is being extended while at great lengths the tension is borne more and more by the collagen until it sustains all the tension. This view was pursued in the German literature, e.g. Wezler and Sinn (1953) and in a valuable review by Burton (1954). By digesting away either the elastin or the collagen Roach and Burton (1957) produced some support for the idea. It is certainly true that the highest values for the elastic modulus of the arteries, e.g. the longitudinal length–tension curve of the saphenous artery in Fig. 10.6B gives a modulus which does approximate to the elastic modulus of collagen but these values are always well outside the physiological range. It may be said that the high tensile strength of collagen is clearly a protection against over-stretching of arteries and is the principle protection against rupture at high pressures.

THE COMPOSITION OF THE ARTERIAL WALL

In view of the diverse elastic properties of the components of the arterial wall it is clearly of interest to know in what proportions they occur. Many estimates have been made, e.g. Hürthle (1920) from a study of histological sections (see Bergel, 1960, for a review of the older literature). From the fibrous nature of collagen and elastin this is of necessity very difficult and the results only approximate. For example, Hürthle gives proportions for the aorta of: collagen, 1/3–1/10; elastin, 1/3–2/5; muscle, 1/3–1/2.

As the chemical composition of collagen and, to a less certain extent, elastin are known, Harkness, Harkness and McDonald (1957) made a chemical analysis of arteries throughout the arterial tree. They first found that, in common with most living tissues, water comprised some 70 per cent of the weight of the wall (comparison of initial weight with the weight after

24 hours in a desiccator). Of the dry weight about 50 per cent was made up of elastin and collagen; the remainder consists of muscle (which was not estimated) and non-fibrous matrix. The distribution between elastin and collagen was strikingly different between the intrathoracic and extrathoracic arteries. This is illustrated in Fig. 10.8; here the elastin is plotted as a fraction

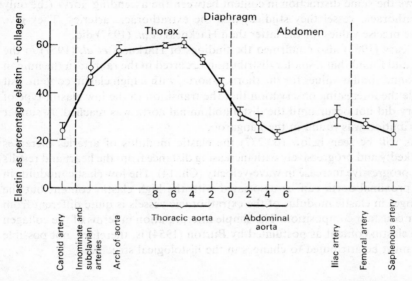

Fig. 10.8. The chemical composition of the fibrous elements of the arterial wall. The ordinant represents the elastin expressed as a percentage of the total elastin and collagen. Note that elastic greatly preponderates in the thoracic aorta while outside the thorax the reverse is the case. The transition from one type to the other occurs over about 5 cm and there is no significant difference in composition among the extrathoracic arteries even though the elastic modulus steadily increases with increasing distance from the heart. (From Harkness, Harkness and McDonald, 1955.)

of total elastin and collagen. In the thoracic aorta the elastin formed 60 per cent of total fibrous element and collagen 40 per cent. In the extrathoracic vessels the composition reversed to elastin 30 per cent and collagen 70 per cent. The transition occurred rapidly over the last 5 cm of the aorta above the diaphragm and over a similar distance in the branches leaving the arch of the aorta. Thereafter, no significant change in composition could be found in any artery. A similar distribution has since been found in the pig.

A similar study has been made by Apter, Rabinowitz and Cummings (1966) for the aorta in which chemical analyses have been compared with histological estimates. This has produced divergent results between two methods used for estimating collagen but are substantially in agreement with Harkness *et al.* (1957). In addition, an attempt was made to estimate the muscle protein although Apter *et al.* (1966) admit that this is subject to error. The values found were: ascending aorta, 35 per cent; thoracic aorta, 44 per cent;

abdominal aorta, 51–61 per cent. The number of muscle cells per mm² were in parallel with these values but no attempt was made to calculate this as a proportion of the cross-sectional area of the aorta. Most estimates approximate 25 per cent as the amount of muscle cells in the aorta. Fisher and Llaurado (1966) have also estimated the collagen and elastin content. This shows the same distinction in content between the ascending aorta (the only intrathoracic vessel they studied) and the extrathoracic arteries. They give more precise values for the latter than Harkness *et al.* (1957) did.

Cleary (1963) also confirmed the findings of Harkness *et al.* (1957) in the dog and found that a similar distribution occurred in the rabbit. In the human he found similar values for the thoracic aorta, with a high elastin content, but made the interesting observation that the transition to the low elastin type of artery did not occur until the distal abdominal aorta was reached. A similar distribution was found in the kangaroo.

As will be seen below (p. 277) the elastic modulus of arteries increases markedly and progressively with increasing distance from the heart and results in a progressive increase in wave-velocity (Ch. 14). The low elastic modulus in the proximal aorta can be associated with the high elastin content but the changes in elastic modulus of the extrathoracic vessels is quite different from their constant composition. The simple interpretation in terms of the collagen and elastin content as postulated by Burton (1954) is, therefore, not possible but must be attributed to changes in the histological structure.

MEASUREMENT OF THE ELASTIC PARAMETERS OF THE ARTERIAL WALL

(a) Poisson ratio

McDonald (1960) deduced from the relationship between the elastic parameters in eqn. 10.17 that the Poisson ratio of arterial wall must be very close to 0·5. Thus, if the elastic modulus, E, is 1×10^6 dyn/cm² and the bulk modulus, K, is that of water, i.e. $2 \cdot 2 \times 10^{10}$ dyn/cm², then the Poisson ratio will be 0·4998. The bulk modulus of the arterial wall had not then been measured, but in view of the fact that 70 per cent of the wall is comprised of water then its modulus was assumed to be very close to that of water. From the relationship given in eqn. 10.17 it was seen that when the Poisson ratio is 0·5 then there is no change of volume on extension. Lawton (1954) extended strips of arterial wall and could find no detectable change in volume; a more detailed study has been undertaken by Carew, Vaishnav and Patel (1968) with more precise methods and shown that extension is indeed isovolumetric. They derived a bulk modulus for the wall of $4 \cdot 35 \times 10^9$ dyn/cm².

The value for Poisson ratio for small strains may, therefore, be taken as 0·5. Such small strains will occur during radial dilatation by the aortic pulse.

(b) The circumferential elastic modulus

A large number of estimations of this parameter have been published in the literature and it is impossible to survey them all here. For reasons given above, those values derived from measurements on aortic strips, e.g. Lawton (1954, 1955) and Hardung (1952, 1962), or on aortic rings, e.g. Remington (1955, 1962a), or more recently, Apter *et al.* (1966), will not be discussed in detail.

Measurements on the whole vessel have fallen into two main groups; those relating the radial expansion to the change in the distending pressure, and those which have derived the elastic modulus from the wave-velocity by means of eqns. 10.55, 10.56 or 10.58. This latter relationship will be treated again in Ch. 14 but is useful in checking the accuracy of values obtained by the first general method when the performance of diameter gauges is in question. The checking of one method against the other in the same animal is clearly desirable.

Bergel (1960, 1961a, b) made a long series of measurements on isolated segments of dog arteries. The vessels were held in air at their *in vivo* length and the pressure within it recorded while the volume was changed. The external diameter was recorded by directing a collimated light beam across the vessel on to a photo-electric tube. Changes in the diameter of the segment caused a variation in the light falling on the tube.

The use of a light beam to measure wall movements has the great advantage that it imposes no restraint on the wall. Earlier attempts to do this by photographic means (McDonald, 1953, Lawton and Greene, 1956) had not proved very accurate and led to a tedious process of analysis. The Bergel method is, however, impossible to apply *in situ*, and difficult to use in a bath of oxygenated solution to maintain the functional activity of the muscle cells.

Bergel performed two sets of experiments. The first involved static, or maintained, distensions, each held for two minutes to allow for the completion of stress relaxation. The first few inflations after the artery had been removed from the body for some time showed marked hysteresis loops, i.e. the descending pressure limb was markedly divergent from the curve for increasing pressure. After these initial cycles there was very little hysteresis on the curves obtained in slow steps.

The average values for the elastic modulus at various pressures is displayed in Fig. 10.9. It will be seen that the points for the abdominal aorta, femoral and carotid arteries fall close together in these static measurements. The thoracic aorta is markedly less stiff in the range from 80 to 180 mm Hg but they become indistinguishable at 200 mm Hg; the thoracic aorta actually appears stiffer than the carotid at 220 mm Hg.

Dynamic elastic modulus. Bergel (1960, 1961b) used the same apparatus to determine the visco-elastic properties of arteries. Instead of incremental

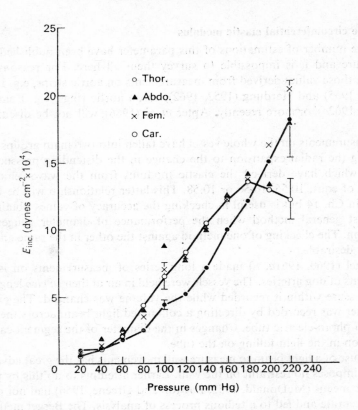

Fig. 10.9. The average static elastic modulus for all specimens tested for arteries from four different sites. (From Bergel, 1960.)

   Symbols: squares—thoracic aorta;
              triangles—abdominal aorta;
              crosses—femoral artery;
              circles—carotid artery.

volume changes a sinusoidal pump oscillated the pressure inside the segments and the variations in diameter were monitored continuously. The mean pressure was held at 100 mm Hg. The ratio of diameter to pressure was analysed into real and imaginary parts and calculated as E_{dyn} and $\eta\omega$ as in eqns. 10.45–10.48. The lowest frequency measured was 2 Hz and it was found that there was a marked increase in the elastic modulus between the static value and that at 2 Hz but thereafter there was no significant rise in modulus up to 20 Hz. The phase lag was between 0·1 and 0·15 radians with the results that the term $\eta\omega$ remained virtually constant over the measured frequency range (Fig. 10.10A and B). This means that the viscosity term η falls inversely with frequency; this is unlike any known viscous material and indicates that the simple conceptual model of a single spring and dashpot should not be regarded as a realistic representation. In an 'orthodox' visco-elastic substance both E_{dyn} and $\eta\omega$ rise steadily with frequency (Fig. 10.11).

A similar investigation was made by the same techniques on human arteries by Learoyd and Taylor (1966). They were classified as young (ages 11–20) and old (36–52). One interesting point of distinction between these and the values for the dog is that in the young group the elasticity of the carotid artery is the same as that of the aorta while that of the femoral artery is much higher, in the human; while in the dog the carotid is very similar to the femoral. The groups of subjects were not very large but it is possible that this difference is connected with the normal upright stance of man.

Learoyd and Taylor (1966) also studied the effect of change of length of the specimen beyond its natural length on the circumferential elastic modulus. When the modulus was plotted against the external radius the effect of lengthening was to increase the circumferential modulus markedly. However, when the modulus was plotted against internal pressure there was little change and indeed there was a tendency for a decrease in modulus. This had

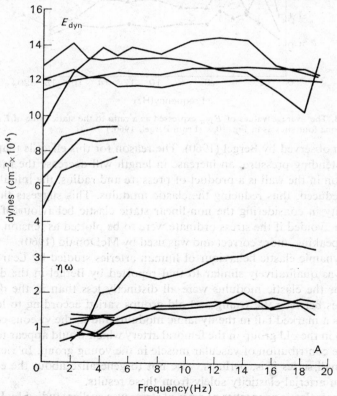

Fig. 10.10A. The values of E_{dyn} and $\eta\omega$ for the abdominal aorta from 2–20 Hz. It can be seen that both variables are virtually constant above frequencies of 2–4 Hz. (From Bergel, 1960.)

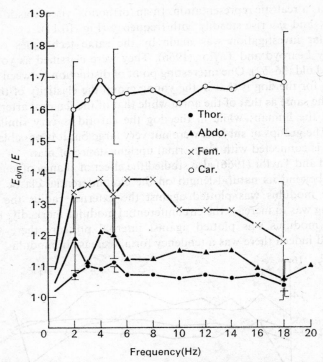

Fig. 10.10B. The average values of E_{dyn} expressed as a ratio to the static value of E in arteries from the same four sites as in Fig. 10.9. (From Bergel, 1960.)

also been observed by Bergel (1960). The reason for this effect is that, at any given distending pressure, an increase in length will decrease the radius. As the tension in the wall is a product of pressure and radius, the initial tension will be reduced, thus reducing the elastic modulus. This suggests that some complexity in considering the non-linear static elastic behaviour of arteries would be avoided if the stress ordinate were to be plotted as tension. This is, strictly speaking, more correct and was used by McDonald (1960).

The dynamic elastic behaviour of human arteries studied by Learoyd and Taylor was qualitatively similar to that reported by Bergel in the dog. The values for the elastic modulus were all distinctly less than in the dog. The differences between the young and old groups varied according to location; there was a marked fall in the dynamic modulus and in the viscous contribution ($\eta\omega$) in the old group in the femoral artery which would appear to be due to a large contribution of vascular muscle in the young group. In view of the rather small series it is, perhaps, wise not to generalize about the effects of ageing on arterial elasticity solely from these results.

The visco-elastic properties of arterial strips was earlier studied by Hardung (1952, 1953) and by Lawton (1955). Qualitatively the results are very similar

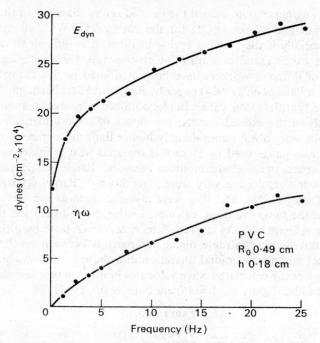

Fig. 10.11. The values of E_{dyn} and $\eta\omega$ for a typical visco-elastic substance—a segment of polyvinyl chloride tubing. Note how both parameters increase in value continuously with increases of frequency in contrast to that of the arterial wall. (From Bergel, 1960.)

to those quoted above and Hardung showed that the rise in modulus from the static value to the dynamic value is complete at a frequency of 1 Hz and almost so by 0·5 Hz. Remington has also done extensive work using arterial strips (e.g. Remington, 1955, 1957). Selections from these results are given in Table 10.7. The values obtained by Apter and Marquez (1968) in which sinusoidal stretches were imposed on aortic rings were calculated for a 2-spring viscous dashpot model and are difficult to compare with these; they also found evidence for a resonance of 4 or 5 Hz which has not been seen by any other workers which suggests that it is an artifact of the apparatus.

Arteries *in situ*. Radial dilatation

Living arteries have been studied by several workers using arterial diameter gauges. Patel and Fry have published a series of papers using a strain-gauge caliper designed by Mallos (1962). Peterson *et al.* (1960) have used a device which moves a metal core in a coil and changes the inductance. Gow (1966) introduced a caliper which uses the same principle and is extremely light in weight. Arndt *et al.* (1968) have used an ultrasound echo device in intact man to measure the carotid artery diameter changes, and Leitz and Arndt (1968)

K

used X-ray angiography to record the carotid artery diameter in the cat and Arndt, Stegall and Wicke (1971) for the cat's aorta. With all mechanical devices, especially if they have a spring in them, it is difficult to determine whether the gauge exercises a restraint on the wall. Discrepancies between the results of different workers have been attributed to this factor, e.g. the discussion on Patel *et al.*'s (1964) paper by Bergel and Scarborough. Although Patel argued that the lower values Bergel obtained were due to an absence of blood supply in the excised vessels; the values of wave-velocity from Patel *et al.*'s results were always considerably higher than those measured *in vivo*. Later the strain-gauge used by Patel was replaced with a lighter one with a resulting decrease in the elastic modulus recorded (Patel, Janicki and Carew, 1969) where the results are very similar to those of Bergel (1961*b*) and of Gow and Taylor (1968), and they were also the same as the wave velocity measured in the same five dogs; calculated value, 548 ± 13 cm/sec, measured foot-to-foot velocity 548 ± 14 cm/sec. Patel *et al.* (1969) have been the first to undertake this highly desirable direct comparison between results derived from the measurement of radial dilatation and the measured wave velocity. Table 10.3 gives the calculated wave velocities in the dog thoracic aorta from various methods (slightly modified from Patel *et al.*, 1969).

TABLE 10.3

	Patel *et al.* (1963) Dynamic; *in vivo*	Patel *et al.* (1969) Static; isolated segment *in vivo*	Bergel (1961*a, b*) static dy- iso- namic lated *in vitro*		Gow and Taylor (1968) Dynamic; *in vivo*	Peterson *et al.* (1960) Dynamic; *in vivo*	McDonald (1968*a*) Measured wave velocity
c (cm/sec)	719	525	506	563	490	743	440–490
$\bar{p}$ (cm H_2O)	142	153	136	136	143	——	——

The majority of the recorded data in the literature falls in the range 400–550 cm/sec at these pressures.

Gow and Taylor (1968) also attempted to measure the visco-elastic components of arteries *in situ* by subjecting the pressure and dilatation curves to harmonic analysis. For the lower harmonics they recorded a small phase lag of radial movement behind the pressure as Learoyd and Taylor and Bergel had found in excised specimens. The behaviour of the small higher harmonics, however, became quite unpredictable. They attributed this to the non-linear behaviour of the arterial wall causing interaction between the harmonic terms and demonstrated that calculated small non-linearities would produce similar effects. The variations in pattern between individual animals was, however, marked and it would be difficult to give a generalized quantitative measure of the non-linear terms.

The direct comparison of values for the elastic modulus for all published accounts is not possible because in many cases the wall thickness was not recorded so that the term E_p introduced by Peterson *et al.* (1960) has been substituted.

$$E_p = \frac{\Delta P . R}{\Delta R}$$ **10.60**

(This value is, for some reason, always given by Patel *et al.* with the force as gm.wt instead of in dynes or newtons.)

E_p can thus be called the elastance, or stiffness, of the whole arterial wall. The comparative values for the results obtained by various workers was graphically illustrated by Gow and Taylor (1968) and are displayed in Table 10.6A.

The circumferential modulus of the pulmonary artery in the dog is reported by Patel (1969) as 7.35×10^5 dyn/cm² as compared to 4.7×10^6 dyn/cm² for the thoracic aorta. In man, Luchsinger *et al.* (1962) reported values for radial dilatation of the pulmonary artery and its two major branches using X-ray angiography at 0.5 second intervals; they also made measurements of the aorta. Greenfield and Patel (1962) made their measurements with a strain-gauge caliper on the pulmonary artery and the ascending aorta during open-heart surgery.

The ultrasonic echo technique used by Arndt *et al.* (1968) in measuring the pulsatile changes in diameter of the carotid artery is of particular interest. This technique shares with optical methods the advantage that no restraint is imposed on the wall. It is, however, quite difficult because the density of the wall is little different from that of the blood and does not always give good echoes. The results they illustrate have, nevertheless, shown very clear-cut signals. They report an average pulsatile change of 14.3 per cent of the diastolic radius with a pulse-pressure of 61 cm H_2O (165/104 cm H_2O) as the average for nine subjects. In terms of mean radius this is ± 7 per cent and is considerably larger than that recorded in corresponding dog arteries. It does, however, correspond well with the wave-velocity of 640 cm/sec which they recorded. The calculated value of E_p is 0.46×10^6 dyn/cm². These values are in striking contrast to those measured in man by Greenfield *et al.* (1964) which recorded only about one-tenth of the pulsatile change in diameter with a corresponding E_p of 4.3×10^6 dyn/cm². Arndt *et al.* (1971) attempt to explain the discrepancy as a result of exposing the artery to attach the gauge and indeed inserting sutures in the wall may produce some local spasm of the vascular smooth muscle. However, it has been pointed out that this type of gauge does cause appreciable restraint of the wall movement and the discrepancy is more likely to be due to this cause. The values for the elastic modulus measured in the human carotid by Learoyd and Taylor (1966) with an optical technique bear this out; it was pointed out above that they showed a marked difference from the dog in that the modulus of the carotid was much different from that of the femoral artery (Table 10.6).

The values recorded in various arteries for the radial dilatation with the pulse pressure wave in Table 10.4 may seem to be small in terms of the apparently obvious expansion seen by the naked eye. It should be remembered, however, that considerable lateral movement of arteries often occurs with each heart-beat. This is especially marked in arteries running in a curved course as, for example, in mesenteric vessels. A rise in pressure in a bent-tube causes it to straighten out (Burdon-gauge effect). The actual radial movement of arteries is small and requires very precise methods for its measurement.

TABLE 10.4. Values of radial dilatation in typical arteries

Artery	$\Delta R/R \times 100$ (%)	Author
Asc. aorta (man)	12·00	Barnett et al. (1961)
Asc. aorta (dog)	5·43	Patel et al. (1963)
Asc. aorta (dog)	5·03	Patel and Fry (1964)
Asc. aorta (cat)	18·5	Arndt et al. (1971)
Desc. aorta (cat)	15·5	Arndt et al. (1971)
Desc. aorta (dog)	3·00	Patel et al. (1963)
Desc. aorta (man)	9·1	Luchsinger et al. (1962)
L. pulm. art. (man)	60·9	Luchsinger et al. (1962)
R. pulm. art. (man)	67·5	Luchsinger et al. (1962)

Artery	$\Delta R/R/$cm $H_2O \times 10^4$	Author
Asc. aorta (dog)	14·72	
Thor. aorta (high)	9·43	
Thor. aorta (middle)	3·39	
Thor. aorta (low)	3·01	Patel et al. (1963)
Abd. aorta (high)	2·11	
Abd. aorta (low)	1·26	
Iliac	0·27	
Brachio-cephalic	2·09	

LONGITUDINAL MOVEMENTS OF THE WALL. THE LONGITUDINAL ELASTIC MODULUS

Lawton and Greene (1956) made measurements of longitudinal movement of the abdominal aorta by cinematographic observation of beads sutured to the surface of the vessel. The movements were very small and they often recorded a shortening of length during the systolic rise in pressure. This was confirmed in a more detailed study by Patel, Mallos and Fry (1961); in the thoracic aorta, however, a small lengthening of the vessel was found. The average value was 0·015 per cent per cm H_2O pressure (mean pulse pressure 51 cm H_2O). The effect in the abdominal aorta was coupled to the movements of the thoracic aorta rather than being due to the pressure rise in the vessel because it persisted after the aorta was occluded at the diaphragm. Respiratory movements of the diaphragm also caused a small longitudinal movement in the aorta; during inspiration the thoracic aorta lengthens by 1·5–2·0 mm and the abdominal aorta shortens. A small movement of the ascending aorta towards the heart and a headward movement in the arch of the aorta was also recorded.

The results of studies in these and other vessels were summarized by Patel
et al. (1964) and are given in Table 10.5.

TABLE 10.5. Changes in length of arteries *in situ*

Blood vessel	(N)	ΔP cm H_2O	$(\Delta L/L) \times 100$
Pulmonary artery; dog	10	15	$+11\cdot6$
Ascending aorta; dog	4	36	$+ 5\cdot3$
Descending thoracic aorta; dog	12	52	$+ 0\cdot8$
Abdominal aorta; dog	9	50	$- 0\cdot2$
Femoral artery; man	6	47	$\pm 1\cdot0$
Carotid artery; man	11	61	$\pm 1\cdot0$

The longitudinal modulus of the thoracic aorta has been measured in a detailed
study of the anisotropic elastic properties by Patel *et al.* (1969). They used
a segment of the aorta *in situ* which was isolated by inserting plugs into each
end and attaching it to a force-gauge (Janicki and Patel, 1968) which also
allowed applied extensions of the vessel to be made. At a mean pressure of
154 cm H_2O the average longitudinal modulus was 10,100 g. wt/cm² ($9\cdot8 \times 10^6$
dyn/cm²). When released from the longitudinal tissue attachments the
modulus decreased by 32 per cent. This reduces it to a value that is similar
to the corresponding circumferential modulus of 7,510 g. wt/cm². This is
designated transverse anisotropy and was also found by Tickner and Sacks
(1967) in excised specimens of the thoracic aorta and femoral artery of dogs
and in human brachial, superior mesenteric and external arteries at internal
pressures of 100–120 mm Hg when extended to around the *in vivo* length.
The stress–strain diagrams of the excised femoral artery published by F. M.
Attinger (1968) are also essentially the same up to strains between 1·5 and 1·6
of the excised dimensions. At greater strains the artery becomes considerably
stiffer in the circumferential than in the longitudinal direction. Anliker,
Moritz and Ogden (1968) have generated axial waves in the carotid artery of
the dog *in situ*. While the axial velocity is about 3 times greater than the
velocity of the pressure wave, the calculated difference would be a factor of 5.
They, therefore, concluded that the longitudinal modulus in this vessel is
smaller than the circumferential modulus. It is possible that, because of the
range of movements of the head, the longitudinal restraint of the surrounding
tissues is less in the carotid than in other arteries. Otherwise *in situ* the tethering of the arteries in longitudinal direction is usually greater than in the
circumferential direction as found by Patel *et al.* (1969), at usual physiological pressures. At much higher pressures, they found the situation reversed.
The shear modulus of arteries has not been measured directly. When the
Poisson ratio is 0·5, then from the relationship in eqn. 10.10, the shear
modulus will have a value of one-third that of the circumferential elastic
modulus and these are the values usually assumed to be true. This modulus is
of little practical value since Patel and Fry (1964) show that the shear strains

in the arterial wall are negligibly small as an artery is distended and hence the structure must be elastically symmetrical.

ANISTROPY OF THE WALL

From the outline of the findings of values for the elastic modulus in different directions it is clear that the arterial wall is not a simple isotropic material. From the complexity of the structure, containing, as it does, a large content of orientated fibrous material, this is not surprising. The principles of defining the elastic constants for an anisotropic tube were given on p. 257 above and are also discussed by Kenner and Wetterer (1963) and by Hardung (1964a, b) who also discussed the problem of homogeneity. Experimental work has been done by Tickner and Sacks (1967) on excised arterial segments and by Patel *et al.* (1969) on the thoracic aorta *in situ* and their values for the relative longitudinal and circumferential moduli are given above. Both set out the theoretical background in some detail. Tickner and Sacks inflated their specimens with air and measured the dimensions by X-ray photography. There is a considerable variation in the values they give between one specimen and another. In addition, they found a wide diversity in the Poisson's ratio measured in the three different directions; the values ranged from $+1\cdot0$ to $-0\cdot2$ for individual components and the physical interpretation of this is difficult to see. They comment that, provided the average of the components in the three orthogonal axes does not exceed $0\cdot5$, the situation is physically possible. In all their experiments the average value was less than $0\cdot5$ so that they conclude that the wall is compressible. This is at variance with direct measurements of compressibility by Carew *et al.* (1968); Patel *et al.* (1969) suggest that the conclusion of Tickner and Sacks is due to evaporation of water from the wall. They find that 13 per cent of the wall weight is easily lost by evaporation—a situation that is likely to occur in the Tickner experiments where the segments were both suspended in, and filled with, air.

At their natural length, and with distending pressures comparable to normal mean arterial pressure, the longitudinal and circumferential moduli are approximately equal. The treatment of the wall as isotropic is, therefore, a reasonable compromise under those conditions.

The analysis of large numbers of elastic constants that need to be defined for a full description of the behaviour of the wall has so far been mainly of theoretical interest. They have been incorporated in a detailed theoretical analysis of wave-transmission by Klip (1969) and by Moritz (1969) and the latter has measured the velocity of various wave modes. This detailed analysis using classical elastic theory is, however, based on the assumption of homogeneity in the substances. Whether a material which, for example, has a large component of water which can be easily lost can be considered as homogeneous has only been tentatively explored (Hardung 1964a, b). The physiological

TABLE 10.6A. Static elastic moduli (as Ep–eqn. 10.60) values

Artery	E_p (dyn/cm$^2 \times 10^6$)	Author
Asc. aorta (dog)	0·77	Patel and Fry (1964)
Asc. aorta (dog)	0·664	Patel et al. (1963)
Asc. aorta (dog)	1·474	Remington (1967)
Asc. aorta (dog)	0·34	Nichols and McDonald (1972)
Asc. aorta (cat)	0·402	Arndt et al. (1971)
Asc. aorta (man)	0·466	Barnett et al. (1961)
Thor. aorta (cat)	0·402	Arndt et al. (1971)
Thor. aorta (dog)	0·488	McDonald (1968a)
Thor. aorta (dog)	1·320	Patel et al. (1963)
Thor. aorta (dog)	0·659	Bergel (1961a)
Thor. aorta (dog)	0·67	Gow and Taylor (1968)
Thor. aorta (dog)	1·55	Peterson et al. (1960)
Abd. aorta (dog)	1·54	Bergel (1961a)
Abd. aorta (dog)	1·77	Gow and Taylor (1968)
Abd. aorta (high) (dog)	2·00	Patel et al. (1963)
Abd. aorta (low) (dog)	3·53	Patel et al. (1963)
Abd. aorta (high)	2·43	Peterson et al. (1960)
Abd. aorta (low)	2·40	Peterson et al. (1960)
Iliac (dog)	9·62	Patel et al. (1963)
Iliac (dog)	3·20	Peterson et al. (1960)
Iliac (dog)	2·76	Gow and Taylor (1968)
Femoral	1·69	Bergel (1961a)
Femoral	2·06–3·41	Gow and Taylor (1968)
Femoral	3·26	Peterson et al. (1960)
Saphenous (dog)	8·80	Gow and Taylor (1968)
Brachio-ceph. (dog)	2·83	Patel et al. (1963)
Carotid (dog)	1·93	Bergel (1961a)
Carotid (dog)	2·10	Gow and Taylor (1968)
Carotid (dog)	3·10	Peterson et al. (1960)
Carotid (man)	0·34	Kober and Arndt (1970)
Carotid (man)	0·44	Arndt (1969)

interpretation of these complex analyses remains, therefore, somewhat in doubt.

THE ROLE OF SMOOTH MUSCLE IN THE ARTERIAL WALL

The contribution of smooth muscle to the functional behaviour of the larger arteries has been a controversial topic. While in the smallest arteries and the arterioles contraction of the vascular muscle causes large changes in the vascular lumen with corresponding changes in the peripheral resistance, sympathetic stimulation or increases in circulatory vasoactive substances like norepinephrine do not produce any very obvious changes in the size of the large arteries. This has been attributed to the fact that the wall-tension due to the distending blood pressure is already very high in a large vessel and it did not seem likely that the tension that the vascular smooth muscle in the wall could generate would be sufficient to alter it significantly. This was the point of view taken by McDonald (1960) but the value for the maximal tension developed by vascular muscle in his argument was, from later evidence, much too low. The figures he used were from Burton (1954) who calculated a Young's modulus for maximally contracted smooth muscle of about $1·0 \times 10^5$

dyn/cm^2 which is more than an order of magnitude less than that of the aortic wall (Tables 10.6 and 10.7). At a time when little other data was available Burton had calculated his value from the experiments of Winton (1926) on the erector penis of the dog. This is a relatively thick, unstriated muscle and it is highly probable that only the outer layers were adequately oxygenated.

TABLE 10.6B

The elastic modulus is $E_p \times R/h$; thus, for Bergel (1961a) above, $E_p = 0.659 \times 10^6$ dyn/cm^2, then elastic modulus $= 4.4 \times 10^6$ dyn/cm^2. Gow and Taylor also give wall thickness ratio. Learoyd and Taylor (1966) show small graphs of $h/2R$ ratio which makes calculation difficult, so modulus values are given below for man; young $= 11$–20 years, and old $= 36$–52 years.

Artery	Modulus (dyn/cm^2) $\times 10^6$ Young	Old	Author
Thor. aorta	5·5	20	
Abd. aorta	10·0	12	
Iliac	29·0	7	Learoyd and Taylor (1966)
Femoral	31·0	14	
Carotid	8·0	11	

TABLE 10.7A. Dynamic elastic moduli

Artery	Mean pressure (mm Hg)	Frequency (Hz)	Modulus (dyn/cm^2 $\times 10^6$)	Author
Thor. aorta (dog)	100	2·0	4·7±0·42	Bergel (1961b)
Thor. aorta (dog)	100	5·0	4·9±0·45	Bergel (1961b)
Thor. aorta (dog)	100	18	5·3±0·80	Bergel (1961b)
Mid. thor. aorta (dog)	84–125	1·26–2·38	3·0±0·33	Gow and Taylor (1968)
Upper thor. aorta (dog)	96–124	2·2–4·5	2·95	Gow and Taylor (1968)
Lower thor. aorta (dog)	101–130	1·73–1·84	5·7	Gow and Taylor (1968)
Mid. abd. aorta (dog)	96–130	1·35–2·80	9·8±1·2	Gow and Taylor (1968)
Abd. aorta (dog)	100	2·0	10·9±0·88	Bergel (1961b)
Abd. aorta (dog)	100	5·0	11·0±0·82	Bergel (1961b)
Abd. aorta (dog)	100	18·0	12·2±0·46	Bergel (1961b)
Iliac (dog)	87–115	1·27–2·5	11·0	Gow and Taylor (1968)
Femoral (dog)	90–130	0·96–2·4	12·3±0·2	Gow and Taylor (1968)
Saphenous (dog)	100	1·08	60·6	Gow and Taylor (1968)
Thor. aorta (cow strip)	——	2·00	2·0	Hardung (1953)
Thor. aorta (strip)	——	13·00	2·0	Hardung (1953)
Aortic strip (dog)	——	5·5	5·76	Lawton (1955)
Thor. aorta (young man)	——	10·0	9·4	Learoyd and Taylor (1966)
Thor. aorta (old man)	——	10·0	30·0	Learoyd and Taylor (1966)
Abd. aorta (young man)	——	10·0	14·2	Learoyd and Taylor (1966)
Abd. aorta (old man)	——	10·0	20·4	Learoyd and Taylor (1966)
Iliac (young man)	——	10·0	35·0	Learoyd and Taylor (1966)
Iliac (old man)	——	10·0	15·0	Learoyd and Taylor (1966)
Femoral (young man)	——	10·0	55	Learoyd and Taylor (1966)
Femoral (old man)	——	10·0	37	Learoyd and Taylor (1966)
Carotid (young man)	——	10·0	15	Learoyd and Taylor (1966)
Carotid (old man)	——	10·0	13	Learoyd and Taylor (1966)

The precision of the Learoyd and Taylor (1966) values is not very great as they were read off graphs on a small scale. There is no clear explanation as to why the human moduli are so much higher than in the dog for the observed and calculated wave-velocities are comparable. The reader is recommended to consult the interesting discussion over the causes in variation with age. (Young = 6 subjects, 11–20 years. Old = 6 subjects, 36–52 years.)

The assessment of the role of contracted muscular tension may be more clearly stated in numerical terms. If we take, for example, the thoracic aorta of a dog with a mean radius of $0\cdot5$ cm and a mean internal pressure of 100 mm Hg, the linear tension in the wall is $P \times R$, i.e. $13,300 \times 0\cdot5$ dyn/cm or $6\cdot65 \times 10^4$ dyn/cm. Assuming a wall-thickness to radius ratio of $0\cdot12$ (see p. 259) then the wall-stress will be $5\cdot54 \times 10^5$ dyn/cm². The earlier values suggested that the maximally contracted muscle would not be able to exert a force of much more than 1×10^4 dyn/cm² and would clearly make little material difference. The actual tension that the muscle can exert is now known to be far greater than this. The physiology of vascular smooth muscle has been reviewed critically and in great detail by Somlyo and Somlyo (1964) and they conclude that the active contractile force that can be developed by vascular smooth muscle is between $1\cdot5$ and $2\cdot5 \times 10^6$ dyn/cm². This is very close to the value of $2\cdot73 \times 10^6$ dyn/cm² calculated from the more recent experimental data on the carotid artery of the dog by Dobrin and Rovick (1969); Lundholm and Mohme–Lundholm (1966) made measurements from which a value of $2\cdot62$ dyn/cm² was obtained for the muscle of the mesenteric artery taking a value of 75 per cent of the cross-sectional area as being due to muscle. The assessment of the effective cross-section of the wall that is due to muscle is somewhat imprecise; it is commonly estimated from the total area of muscle in histological section but Dobrin and Rovick derived it from estimates of the intracellular space and Apter (1966) estimated it from the protein content. The value for the thoracic aorta has been variously estimated from 25 to 35 per cent; if we take 1/3 as the value then the tension at maximal contraction will be $8–9 \times 10^5$ dyn/cm² in the aortic wall. If the elastic tension is $5\cdot5 \times 10^5$ dyn/cm² it is clearly possible to double the tension in the wall even when the muscle is contracting less than maximally. With arteries of smaller radius the effect will be even greater because the initial wall tension will be correspondingly less.

The reason that there has been controversy over the constricting effect of vascular smooth muscle appears to have been due to the fact that as circulating norepinephrine, for example, will increase the peripheral resistance due to the concomitant arteriolar constriction there is a rise in blood-pressure which counteracts the constrictor effect in the artery. It is only in recent years that due emphasis has been placed on separating these two effects. A pressure-stabilizing device, or 'barostat', for the arterial pressure has been used in my laboratory in which one femoral artery is connected to a reservoir in which the pressure has been kept at a constant pressure from a compressed air source with a leak through a mercury manometer of adjustable height. Using a Pieper intra-arterial gauge (Pieper and Paul, 1969) a diminution of aortic diameter with vaso-constrictor substances can be measured. Using a similar device, Gerova and Gero (1967) also showed that sympathetic stimulation can significantly reduce the diameter of the dog femoral artery but when the pressure was allowed to rise this effect would be abolished. Using radioangiography Leitz and Arndt (1968) showed that norepinephrine caused marked narrowing of the carotid artery of the cat and Dobrin and Rovick showed the same effect in excised segments of the dog carotid artery up to pressures of 300 mm Hg. In canine pulmonary artery, Somlyo and Somlyo (1964) showed that arterial strips would shorten up to 30 per cent under an isotonic load of $1 \cdot 6 \times 10^5$ dyn/cm^2 which was in excess of the circumferential wall tension under physiological distending pressures.

It is manifest that the contractile tension of the smooth muscle is capable of decreasing the diameter of even the largest arteries. The smooth muscle, however, does not appear to be able to contract beyond 25 and 30 per cent below its resting length (Lundholm and Mohme-Lundholm, 1966) which limits the constriction that can be achieved.

The effect that contraction of the smooth muscle has on the elastic modulus has been interpreted in diametrically opposite ways. Wiggers and Wegria (1936) and later Alexander (1954) found that the distensibility of the aorta was increased by muscle contraction and this would normally be interpreted as a reduction of elastic modulus. The addition of a tensile force in parallel to the elastic fibres would be *a priori* expected to make the wall stiffer, i.e. to increase the elastic modulus. This has been found by Gerova and Gero (1967) and, in the 'barostat' experiments described above, we have found that vasoconstrictive agents cause a rise in the wave-velocity as did Bargainer (1967) in the pulmonary artery. The difference in interpretation is undoubtedly due to the conditions under which the measurements are made.

The earlier workers tended to use distensibility as the ratio of the actual radius or volume rise to the accompanying rise in pressure. Thus Burton (1965) defines an 'absolute distensibility' $= \Delta R/\Delta P$. The strain properly defined is the ratio of the increment ΔR to the initial radius R_0 (p. 240). Under these conditions the value of the distensibility is arbitrary if the starting dimensions are unknown. In published work where the elastic tension and strain are recorded there seems little question that a greater increase of tension is required to distend an artery at any given arterial size when the muscle is stimulated to contract. This defines an increase in the incremental elastic modulus (p. 259) and represents the physiological condition when the artery is *in situ* and the muscle is largely contracting isometrically (Gerova and Gero, 1967). When excised specimens are used with a starting condition of zero distending pressure the application of norepinephrine will cause a marked shortening of the circumference. Again, a given increase in length will, therefore, represent a greater fraction of the initial length, i.e. a larger strain and the modulus calculated in this way will have decreased. This is apparent from the tension–length diagrams published by F. M. Attinger (1968) for the excised femoral artery which increase in slope after the application of norepinephrine and so have an increased elastic modulus. The curves are then recalculated in terms of the reduced initial length and are termed 'corrected'.

Under those conditions, the modulus would be reduced. The divergence of interpretation has been clearly discussed by Dobrin and Rovick (1969) in terms of their experimental data on the dog carotid artery. Where the value of the modulus is plotted in terms of the internal pressure the modulus is reduced after norepinephrine. When the modulus is plotted against the strain it is increased with muscle contraction as compared to a control vessel treated with potassium cyanide to eliminate all muscle contraction (Figs. 10.12 and

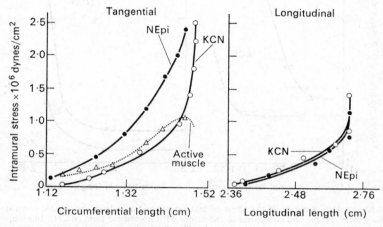

Fig. 10.12. The stress–strain diagrams for the carotid artery of the dog comparing the vessel when all muscle tone is abolished by potassium cyanide (KCN curve) and when it is in a strong stage of contraction due to norepinephrine (NEpi curve). The broken line is calculated from the difference between the 2 curves to indicate the force developed by the muscle. It will be seen that there is no muscular force developed in the longitudinal direction. The apparent elastic modulus therefore will be increased when the stress is (as it should be) calculated against the strain. If it is calculated against the pressure then the modulus appears to decrease with muscle contraction because the contracting muscle reduces the circumference and reduces the strain. This apparently paradoxical effect of muscular contraction reducing the stiffness of the wall is to be explained by the elastin and collagen fibrous elements being in a meshwork and the stress falls progressively on the much stiffer collagen fibres as the strain is increased. (Courtesy of Dr. Philip Dobrin.)

10.13). At very high strains, however, the modulus of the control vessel exceeds the vessel with contracting muscle; this may be interpreted as being due to the muscle fibres sustaining the stress rather than the collagen fibres whose high elastic modulus largely determines the elastic properties of an artery at large distensions.

The incremental modulus at a given arterial diameter which increases with muscle contraction would seem to be the most desirable value to use in functional terms for it is consonant with increase in the velocity of wave-propagation which we have seen also occurs under these conditions. Anliker *et al.* (1966, 1968) have also shown that the velocity of an impact pressure wave in veins is increased by vasoconstrictor drugs. This has also been found in my own laboratory both with artificially generated waves in the thoracic vena cava, and with the venous pressure pulse generated by the heart. Available data on the wave-velocity found in the arterial tree is discussed more fully in Ch. 14.

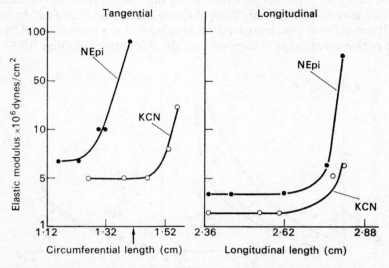

Fig. 10.13. Another example of the effect of making arterial muscle in the carotid contract with norepinephrine (NEpi) and compared to the artery with no muscle tone (KCN). In comparison with Fig. 10.12 there is an appreciable muscle effect in the longitudinal direction. (Courtesy of Dr. Philip Dobrin.)

11
Pulsatile Flow in an Elastic Tube

We have already seen, in Chs. 5 and 6, that the hydrodynamic problems of pulsatile flow are considerably more complicated than those of steady flow even in pipes of unvarying diameter. The figures presented in Ch. 6 showed that we can make quite reasonable approximations while ignoring the movement of the arterial wall, yet it is clearly unsatisfactory to leave the physical analysis at this stage. In this chapter, it is proposed to give an account of the hydrodynamic properties of oscillatory flow in an elastic tube system with an indication as to how valid it seems to be when applied to arteries. In view of the incompleteness of our knowledge of the complex elastic properties of arteries that was shown by the review of existing knowledge in Ch. 10, it is clear that we are inevitably some way from a complete solution.

As always, it is necessary to consider what approximations may reasonably be made and what is the most realistic physical model of an artery. The model that has usually been regarded as the most appropriate is that of a thin-walled tube with walls that are perfectly elastic. This is because we think of arteries as independent pipes running through the body, and the behaviour of such a model must be considered. Anyone who has attempted to define an artery by dissection, however, is aware that it is difficult to define precisely where the adventitia ceases and the surrounding tissue begins. In terms of the intact animal one can make out a very good case for regarding the arteries as tubes drilled through the body mass. The mathematical model for this is a cylindrical hole in an infinite elastic body, and in certain cases has been studied in detail, as in the properties of oil-wells. Womersley (unpublished) used this model in an exploratory way but the analysis has not been pursued because it does not seem the most realistic model for the circulation and because the mathematical forms are rather intractable.

From the consideration of the relation of the arterial wall, which was described as 'tethering' in Ch. 10, and in view of the fact that arteries are surrounded by tissue masses, Womersley (1957b) has developed a further model. This is essentially that of an elastic tube which is subjected to a longitudinal restraint (the 'tethering') with walls that are loaded by additional mass. This appears to be the most realistic model that has been studied fully

283

up to the present time. An extension of this model to include visco-elastic properties of the wall has also been made (Womersley, 1957*a*) and was tested in detail by Taylor (1959*b*) on a rubber-tube model.

In work in this field over the past century it is convenient to follow Taylor's (1959*c*) subdivision of the work on wave-propagation in elastic tubes, filled with liquid, into three stages.

(a) Those in which the viscosity of the liquid is neglected and hence there is no consideration of the longitudinal movement of the wall; the wall material is assumed to be perfectly elastic.

(b) Those in which fluid viscosity is included but the viscous drag on the wall is neglected although longitudinal movement of the wall is included; again the wall is assumed to be perfectly elastic.

(c) Those in which both fluid viscosity and the viscous drag on the wall are considered; in these, the wall has been treated both as elastic and as visco-elastic. This chapter will be principally concerned with the more sophisticated analyses of this group. The elastic models for the wall have proliferated during the past decade, e.g. Mirsky's papers (1967, 1968) on the orthotropic elastic tube, but these are not considered in detail unless they have been used as a basis for experimental work on the arterial system.

In the first group belong a number of early studies which, as noted in Ch. 10, have been well reviewed by Lambossy (1950). This is the simplest case and we have seen (Ch. 6) that in large vessels, or at higher frequencies, the effects of viscosity are small. From the work of Young (1808, 1809), Weber (1850), Resal (1876), Moens (1878), and Korteweg (1878) we have obtained eqn. 10.56:

$$c_0 = \sqrt{\frac{E.h}{2R\rho}}$$

From this analysis we also obtain the water-hammer equation of Allievi (1909) which was applied in circulatory analysis by Frank (1930) and Broemser (1930). The simplest form of this is

$$P = \rho \bar{V} c_0 = \frac{\rho}{\pi R^2} . Q . c_0 \qquad \qquad \textbf{11.1}$$

where P is the pressure, ρ the density of the liquid, $\bar{V}$ its average velocity across the tube or Q its volume, and c_0 the velocity of wave-propagation. In an elastic tube, this velocity is determined by the properties of the vessel wall for, by comparison, the fluid is incompressible. In the more familiar experience of a 'water-hammer' in the domestic water supply with rigid metal tubes the value of c_0 is very high, being of the order of the velocity of sound in water, and it can be seen why high pressures are developed. The same factors operate in the production of cavitation, e.g. around ships' screws.

In spite of the approximation involved in neglecting viscosity this simple formula forms a useful guide to the pressure developed by the rapid injection of liquid into an elastic tube such as the aorta. In the absence of wave-reflection from nearby points the pressure curve follows the flow velocity almost exactly. In experiments using transient impulse excitation of the system as in those of Peterson (1954) where he injected a rectangular pulse of liquid into the proximal aorta the initial rise of pressure can be predicted quite closely by this equation. Similarly in Starr's (1957) studies of the pressure resulting from the injection of a single slug of blood into the arterial system of the cadaver this equation actually fits the results better than the other, more complex, ones derived from *Windkessel* theory that he tested.

Nevertheless, it is clear from the simple theory set out in Chapters 5 and 6 that the effects of viscosity are far from negligible in pulsatile flow in tubes of the calibre of arteries. We then pass on to analyses which fall into group (b) above.

The mathematical analysis of the oscillatory motion of a viscous fluid in a free elastic tube was studied by Lamb (1898) and in especial relation to the arterial tree by Witzig (1914) and by Frank (1920). General studies were made by Tyler and Richardson (1928), Sexl (1929, mainly relating to gases), Iberall (1950), Lambossy (1951) and Evans (1962). The analyses under group (c) were heralded by that of Morgan and Kiely (1954), followed a few months later by an independent treatment with essentially the same result by Womersley (1955c). As the latter considered the motion of the liquid as well as wave-propagation and was more specifically related to the dimensions of the arterial system, its conclusions will be described here. Although, as noted above, the free elastic tube is not entirely satisfactory as an arterial model, it is necessary to consider its physical behaviour to test it against other models and the circulatory system *in situ*. The primary assumptions made in the treatment are (1) that the wall is perfectly elastic, unrestrained and that the wall is thin in comparison to the diameter of the lumen; (2) that the wave-length λ is long in comparison to the circumference of the tube, specifically that the dimensionless parameter $\omega r/c_0$ ($= 2\pi r/\lambda$) is small, and (3) that the tube is extended infinitely on either side of the region studied, i.e. that the motion is established and that there are no entrance effects and no end-effects in the form of reflections of the wave. In terms of the arterial system, the assumption of the thinness of the wall is fairly reasonable, as noted above (p. 259) the ratio $h/2R$ ranges from about 0·05 to 0·08. The condition of long wave-lengths is also reasonably satisfactory; the mean wave-velocity of the whole arterial system is about 700 cm/sec so that a component at 2 Hz will have a λ of 350 cm and even at 20 Hz (about the highest frequency that we consider in practice) λ is 35 cm compared to the circumference of the proximal aorta which is about 6–7 cm. The assumption (1) of perfect elasticity is, on the other hand, certainly untrue (Ch. 10) and far from being infinitely extended the arterial system is short and both entrance effects and wave-reflections do occur.

The full mathematical treatment given by Womersley (1955c, 1957b) is too complex to be repeated in full here and only a brief résumé and a consideration of the physical results predicted will be given here. These may be considered under the following headings:

A. Movements of the wall.
    1. The longitudinal movement due to the viscous drag of the liquid.
    2. The radial dilatation.
B. The change in the pressure-flow relationship compared with that of the simple theory (Ch. 5).
C. The properties of the propagated wave.
    1. The wave-velocity and its dependence on the frequency.
    2. The damping of the wave.
D. Non-linearity of the equations.

A. Movement of the wall

1. *The longitudinal movement.* An important effect of the viscosity of the liquid is that the resulting drag pulls the wall in a longitudinal direction. The magnitude of this effect is sensitive to changes in Poisson's ratio and, as Womersley has calculated its value for various values of $\alpha = R \sqrt{(\omega/\nu)}$ it might serve as a means of studying the elastic properties of the arterial wall under dynamic conditions. With parameters analogous to those of the dog's femoral artery ($\alpha = 3.34$ and $\sigma = 0.5$) the computed value of the velocity of movement of the wall is approximately 0·12 of the average velocity of the liquid, which is surprisingly high. Also the velocity of movement of the wall leads the average velocity in phase; in the fundamental component of the example quoted, by 74° (Fig. 11.1). This phase effect may be understood by reference to the diagrams of the velocity profiles (Figs. 5.3 and 5.4) where it can be seen that change in direction of flow begins at the wall of the pipe. This longitudinal movement has not previously received much attention but it can easily be seen when an oscillating flow is created in a rubber tube. I have, however, failed to observe any longitudinal movement of a comparable magnitude (Fig. 11.1 predicts an excursion of c. 1·0 cm in the femoral artery) in the wall of any arteries studied with high-speed cinematography. Lawton and Greene (1956) also found that any movement of the wall, which they found to be only of the order of a few μm, was in the sense of a shortening as the vessel dilated. Patel and Fry (1966) used a longitudinally oriented gauge attached to the wall and made similar findings. This adds further evidence to the suggestions that the outside of an artery is subjected to a longitudinal tethering or constraint and will be discussed further when the behaviour of the 'tethered' tube is considered.

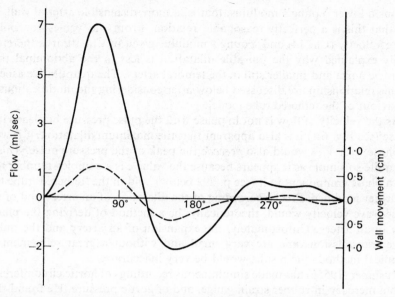

Fig. 11.1. The flow curve for the femoral artery (ordinate on left) with computed curve that the wall would make if it behaved like a free elastic tube (broken line—ordinate on right). This longitudinal movement is due to the viscous drag of the liquid within it. It can be seen that the total excursion would be of the order of 1 cm whereas in fact none can be observed at all. This is additional evidence that the artery is strongly constrained by its connections with the surrounding tissues.

For the fundamental component the velocity of the wall leads the corresponding flow by about 74° but the total movement (plotted here) lags by 16°.

2. *The radial movement.* The second relation that emerges from this work is of greater practical importance. It is shown that the radial dilatation is related to the velocity of flow and not directly to the pressure. The relation is a very simple one

$$\frac{\bar{V}}{c_0} = \frac{2\zeta}{R}$$

11.2

where again $\bar{V}$ is the average velocity, c_0 the wave-velocity, 2ζ the radial expansion, i.e. $\pm\zeta$ about R the 'resting' radius, that is, the radius at the mean pressure.

At first sight, this seems a most surprising conclusion because we are accustomed to regarding the pulse-*pressure* as the prime distending force in an artery. Further thought will make it clear, however, that in pulsatile flow in an elastic tube, any short section that we consider will, during the acceleration of flow, have more fluid entering it than there is leaving it, and, hence, the distension of the segment is due to the increase in the amount of fluid in this segment. From the equation we see at once that for a given velocity of flow, the slower the pulse wave, the greater the dilatation. As a slow pulse wave means a lower Young's modulus, that is, a more distensible arterial wall, we see that this is a perfectly reasonable relation. From the values for pulse-wave velocity (Ch. 14) and Young's modulus given in Ch. 10, it is therefore easily explained why the pulsatile dilatation is less in the abdominal than thoracic aorta and smaller still in the femoral artery. The quantitative aspects of this relationship are discussed below after considering the modifications in behaviour of the tethered tube model.

As the velocity of flow is not in phase with the pulse pressure but leads it in phase (see Fig. 6.1) it is also apparent that the maximum dilatation, if it were in phase with $\overline{V}/c_0$ would also *precede* the peak of the pressure pulse. This is not quite so simple as it appears because the value c is a complex number and has a phase component in it (see p. 292 below), and in the 'tethered' tube this is further modified. Precise recording of the dilatation of an artery and of the pulse-wave velocity would, theoretically, be a method of deriving the phasic flow in an artery. Unfortunately, the expansion of an artery and the pulse-wave transmission time are very small and without a great refinement of technical methods the results would be very inaccurate.

Rushmer (1955*b*) has made simultaneous recordings of aortic circumference with a mercury-in-rubber strain gauge, and of aortic pressure. He found that in the living animal the maximum dilatation *preceded* the pressure peak. In the excised aorta that was distended, on the other hand, and also in a rubber tube he found that the dilatation either moved with the pressure (as in the rubber) or lagged slightly behind in the case of the aorta (which was to be expected from the hysteresis phenomenon in a visco-elastic tube discussed above, p. 247, Ch. 10). The difference between the living animal and excised aorta fits the prediction that the dilatation is following the changes in velocity of flow. Most studies of radial dilatation are made in the aorta where the lead of flow over pressure is small and, with the phase-lag in wall movement due to its visco-elastic nature, the curve of the dilatation in fact follows the time and relations of the pressure-curve quite closely. This can be seen from the papers of Patel and his colleagues (e.g. Patel *et al.*, 1963), and Gow and Taylor (1968). If a diameter gauge restrains the radial movement of the wall the mural tension will be activated by the distending pressure, rather than solely by wall-movement. From the fact that the elastance of arteries measured by strain gauge techniques is higher than those from other methods, there is a suspicion that this effect was modifying the records of wall-movement recorded by Patel *et al.* (1963) and the later gauge used by Patel *et al.* (1969) appears to confirm this view.

B. The pressure–flow relationships in the free elastic tube

Expressing the pressure–flow equation for the elastic tube in terms comparable with those used for the simple tube we can write down the following relations.

For the mathematical derivations and the full definition of the functions reference should be made to Womersley (1955c).

If we take a sinusoidal pressure gradient per unit length of the form

$$\Delta P = A^* e^{i\omega t} \qquad \textbf{11.3}$$

of which the real part is

$$\Delta P = M \cos (\omega t - \varphi) \qquad \textbf{11.4}$$

it will be recalled that, from eqn. 5.14,

$$w = \frac{MR^2}{\mu} \cdot \frac{M'_{10}}{\alpha^2} \sin (\omega t - \varphi + \varepsilon'_{10}) \qquad \textbf{11.5}$$

where $\alpha = R\sqrt{(\omega/\nu)}$, i.e. is a function of the radius (R) of the tube, the circular frequency of the motion (ω) and the kinematic viscosity of the liquid (ν). M'_{10} and ε'_{10} are dependent solely on α. w is the velocity in the direction of the z-axis.

The corresponding equation for the elastic tube may be written

$$w = \frac{MR^2}{\mu} \cdot \frac{M''_{10}}{\alpha^2} \cdot \sin (\omega t - \varphi + \varepsilon''_{10}) \qquad \textbf{11.6}$$

In this equation, M is the modulus of the pressure-gradient; M''_{10} and ε''_{10} are, like their analogous factors M'_{10} and ε'_{10} in eqn. 11.5, dependent on the parameter α, but also on the Poisson's ratio (σ) and on the relative thickness of the tube (h/R). This last ratio is called K which is useful, for the modifications due to tethering and loading of the tube may be all combined into modifications of this factor. The values of M''_{10} and ε''_{10} have been tabulated (Womersley, 1957a). It is found that for most conditions M''_{10} is slightly larger than M'_{10} and ε''_{10} slightly smaller than ε'_{10} at the same α. This means that both amplitude and phase-lag are increased. For example, taking the Poisson ratio as 0·5, which is a close approximation to that in arteries (see p. 266) and $K = 0·1$ (which is a little low for arteries, $K = 0·16$ is more generally correct (p. 259)), we find over a typical range for the femoral artery:

TABLE 11.1

α	M''_{10}	M'_{10}	ε''_{10}	ε'_{10}
3·34	0·7373	0·6551	29·26°	30·98°
6·77	0·8471	0·8096	11·59°	13·49°

With lower values for σ the effect is decreased until when $\sigma = 0$ it is reversed* and M''_{10} is actually smaller than M'_{10} and ε''_{10} is larger than ε'_{10}.

In calculating a flow curve accurately it is also necessary to introduce an

* Cork is the only material for which $\sigma = 0$.

allowance for the pulsatile variation in diameter—this, in effect, means substituting $(R + \zeta)$ for R into the equations where the dilatation (ζ) is defined by the relation in equation 11.2 above. The effect of these corrections is shown in Fig. 11.2 applied to one set of data in the femoral artery reported by

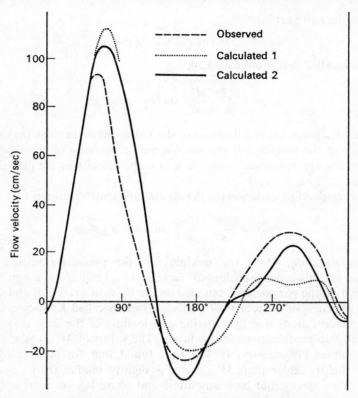

Fig. 11.2. A flow velocity curve ('observed') in the femoral artery measured by high-speed cinematography compared with two calculated curves. 'Calculated 2' is computed from the equation of motion in a perfectly free elastic tube (see text) compared with 'Calculated 1' computed from eqn. 5.13 in which it is assumed that there is no movement of the wall.

It can be seen that the corrections do not alter the pattern very much but do tend to improve the fit with the observed curve—especially in the period of diastolic flow. (Diagram from Womersley, 1955c.)

McDonald (1955a). It will be seen that the modifications of the original calculated curve are small but alter the curve in the right direction in relation to the observed curve. The peak systolic flow rate is slightly decreased and the diastolic flow increased. In other cases, the curves calculated from the simple theory are the better fit. The differences in these parameters are small compared with the probable errors in the flow measurement so that the exact form of the flow curve is not a critical test of minor variations in the physical relationships.

For ease of mathematical manipulation the equations expressed above are better kept in their complex form. A travelling pressure-wave (P) which at the origin is $A^*e^{i\omega t}$ will be represented in general as

$$P = A^*e^{i\omega(t-z/c)} \qquad \textbf{11.7}$$

at any point a distance z along the tube.

The velocity of flow (cf. eqn. 11.6) is then

$$w = \frac{A^*}{\rho c} \cdot e^{i\omega(t-z/c)} M''_{10} e^{i\epsilon''} \qquad \textbf{11.8}$$

and as the rate of flow, $Q = \pi R^2 . w$ the corresponding equation for flow may easily be written.

The presence of the factor $1/c$ recalls that the pressure-gradient, dp/dz, along the tube (eqn. 6.7) for a sinusoidal oscillation, in the absence of refections is given by

$$-\frac{dp}{dz} = \frac{1}{c} \cdot \frac{dp}{dt}$$

where c is a complex quantity.

This emphasizes once more that in the hydrodynamics of elastic tubes, of whatever properties, the wave velocity is one of the most important parameters.

C. The characteristics of the propagated wave

1. The velocity of propagation. 2. Damping (Attenuation).

When a wave is propagated in a viscous medium it will be progressively attenuated and its amplitude will diminish exponentially as it travels. This is apparent from the nature of viscosity as discussed in Ch. 2.

A travelling wave may be expressed mathematically as by eqn. 11.7 when we write

$$P_{(z)} = P_0 e^{+i\omega(t-z/c)} \qquad \textbf{11.9}$$

if it is understood that, in a viscous medium, the velocity c is a complex quantity. The commoner way to express this, e.g. in electrical transmission line theory, is by defining a *propagation constant*, γ. We may then rewrite eqn. 11.9 as

$$P_{(z)} = P_0 e^{-\gamma z} . e^{i\omega t} \qquad \textbf{11.10}$$

Hereafter we will omit the term $e^{i\omega t}$.

The propagation constant is complex and may be written

$$\gamma = a + ib \qquad \textbf{11.11}$$

so that eqn. 11.10 can be expanded as

$$P_{(z)} = P_0 e^{-az} \cdot e^{-ibz} \qquad\qquad \textbf{11.12}$$

If we define c_1 to be the phase velocity, then we have

$$b = \frac{\omega}{c_1} \text{ or } c_1 = \frac{\omega}{b} \qquad\qquad \textbf{11.13}$$

so that the velocity of propagation can be found from the imaginary part of γ, while the attenuation per unit length is given by the real part a. The amplitude of an oscillation after a distance z is thus

$$|P_{(z)}| = |P_0| e^{-az} \qquad\qquad \textbf{11.14}$$

and after travelling one wavelength, λ, is thus,

$$|P_0| e^{-a\lambda} = |P_0| e^{-ac/f} = |P_0| e^{-2\pi a/b} \qquad\qquad \textbf{11.15}$$

In Womersley's treatment he did not immediately use the propagation constant, but employed a complex wave velocity, c, such that

$$\frac{c_0}{c} = X - iY \qquad\qquad \textbf{11.16}$$

where c_0 is the velocity defined by the elastic properties of the artery, containing a non-viscous liquid; in equation 10.56, $c_0 = (Eh/2R\rho)^{1/2}$.

If, in eqn. 11.9, we now replace $1/c$ by $(X - iY)/c_0$, then we have

$$P_{(z)} = P_0\, e^{i\omega\,[t - Xz/c_0 + iYz/c_0]} = P_0\, e^{-\omega Yz/c_0}\, e^{-i\omega Xz/c_0}\, e^{i\omega t} \qquad\qquad \textbf{11.17}$$

Now, by comparison with eqns. 11.12 and 11.13, we may identify the phase velocity c_1 as c_0/X, while the attenuation constant a is seen to be $\omega Y/c_0$.

An oscillation, after travelling one wavelength, is thus attenuated by the factor (eqns. 11.15, 11.16)

$$e^{-2\pi Y/X} \qquad\qquad \textbf{11.18}$$

which Womersley refers to as the 'transmission per wavelength'.

The transmission may be regarded as the complement of the attenuation and is the amplitude that remains after a defined distance so that the attenuation is (1 – transmission).

The values of c_1/c_0 are illustrated graphically in Fig. 11.3 and they vary with the value of the parameter α. α, it will be recalled, is $R\sqrt{(\omega/\nu)}$, that is, it

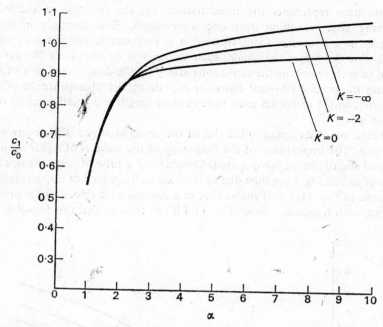

Fig. 11.3. Curves illustrating the variation of the phase velocity of a wave in a perfectly elastic tube filled with viscous liquid as the value of α varies. Ordinate—ratio of phase velocity, c_1, to the wave-velocity, c_0, given by the Moens–Korteweg equation (10.56). The term K is defined by eqn. 11.22 representing the longitudinal restraint. The fall in velocity where $\alpha < 2$, i.e. in small arteries, is marked in all cases. In the femoral artery α is approximately 2·5 for the fundamental, so that it can be seen that in a free tube of this or larger size the viscosity of the liquid has little effect on the wave-velocity; the ratio is within 10 per cent of the limiting value of 1·0. Longitudinal tethering increases the limiting value to 1·16 but even so the effect of size or frequency is not very great for $\alpha > 3$.

In a visco-elastic tube Taylor (1959b) has shown that for values of α up to 90 the phase velocity fits very well for the Womersley curve with limiting longitudinal constraint $K - \infty$ (see Fig. 11.7).

increases directly with the calibre of the tube and the square root of the frequency. With values of α about 3 which corresponds to the fundamental in a vessel of the size of the femoral artery, c_1 is about 90 per cent of the ideal velocity and in larger vessels, or at higher frequencies, it gradually increases to a value of about 95 per cent. In the large vessels, the slowing effect of viscosity, therefore, is relatively small. It is of interest that Moens (1878) added this value of 0·9 as an experimental constant to the formula for the wave-velocity in an ideal fluid. The part of the curve that is highly significant in circulatory physiology is the steep fall of actual velocity at values of α less than 3. With an α of 1·0 it is only half the ideal value and at smaller values becomes so small as to be virtually uncomputable.

This slowing of the pulse-wave velocity must be associated with increased damping. In Fig. 11.4 the value of $e^{-2\pi Y/X}$ is shown also in relation to α. The ordinate here represents the transmission, i.e. the fraction of the wave remaining after travelling over one wave-length. This damping increases markedly as α decreases from 10 until it is very nearly 100 per cent when $\alpha = 1 \cdot 0$. For the larger mammals, such values will be found for the fundamental in such vessels as the saphenous artery (in the dog, $\alpha = 0 \cdot 8$ to $1 \cdot 0$) and indicates the precise physical basis for explaining the disappearance of the pulse wave in the arterioles even though their length is a small fraction of a wave-length.

The relation of damping to the size of the vessel involved is therefore very important. The importance of the frequency of the wave is of equal significance and slightly more complicated. Considering a tube of constant size the effects of increasing α are then due to increase of frequency of the oscillation. The curve in Fig. 11.3 thus shows that in a viscous fluid velocity of propagation rises with frequency. From Fig. 11.4 it can be seen that the damping *per*

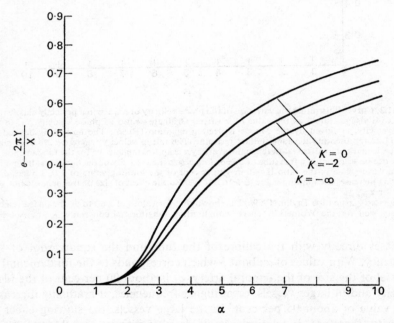

Fig. 11.4. Curves describing the damping, or attenuation, of a wave travelling in an elastic tube under the same conditions as in Fig. 11.3. Ordinate here is the proportion of the wave remaining after travelling one wave-length, i.e. damping is virtually 100 per cent when $\alpha < 1 \cdot 0$. Tethering the tube increases damping. When the increase in α is due to an increase in frequency the damping *per unit length* increases because the wave-length becomes shorter. The attenuation in a rubber tube is shown in Fig. 11.6.

wave-length also decreases, but with increasing frequency the wave-length becomes shorter. As the wave velocity is the product of the frequency and the wave-length this is not quite so simple as, for example, the calculation of the wave-length of radio waves, because the velocity also changes with the frequency. The net effect is, however, that the wave-length always decreases with frequency. (The wave-length also is shorter in large arteries such as the thoracic aorta, which have a lower wave-velocity because the wall has a lower elastic modulus.) As damping in practical terms needs to be considered in terms of distance the result is that over a length of tube of, say, 10 cm, the percentage damping increases with the frequency even though the wave-velocity increases and hence shortens the transmission time (Fig. 14.13). Thus, for an $\alpha = 3.34$, Womersley (1955c), in the free elastic tube, has computed that the wave-velocity is 91·4 per cent of the ideal and the amplitude is damped to 27 per cent of its initial value in one wave-length. This represents a damping of 5·4 per cent in a 10 cm length. For the fourth harmonic, i.e. at four times the frequency ($\alpha = 6.67$), c_1 is 94·2 per cent of c_0, and the amplitude of the wave is only reduced to 63·5 per cent *in one wave-length*, but the damping per 10 cm length is increased to 7·5 per cent. Experimental measurements in arteries are illustrated in Ch. 14. These values are, of course, for the simple free elastic tube model.

This effect must be considered in the transmission of the pulse-wave generated by the heart which is a mixture of harmonic frequencies. The higher frequencies will travel somewhat faster than the lower, and hence the phase relations of the harmonic components will change and alter the shape of the wave by dispersion. At the same time, however, the higher frequencies will be damped out first so that the pulse as it travels peripherally will lose high frequency components, for example, the incisura of the central aortic pulse becomes damped out rapidly (Fig. 12.12).

With a complex wave, which clearly still has a corporate existence even though it alters in shape, the term *group-velocity* is used to express the modal velocity of the group of components which have velocity dispersion. The velocity of individual harmonic waves is referred to as their *phase-velocity*. It is difficult to make a measurement of the group-velocity of a wave like the pulse-wave that would satisfy a mathematician and it is doubtful what value this concept has in the presence of reflections, so that no attempt is made to define it here.

Müller (1951) has measured the phase-velocity, and what he calls the group-velocity, of sinusoidal waves in a rubber tube using both water and a glycerine solution. Group-velocity was here measured from the foot of the first wave he generated, but this is more probably the velocity of the highest frequencies because at such a discontinuity there would be, theoretically, a complete spectrum of frequencies. It is, in fact, seen from his results that the phase-velocity, which increases with frequency, becomes virtually the same as the 'group-velocity' at 20 Hz. The phase-velocity was measured from the waves when they had settled down to a steady state oscillation. His illustrations show vividly the changes in wave-velocity and damping with frequency qualitatively

similar to those predicted by Womersley. Womersley has calculated in that
arteries with $\alpha > 3$ the difference between phase- and group-velocity would not
be more than 2 to $2\frac{1}{2}$ per cent.

D. Non-linearity in the equations

It has been assumed throughout all the previous discussion that there is a
simple relation between individual harmonic components of the pressure and
flow waves. Thus, the Fourier series for the pressure-gradient can be transformed into flow term by term. This is the principle of superposition, and for
the simple theory in the 'rigid' tube this is true. In the elastic tube, however, this
is no longer strictly accurate and the harmonics will show an interaction. The
mathematical reason for this is that the non-linear terms of the full equations
are no longer negligible. The physical basis of this is that (1) as a result of the
changes in radius there is a radial component of flow, and (2) the non-linear
inertia terms. In addition, (3) the interaction between the oscillatory and the
steady flow term (taken in Ch. 5 as simply additive) has to be considered. (1)
was computed in the paper dealing with the free elastic tube (Womersley,
1955c) and found to be small as also are the inertia terms (Womersley, 1958a).
At greatest they are only a few per cent. The interaction between steady and
oscillatory flow was also studied by Womersley (1955a) but much more fully
by Womersley (1957a). (3) An earlier treatment of a small oscillatory motion
in a large steady flow was investigated by Morgan and Ferrante (1955).
Womersley concluded that in a situation such as the femoral artery the
oscillatory terms might alter the steady flow by as much as 14 per cent which
is far from negligible. In terms of a phasic flow curve the steady flow is very
small compared with the oscillating components and it is difficult to detect
whether this amount of alteration occurs. The 'steady' pressure-gradient is, as
observed in the discussion of the calculation of the flow curve (p. 127) so
small that it cannot be measured accurately. The presence of the interaction
means that Poiseuille's law cannot strictly be applied even to the steady
pressure-gradient and flow in the presence of oscillatory terms.

The presence of a steady flow also modifies the wave-velocity. This has been
studied mathematically by Morgan and Ferrante (1955) and Womersley
(1955a). It may be taken that the wave-velocity in the presence of a steady
flow is the algebraic sum of the normal wave-velocity and the steady flow
velocity. Some experiments of Müller (1950) appeared to show that there was
a slightly different effect when the wave was 'with' or 'against' the stream but
there seems to be no physical reason for this and the observation is slightly
suspect because he used transient waves and did not allow for dispersion
which alters the wave-form as it travels (see Fig. 12.1). The *steady flow*
component in arteries is so small in comparison with the pulse-wave velocity
that these effects would appear to be of little practical importance. When one
is measuring the phase-velocity of a sinusoidal wave of long wave-length it is

clearly the average stream velocity throughout the cycle that we must consider. When, however, the wave-velocity of a short transient is considered, as
in the experiments of Anliker, who used a short train of sinusoidal oscillations
in the frequency range 40–200 Hz the local stream velocity at the time of the
transient is more relevant. As the peak flow velocity in systole is of the order
of 100 cm/sec this effect can greatly affect the measured velocity of a transient
imposed during systole (Ch. 14).

The results of the theoretical treatments in regard to damping are somewhat confusing. Womersley (1957a) predicted that the presence of a steady
stream velocity would produce a small increase in the damping. Morgan and
Ferrante (1955), on the other hand, predicted a decrease in the damping of a
wave propagated in the direction of the stream and an increase in the damping
when propagated upstream. The latter authors, however, were considering a
situation where the flow oscillations were small ones superimposed on a large
stream velocity and Womersley considered a situation analogous to that in
arteries where the oscillations were large in amplitude compared to the mean
stream velocity so that both solutions may be correct under their different
conditions.

The change in the elastic properties of the wall with increasing strain which
is found in arteries (Ch. 10) and which is a property common to elastomeric
substances which are capable of undergoing large strains, is not, strictly
speaking, relevant here with the consideration of the perfectly elastic tube.
But in practice, when one is putting the theoretical derivations to experimental test where the tubes will have this type of non-linearity, it is very difficult to separate this from the other causes for non-linearity noted above.

Taylor (1959c) used a transmission line analogy, using a non-linear
capacitor representing the wall, to analyse the non-linearity, in a rubber pipe.
His final equation for the amplitude of the second harmonic created by the
sinusoidal excitation of the line was

$$E_2(z) = \frac{1}{c_2} \cdot \frac{I_1^2{}_{(0)}}{\omega^2} \cdot \frac{\gamma_1^3}{4\gamma_1^2 - \gamma_2^2} \cdot (2\gamma_1 e^{-2\gamma_1 z} - \gamma_2 e^{-\gamma_2}) \qquad \textbf{11.19}$$

where $E_2(z)$ is the voltage (analogous to pressure) of the second harmonic at a
distance z from the origin and $I_{1(0)}$ is the current of the imposed (fundamental) oscillation at the origin. Current is analogous to the linear velocity of
the flow. The propagation constants of the first and second harmonics are
γ_1 and γ_2 respectively.

From this equation, we can see that the amplitude of the second-harmonic
component of the pressure will not be maximal at the origin but instead it
rises to a maximum along the line and then declines. An example computed
from equation 11.19 is illustrated in Fig. 11.5 where it can be seen that the
second harmonic creates a maximum distortion at about 1·5 wave-lengths (of

the fundamental) from the origin. The results of an experiment in a rubber tube are shown in Fig. 11.6 and are in general agreement with the theoretical prediction in that the second harmonic was at a maximal value from about 2/3 to 4/3 of a wave-length from the origin. In this experiment the mean pressure within the tube was atmospheric so that during half of each pump cycle the

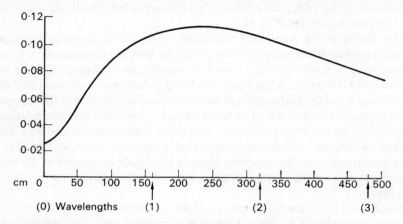

Fig. 11.5. The computed behaviour of the modulus of the bracketed part of the function in eqn. 11.19, i.e. the variation of $E_2(z)$ with z. For purposes of illustration, two values, $\gamma_1 = 0.0206 + i$ 0.368 and $\gamma_2 = 0.0465 + i\, 0.718$ were used; these had been determined in two independent experiments on a rubber tube.

The abscissa gives the distance from the origin in cm and in terms of wave-length for the fundamental oscillation. The maximum amplitude here is at about 1.5 fundamental wave-lengths from the origin. (From Taylor, 1959c.)

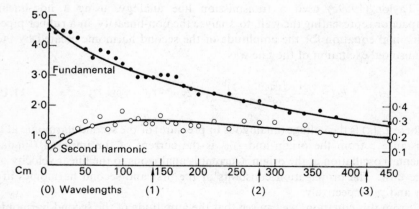

Fig. 11.6. Experimental results in the non-linear rubber tube described in the text. The amplitude of the fundamental oscillation (scale in arbitrary units at the left) and for the second harmonic (scale at the right) shown as functions of distance (cm and fundamental wave-lengths as in Fig. 11.5). The fundamental frequency was 10 Hz and the second harmonic 20 Hz.

The fundamental oscillation shows some degree of second harmonic modulation on an otherwise declining amplitude; the second harmonic increases in amplitude by about 3 times over the first fundamental wave-length and thereafter declines slowly. (From Taylor, 1959c.)

pressure was below atmospheric and the tube tended to collapse. This visibly increases the non-linear distortion of the wave. In addition, in some experiments an attempt was made to imitate the non-linear elastic behaviour of arteries by wrapping a double helix of strong adhesive tape around the tube. There was no measurable difference in the amount of second harmonic developed so that Taylor considered that the distortion found was probably due to the hydrodynamic terms in the equation. In the normal situation in an artery where the pressure never falls below atmospheric the amplitude of these non-linear terms will be small. From equation 11.19 it can be seen that they will be of the order of $(\gamma/\omega)^2$ or $(1/c^2)$. The experimental findings of Dick *et al.* (1968) referred to in Ch. 7 bear out this theoretical prediction, and reinforce the other findings (Chs. 7 and 13) that in terms of pressure–flow relations the non-linear distortion is small. In relation to the study of wall-motion we have noted that Gow and Taylor (1968) concluded that non-linearities need to be considered (Ch. 10); the role of non-linearities in the study of the propagation-velocity of superimposed transients by Anliker is discussed in Ch. 14.

THE EFFECTS OF EXTERNAL RESTRAINT.
THE TETHERED AND LOADED TUBE

In the discussion, at the beginning of the chapter, of the most realistic mathematical model of an artery, it was pointed out that the anatomical attachment of the arterial wall to its surroundings suggested that the tube was tethered, i.e. subject to an external restraint. The evidence from the amount by which an artery retracts when it is freed from these attachments has already been discussed in Ch. 10. The fact that a free elastic tube would exhibit a large longitudinal movement due to the viscous drag of the liquid while, in fact, such a movement does not occur (p. 286) *in situ* again indicates that they are not free to move longitudinally. By elegant experimentation Patel and Fry (1966) have made quantitative measurements of the degree of 'tethering'.

Womersley (1957b) has treated this mathematically by introducing a factor into the constant K, which in the free tube represented the relative thickness of the wall. The constraint is assumed to act purely in the longitudinal direction and has a natural frequency, m. The factor he introduces is

$$\left(1 - \frac{m^2}{\omega^2}\right) \qquad \text{11.20}$$

where ω is the circular frequency of the oscillation.

The 'loading' of the tube adds to the wall a mass that takes no part in the elastic deformation. This increases its inertia. The factor used in this case is the same as that introduced by Morgan and Kiely (1954) as a mathematical means of describing the effects of surrounding tissue masses on the artery.

The thickness of the wall of the tube, h, in the original equations is replaced by the term H' such that

$$\frac{H'}{h} = \left(1 + \frac{h_1 \rho_1 R_1}{h \rho R}\right) \qquad \textbf{11.21}$$

where h_1, ρ_1, and R_1 are the thickness, density and radius of the added mass and h, ρ, and R that of the tube wall.

Combining these two factors Womersley (1957b) defines K as

$$K = \left(1 + \frac{h_1 . \rho_1 . R_1}{h . \rho . R}\right) \left(1 - \frac{m^2}{\omega^2}\right) \qquad \textbf{11.22}$$

From this it can be seen that with a fairly stiff constraint, $m > \omega$ then K will be negative. With a very stiff constraint, $m \gg \omega$, $K \to -\infty$. If $m = \omega$ then $K = 0$ and the wall behaves as though it has no mass.

With this alteration in the definition of K the mathematical equations are of exactly the same form as those for the free elastic tube discussed above (eqns. 11.6, 11.8). The values of M''_{10} and ε''_{10} are dependent, as before, on the parameter α, the Poisson ratio and on K. These have been tabulated (Womersley, 1957a) for values of K from 0·4 to $-\infty$. There is no direct way of evaluating K at the present time, that is, the dimensions of the 'added mass' and the natural frequency cannot be measured directly.

From the evidence of the tethering effect it would appear to be stiff and hence we should expect K to have a fairly large negative value. The most interesting fact that emerges from the tables is that when $K \to -\infty$ then $M''_{10} \to M'_{10}$ and $\varepsilon''_{10} \to \varepsilon'_{10}$, i.e. the values used in the simple theory using the rigid tube model (Chs. 5 and 6). These values are very nearly the same with values of K of -10 or greater.

We may consider briefly the physical behaviour of oscillatory flow in such a tethered and loaded elastic tube under the same headings as for the free elastic tube.

Movements of the wall

1. *Longitudinal.* The condition of external constraint that has been postulated naturally tends to prevent any longitudinal movement. It was my own observations that virtually no such movements occur that led to the suggestion that such a longitudinal constraint existed. Hosie (1957) has made similar observations. Lawton and Greene (1956) have reported small variations in length but they appear to be in the opposite direction to that which might be anticipated, i.e. there is a contraction of length in systole. The movement is, however, very small. Evans (1956) has suggested that this must be due to anisotropism in the wall, but this may be regarded as a special case of constraint in the longitudinal direction. The findings of Patel and colleagues,

however, indicate that the difference between the longitudinal and circumferential moduli would not be enough to account for this and, as noted above, Patel and Fry (1966) have made direct estimates of the longitudinal restraint.

The presence of a longitudinal constraint must be conceived physiologically as due largely to the connective tissue attachments on the outside of the artery. The viscous drag on the inside of the wall will still tend to move it and so will create a shearing force in the wall. In such a thin wall it is unlikely that the inner side would be able to move more than a fraction in excess of the permitted movement of the outer side. Nevertheless there must be a continuous oscillating shear in the wall with each heart beat. As some present-day investigators of arteriosclerosis, such as Duguid (e.g. Duguid and Robertson, 1957), are stressing the role of mechanical factors in its causation, this shearing force is probably one of the most important. Its magnitude is mainly dependent on the degree of pulsatile variation in flow velocity and the degree of tethering. It would, therefore, be interesting to seek for a correlation between regions of the arterial tree where these are maximal and the commonest sites of arteriosclerotic degeneration. This has been discussed in the light of the work of Fry and others in Ch. 5 (pp. 115–19).

2. *The radial movement.* From the equation relating dilatation to flow velocity (eqn. 11.2) and the equation (11.8) relating the velocity to the pressure, it is easy to relate the pressure to the flow, thus

$$\frac{2\zeta}{R} = \frac{P}{\rho c_1^2} \cdot M''_{10} e^{i\varepsilon''}{}_{10} \tag{11.23}$$

$$= \frac{P}{\rho c_0^2} \cdot \left(\frac{c_0}{c_1}\right)^2 \cdot M''_{10} \cdot e^{i\varepsilon''}{}_{10} \tag{11.24}$$

where c_0/c_1 is the reciprocal of the velocity ratio plotted in Fig. 11.3. For all finite values of K this means that the expansion always leads the pressure in phase but the lead becomes progressively smaller with increasing negative values of K. When $K \rightarrow -\infty$ the limiting form is

$$\frac{2\zeta}{R} = (1 - \sigma^2) \frac{P}{\rho c_0^2} \tag{11.25}$$

or for $\sigma = 0.5$,

$$\frac{2\zeta}{R} = \frac{3}{4} \frac{P}{\rho c_0^2}$$

and pressure and frequency are in phase at all frequencies. When the wall is visco-elastic (Ch. 10), however, the wall movement will lag *behind* the pressure.

Womersley (1957a) applied this form of analysis to the data on expansion and pressure measured simultaneously in the abdominal aorta by Lawton and Greene, some of which are illustrated in their 1956 paper. Potentially, this provides a good method of testing the theory. In the present case there were inconsistencies in the results but it appeared that the phase lead of expansion over pressure, if present, was small, certainly less than 10° and often lagged a small amount behind it. It is, therefore, suggested on present evidence that the mathematical theory of stiff constraint, which also has the simplest form, is the best description of the situation.

The measurements of pulsatile dilatation of Lawton and Greene (1956) were made from cinematograph film. This method was also used by Hosie (1957).

The wave-velocity and the damping

The addition of a longitudinal constraint has, as we might expect, a stiffening effect on the wall and this results in a relatively greater wave-velocity compared with the free elastic tube. This is shown in the upper curve of Fig. 11.3 which represents the limiting curve for a stiff constraint ($K \to -\infty$). It will be seen that the form of the curve is similar to that of the free elastic tube. The limiting value of c_1/c_0 in this case, however, is not unity as in the case of the free tube, but is

$$\begin{array}{ll} \text{Limit} \\ \text{K} \to -\infty \end{array} \qquad \frac{c_1}{c_0} = \left(\frac{M'_{10}}{1-\sigma^2} \right)^{\frac{1}{2}} \sec \frac{\varepsilon'_{10}}{2} = 2/\sqrt{3} = 1 \cdot 16 \qquad \textbf{11.26}$$

If the data on the elastic constants of arteries were accurate enough to predict c_0, the fact that a stiff longitudinal restraint leads to wave-velocity values up to 16 per cent greater could be used as a test of the model.

Stiffening the tube also has the effect of increasing the damping. This is also illustrated in comparison with the free elastic tube in Fig. 11.4. The degree of damping this appears to predict may seem high, but it must be appreciated that the arterial system is a fairly short one in terms of wave-length. In fact, as noted below, the viscous behaviour of the wall increases the damping further.

The pressure–flow relationship in the constrained tube

The essence of the modifications into the flow equation has already been discussed in considering the radial dilatation. If the constraint is such that K has a large negative value, and the evidence noted above indicates that it has, then the form of the equation becomes identical with that for the simple rigid tube theory (eqn. 6.4). The curves calculated using the formula (Ch. 5) and the applications to the measurement of cardiac output (Ch. 15) stand as evidence that the physical model is a reasonable one.

WAVE–VELOCITY AND ATTENUATION IN THE VISCO–ELASTIC TUBE

The modifications of the Womersley equations to allow for a visco-elastic wall were given in eqns. 10.49 and 10.50 when the elastic modulus and Poisson's ratio were given complex values. The equation for the complex wave-velocity, c, derived by Womersley (1957b) then became

$$\frac{c_0}{c} = \left(\frac{1-\sigma^2}{M'_{10}}\right)^{\frac{1}{2}} e^{-i\varepsilon'} 10^{/2} \left\{1 - i\omega\left(\frac{\Delta E}{2} + \frac{\Delta\sigma}{3}\right)\right\}$$ **11.27**

which adds a second term on the RHS of the earlier equation. As the term in the braces is less than 1, we can see that the velocity and the attenuation will be increased.*

The conclusions were tested by Taylor (1959b) in a rubber tube, and he also analysed in detail the components of the longitudinal and transverse impedances. This paper also discussed at length the validity of electrical analogues in representing the hydrodynamic situation and, in view of the common use of electrical line models to represent the arterial system, is a very important analysis of this approach.

The experimental set-up consisted of a sinusoidal pump attached to a rubber tube which was of such a length that reflections could be eliminated. Measurements of the characteristic impedance (Z_0) and propagation constant (γ) were made over a range of frequencies from 2 to 30 Hz using a variety of liquids within it ranging from pure glycerine through a variety of glycerine–water mixtures to water so that the range of values of the parameter α was from about 1–90 (see Fig 11.7). In electrical terms, the tube and liquid were represented by a four-element circuit; the inertia and viscous drag of the liquid by an inductance and resistance in series, the elasticity and the viscous element of the wall by a capacitance and resistance in series. As both the impedance and the propagation constant are complex they provide four components from which to derive the four unknowns. This model was a combination of the three-element models used by Landes (1949) and Ronninger (1954) which both assumed a perfect elastic wall and had a single capacitance to represent the wall and the three-element model used by Hardung (1952) which assumed a visco-elastic wall but neglected the viscosity of the liquid and had a series inductance alone (Westerhof and Noordergraaf, 1970).

From the telegraph equations one can write

$$\gamma = [(Rx + i\omega L)(i\omega C)/(1 + i\omega RyC)]^{\frac{1}{2}}$$

and

$$Z_0 = [(Rx + i\omega L)(1 + i\omega RyC)/(i\omega C)]^{\frac{1}{2}}$$ **11.28**

so that

$$Rx = Re\{\gamma Z_0\}; \qquad L = \frac{1}{\omega} Im\{\gamma Z_0\}$$

* In Womersley's monograph there is a typographical error that makes it seem that these two terms will change in opposite senses; this error was pointed out by Taylor (1959b).

L

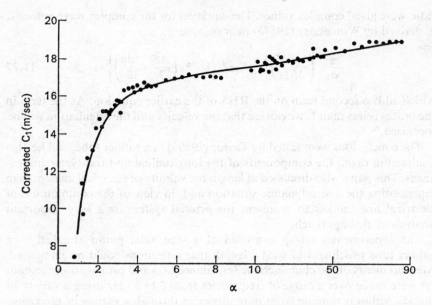

Fig. 11.7. A study of wave-velocity in a rubber tube with a range of α from 1–90 which we achieved by using six different glycerine–water mixtures. The ordinate gives the phase velocity in m/sec (corrected for the density of the different liquids) as a function of α (abscissa). Note that the scale has been compressed above $\alpha = 10$. The solid line is the behaviour predicted by Womersley's equations for an elastic tube in a condition of limiting longitudinal constraint. The only constraint the tube was actually under was its connection to the pump and the friction with the thin supports at 10 cm interval along its length. (From Taylor, 1959*b*.)

$$Ry = Re\{Z_0/\gamma\}; \qquad\qquad \frac{1}{C} = -\omega Im\{Z_0/\gamma\} \qquad\qquad \textbf{11.29}$$

The impedance was calculated as the ratio of pressure to flow velocity, taking velocity, and not volume flow, as the analogy of current.

The general behaviour of the inductance and fluid resistance in Taylor's (1959*b*) models were similar in kind to those for a rigid tube (Fig. 6.13). The effective elasticity showed a marked fall in the low α region for the free tube but remained virtually constant throughout the frequency range for the 'tethered' tube. The wall resistance ratio is of especial interest because it is negative—a condition that cannot be realized in a circuit with passive units. This may be considered as an analogue of the fact that the vessel wall dilates and that this dilatation leads the pressure (p. 287 above) in the free-tube. With a longitudinal restraint this 'negative' resistance disappears except at very low values of α which are difficult to realize experimentally. From the experimental results it was seen that the visco-elastic rubber tube behaved very like the longitudinally-restrained tube—a similarity also seen in the variation of

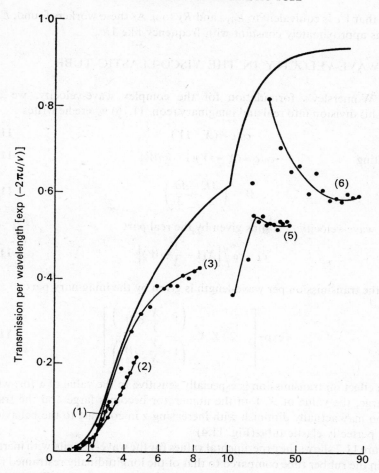

Fig. 11.8. The ordinate gives the transmission per wave-length as a function of α (abscissa), the same experiment used in Fig. 11.7; as before, the scale is compressed above α=10. The heavy solid line is the behaviour predicted by Womersley's equations for an elastic tube under limiting longitudinal constraint. The experimental values are grouped together, and identified by numbers which represent liquids of different viscosity because in a visco-elastic tube the transmission is in part determined by frequency alone, and the parameter α is determined by both density and frequency. (From Taylor, 1959b.)

velocity with frequency (Fig. 11.7)—although the tube was only restrained by the necessary conditions of its attachments to the pump at the origin, and by its contact with the spaced supporting rods. We may, therefore, conclude that the influence of wall-viscosity is very similar to that of tethering, presumably because the internal viscosity impedes the longitudinal movement of the wall.

Comparing these results with the analyses of Bergel and Hardung (Ch. 10) we see that $1/c$ is equivalent to E_{dyn} and Ry to η. As these workers found, E_{dyn} remains approximately constant with frequency like $1/c$.

THE WAVE-VELOCITY IN THE VISCO-ELASTIC TUBE

From Womersley's formulation for the complex wave-velocity, we can follow his division into real and imaginary (eqn. 11.16) where he writes

$$c_0/c = (X - iY) \qquad\qquad \textbf{11.16}$$

by writing

$$c_0/c = (X - iY)(1 - i\omega W) \qquad\qquad \textbf{11.30}$$

where

$$W = \left(\frac{\Delta E}{2} + \frac{\Delta\sigma}{3}\right) \qquad\qquad \textbf{11.31}$$

The wave-velocity c_1 is thus given by the real part

$$c_1 = c_0 \bigg/ \left[X\left(1 - \frac{Y}{X}\omega W\right)\right] \qquad\qquad \textbf{11.32}$$

while the transmission per wave-length is given by the imaginary part

$$\exp\left[-2\pi Y/X . \frac{\left(1 + \frac{X}{Y}\omega W\right)}{\left(1 - \frac{Y}{X}\omega W\right)}\right] \qquad\qquad \textbf{11.33}$$

The effect on transmission is especially sensitive to the value of α for, when α is large, the value of X/Y in the numerator becomes large and the transmission may actually diminish with increasing α in contrast to the behaviour in the perfectly elastic tube (Fig. 11.4).

Figure 11.7 shows the experimental values for the wave-velocity with increasing α in the rubber tube compared to that of the longitudinally restrained tube and we see that there is no significant difference between them. This emphasizes again that one of the effects of a viscous element in the wall is to restrain longitudinal movement.

Figure 11.8 shows the results that Taylor (1957a, 1957b, 1959c) obtained for transmission in the rubber tube with increasing α; it will be seen that, as predicted, the transmission declines for $\alpha > 20$ with an increase in frequency.

One final important conclusion in this paper is that whereas wave-transmission in a visco-elastic tube can be modelled by an electrical transmission line made of passive elements (though it cannot for a perfectly elastic tube) this analogue is only accurate for one specific frequency; a change in frequency requires a change in the values of at least some of the components. Therefore, it can only be approximate in representing an analogy for a pulse-wave which contains a number of component frequencies.

THE FREQUENCY DEPENDENCE OF WAVE-VELOCITY AND ATTENUATION IN ARTERIES

It was noted in Ch. 10 that Bergel (1961b) was able to derive values for the wave-velocity expected in arteries from the real and imaginary parts of the complex elasticity. The direct measurement of these parameters in arteries *in situ* is made very difficult by the presence of reflected waves. It was pointed out by Taylor (1959c), however, that this could be done by measuring the pressure at three points equally spaced in a homogeneous artery. This was extended by McDonald and Gessner (1968) as follows:

If the distance between the pressures P_1 and P_2 and P_2 and P_3 (farthest downstream) are both x cm and the pressure P_2 is the sum of a forward (or centripetal) wave of amplitude P_f and a retrograde (or centrifugal reflected) wave of amplitude P_r then

$$P_2 = P_f + P_r \qquad\qquad \textbf{11.34}$$

and we can write

$$P_1 = P_f e^{+\gamma x} + P_r e^{-\gamma x} \qquad\qquad \textbf{11.35}$$

and

$$P_3 = P_f e^{-\gamma x} + P_r e^{+\gamma x} \qquad\qquad \textbf{11.36}$$

so that it is easy to see that

$$\cosh \gamma x = \frac{P_1 + P_3}{2P_2} \qquad\qquad \textbf{11.37}$$

or

$$\gamma = \frac{1}{x} \cosh^{-1} \left(\frac{P_1 + P_3}{2P_2} \right) \qquad\qquad \textbf{11.38}$$

The pressures are all expressed in complex form, i.e. if $P = A \cos \omega t + B \sin \omega t = A - iB$ (Ch. 7) and the complex propagation constant $\gamma = a + ib$ then we may write

$$\left(\frac{P_1 + P_2}{2P_2} \right) = Q e^{i\phi} \qquad\qquad \textbf{11.39}$$

and it can be shown that

$$\frac{a}{b} = \begin{matrix} \cosh^{-1} \\ \cos^{-1} \end{matrix} [Q^2 \pm (1 + Q^4 - 2Q^2 \cos 2\varphi)^{\frac{1}{2}}] \qquad\qquad \textbf{11.40}$$

or, more easily, using the logarithmic form for the inverse hyperbolic cosine

$$a = \ln Q / x$$

and
$$b = \frac{\varphi + 2\pi N}{x}$$
11.41

Then, as noted above (p. 292) the attenuation is given by e^{-ax} or the transmission per wave-length as $e^{-2\pi a/b}$ and the wave-velocity $c_1 = \omega/b$.

The values found for the wave-velocity were compatible with those derived from the elastic constants of the wall using the standard wave-velocity equations, as Taylor found for the rubber-tube. The values of the attenuation are given in Ch. 14 where the experimental data for arteries are collected together. McDonald and Gessner (1968) used either isolated lengths of thoracic aorta or common carotid artery perfused with oxygenated Krebs' solution or the common carotid artery *in situ*. Both they and Bergel found a greater attenuation in arteries than was predicted from the viscous dissipation due to blood viscosity alone. This confirms the prediction that the viscous element in the wall will increase the damping. In addition, McDonald and Gessner found a greater attenuation than Bergel; this they attributed to the fact that in their experiments the muscular component of the wall was in a more active state, and that a large part of the viscous behaviour is to be attributed to this component. Bergel had also made the latter deduction from the fact that the carotid and femoral arteries had a larger viscous component than the aorta and that they also contained more muscle. The 'three-point' analysis has also been used by Gabe in an analysis of wave-transmission in the thoracic aorta. The results from these experimental studies are discussed in Ch. 14 (pp. 409–12).

12
Wave Reflection

So far we have considered pulsatile flow in arteries as though they were long tubes with a remote end. The actual situation with the repeated occurrence of branches ending in the capillary bed makes it necessary to consider what effect, if any, changes in the vessel beyond the point of observation will have on the pressure and flow. Any such effect will be due to the creation of reflected waves and it is generally agreed that such waves occur. The only point of dispute is 'how important is wave reflection in arterial dynamics?'

A travelling wave such as the pulse wave will be reflected to some extent wherever there is a discontinuity in the system. The extreme cases are where a tube is either completely blocked or opens into a large reservoir, either of which cause total wave-reflection though in the latter case it is in the opposite sense, i.e. 180° out of phase with the former. In the circulation we are obviously dealing with intermediate conditions causing only partial reflection but the terms 'closed' or 'open' are convenient to describe their character. The discontinuity may be a change in calibre as at a point of branching or merely a change in the elastic properties of the wall. It might, therefore, seem obvious that the arterial tree which has many discontinuities of this sort would create large reflections and that there are no grounds for argument. The case for the contrary is probably best summed up by the remark that Womersley made when he was first confronted with the problem—'If you wanted to design a perfect sound-absorber you could hardly do better than a set of tapering and branching tubes with considerable internal damping such as the arterial tree.' The experiments of Peterson and Shepard (1955) furthermore appear to bear this out because they showed that a large pressure wave created by a rapid injection pulse of blood retrogradely into a femoral artery caused no detectable effect in the pressure-curve recorded at the root of the aorta. Their interpretation was that any reflected waves created in the periphery, which would undoubtedly be very much smaller than their experimental ones, would be very rapidly damped out. This bore out the earlier findings of Peterson (1954) that the pressure curve due to an injection pulse in the arch of the aorta contained no components which could be attributed to discrete reflected waves. Wehn (1957) quotes several authorities who have questioned the importance of reflections. On the other hand the fact that the pulse wave normally develops secondary humps such as the dicrotic wave as it travels peripherally is usually ascribed to the presence of reflected waves. Indeed, much of the analysis of arterial dynamics is based on the assumption that not only are there centripetal reflected waves but that these are in turn reflected at the aortic valves and re-traverse the system, setting up a condition of 'resonance';* this is an integral idea in the development of the *Windkessel* hypothesis and is used as a basis for estimating the length of the *Windkessel* (Wezler and Boger, 1939; Wetterer, 1956). Allied to this is the description of 'a standing wave' in the arterial system (Hamilton and Dow, 1939). There have been so many conflicting opinions of these points that it is desirable that the elementary properties of reflected waves should first be considered.

THE REFLECTION OF A TRANSIENT PULSE

The simplest case to consider is that where a single short pressure pulse is created by an injection of fluid into one end of a long rubber tube filled with water. The amplitude of the pulse will be determined approximately, by the 'water-hammer' relation, $P = \rho \bar{V} c$ (eqn. 11.1) where $\bar{V}$ is the velocity of the injection and c the wave-velocity determined by the elastic properties of the tube. This pulse will travel away from the origin of this tube with this velocity but diminishing in amplitude, due to viscous dissipation of energy, as it travels. When it reaches the end of the tube it will be reflected and will not be recorded again at the origin until it has completed a second transit time. If the termination is closed it will be returned as a positive pressure wave; if the end opens into a large reservoir (an 'open' end) it will be returned as a negative wave. This second concept is often found difficult to understand but it is clear that once the fluid flow reaches a reservoir, which is large in comparison to the volume injected, there will be no pressure variation in that reservoir. The energy of the transmitted wave cannot, by the law of the conservation of energy, disappear; thus a wave equal in amplitude but opposite in sign is created. This can be easily demonstrated in a simple laboratory model.

In the arterial system we are concerned with a set of tubes terminating in an outflow of many very fine tubes at the far end which have a fluid resistance which is very high compared to that of those at the origin. An injection of blood into it by systolic ejection leads to a rise in pressure which persists longer than the period of the injection. We speak of the system as being 'filled' with the subsequent decay of pressure as due to 'run-off' or 'leak' through the 'resistance vessels'. Thus, it is of the nature of a system with a closed end, and so will give rise to positive reflections. In the model (Fig. 12.1) the interaction between the original and reflected waves is seen to be a function

* This may be a mistranslation of Otto Frank's term *Grundschwingung* (see footnote, p. 11, Ch. 1).

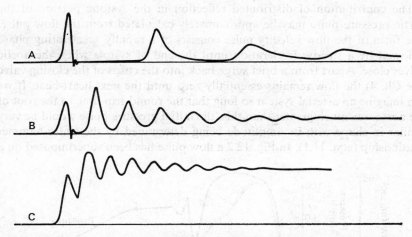

Fig. 12.1. The behaviour of a pressure pulse due to a sudden injection of liquid, travelling in a long pipe. A. Note the return to base-line pressure until the first reflection arrives, the progressive spreading of the pulse, and the stepwise approach to the final pressure level.

B. Reflections in a shorter pipe; again the pressure returns to the base-level before the first reflection arrives, and the more rapid succession of reflections gives the appearance of oscillations.

C. In this example the reflection arrives during the initial impulse. (From McDonald and Taylor, 1959.)

of the duration of the pulse and time it takes to travel to the end and back (round-trip time). In the upper trace the tube is clamped at a considerable distance away so that the initial pulse is completed and the pressure has returned to its initial level before the reflected pulse returns. It is then reflected again from the origin but now the effective level has increased by a small amount and again at the next return; finally, by the time the wave has died out, the pressure in the tube is increased by an amount corresponding to an increase equivalent to that caused by a gradual injection of the original volume. The second trace shows the effect of clamping the tube closer to the origin and the returning wave arrives before the original pulse is completed. When the tube is shortened further, as in the lower trace, it can be seen that the reflected waves are fusing with the initial wave; if there were many terminations at varying distances from the origin it would be easy to visualize that this fusion would result in a smoothly rising curve which would resemble that of the systolic pressure curve in the aorta. Indeed, in any tube system where we can talk of a 'filling' curve there must clearly be an end, and hence end-effects in the form of reflections. The old debate as to whether there are, or are not, 'reflections' is, therefore, unreal. What the protagonists were debating, in essence, was whether any single components were large enough to contribute a discrete deformation of the wave recorded in the ascending aorta or whether the components were so scattered in time as to be indistinguishable—the condition of 'distributed' reflections. Such models in considerable variety are illustrated and discussed in detail by Wetterer and Kenner (1968).

The contribution of distributed reflection in the systolic portion of the aortic pressure pulse may be approximately calculated from the flow pulse. The form of the flow velocity pulse consists of a rapidly accelerating phase followed by a steady deceleration until the end of systole when the aortic valves close. Apart from a brief surge back into the cusps of the closing valve (see Ch. 4) the flow remains essentially zero until the next heart-beat. If we can imagine an arterial system so long that the round-trip time to the root of the aorta was much greater than this, the initial pressure pulse would be very similar in shape with its amplitude being determined by the water-hammer relationship (eqn. 11.1). In Fig. 12.2 a flow pulse has been superimposed on a

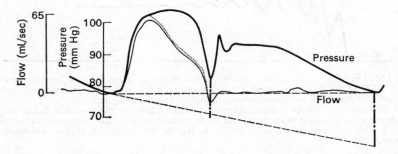

Fig. 12.2. The pressure curve in the ascending aorta with the aortic flow curve superimposed but scaled so that the height of each curve is the same. If there were no reflections in the arterial system then the pressure curve would approximately follow the flow as indicated by the dotted line. The fact that the pressure is sustained can only be attributed to 'distributed' reflected pressure waves from the periphery. (See text for a fuller discussion.) The dashed lines below the flow curve indicate the presumed drainage from the system during the duration of the cardiac cycle. (From Kouchoukos *et al.*, 1970.)

recorded pressure pulse and the initial pressure created is indicated by a broken line. The rise in pressure during systole which persists beyond this must be due to distributed reflection. A comparison of the areas gives an estimate of the amount of this reflection; in this case it amounts to some excess of pressure of 38 per cent. Frank (1930) considered that some 30–40 per cent of the aortic pressure pulse in systole was due to reflection and appears to have derived the range of values from the same line of reasoning. There has thus never been any serious doubt that reflected waves make a large contribution to the arterial pressure pulse but the contribution of discrete wave-reflection and its detection remains to be considered.

The experiments of Peterson (1954) show a similar phenomenon. An artificial square pulse, of the volume and duration of cardiac systole, was injected into the proximal aorta at arbitrary times during the cycle. An initial step in pressure is seen followed by a steady build-up of pressure for the duration of the injection. This is clearly due to distributed reflection from the terminations.

Dispersion of waves. A second feature of a transient wave travelling in a viscous medium is also illustrated in Fig. 12.1. It will be seen that the reflected wave is somewhat altered in shape as well as in amplitude when it returns. It is less sharply peaked and more spread out in time. From the consideration of the frequency components of a transient pulse in Ch. 7 it was noted that such a pulse is made up of a wide spectrum of frequencies. In a viscous medium it was seen in Ch. 11 that the wave velocity will vary somewhat with frequency. In travel over a considerable distance, as in the upper trace in Fig. 12.1, this leads to the spreading of the pulse that is seen. This phenomenon is known as 'dispersion'. In a short tube, as in the lower trace, it does not normally have much effect and does not appear to play a significant role in determining the form of the travelling pressure wave because at the frequencies normally involved, the significant components of the arterial pulse wave all travel at approximately the same velocity (see Ch. 14).

REFLECTED WAVES IN A STEADY-STATE OSCILLATION

For the arterial system where the heart beats regularly we need to consider steady-state oscillation rather than the behaviour of a single transient. Let us consider a wave in the form of a simple harmonic oscillation which is not being damped and which is completely reflected at a closed end. There are two components, an incident, or centrifugal wave, travelling away from the origin and the reflected, or centripetal, wave travelling towards the origin. At the point of reflection they are in phase and the amplitudes of the two oscillations sum together. If we move one-quarter of a wave-length from the end this will be a point one quarter, or 90°, earlier for the centrifugal wave but 90° after the point of reflection for the centripetal wave. They will therefore differ in phase by 180° or one half-cycle and will cancel each other out. No pressure oscillation will occur at this point. At a half wave-length distance from the end they will be one cycle apart, i.e. in phase once more and they will sum together. A series of maxima and minima will be spaced at quarter wave-length intervals from the end of the tube. The points of minimum oscillation are termed nodes and the maxima termed antinodes. If the wave is less than 100 per cent then the amplitude of the oscillation at the node will be the difference between the incident and reflected waves and the amplitude at the maxima will be their sum (Fig. 12.3).

If the length of the tube is such that it is a multiple of a half wave-length this summation will build up at each beat and, in the absence of any damping, the maxima would get infinitely large while the nodes will remain at zero amplitude. This is the condition of resonance. If the frequency is such that the tube is a wave-length long, for example, there will be a very large oscillation of pressure at both ends and in the middle of the tube—the antinode and two intermediate nodes of virtually zero oscillation spaced between them. The demonstration of this is familiar in the standard classroom demonstration

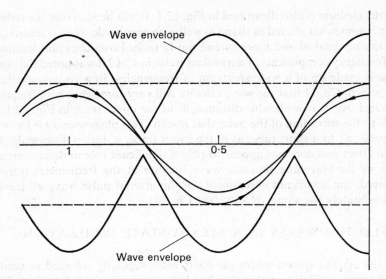

Fig. 12.3. A diagram to show the interaction of a centrifugal and a reflected wave at a closed end (vertical line on right). For clarity it is assumed that only 80 per cent of the wave is reflected (i.e. reflection coefficient = 0·8). The individual components are shown, at one instant of time, with arrows to identify them. The abscissa is marked in fractions of a wave-length. At the point of reflection both waves are in phase and sum together. With reference to a point one quarter wave-length away, the incident wave is 90° earlier and the reflected wave 90° later so that they are 180° out of phase and cancel. This point is a node and the only oscillation is the difference between their maximum amplitudes. At one half wave-length they are separated by a full cycle (360°) and so in phase again and the wave sum together for another maximum—an antinode.

The total excursion throughout the cycle is represented by the wave envelope (heavy outer lines). If there were no reflections and no damping, as we have here, this would be a straight line (broken lines). In all subsequent figures only half the envelope is shown as 'the amplitude (or modulus) of the oscillation'.

If reflection was complete the nodes would be at zero and the antinodes twice the amplitude of the incident wave. Repeated reflection from the origin, as shown here, would not increase this. If, however, the origin were one-half or one wave-length from the end, summation would occur here as well and then be repeated again at the far end. Thus, theoretically, the antinodes could become infinitely large—for this is the condition of resonance.

In the presence of damping the incident wave would be larger nearer the origin and the reflected wave would be growing smaller towards the origin and mutual interaction would be progressively smaller—as shown in Fig. 12.4.

in acoustics of the Kundt's tube (where lycopodium or cork dust that is scattered on a resonating tube only collects at the nodes). The oscillations at the antinodes will be exactly synchronous everywhere and so the phenomenon is called a stationary, or standing, wave.

When we consider flow rather than pressure, it is clear that there is no oscillation at the closed end and the incident and reflected flow waves must be in opposite phase. By the same reasoning as for the pressure waves the flow oscillations will therefore be in phase at a quarter wave-length distance to form a flow antinode and in opposite phase at a half wave-length to form another node of flow. That is, a point which is an antinode of pressure will be a node of flow and vice versa. If the end is *open* there will be a maximal flow oscillation there but a node of pressure. At a quarter wave-length distance from this point will now be a pressure antinode and at a half wave-length another node. With an open-ended tube resonance will thus occur when the tube is an odd-number multiple of a quarter wave-length in contrast to the closed end tube where it occurs when the tube is an even-number multiple. The position of nodes and antinodes is always determined by the distance in terms of wave-length from the termination.

When dealing with tubes filled with liquid we must, however, take into account the effect of damping. In this situation the amplitude of a propagated wave diminishes exponentially as it travels (Ch. 11); this applies equally to the reflected wave. Therefore, even with complete reflection the reflected wave will always be smaller than the centrifugal wave in amplitude (with the exception of the point of reflection where they will be the same). This discrepancy will increase the further away from the point of reflection that we move. Therefore, there can never be complete cancellation even at the first node from the end and each successive node will have an increasing, though relatively small, amplitude. The nodes and antinodes in this situation are more properly called relative nodes and antinodes. The condition of a standing wave also cannot be achieved, in the strict sense of the phrase, because adjacent portions of the wave will never be completely synchronous and there will be an apparent movement of the wave. At a relative antinode the amplitude is large but the phase shift is small; expressed as a velocity this gives a high apparent phase velocity. At the nodes the phase shift is large and the apparent phase velocity, c', like the amplitude, is very low.

The conditions for reflection also have a phase element when they are incomplete. In the ideal, or undamped, situation, we have seen that with a closed end there is zero phase shift between the incident and reflected wave and with an open end there is 180° phase shift between them. This also applies to partially closed and partially open terminations; the change from one to the other occurs abruptly at zero reflection. With damping the conditions of zero and 180° only occur with completely closed or completely open reflections.

This attempt to describe the interaction of incident and reflected waves in simple conceptual terms is given as an introduction to a problem that is unfamiliar in biology but is inadequate for more precise analysis. It is thus necessary to formulate it mathematically.

REFLECTIONS IN A TRANSMISSION LINE

The mathematical analysis has been set out by Taylor (1957a) by a treatment of the analogy of an electrical transmission line. The analogies taken are that voltage is equivalent to pressure and current to flow. The solutions were verified by testing on a simple hydraulic model (Taylor, 1957b). From the treatment discussed in Ch. 11 (eqns. 11.7 to 11.14) we can define a propagated wave $P_{(z)}$, using the propagation constant γ, as

$$P_{(z)} = P_0 e^{-\gamma z}$$

where P_0 is the wave at the origin and $P_{(z)}$ at any distance z along the tube. If the length of the tube is l and the reflection coefficient is R_f, the reflected wave at a distance z will be

$$P_{(z)} = R_f P_0 e^{-\gamma(2l-z)} = P_0 \cdot R_f e^{\gamma(z-2l)} \qquad \textbf{12.1}$$

and the composite term will be

$$P_{(z)} = I_0 Z_0 \left(\frac{e^{-\gamma z} - R_f e^{\gamma(z-2l)}}{1 + R_f e^{-2\gamma l}} \right) \qquad \textbf{12.2}$$

where I_0 is the flow at the origin and Z_0 is the characteristic impedance of the tube (Ch. 6).

If the end is completely closed the reflection coefficient R_f may be written as $-1\cdot0$. (In this derivation, Taylor departed from common usage where R_f is usually defined for pressure rather than flow but his form will be used in this immediate section.)

Equation 12.2 then becomes

$$P_{(z)} = I_0 \cdot Z_0 \left(\frac{e^{-\gamma z} + e^{\gamma(z-2l)}}{1 - e^{-2\gamma l}} \right) = \frac{I_0 Z_0 \cdot \cosh \gamma(l-z)}{\sinh \gamma l} \qquad \textbf{12.3}$$

and

$$P_0 = I_0 \cdot Z_0 \cdot \coth \gamma l \qquad \textbf{12.4}$$

Since

$$\gamma = a + ib \qquad \text{(eqn. 11.11)}$$

equation 12.3 can be expanded and the amplitude $|P_{(z)}|$ of the pressure then is given by

$$|P_{(z)}| = |I_0 \cdot Z_0| \left\{ \frac{\cosh 2(l-z)a + \cos 2(l-z)b}{\cosh 2la - \cos 2lb} \right\}^{\frac{1}{2}} \qquad \textbf{12.5}$$

Input impedance, Z, of a line of length l, closed at the end then is expressed in relation to the characteristic impedance Z_0 when there are no reflections as

$$\frac{|Z|}{|Z_0|} = \left(\frac{\cosh 2la + \cos 2lb}{\cosh 2la - \cos 2lb} \right)^{\frac{1}{2}} \qquad \textbf{12.6}$$

The form of the variations of voltage at various points along a transmission line calculated from eqn. 12.5 are shown in Fig. 12.4A and the corresponding variations of the pressure oscillation along a rubber tube at two different frequencies are shown in Fig. 12.4B. The effect of damping creates an oscilla-

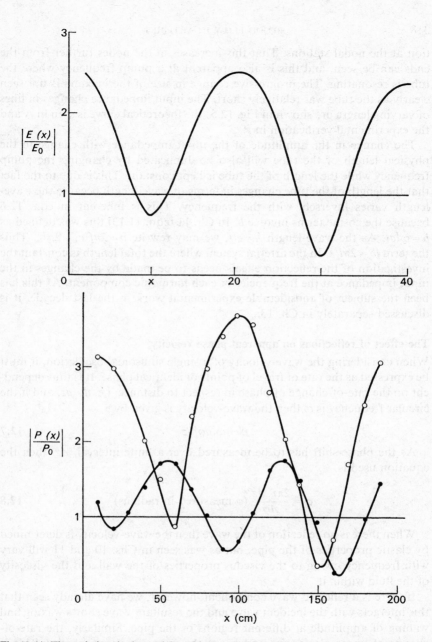

Fig. 12.4A. The variations in the modulus of voltage calculated for a transmission line terminating at $l=40$ units; expressed as a ratio of the voltage in a non-terminating line. (From Taylor, 1957*a*.)

B. In A voltage was taken as the analogue of pressure. Here, the actual pressure amplitudes in a rubber tube closed at 200 cm from its attachment to a pump of sinusoidal output. The wave-velocity of the tube was c. 7,400 cm/sec so that at 7 Hz (O) it was one wave-length long and analogous to the curve in A. This is a resonating length and the amplitudes should be compared to the curve at 10 Hz (●). (From Taylor, 1957*b*.)

tion at the nodal stations. That this increases in the nodes further from the ends can be seen, and this is also apparent at a pump frequency where the tube is resonating. The progressive change in size of the maxima is not seen clearly as the tube was relatively short. The input impedance changes in lines of varying length are shown in Fig. 12.5; the theoretical curve is seen in A and the experimental verification in B.

The change in the amplitude of the input impedance with change in the physical length of the tube will also be duplicated by changing the pump frequency while the length of the tube is kept constant. This is due to the fact that the length of the tube changes in terms of wave-length because the wave-length varies inversely with the frequency. This is inherent in eqn. 12.6 because the cosine terms involve b. In Ch. 11 (eqn. 11.13) this was defined as $b = \omega/c_1$. As the wave-length $\lambda = c/f$, we may rewrite $b = 2\pi f/c_1 = 2\pi/\lambda$. Thus the term $lb = 2\pi l/\lambda$. In the arterial system where the total length is constant the investigation of the reflection effects needs to be made by the changes in the input impedance at the frequencies of each harmonic component. As this has been the subject of considerable experimental work in the last decade, it is discussed separately in Ch. 13.

The effect of reflections on apparent phase velocity

When considering the wave velocity of a single sinusoidal oscillation, it must be expressed as the rate of travel of points of identical phase. It is thus dependent on the rate-of-change of phase in respect to distance, i.e. $d\varphi/dz$, and if the circular frequency is ω then the wave-velocity is given by

$$c' = \omega/d\varphi/dz \qquad \textbf{12.7}$$

As the phase-shift has to be measured over a finite interval, Δz, then the equation used is

$$c' = \frac{2\pi f \cdot \Delta z}{\Delta \varphi} \ (\varphi \text{ measured in radians}) \qquad \textbf{12.8}$$

When there is no reflection of the wave then the wave-velocity is determined by elastic properties of the pipe, but as was seen in Chs. 10 and 11 will vary with frequency owing to the viscous properties of the wall and the viscosity of the fluid within it.

If there is a reflected wave component, however, we have already seen that this interacts with the incident wave and the resultant wave shows waxing and waning of amplitude at different regions of the pipe. Similarly, the rate-of-change of phase also varies and hence the *apparent* phase-velocity. This is termed the apparent phase-velocity to distinguish it from the *true* phase-velocity, which is determined by the physical properties of the wall and the contained liquid. The appreciation of the modification of phase shift due to reflections is not easy to see intuitively, but was determined mathematically

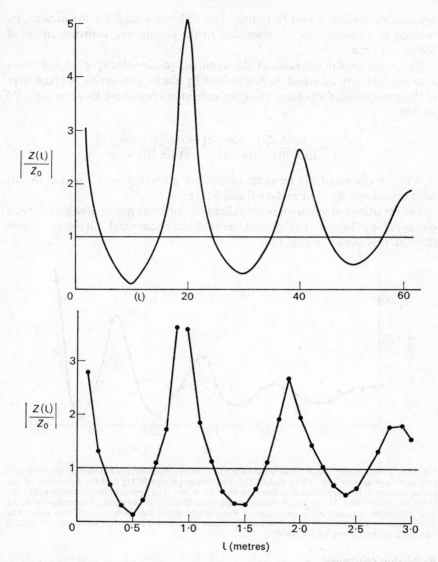

Fig. 12.5A. The input impedance in terms of the characteristic impedance calculated for a transmission line. Forty units on the abscissa represent a wave-length. (From Taylor, 1957*a*.)

B. The input impedance in the same rubber tube as in Fig. 12.4B. The pattern is the same as the theoretical curve in A. The frequency used was 7 Hz so the wave-length is 2·0 metres. Note that the deviation of the nodes and antinodes diminishes progressively with distance from the pump; this is due to damping. (From Taylor, 1957*b*.)

by Taylor (1957*a*). He found that the apparent phase-velocity in the presence of reflections varied in the same way as the amplitude of the pressure oscillations, with the exception that close to an open end it continues to rise when the pressure oscillation would be falling. This difference may, for the present, be ignored as we appear to be concerned, in the circulation, with reflections of the closed type.

The equation for the ratio of the apparent phase-velocity c' to the characteristic velocity c_0, which is determined by elastic properties, is given here in the generalized form for a complex reflection coefficient $R_f = \exp 2(a + ib)$ so that

$$\frac{c'}{c_0} = \frac{\cosh 2[(l - z)a - a] - \cos 2[(l - z)b - b]}{\sinh 2[(l - z)a - a] - (a/b) \sin 2[(l - z)b - b]}$$

With an open end the terminal impedance $Z_T = 0$, $R_f = +1$ and $a = b = 0$; for a closed end $R_f = -1$ and $a = 0$ and $b = \frac{1}{2}\pi$.

The variations of apparent wave-velocity at different points along a tube was measured by Taylor (1957b) and verified the theoretical curves in Taylor (1957a). It is shown in Fig. 12.6.

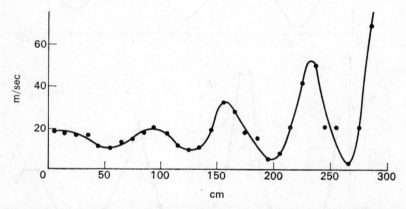

Fig. 12.6. The apparent phase velocity measured in a rubber pipe occluded at 300 cm from the end (the same model as in Figs. 12.4B and 12.5B). The frequency was 10 Hz and the true value of the phase velocity in the pipe without reflections was 14·1 m/sec. The apparent phase-velocity, like the input impedance (Fig. 12.5B), oscillated about the value found in the absence of reflections with the first minimum approximately one quarter wave-length from the distal end of the pipe. The diminution in these variations in velocity, as measurements are made further from that end, is due to damping. (From Taylor, 1957b.)

Reflection coefficient

Reflection of a travelling wave in a viscous liquid will occur to some degree whenever there is a change in the impedance of the tube down which it is propagated. We have already defined the characteristic impedance of an elastic tube in Ch. 6 (eqn. 6.26).

$$Z_0 = \frac{\rho c_0}{(1 - \sigma^2)^{\frac{1}{2}} . (M'_{10})^{\frac{1}{2}}} . e^{-i\epsilon/2}$$

Thus, it can be seen that a change in the wave-velocity, c_0 (which depends on the elastic properties and relative thickness of the wall) and/or a change in the value of the parameter, α, on which the values of the Bessel function terms M'_{10} and ε_{10} depend, will change the impedance. As $\alpha = R(\omega/v)^{1/2}$ this change in the value of α will be brought about by a change in radius as the angular frequency (ω) and the kinematic viscosity (v) are the same throughout. If we treat a discontinuity at which a change in wave-velocity or a change in radius occurs as a 'termination' and symbolize the impedance from that point onwards as Z_T then the usual convention for defining the reflection coefficient, R_f, is

$$R_f = \frac{Z_T - Z_0}{Z_T + Z_0} = \frac{1 - Z_0/Z_T}{1 + Z_0/Z_T} \qquad \textbf{12.9}$$

When the end is completely closed, then the terminal impedance will be infinitely large $(Z_T = \infty)$ and the coefficient will be $+1$, i.e. the wave will be 100 per cent reflected. When the end is open $Z_T = 0$ and the coefficient will be -1, i.e. the reflection will be of a wave $180°$ out of phase with the incident one.

(In the derivations from Taylor (1957a) above, he was defining the reflection coefficient in respect to flow, and, for convenience, wrote the upper line of eqn. 12.9, $Z_0 - Z_T$ so that a complete reflection had a coefficient of -1. Henceforth the more common convention will be used and it is easier to follow when considering pressure waves.)

For any given discontinuity, as characterized above, where partial reflection occurs then the remaining fraction of the wave will continue past the reflection point. Thus, if we call the amplitude of the centrifugal pressure wave A_1 and the amplitude of the reflected wave A_2 then the amplitude of the transmitted wave A_3 will be such that

$$A_1 = A_2 + A_3 \qquad \textbf{12.10}$$

and as the reflection coefficient is the ratio A_2/A_1, then the ratio of the transmitted wave to the original wave is A_3/A_1 and is termed the *transmission coefficient*, and will be the complement of the reflection coefficient.

As a numerical example we can take a situation where the impedance increases by a factor of two so that $Z_T = 2Z_0$. From eqn. 12.9 the reflection coefficient will be

$$R_f = \frac{1 - \frac{1}{2}}{1 + \frac{1}{2}} = +\frac{1}{3}$$

and the transmission coefficient will be 2/3. If the transmitted wave is reflected at a subsequent termination it will, naturally, return to the same discontinuity from the opposite direction and the impedance of the first segment of the tube, Z_0, will be, in effect, the terminal impedance. The value of R_f approaching from that side will be $(1-2)/(1+2)$ or $-1/3$, i.e. will behave as a partially open reflection and 1/3 of the wave will be reflected in an opposite phase.

In a system like the arterial tree where there are a succession of branching points as the pressure waves travel away from the heart this possibility of repeated reflections of this type makes a precise analysis extremely difficult. Remington (1965) attempted to do such an analysis for the individual branching points of the arteries of the fore-part of the dog by following discrete portions of the pulse pressure-wave recorded at several different points (based on the measurements of Meisner and Remington 1962). The labour involved was very great and, even so, the values obtained are doubtful in the absence of good evidence of such factors as wave-attenuation. Taylor (1966a, b) approached the same problem with computer simulation by setting up a 'model' of branching lines. As he was more concerned with describing the input impedance at the root of the aorta this analysis is more properly discussed with the consideration of arterial impedance in Ch. 13. For the present, we will confine ourselves to assessing the reflection coefficient at points of simple arterial branching.

THE REFLECTION AT A SINGLE ARTERIAL JUNCTION

In the simplest case we may neglect the effects of viscosity as was done by Karreman (1952). For convenience we will write $\delta = Z_0/Z_T$ so that from eqn. 12.9

$$R_f = \frac{1-\delta}{1+\delta} \qquad\qquad 12.11$$

Then for a tube of radius r_1 and wave-velocity c_1 making a junction with a tube of radius r_2 and wave-velocity c_2, from the 'water-hammer' equation (11.1), we obtain $Z_0 = \rho c_1/\pi r_1^2$ and $Z_T = \rho c_2/\pi r_2^2$ so that

$$\delta = (r_2^2/r_1^2) \cdot (c_1/c_2) \qquad\qquad 12.12$$

or, in the case of a bifurcation into two equal branches

$$\delta = 2(r_2^2/r_1^2) \cdot (c_1/c_2) \qquad\qquad 12.13$$

Now, if $c_1 = c_2$, i.e. the elastic properties of the vessel wall do not change, it can be seen that δ is the ratio of the cross-sectional areas of the vessels on either side of the junction. As when $\delta = 1$, the reflection coefficient is zero and no reflection occurs, then, in the simplest case, partial reflection of a closed type will occur when the cross-sectional area increases. In practice, however, the wave-velocity in arteries always appears to increase as arteries pass peripherally, i.e. $c_2 > c_1$ so that the condition of zero reflection is at a bifurcation with an area-ratio greater than 1 (as shown in Table 2.2). Karreman

(1952) calculated this assuming that the wall thickness remained unchanged, so that from the Moens equation (10.56)

$$c_1/c_2 = (r_2/r_1)^{\frac{1}{2}}$$

and then the point of zero reflection is at an area-ratio, for a bifurcation, of approximately 1·15.

Womersley (1958) extended this analysis by incorporating the full equation (6.4) of the impedance for a viscous liquid when, for the tethered elastic tube, he showed that from the impedances calculated from eqn. 6.26.

$$\delta = 2 \left(\frac{r_2}{r_1}\right) \cdot \frac{c_1}{c_2} \left[\frac{M'_{10}(\alpha_2)}{M'_{10}(\alpha_1)}\right]^{\frac{1}{2}} e^{i \cdot \frac{1}{2}[\epsilon\alpha_2 - \epsilon\alpha_1]} \qquad \textbf{12.14}$$

where $M'_{10}(\alpha_2)$ is the appropriate value of M'_{10} for the value of α of the branch and correspondingly for the other values. The expression can be seen to be similar to that of Karreman with the additional factor to the right of c_1/c_2 which represents the effect of viscosity. Figure 12.7 shows the resultant curves for values of α of 5 and 10 in the parent branch, values that are appropriate to the abdominal aorta of the dog or man. The assumption made again is that $c_1/c_2 = (r_1/r_2)^{1/2}$ as in Karreman's (1952) paper, and the latter author's curve ($\alpha = \infty$) is also included for comparison. The general impression is that for relatively large values of α, e.g. $\alpha = 10$, the reflection conditions for blood are not very different from those in a non-viscous fluid, but the effect of viscosity is to shift the curves to the right. Points of considerable interest are: (1) With a viscous fluid modulus and phase of the incident and transmitted waves change in such a way that there is never exact matching of the systems although the minimum reflection at the point of 'impedance matching' is only a few per cent. (2) The area-ratios of major branches that are found in the body which are about 1·15 to 1·25 (see Ch. 2) represent very small reflection coefficients in vessels of the calibre of those at the aortic bifurcation. (3) The phase change from a 0° to a lag of 180° occurs more gradually in vessels containing a viscous liquid, so that in the vicinity of the minimal reflection conditions of intermediate phase shift can occur. (4) If we regard α as a function of frequency it can be seen that the amount of reflection is not markedly frequency-dependent. There are marked proportional differences in the region of the minimum but the amplitude is so small here that this is of doubtful physiological significance.

It should be emphasized once more that this calculation is an abstraction concerned only with a single junction with the assumption that the branches are infinitely long tubes so that no subsequent reflection occurs. It does, however, emphasize that in large elastic tubes very little reflection will occur unless the change in cross-sectional area is very considerably different from those found in the body. With smaller tubes the effect of viscosity becomes much more apparent and Fig. 12.8 shows corresponding curves for

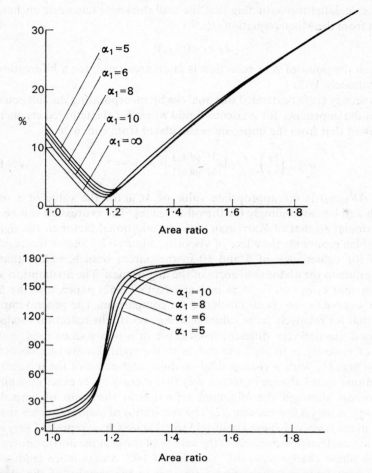

Fig. 12.7. The magnitude of reflections at the point of division of a tube into two equal branches. The radius of the single trunk is R and that of the branches is r. The corresponding wave-velocities (c_1 and c_2) are taken in this case as varying inversely with the square root of the radius, i.e. $c_1/c_2 = (r/R)^{1/2}$. Curves are drawn for four values of α, in the incident tube ($\alpha_1 = 5$, 6, 8 and 10) for tubes with limiting longitudinal restraint filled with a viscous liquid, and also for a non-viscous liquid ($\alpha_1 = \infty$). The abscissa is the ratio of the cross-sectional area of that of the two branches to that of the incident tube, i.e. $2r^2/R^2$.
Upper: the amplitude of the reflected wave expressed as a percentage of the incident wave.
Lower: The phase-lag of the reflected wave. For the non-viscous tube this changes from $0°$ to $180°$ at the point where the amplitude ratio is zero in A. A phase lag of $0°$ is a 'closed' type of reflection and $180°$ is an 'open' type. (From Womersley, 1958.)

bifurcations in which the parent branch as an $\alpha = 0.5$ (in the dog this represents the fundamental component in an artery of the order of the saphenous artery) and $\alpha = 2.0$. The same ratio for c_1/c_2 has been taken arbitrarily, in the absence of an exact knowledge, because this approximately offsets the retarding effect on wave-velocity that viscosity has in small tubes (Fig. 11.4). The

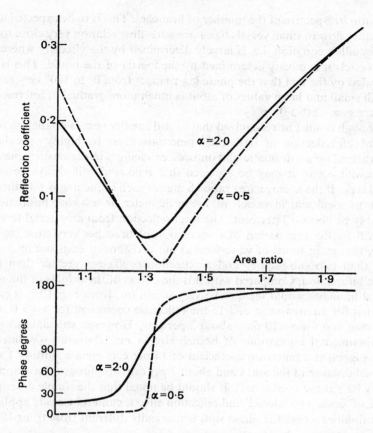

Fig. 12.8. Theoretical curves of the reflection conditions at a bifurcation calculated in the same way as those of Womersley in Fig. 12.7 but for smaller vessels. One curve is for $\alpha=2\cdot0$ in the main artery and one for $\alpha=0\cdot5$; the same wave-velocity assumptions are made. Ordinate—modulus of reflection-coefficient above; phase of reflection below. Abscissa—as in Fig. 12.7 the ratio of total cross-sectional areas of branches to that of main artery.

In the small artery it can be seen that the point of minimum reflection (or closest matching of impedances) is at an area ratio of 1·35 and the reflection is only 1 per cent. The limiting case as the vessels get smaller will be at the area ratio for matched resistance, i.e. 1·414 (see Ch. 2). The phase also changes rapidly from 0° to nearly 180°. The larger artery shows a more imperfect matching of impedance at the minimum although reflection is still only 2·3% at this point; the reversal of phase is, however, much more gradual (cp. curve for $\alpha=5$ in Fig. 12.7).

point of minimal reflection is shifted once more towards larger area-ratios; for $\alpha=0\cdot5$ this is now approximately 1·35 and any change in area at a junction smaller than this will cause a closed type of reflection. This value, it will be seen, is approaching that of the area-ratio for identical fluid resistance of steady flow across a bifurcation which is 1·414 (see Ch. 2). Just as it was shown that the resistance changes increase with the number of branches so will the impedance change increase. This effect is much less with larger branches and if viscosity is neglected as in eqn. 12.12 the reflection is determined by the area-ratio irrespective of the number of branches. This is to be expected as the oscillatory flow in small vessels has a pressure–flow relation very close to that of Poiseuille's equation, i.e. is largely determined by the viscosity whereas in large vessels it is mostly determined by the inertia of the liquid. This is also illustrated by the fact that the phase lag changes from 0° to 180° very rapidly at both small and large values of α but is much more gradual at intermediate values, e.g. $\alpha = 2\cdot0$, $5\cdot0$.

Although it must be recognized that in still smaller vessels prediction of the amount of reflection at individual junctions must be highly speculative, nevertheless, unless dramatic and unforeseen changes in the elastic behaviour of the wall occur, it may be expected that reflection will always be of the closed type. If the average area ratio change at each branching is $1\cdot15$ then the reflection coefficient in vessels of 1 mm diameter or less that bifurcate will probably be about 13 per cent. The total reflection from an arterial termination will be the summation of a succession of branches very close together (close, that is, in terms of wave-length) but divisions at each site into many more than two subsidiaries and a reflection coefficient greater than for a simple bifurcation. Compared with this the effects of the origins of the major arterial branches would seem to be very small, for, from Fig. 12.5, it can be seen that for an area-ratio of $1\cdot15$ the reflection coefficient for $\alpha = 5$ is about 4 per cent and for $\alpha = 10$ only about 2 per cent. However, calculations based on experimental estimations of branch size in my laboratory (Womersley, 1958) suggested a reflection coefficient of 14 per cent (phase shift 40°) at the terminal division of the aorta and about 7 per cent amplitude (phase approximately 90°) at the coeliac axis. It should be noted that the simple description above, of 'open' and 'closed' end reflection effects, cannot be easily applied to discontinuities where the phase shift is markedly different from 0° or 180°.

REFLECTIONS DUE TO A CONTINUOUS CHANGE IN ELASTIC PROPERTIES

As has been discussed in Ch. 10, the modulus of elasticity of arteries increases with the distance from the heart. This causes a progressive increase in wave-velocity rising, in the dog, from a value of about 4 m/sec in the ascending aorta (Nichols and McDonald, 1972) to some 14–15 m/sec in the tibial artery of the distal part of the hind leg (McDonald, 1968a), a phenomenon that is discussed in more detail in Ch. 14. As this clearly will cause a change of impedance it can be expected to give rise to wave reflection. Initially it may be thought of as a large series of small discontinuities spaced closely along a tube but this is cumbersome to analyse. Taylor (1964, 1965) has, instead, treated it as analogous with a non-uniform electrical transmission line and, in these initial papers, neglected viscous effects. In his later computer model of an array of branching tubes the viscosity terms were incorporated (Taylor

1966a, b). Fich, Welkowitz and Hilton (1966) have also analysed an electrical analogue model of the aorta which treats it as a single tube which tapers with a diminishing diameter and the net effect is similar.

The mathematical treatment is essentially the same as that used by Taylor (1965), which has been discussed above, but becomes too complex to be usefully incorporated here. Taylor has illustrated the effects by computing the effects for a line in which the impedance (and the wave-velocity) increases by a factor of three from the origin to the end. When the line then terminates in a matched impedance, so that no reflections will arise at this termination alone, it is interesting to note that the amplitude of the pressure wave will, nevertheless, rise and fall as if through the creation of nodes and antinodes (Fig. 12.9).

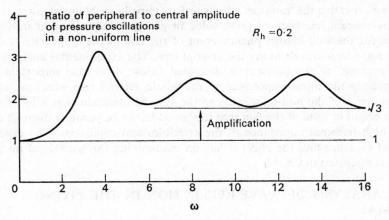

Fig. 12.9. The behaviour of the amplitude of reflections in a non-uniform line; the wave-velocity, in this example, increases by a factor of 3 from the origin to the termination. At the higher frequencies the minimum amplitude becomes $\sqrt{3}$ because this is the ratio of the square root of the characteristic impedances at the two ends of the tube, i.e. $(Z_0(x)/Z_0(0))^{1/2}$. (From Taylor, 1964.)

These are, however, superimposed on a general rising trend of amplitude along the tube. The final level of the mean pressure oscillation in this example (where the impedance increases by a factor of 3) rises to $\sqrt{3}$ times that at the origin. The rate of rise in wave velocity along the tube was represented by a cosine curve so that the velocity, c, at any distance, z, from the origin was

$$c(z) = c(0) . (2 - \cos \pi z) \qquad \textbf{12.15}$$

as the value of c rose smoothly from $c(0) = 1$ to $c(l) = 3$ the elastic modulus correspondingly would rise by a factor of 9 from the Moens-Korteweg equation (10.56) if it was assumed that the wall-thickness/diameter ratio remained constant.

When, in addition, there is superimposed a terminal reflection the formation of clear maxima and minima of pressure oscillations are seen (Fig. 12.9) at the origin with changes of frequency and similarly at varying distances along the tube. In a uniform line tube we have seen that these are spaced at regular intervals of a quarter wave-length from the termination. When the wave-velocity is increasing with distance from the origin this changes the wave-length, and so the spacing between a maximum and a minimum, and they are separated by longer intervals at the end of the tube than they are nearer the origin. These maxima and minima are, furthermore, superimposed on the same rising trend of pressure oscillation as occurs when there is no terminal reflection. In the latter case the pressure amplitude is determined by the relation at any distance z from the origin

$$P_{(z)} = P_{(0)} \, | \tilde{Z}_{0(x)} / \tilde{Z}_{0(0)} |^{\frac{1}{2}}$$ **12.16**

where $\tilde{Z}_0$ is called the 'nominal' characteristic impedance at any point.

This concept has been of great value in giving a deeper insight into the causes for the well-known phenomenon of the rise in the amplitude of the pulse wave as it travels along the arterial tree. The experimental analysis of this 'peaking' of the pressure is discussed below. It is also important in interpreting the input impedance of the whole arterial tree which is, as a consequence of the non-uniformity of the system, maintained at a low level at the origin in spite of the fact that the blood has to be pumped through the very high terminal impedance of the arterioles and capillaries. The experimental evidence and the effect it has on maintaining the work-load on the heart is discussed in Ch. 13.

THE ANALYSIS OF WAVE-REFLECTION IN THE LIVING ANIMAL

Thus far in this chapter we have discussed the behaviour of a single simple harmonic oscillation of pressure in a tube with a defined termination. The evidence from a theoretical analysis of vessel branching indicates that much larger reflection will occur where there is multiple branching into small branches such as occurs at the origin of the arteriolar and capillary bed than from the origin of single large branches from the main trunks. Nevertheless, every organ has an arteriolar bed and so, if there is to be a dominant region where discrete reflections arise, it is necessary to see if we can determine where this is. In a recent report on forward and backward waves in the arterial system, Westerhof *et al.* (1972) found that one may distinguish between reflections at bifurcations of the large vessels and reflections at the arteriolar part of the arterial tree. The former contribute a small, rather constant amount to the returning wave, while the latter reflects a strongly variable amount. In addition, the pulse-wave is compounded of a range of harmonic components so that the behaviour of each one needs to be analysed separately (Ch. 7) to be able to apply the results of the analysis of the previous part of this chapter. As the wave-length for each component is inversely related to its frequency the spacing of nodes and antinodes will be different for each component and the position of the first node will be spaced differently from the common reflecting site for all of them. A diagrammatic representation of the pressure-amplitude of such a set of four harmonic terms in the presence of damping in transmission is shown in Fig. 12.10 assuming an arbitrary

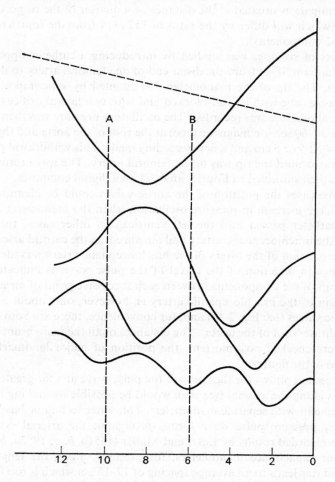

Fig. 12.10. A diagram of the amplitude changes with distance from a reflecting termination at the right of the diagram. Abscissa, distance from termination; ordinate, relative amplitude. Four harmonic components of a wave are shown and it can be seen that the first node at one quarter wave-length becomes progressively nearer the termination at 0. A reflection coefficient of 0·33 is assumed. (Compared to Fig. 12.3 only the upper half of the wave envelope is drawn, and a different base-line for each harmonic is imagined to avoid super-imposition of the waves.)

This is the case for a uniform elastic tube filled with a viscous liquid. As a result the antinodes get progressively bigger as they get nearer the origin—to the left. For the dog analysed in Fig. 12.11 the wave-length relations are such that the aortic root would be at the dashed vertical line A. The dashed line B is the corresponding position of the origin in the dog analysed in Fig. 12.13.

value of the reflection coefficient of $R_f = 0.33$. The first point to note is that close to the termination the amplitudes of all the components are rising together and that this is the only region where this is the case. This provides us with the means for identifying a site from which discrete reflections are arising and its location can be checked by testing whether any site allows for the same termination situated at the distance of a quarter of the respective wavelengths (which will differ by the ratio of $1:2:3:4$ from the fourth to the first harmonic components).

A series of six dogs was studied by introducing a catheter-tipped manometer (Statham SF-1) from the distal end of one femoral artery to the root of the aorta. The tip of the manometer was adapted by superimposition of a short plastic tube with its end blocked and with two lateral orifices so that a true lateral pressure was recorded. The oscillatory pressure was then recorded for some 30–60 sec (on magnetic tape) at the root of the aorta and the catheter withdrawn 2·5 or 5 cm and a new recording made. This withdrawal procedure was repeated until the tip was in the femoral artery. The wave forms at each site were then subjected to Fourier analysis on a digital computer.

In some cases the position of the aortic valves could be identified by the sudden large increase in pressure oscillation when the manometer at the tip of the catheter passed into the left ventricle. In other cases, the catheter entered the brachiocephalic artery and advanced up the carotid artery. In this case, the position of the origin of the brachiocephalic artery was identified by the change in direction of the travel of the pulse wave as indicated by the phase-shift of the components between each successive point of measurement. The origin of the brachiocephalic artery is, however, only about 3 cm from the aortic valves (see Fig. 2.10) and, for convenience, these are both described by the phrase 'root of the aorta'. The distances of all the main branches of the aorta were checked post-mortem; the position of major landmarks is also indicated in the figures.

This method allows for the study of the pulse-wave at a far greater number of points along the arterial tree than would be possible by making individual measurements with separate manometers. This latter technique has been used to survey pressure pulse wave forms throughout the arterial system with valuable recorded results by Laszt and Müller (1951a, b, c; 1952a, b, c). They used four capacitance manometers, for example, along the length of the aorta and this leads to an average spacing of 12–15 cm which is too far distant to distinguish with any certainty many of the possible nodes and antinodes that may be formed. They used special needles which were bent at 90° 1–2 cm from the tip which could be inserted through the wall and clamped to the inner side. A true lateral pressure was thus recorded and the obstruction to the lumen was negligible. Some of their records were submitted to Fourier analysis by McDonald (1960) and are shown later in Figs. 12.11, 12.13, 12.16, 12.17, to compare with the results obtained with the tech-

Dog 5: Pulse frequency 3·65∓0·01 c/sec

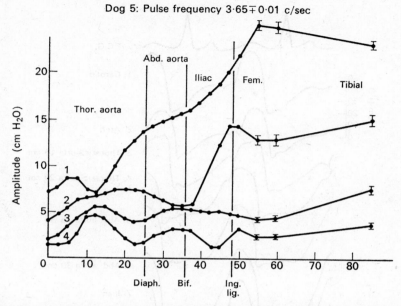

Fig. 12.11. The points here represent the modulus of pressure of the first four harmonics of the pulse-wave recorded every 2·5 cm from the aortic valves (0 cm) to the inguinal ligament at 50 cm. (For anatomical terminology refer to Fig. 2.10). The remaining points in the femoral and tibial arteries show the amplitudes (with bar representing the SE) recorded by manometers at constant positions throughout the experiment; the heart rate was $3·65 \pm 0·01$ Hz throughout.

The discussion of the position of nodes and antinodes is given in the text, e.g. in the 4th harmonic there is a node between $42·5 - 45·0$ cm and at $22·5$ to $25·0$ cm with an antinode between. The spacing of the first node progressively nearer the aortic root may be compared to the theoretical diagram in Fig. 12.10. There is one big discrepancy, however, for the antinode at the reflecting site at the inguinal ligament is not smaller than the more proximal antinodes as they are in a uniformly elastic line. The modification of wave-behaviour in a non-uniform line is shown in Fig. 12.14.

nique of successive withdrawals of an intra-arterial catheter-tipped manometer.

The introduction of a catheter will produce some reduction of the lumen and hence a change in cross-sectional area at the tip. This will itself give rise to some wave-reflection. If the radius of the artery is R and the radius of the catheter, r, then, at the tip of the catheter the cross-sectional area will diminish from πR^2 to $\pi(R^2 - r^2)$. If r is much smaller than R we may neglect viscous effects and use the simplified equation of 12.12 so that

$$Z_0 = \rho c/\pi R^2 \text{ and } Z_T = \rho c/\pi(R^2 - r^2)$$

and

$$\delta = Z_0/Z_T = (R^2 - r^2)/R^2$$

and

$$R_f = (1 - \delta)/(1 + \delta) \qquad\qquad \textbf{12.11}$$

The radius of the catheter was 0·11 cm approximately. In the descending thoracic aorta where R is approximately 0·5 cm this gives a calculated value

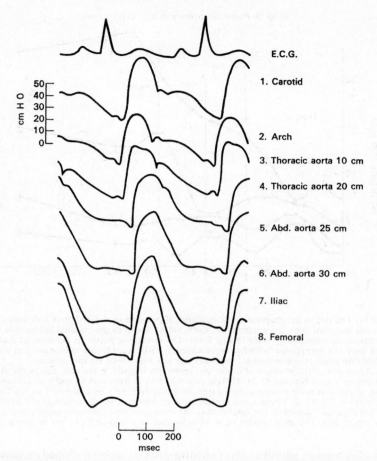

E.C.G.

1. Carotid

2. Arch

3. Thoracic aorta 10 cm

4. Thoracic aorta 20 cm

5. Abd. aorta 25 cm

6. Abd. aorta 30 cm

7. Iliac

8. Femoral

cm H O

50
40
30
20
10
0

0   100   200
msec

Fig. 12.12. The form of the pressure pulse-wave recorded by a high-frequency catheter-tip manometer inserted from the femoral artery up to the carotid artery (trace 1) and progressively withdrawn. The curves are all drawn relative to the ECG trace to indicate the transmission time between locations. The features of the pulse-wave are discussed in the text, e.g. the sharp 'incisura' in the arch of the aorta which has virtually disappeared after 20 cm travel in the aorta or 10 cm in the carotid. The peaking of the pulse in the femoral (the pulse amplitude here is almost double that in the arch) and the formation of a dicrotic wave from the distal abdominal aorta (Trace 6 at 30 cm) outwards can also be seen.

of $R_f = +0.023$ or $+2.3$ per cent and may be regarded as negligible. In the distal abdominal aorta where R is approximately 0.3 cm the value rises to $+6.7$ per cent. Thus, the presence of the catheter would cause a spurious rise in measured pressure oscillation of $+4.4$ per cent. In smaller vessels the artifact increases rapidly and in a vessel where $R = 0.2$ cm such as the femoral artery, the reflection coefficient will be about $+16$ per cent and becomes an appreciable source of error. Measurements with this manometer were, therefore, confined to the aorta and iliac arteries.

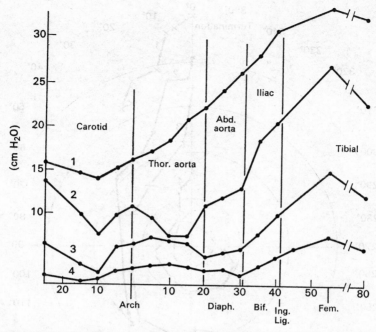

Fig. 12.13. A plot of the amplitude of the first four harmonic components of the pressure pulse recorded at 5 cm intervals from the carotid artery to the femoral artery as in Fig. 12.11. The dog, in this case, is the one whose pressure waves were displayed in Fig. 12.12. The heart-frequency was $2 \cdot 78 \pm 0 \cdot 017$ Hz in this animal; thus the first node of pressure, e.g. at 40 cm in the 4th harmonic, is further from the inguinal ligament because the wave-length is longer. The fundamental component has no node in the aorta. The idealized position of nodes and antinodes is shown in Fig. 12.10 if the arch of the aorta was at dashed line B.

The main biological source of distortion arises from variations in the force of the ventricular ejection over the period of time necessary to make the successive records together with changes in pulse frequency and constancy of the peripheral impedance. Analyses were, therefore, limited to dogs that could be maintained in extreme cardiovascular stability for periods of an hour or more. In order to minimize the effects of surgical trauma the dogs had closed chests and abdomens and respiratory variations of mean arterial pressure and heart rate were kept very small by ensuring a clear airway with an intra-tracheal tube. The animals were maintained in fairly deep anaesthesia with intravenous pentobarbital. The variations in pulse frequency were small as indicated by the SE calculated for the whole period over which the pressure measurements were made. Thus, in the animal analysed in Fig. 12.11 the mean pulse frequency was $3 \cdot 65 \pm 0 \cdot 047$ Hz and for that illustrated in Fig. 12.13 the mean frequency was $2 \cdot 78 \pm 0 \cdot 078$ Hz.

The variations of the force of ejection were monitored approximately by maintaining pressure measurements at the same sites in the arterial system

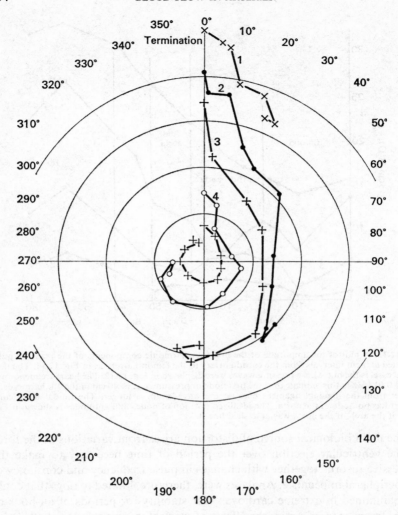

Fig. 12.14. A polar diagram in which both the amplitude and phase of the analysis shown in Fig. 12.13 is shown. From the calculation shown in the text the 'termination', in the sense of the source of a discrete reflection is placed at the top of the diagram, 0° and phase shift due to transmission is plotted clockwise. Thus, at 90° for the second and third harmonics the amplitudes are minimal but the phase-shift is maximal. Due to the latter effect the apparent phase-velocity is also minimal. The first harmonic, however, travels over less than a quarter wave-length. The first point in the carotid artery is shown so that the arch of the aorta is indicated when the phase reverses.

throughout the experiment. The strain-gauge manometers measured the pressure in one common carotid artery through a short cannula inserted into the superior thyroid artery; in addition, a needle of the type used in Laszt and Müller's studies was inserted into the femoral artery not being used to insert the catheter-tip manometer and another pressure was recorded in the femoral

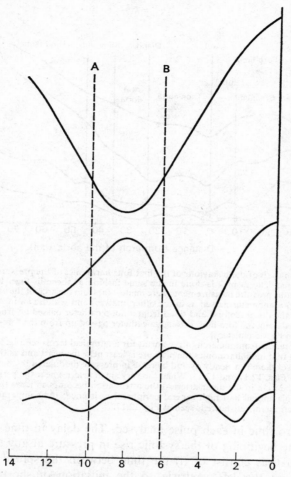

Fig. 12.15. An idealized diagram (to be compared with Fig. 12.10) of the behaviour of four harmonics in a non-uniform tube, i.e. one that gets progressively stiffer as it approaches the termination at the right. Reflection coefficient 0·33 as before; vertical lines A and B marking situation of arch of aorta in Figs. 12.11 and 12.13 respectively.

Now it can be seen that, as in the experimental plots of Figs. 12.10 and 12.11, the antinode at the termination is the largest one.

bed through a distal branch. Finally, a pressure was recorded at the angle or the foot in the distal end of the tibial artery or the dorsalis pedis artery. The SE of these last three recorded pressures are shown in Fig. 12.11. The source of error from this variation in oscillatory pressure was minimized by normalizing the harmonic components measured at each successive site against the corresponding carotid artery pressure for that cycle.

The phase shift between the pressure recorded at each site in the aorta was measured by using the QRS spike of the electrocardiogram as the reference

M

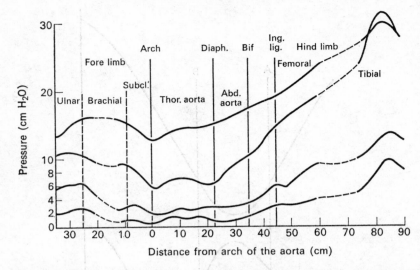

Fig. 12.16. An analysis of the behaviour of the first four harmonics of the pressure pulse over the whole arterial tree. The display is done in the same fashion as those in Figs. 12.11 and 12.13. Three simultaneous pressure measurements were made—(a) from the arch of the aorta the femoral by a catheter-tip manometer passed as in the other analyses and withdrawn in 2·5 cm steps, (b) pressures along the distal femoral and tibial from a no. 5 catheter passed up from the hind-foot and (c) pressures along the fore-limb through a catheter passed up from the fore-foot (with these latter withdrawn by 1·5 cm steps).

Abscissa—distances from the arch of the aorta; for anatomical terms see Fig. 2.10.

It can be seen that in all harmonics the pressure is least near the heart and as the distance from the heart increases there is a steady overall increase in pressure modulated by fluctuations similar to those seen in Figs. 12.11 and 12.13. When the very small arteries near the periphery (at 80 cm in the tibial and 25 cm in the ulnar arteries) the attenuation becomes so large that the pressures begin to fall. This animal had high general peripheral resistance; the comparable picture in a dog with low peripheral resistance is seen in Fig. 12.17.

point for zero time in each pulse analysed. The delay in time between this point and the beginning of the systolic rise in pressure at any given arterial location will thus consist of (i) the time between the spread of electrical excitation over the left ventricle to the initiation of shortening of the muscle fibres; (ii) the time from the initiation of ventricular contraction which closes the atrio-ventricular valve to the point when the intraventricular pressure exceeds the aortic pressure and opens the aortic valves (the period of isovolumic ventricular contraction) and (iii) the time taken for the pressure-wave to propagate from the ascending aorta to the point where the arterial pressure measurement is made. With a heart that is beating at a constant rate, it must be assumed that the components (i) and (ii) are constant and un-doubtedly they will vary very little. Thus, changes in the phase (or true delay from the arbitrary point of zero time) of each harmonic component are attributed entirely to apparent travel time of the pressure wave from the heart. This is a good approximation but, nevertheless, the measurement of successive increments of phase delay in the pressure pulse is a less accurate

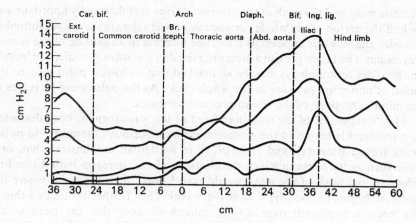

Fig. 12.17. An analysis of the first four harmonics similar to that in Fig. 12.16; the anterior pressures are here measured in the carotid system rather than in the fore-limb. This dog had a low peripheral resistance; the oscillatory pressures and the mean pressure were much lower than in Fig. 12.16.

The main difference is that the 'peaking' of the pressures in the hind-part of the tree ceases in the proximal hind-limb; similarly in the common carotid there is a downward trend with one 'peak' in the external carotid in the first two harmonics. Thus, without marked reflections from the distal arteriolar beds the attenuation in the peripheral arteries 'overcomes' the other effects such as increasing stiffness of the arteries that cause the pressure to climb as it travels away from the heart.

means of measuring phase velocity than the recording of the same pressure wave simultaneously at two points a known distance apart.

The shape of the travelling pulse wave

The transformation of the arterial pressure wave as it travels away from the heart is illustrated in Fig. 12.12. This is a typical selection of wave forms shown in relation to the ECG, from the waves analysed in Fig. 12.13 (where the pressure was recorded at 5 cm intervals along the aorta and iliac artery). It can be seen that the total pressure swing, or pulse pressure, doubles in amplitude between the arch of the aorta and the femoral artery and is also increasing in travelling up the carotid artery. In addition, the wave changes markedly in shape. The dome-shaped systolic portion in the arch becomes more square, with an appearance of a double hump in the distal thoracic aorta and rapidly changes to the peaked form of the peripheral pulse by the time it reaches the bifurcation of the aorta. The sharp notch which marks the closure of the aortic valves (the *incisura*) in the proximal aortic pulse diminishes rapidly in amplitude due to attenuation of its higher frequency components, although traces of it persist to the end of the aorta. The diastolic portion of the wave which is slightly curved upward in the arch flattens and becomes concave in the abdominal aorta. This dip becomes greater in the iliac and femoral arteries and is succeeded by a secondary diastolic rise of pressure with a rounded top (the dicrotic wave). The period between the peak of the dicrotic wave and the peak of the pressure during systole usually approximates to half the period of the whole cardiac cycle; when the curves are submitted to Fourier analysis this appears as a marked increase in amplitude of the second harmonic. The fall in pressure preceding the dicrotic wave (the dicrotic 'notch' in the older terminology) may be so marked that its lowest point may be the point of minimum pressure in the whole cycle. As the pulse wave increases in amplitude the slope of the rise in pressure increases.

This 'steepening' of the travelling front of the wave form as been discussed at considerable length in the extensive earlier descriptive literature on pulse-wave forms. Bramwell and Hill (1923), in particular, emphasized that, in a tube such as the aorta in which the elastic modulus increases with distending pressure, the peak of the wave would travel faster than the point where the pressure begins to rise (the *foot* of the wave). They further postulated that if the process continued over a long enough distance that the peak would overtake the foot and that 'breakers' would form analogous to those formed by ocean waves approaching a shelving shore. It was pointed out by McDonald and Taylor (1959) that the analogy between a pressure wave in an enclosed tube and surface waves in an open canal was not a good one. Furthermore, the 'steepening' of the wave is in large part attributed to increase in amplitude and the time from the beginning of the pressure rise to its peak does not, in fact, vary very much. The effect of elastic non-linearity on the slope of the wave front was investigated mathematically in some detail by Barnard *et al.* (1966) who found that there would be some increase in slope but that the change was not very marked. These aspects of the apparent differences in velocity of the various regions of the pulse-wave are discussed further in Ch. 14.

THE CHANGES IN AMPLITUDE OF THE HARMONIC COMPONENTS OF THE PULSE-WAVE

The amplitude of the first four harmonics of the pressure-wave from one experiment is displayed in Fig. 12.11. The pressure was recorded at intervals of 2·5 cm from the aortic valves. Looking at the individual harmonics, the amplitude of the first, which is initially 7 cm H_2O, rises somewhat to a local maximum at 5–7·5 cm distance and then decreases again to a value of c. 7 cm H_2O at a distance of 12·5 cm and thereafter continues to rise to a value of c. 23 cm H_2O in the proximal femoral artery and then falling slightly towards the end of the hind-limb. The second harmonic also increases slowly up to a maximum value at about 20 cm distance and then falls to a distinct local minimum between 32·5 and 37·5 cm in the region of bifurcation of the aorta; it then rises steeply to a distance of about 50 cm, dips slightly in the femoral artery and rises a little at the foot. The amplitude of the third harmonic reaches a local maximum at 15 cm then dips and rises slightly again but thereafter shows no very marked change. The fourth harmonic, however, shows a clear series of two maxima and two minima; the former between 10 and 15 cm and between 32·5 and 37·5 cm, with minima at 22·5 cm and between 42·5 and 45 cm.

The presence of minima at 12·5 cm in the first harmonic, 35 cm in the second harmonic and 45 cm in the fourth, i.e. progressively closer to the distal end of the abdomen, suggests a parallel to the position of the node nearest the termination in the diagram in Fig. 12.10.

The hypothesis that the spacing of these minima is that of node formation by a single site of reflection can be tested arithmetically. Let this site be situated at T cm from the origin and let a quarter wave-length at the frequency of the first harmonic be indicated by L cm. The node nearest the termination will be at a distance of $(T-L)$ cm from the origin for the first harmonic. The corresponding node for the second harmonic will be $(T-L/2)$ cm from the origin because its wave-length is half that of the first harmonic. Similarly, this node will be $(T-L/3)$ cm from the origin for the third harmonic and at $(T-L/4)$ cm for the fourth harmonic. At the distance of $(T-L/2)$ cm the fourth harmonic will be at a half wave-length maximum while the second is at a minimum (as in Figs. 12.10 and 14) and at $(T-L)$ cm the minimum of the first harmonic should correspond to a maximum of the second harmonic (half wave-length) and of the fourth harmonic (whole wave-length) and these relations can be seen in Fig. 12.11.

Because the spacing of the measuring points makes fine discrimination impossible we may simplify the calculations by averaging the wave-velocity along the whole aorta. In the dog analysed in Fig. 12.11 this mean velocity was 517 cm/sec and the pulse-frequency was 3·65 Hz. The wave-length of the first harmonic is, therefore, 141·6 cm and a quarter wave-length (L) is 35·4 cm. As the minimum in this harmonic is 12·5 cm from the origin $(T-35·4) = 12·5$ cm so that $T = 47·9$ cm. For the second harmonic $(T-17·7) = 32·5$ cm giving $T = 50·2$ cm; for the fourth $(T-8·9) = 42·5$ cm giving $T = 51·4$ cm. These distances only differ by 3·5 cm overall, which is within the range of error when calculated from points 2·5 cm apart, and indicate a reflecting site in the region of the inguinal ligament, which was 49 cm from the aortic valves in the dog. Minima in the fourth harmonic are seen at 42·5, 22·5 and 2·5 cm from the origin—an internodal distance of 20 cm which is quite close to the half wave-length of 17·7 cm. The distance between the minima of the first and second harmonics is also 20 cm (when again it should be 17·7 cm but within the possible error in measurement).

Applying the same calculations to the data in Fig. 12.13 the mean aortic wave-velocity was here 700 cm/sec and the pulse frequency 2·78 Hz so that the fundamental wave-length in this case was 251·8 cm. The length L was thus 63 cm and from the minimum in the second harmonic between 10 and 15 cm we derive T as between 41·5 and 45·5 cm. The value of T from the third harmonic is from 40 to 45 cm, and from the fourth harmonic $T = 44$ cm. In this dog, the distance from the arch to the inguinal ligament, at the junction of the iliac and femoral arteries was 41·5 cm. From these calculations it can be seen that no minimum for the fundamental harmonic occurs in the aorta because the length T is shorter than a quarter wave-length.

In the other experiments in this series the minimum in the second harmonic was the only one that could be distinguished clearly.

This agreement, between all the intercorrelated determinations that we have made here, shows that there must be a fairly discrete reflection from a single site. No other hypothesis will explain the variations in amplitude of the harmonic components of the pressure wave along the aorta. When measurements are made at 5 cm the 'resolution' in the predicted distance cannot be more accurate than $\pm 2 \cdot 5$ cm.

The interpretation of the anatomical site, from which these reflections occur, is in terms of the number of arteriolar beds at this distance from the heart. Reference to Fig. 2.10 will show that these comprise the beds of the pelvic organs and those of the thigh muscles (which constitute by far the greatest fraction of the muscle of the hind-limb in the dog); in addition, the arteriolar beds of the small intestine supplied by the superior mesenteric artery average out at about the same distance from the heart. The effect will, of course, be masked to a considerable extent by reflections from other regions but many of the abdominal organs have their arteriolar beds relatively close to the aorta which is the probable reason that no distinctive patterns arise from them.

Close to the heart interaction will also occur with reflections occurring in the forepart of the body and no coherent pattern can be distinguished in the carotid artery region in Fig. 12.13. This interaction can be more conveniently discussed in terms of the input impedance and is discussed further in Ch. 13.

The phase relations along the aorta

If the interpretation of the variations in amplitude of the harmonic components given above is correct then it should be accompanied by corresponding changes in the phase relations. In a reflecting system in the region of a node in amplitude the shift in phase will be large (i.e. the apparent phase velocity will be at a minimum also). These changes in amplitude and phase can be shown by plotting both together on a polar diagram. Fig. 12.14 shows such a plot for the data presented in Fig. 12.13. The calculated distance of the reflecting site is set at 0° (termination—at top of diagram). The first harmonic is large in amplitude but diminishes as the distance from the termination increases but the phase shift between points is relatively small and the maximum value is 27°. This represents the arch of the aorta, for the phase shift then reverses as the catheter tip moves into the carotid artery. The second harmonic moves to 145° before the reversal indicating where the origin of the carotid artery occurs. The progressive phase shifts backwards from the termination and progressively increases to the region around 90° (i.e. at a quarter wave-length) at the same time as the amplitude decreases so that the polar plot forms almost a vertical straight line. The same behaviour is seen for the third harmonic but the total phase increases to 195° before reversing; in the meantime, the amplitude has again increased at the half wave-length position, 180°. A similar pattern can be seen for the fourth harmonic but the minimum of amplitude has been displaced to around 110°. (The non-uniform wave-velocity along the arterial tree introduces complications in fine detail of interpretation on this type of diagram.) The fifth harmonic finally shows a typical behaviour at a frequency when the effect of damping becomes dominant; the amplitude progressively decreases as the phase moves through a 360° cycle and the plot takes on a spiral form.

The behaviour of the phase thus lends strong support to the hypothesis that much of the changes in amplitude is due to reflections arising from the distal end of the abdomen.

Measurements of the amplitude of the harmonic components of the pressure wave have also been made in man by Luchsinger et al. (1964). The trend was very similar but the presence of minima were less distinct; this may be attributed in part to the fact that it was necessary to space the measurements a greater distance apart, and to the fact that their graphs represent values averaged from several patients whose heart rates varied considerably. Taylor (1964) has measured changes in amplitude in the rabbit and O'Rourke (1965, 1967b) in the dog and in the wombat (an Australian marsupial). While the dog and the rabbit are similar, the patterns in the turkey and wombat are distinctly different. In the turkey, the amplitude of the first four harmonics remains relatively constant (with a slight tendency to rise) along the length of the aorta (Taylor, 1964). In the wombat, there is a marked rise in amplitude in all harmonics suggesting a marked reflection at the end of the squat body in a system which is short in terms of wave-length.

O'Rourke (1967a) made some very interesting studies in dogs by stiffening the proximal aorta artificially to mimic arterial disease which increased moduli of pressure there and so diminished the increase towards the periphery. O'Rourke et al. (1968) studied human subjects of varying ages and found a similar effect in the older subjects with atherosclerosis.

THE ROLE OF ELASTIC NON-UNIFORMITY IN THE PRESENCE OF DAMPING

The simple treatment of a tube with elastic non-uniformity, i.e. becoming progressively stiffer away from the origin (discussed earlier, p. 327) reveals that a centrifugal wave increases in amplitude as it travels. Conversely a reflected wave travelling towards the origin will diminish in amplitude. Viscous damping will, on the other hand, attenuate travelling waves by the same amount irrespective of direction. The effect of the interaction of a centrifugal with a reflected wave in respect of the amplitude of the nodes and antinodes has already been discussed (p. 313) and illustrated in Fig. 12.3.

In the aorta where there is both viscous attenuation and a progressive increase of elastic stiffness the two factors acting in an opposite sense to each other will tend to cancel out. The attenuation due to the viscosity of blood in a perfectly elastic tube can be calculated from the equations of Womersley (1957a, b). With the parameter $\alpha = 10$ the attenuation, due to blood viscosity alone, has a value of approximately $e^{-0.4}$ per wave-length. As the wave-length diminishes progressively with the frequency of the harmonic components the attenuation over a measured distance increases with harmonic order. Assuming a mean value of α along the aorta as 8 the calculated attenuation due to *blood viscosity* alone over the 40 cm length from the aortic valves to the bifurcation of the aorta for the first four harmonics is, approximately, (1) 10 per cent, (2) 16·5 per cent, (3) 20 per cent, (4) 22 per cent. In arteries the visco-elastic properties of the wall add markedly to the damping and the total attenuation is about double this value. The values found in the thoracic aorta over the frequency range found in the arterial pulse was from $e^{-0.7}$ to $e^{-0.8}$ per wave-length. Anliker *et al.* (1968) derived the similar values of $e^{-0.75}$ to $e^{-0.89}$ in the frequency range of 40–150 Hz. (The methods for measuring attenuation and the results obtained are discussed in Ch. 14.)

In the six experiments analysed in this series the average measured increase in wave-velocity from the thoracic aorta to the femoral artery was from 6·0 to 8·3 m/sec. We see that the predicted amplification is approximately $(c_1/c_0)^{1/2} = (8·3/6·0)^{1/2} = 1·18$. In one animal the increase has been greater, from 4·5 m/sec to 10·0 m/sec which would give an amplification of $(10·0/4·5)^{1/2} = 1·42$, and these values are in agreement with the more direct measurements by Nichols and McDonald (1972) (Fig. 14.3). The rise in amplitude between the proximal aorta and the femoral artery due to the elastic non-uniformity may therefore be anticipated as being between 20 and 40 per cent. As we have seen that the attenuations due to blood viscosity and wall viscosity will be about double those calculated above, i.e. from 20 to 44 per cent for the first harmonics, it is apparent that the two effects will indeed more or less cancel each other out in the centrifugal wave. The effects will, however be, *additive* for the reflected wave which will diminish along the length of the aorta by 0–80 per cent. The interaction between the centrifugal and centripetal waves will, therefore, produce a similar ratio in *relative* amplitude at the nodal and antinodal positions as in the case without elastic 'taper'. The actual magnitudes will, on the other hand, vary in such a way that the antinodes towards the termination will be larger and the amplitude at the nodes will remain more nearly constant. This is illustrated in Fig. 12.15. This diagram is calculated for the same damping and reflection coefficient (i.e. 0·33) as the previous diagram in Fig. 12.10, but an amplification due to elastic non-uniformity equal and opposite to the viscous damping has been added. The vertical broken lines marked A and B indicate where the root of the aorta would fall for the experiments analysed in Figs. 12.11 and 12.13 respectively in consideration of their differing pulse-frequency and wave-length relations. It can be seen that the overall diagram gives quite a reasonable, if idealized, picture of the way that reflections set up in a non-uniform system, such as that of the aorta and its major branches, do affect the amplitudes of the constituent harmonic components of the pulse-wave at different points along the system.

The coefficient of reflection

Where we can measure the oscillatory amplitudes of a pressure at a number of points towards a region where discrete reflection occurs it is possible to calculate the reflection coefficient from the relative amplitudes at the antinodes and the nodes. In a uniform elastic tube without damping illustrated diagrammatically in Fig. 12.3 this ratio remains constant. The amplitude at the terminal antinode was the sum of the amplitudes of the incident wave and the reflected wave; the amplitude at the node was the difference of these two waves.

If we call the amplitude of the centrifugal wave P and designate a reflection coefficient of R_f then the amplitude at the antinode (AN) is $(P + R_f.P)$ and the amplitude at the node (N) is $(P - R_f.P)$. The ratio, therefore, is

$$\frac{AN}{N} = \frac{(P + R_f.P)}{(P - R_f.P)} = \frac{(1 + R_f)}{(1 - R_f)}$$

For simplicity, let this ratio be n, then

$$n = \frac{(1 + R_f)}{(1 - R_f)}$$

and

$$R_f = \frac{(n - 1)}{(n + 1)} \qquad \textbf{12.17}$$

The ratio, n, is often named, in transmission line terminology, the *standing-wave ratio*, or the partial standing-wave ratio. The latter name indicates that the phenomenon may be thought of as a situation where part of the wave is totally reflected and forms a standing-wave.

If elastic non-uniformity causes an amplification of a per cm, then, by similar reasoning, it is easy to show that (in the absence of damping) the reflection coefficient is approximately given by

$$R_f = \frac{(n - ax)}{(n + ax)}$$ **12.18**

where x cm is the distance between the node and the antinode.

In a uniform tube with damping characterized by a propagation constant γ the corresponding equation is

$$R_f = \frac{(ne^{\gamma x} - 1)}{(ne^{-\gamma x} + 1)}$$ **12.19**

which, in the presence of damping and elastic non-uniformity, becomes

$$R_f = \frac{(ne^{\gamma x} - ax)}{(ne^{-\gamma x} + ax)}$$ **12.20**

It will be seen from these formulations that the value of the reflection coefficient calculated will be, relative to the simple uniform undamped case, decreased by the presence of amplification due to elastic 'taper' and increasing by allowing for the damping.

In the series of experiments of which Figs. 12.11 and 12.13 are examples the average reflection coefficient was calculated for all the harmonic terms ($N = 13$) where a clear distinction of a node in the aorta could be seen. The values were as follows, according to the assumptions made:

(i) uniform tube without damping $R_f = 0.42 \pm 0.09$ SD
(ii) non-uniform tube without damping $R_f = 0.33 \pm 0.08$ SD
(iii) uniform tube with damping $R_f = 0.65 \pm 0.11$ SD
(iv) tube with non-uniformity and damping $R_f = 0.54 \pm 0.12$ SD

The damping assumed for these calculations was $e^{-0.7}$ per wave-length and the elastic taper amplification was 0·5 per cent per cm (assumed to be linear). Both of these values are probably at the lower end of the normal range,

From the value calculated from eqn. 12.20 and listed under (iv), we can thus say that there is approximately 50 per cent reflection arising in the system of the dog from the region of the junction of the trunk with the hind-legs. From impedance data, that is discussed further in Ch. 13, O'Rourke and Taylor (1966) concluded that the reflection coefficient at the terminal arterioles of the femoral bed was of the order of 0·8 under normal conditions but could vary between 0·95 with marked arteriolar constriction and virtually zero with maximum vasodilatation.

The variations in input impedance at the origin of the femoral bed are part of the 'terminal' impedance of the aortic system. The variations of impedance with frequency that such reflections will cause will alter the apparent reflection seen in the aorta and is part of the cause of the scatter indicated by the Standard Deviation of the calculated values of the reflection coefficients given above. For example, at the frequency of the third harmonic shown in Fig. 12.13 the input impedance of the femoral bed was at a minimum and thus accounts, in part, for the virtual absence of reflection in this component as indicated by the absence of a node in the distal aorta.

This is but one simplified case of the complexities of interpreting with any precision the apparent values calculated for a reflection coefficient except in a situation where there is only one reasonably clearly defined termination. What the propagated wave 'sees' in the aorta is a mixture of reflections from arteriolar beds close to it and the reflections from the interactions with impedances of longer beds arising from it. Nevertheless, in terms of modifying the amplitude and phase of the harmonic components of the wave along the aorta we have seen that the effective reflection coefficient is of the order of 50 per cent.

The situation of the terminations of the arteries supplying the anterior part of the body average a distance of about half that of the main reflecting sites for the aorta in the hind-part of the body. It is thus more difficult to obtain a long enough distance to detect node formation in the lower frequency harmonics of relatively large amplitudes. In such studies as have been done it would appear that reflections that arise from the fore-limbs are approximately the same as for the hind-limb but in the carotid system are considerably lower. This latter effect is due to the relatively low resistance in the cerebral circulation. It appears that, 'seen' from the arch of the aorta, the overall reflection coefficient is about 40–50 per cent and thus similar to that at the distal aorta.

THE DISTRIBUTION OF PRESSURES THROUGHOUT THE SYSTEMIC ARTERIES

A series of experiments has been performed in my laboratory which were an extension of those tracking the pressure wave along the aorta illustrated above in Figs. 12.11 and 12.13. In these studies, catheter-tip manometers were introduced into the aorta from the femoral artery as before; in addition, a fine (no. 5, French) catheter was introduced into the dorsalis pedis artery on the foot of the other leg and threaded through until its tip was in the iliac artery. A third catheter (no. 4 or 5 French) was introduced either into a distal branch of the external carotid system at the level of the mandible or into an artery on a paw of a fore-limb and threaded through to the arch of the aorta. As before, the signal for synchronization of all pressure measurements was the QRS spike of the electrocardiogram; also pressures were recorded throughout at fixed sites in the carotid and femoral artery to check the constancy of the pressure created at the heart-beat over the whole compartment.

The results from two of these experiments are illustrated in Figs. 12.16 and 12.17. In the first, there was a much higher mean pressure with a larger peripheral resistance indicating generalized arteriolar constriction. It is immediately apparent that the amplitude of pressure oscillation in the arch of the aorta close to the heart is the smallest throughout the major arteries and builds up both in fore- and hind-parts of the body. However, as the small arteries at the ends of limbs are reached the high attenuation in small vessels begins to dominate the effects of reflected waves and the increasing elastic stiffness and the amplitude begins to fall. In the hind-limb this fall is not apparent until the distal part of the tibial artery; in the fore-limb the pressures have reached a plateau in the brachial artery and diminish throughout the ulnar artery. The experiment illustrated in Fig. 12.17 shows a case where there was a more general vasodilatation and lower pressures throughout the arterial tree. The change in the pressure distribution in the hind-part of the body was markedly different. The build-up of harmonic amplitudes in the aorta is still considerable for the first two harmonics; the third harmonic, however, shows no marked rise until the iliac artery while the fourth harmonic shows relatively little overall rise. These observations are consistent with the fact that the damping over any given distance will increase markedly with frequency. In the hind-limb the pressure amplitudes all fall until at the hind-paw only the amplitude of the first harmonic is significantly higher than that at the arch of the aorta. In the carotid system there is a small upward trend in the common carotid which increases in the proximal external carotid artery but falls again as the smaller branches are reached. The second harmonic varies with distance around a fairly steady level while the third and fourth harmonics diminish continually.

These two cases show the extremes that were found in the limited series of experiments. The more usual finding is seen in the data used by McDonald (1960) and shown in Fig. 12.18 in which the amplitude reached at the proximal femoral artery shows only a slight further rise (or in the first two harmonics a relative constancy) along the hind-limb. But it can be seen that while the behaviour of the pressure wave in the peripheral arteries can vary widely with changes in arteriolar constriction the pressures that are generated at the heart show relatively little change so that the changes in the pulsatile load imposed on the heart are minimized and always remain low in terms of the terminal impedance.

SECONDARY REFLECTION OF THE REFLECTED WAVES AT THE HEART

Concepts of a 'standing wave' in the aorta (Hamilton and Dow, 1939) and 'the natural frequency' of the arterial system (Alexander, 1953) imply a condition of resonance. This requires that a reflected wave reaching the heart will be

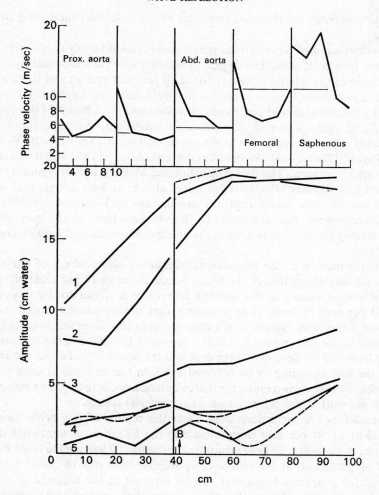

Fig.12.18. A plot of the first 5 harmonics of the travelling pulse-wave which is intermediate in pattern between the high peripheral resistance condition shown in 12.16 and the low resistance pattern seen in Fig 12.17.

reflected anew and once more travel to the periphery, be reflected again and so on. For waves of suitable frequency in terms of their wave-lengths the antinodal maxima will build up in contrast to their nodal minima and will dominate the harmonic components of the pulse-wave. These concepts have been revived by O'Rourke (1967b) in relation to his data on the wombat and apparently largely predicted on the finding of a shallow node in the thoracic aorta in the third harmonic with a frequency of 3·17 Hz which is close to the 'natural frequency' which he states is 3·1 Hz. He modifies the previous arguments by suggesting that no reflections occur at the heart but the repeated rcfleetion is from the terminal arterioles of the fore- and hind-parts of the body.

The discussion of these various points must remain largely speculative and thus are kept brief here. The degree to which a wave is attenuated over one round-trip of the arterial system is not at all precisely known and is the hinge of the argument. O'Rourke suggests that McDonald and Taylor (1959) when denying the possibility of resonance overestimated the amount of the attenuation, and underestimated the reflection coefficient. As seen above, the estimated reflection coefficient at the arteriolar bed of 75 per cent (O'Rourke and Taylor, 1966) is much higher than that calculated in 1959 which was taken as about 35 per cent. The damping estimated by Bergel (1961b) and by McDonald and Gessner (1968) are (as noted above) at least double that value which was assumed earlier from the calculations by Womersley (1955b), for the larger vessels. The effects due to the visco-elasticity of the wall will be considerably higher than this when the amount of muscle in the wall increases greatly.

The attenuation of the fundamental frequency along 40 cm of aorta due to the viscous dissipation of the blood is calculated as 10 per cent; allowing for the visco-elasticity in the wall the true value is about double this value, i.e. 20 per cent at least. Even assuming that it remains unchanged in the leg (and it increases rapidly with a decrease in radius) over the distance from the heart to the feet and back, which is normally 180–200 cm, the attenuation at the least will be close to 100 per cent and the possibility of a wave reflected from the feet returning to be reflected again in the terminal arteries of the forepart of the body is remote, for this calculation needs to assume a reflection of 100 per cent at the extreme ends of the arterial system.

Considering the reflections seen from the region of the pelvis (with a coefficient of 50 per cent approximately) the situation is somewhat more possible. A wave of c. 2 Hz of arbitrary amplitude 100 leaving the heart would be of amplitude 60 at the pelvis. (The amplification due to elastic taper is ignored for simplicity because it will be reversed in the reflected wave.) If 50 per cent is reflected there the returning wave will have an amplitude of 30, and of 18 when it reaches the arch of the aorta. If it was unchanged there, and if the attenuation in the fore-limb vessels is assumed to be no greater, at the termination of the vessels, approximately 30 cm distant, it would be only of amplitude 11, or approximately one-tenth of its initial amplitude. With incomplete reflection and a more realistic attenuation taken in the smaller vessels it can be seen that the possibility of a reflected wave surviving more than one return trip around the arterial system is very small, and hence the possibility of creating a resonance phenomenon such as a standing wave at such a low frequency. For example, in the fourth harmonic the attenuation will be more than double this value. This conclusion is consonant with the findings of Starr (1957) in human cadavers. He created a single transient wave in the aorta of an amplitude approximately the amplitude of the pulse wave. A reflected wave is just detectable at the arch but there is no sign of a secondary reflection.

The assumption is usually made that secondary reflection would occur at the heart. This was made by McDonald and Taylor (1959) on the analogy of the hydraulic models used with a mechanical pump which will create a 100 per cent reflection at the origin. The analogy appears realistic in that, during diastole, the aorta is closed by valves while, during systole, the contracting ventricle will present a firm closed end. This last term would be represented by the source impedance of the heart. Robinson (1965) came to the conclusion that this would be about six times higher than the input impedance of the aorta. This would give rise to a reflection coefficient of 5/7 or approximately 70 per cent. Further consideration by McDonald (1968b), however, suggested that the concept of the source impedance of the heart is a confused one and while it would be high at the time of opening of the valves it would fall rapidly to a very low value by the time that the ejection phase was ending.

Experimentally, I have studied dogs in which the arterial system was perfused by a heart-oxygenator by-pass pump. This maintains a steady pressure without pulsation imposed by the heart. By attaching a sinusoidal pump to the distal aorta it was possible to study the behaviour of centripetal waves in the region of the heart. No evidence of reflection in the region of the aortic arch could be found even although the valves were closed. This was attributed to the fact that the impedance presented by the large vessels arising from the arch together with the heart (in this case the valves were closed continuously) closely matched the impedance of the aorta. The possibility of an appreciable secondary reflection of waves in the region of the heart seems, therefore, to be excluded.

This reinforces the conclusions reached earlier by McDonald and Taylor (1959) and McDonald (1960). A search by McDonald and Taylor (1956) for a 'natural frequency', or resonance, in the arterial system at frequencies below 6 Hz had produced negative results. This investigation attached a sinusoidal pump to the proximal subclavian artery and superimposed oscillatory pressures of varying frequencies on the natural pulse wave. No evidence of a preferred amplification of any frequency was found. A further line of reasoning can be pursued from the time taken for a 'steady state' to be reached after a sudden disturbance.

Steady state oscillation was discussed briefly in Ch. 7 in relation to the validity of applying Fourier analysis to the arterial system. When an oscillatory pressure is first imposed on a system there is a transient response which decays; not until this has disappeared will each cycle be truly repetitive, i.e. in steady-state. Clamping of a large artery with its subsequent release will provide such a transient. It is found that on release the arterial system reaches a steady-state within one cardiac cycle—approximately 0·5 sec in the dog

(Fig. 7.9). This indicates a heavily damped system. And as the period is of the order of the time it takes a pressure wave to make a round-trip of the whole system it further reinforces the conclusion that, while reflected waves play a significant role on their first centripetal travel, they do not persist longer than this.

13
Arterial Impedance

As its name implies, the term 'impedance' is the measure of the opposition to flow presented by a system. By conventional use in physics, and in its most familiar form in the terminology of electric current theory, the term is confined to oscillatory motions or alternating current. Thus usage is not confined to electrical current but is also used as 'mechanical impedance' in vibrating solid systems and as 'acoustic impedance' in gas-filled systems. Etymologically, the term resistance conveys the same sense as impedance but is, by conventional definition, confined to non-oscillatory, or steady, motions. Resistance may thus be considered as the impedance at zero frequency.

The use of the concept of impedance in the study of pulsatile liquid flows in relation to the pressure-gradient was apparently first made by Womersley in 1955 when he drew attention to the way in which the ratio of the pulsatile flow determined by his equations to the oscillatory pressure-gradient could be written in real and imaginary parts (Ch. 6). Recapitulating briefly we write, by analogy with the equation for electrical impedance,

$$Z = R + i\omega L \qquad\qquad \textbf{6.18}$$

in a circuit of resistance R and inductance, L, then R can represent the fluid resistance and L can represent the inertia of the liquid. In Ch. 6 we derived the components in terms of linear velocity (see page 143). Expressed for volume flow these become

Fluid resistance

$$(R) = \frac{\mu\alpha^2}{\pi R^4 M'_{10}} \sin \varepsilon_{10} \qquad\qquad \textbf{6.19}$$

or (expanding α)

$$(R) = \frac{\omega\rho}{\pi R^2 M'_{10}} \cdot \sin \varepsilon_{10} \qquad\qquad \textbf{6.21}$$

and fluid reactance

$$(\omega L) = \frac{\mu\alpha^2}{\pi R^4 M'_{10}} \cdot \cos \varepsilon_{10} \qquad\qquad \textbf{6.20}$$

351

or

$$\omega L = \frac{\omega \rho}{\pi R^2 M'_{10}} \cdot \cos \varepsilon_{10} \qquad \textbf{6.22}$$

Hence the fluid inductance

$$(L) = \frac{\rho}{\pi R^2 M'_{10}} \cdot \cos \varepsilon_{10} \qquad \textbf{6.23}$$

The variations of the terms R and L with α are illustrated in Fig. 6.13. The complex impedance

$$Z = \frac{i\omega\rho}{\pi R^2 M'_{10}} e^{-i\varepsilon_{10}} \qquad \textbf{6.16}$$

is the impedance per unit length of the pipe with an oscillatory flow of angular frequency ω, because the pressure term used was the pressure change over 1 unit (the pressure-gradient). It is termed the *Longitudinal Impedance*.

When we are considering a conducting system (i.e. an elastic pipe) of some length the ratio of the oscillatory pressure and the oscillatory flow is termed the *Characteristic Impedance* if only centrifugal flow waves are present at the origin, i.e. if no reflected waves are present, or, if created at the termination of the system, the system is of such a length that they are completely attenuated before they can return to the origin.

The relation of the characteristic impedance Z_0 to the longitudinal impedance Z is, by analogy with transmission line theory, expressed as

$$Z_0 = Zc/i\omega \qquad \textbf{6.24}$$

so that we obtain

$$Z_0 = \frac{\rho c}{\pi R^2 M'_{10}} \cdot e^{-i\varepsilon_{10}} \qquad \textbf{6.25}$$

where c is the complex wave velocity of Womersley's terminology (eqn. 11.16).

Assuming that, for an artery, we are considering a longitudinally constrained tube we substitute for c the form in eqn. 11.26, and we obtain

$$Z_0 = \frac{\rho c_0}{\pi R^2 \sqrt{(1 - \sigma^2)}} \cdot \frac{1}{(M'_{10})^{\frac{1}{2}}} \cdot e^{-i\varepsilon/2} \qquad \textbf{6.26}$$

where c_0 is the wave velocity given by the Moens-Korteweg equation (10.56).

The situation when there are reflected waves present has been considered in Ch. 12 and has been seen to be more complicated owing to the formation of nodes and antinodes. To distinguish the impedance at the origin modified by reflected waves from that due to the transmission properties of the artery alone (the characteristic impedance), we term this the *Input Impedance*.

The *input impedance* of any region of the circulatory system is thus the ratio in that region of the single harmonic term of the pressure at the input to that of the corresponding harmonic term of flow. Thus the ratio of the pressure and flow in the ascending aorta determines the input impedance of the arterial system as a whole. Similarly, the ratio measured in the femoral artery expresses the input impedance of the arterial bed supplied by that artery.

Expressing each complex harmonic term in modulus and phase form we thus need to express the input impedance as a set of terms of the values of the modulus and the phase at each frequency determined by the Fourier analysis. The modulus of the input impedance $|Z|$ is given by

$$|Z| = |P|/|Q|$$ **13.1**

and the phase, Z_{ph}, by

$$(Z)ph = P(\text{phase}) - Q(\text{phase})$$ **13.2**

The phase of the impedance will be negative when the flow leads the pressure and positive when pressure leads the flow.

A detailed review of the concepts of vascular impedance has recently been published by Gessner (1972).

VARIATIONS IN THE MODULUS AND PHASE OF THE INPUT IMPEDANCE

The simplest way to illustrate the relative variations in the modulus and phase of the input impedance is by the use of a simple hydraulic model. In Fig. 13.1A these two components are shown as measured at the origin of a single line of rubber tubing, filled with water, which is clamped at the far end. As shown in Fig. 12.5, the modulus is high at low frequencies but falls rapidly with increased frequency until it reaches a minimum when the length of the tube is one-quarter of a wave-length. It then rises to a maximum at double this frequency, when the tube is one-half of a wave-length and then falls to another minimum at three-quarters of a wave-length. This pattern is the same as the corresponding one of the nodes and antinodes of the pressure oscillation which was discussed in detail in Ch. 12.

The variations in the phase of the input impedance oscillate in a similar manner. At the lowest frequency measured the phase is markedly negative. With a pump capable of going down to extremely low frequencies this negative phase (or phase lead of flow) would increase to approximately 90° but would be reduced rapidly very close to zero frequency, for at zero frequency, i.e. steady flow, there is no phase difference.

With increase of frequency the negative phase increases rapidly and is approximately zero at the quarter wave-length situation. (More strictly

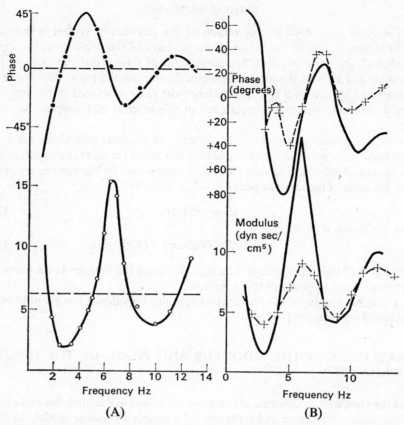

Fig. 13.1A. The modulus and the phase angle (in degrees) of the complex input impedance measured at the origin of a water-filled tube which was completely blocked at the distal end. The tube was attached at the origin to a pump with a sinusoidal output of variable frequency. The modulus shows a high value at low frequencies, falling rapidly to a minimum at c. 3 Hz. The horizontal dashed line represents the characteristic impedance of the tube, i.e. without any reflected waves returning from the distal end. The phase of the impedance is markedly negative at the lowest frequency but rapidly changes so that it is 0° at the frequency when the modulus is at a minimum (actually at the phase of the characteristic impedance—which is close to zero). When the modulus is equal to the characteristic impedance the phase is at a maximum positive value. At 6 Hz the modulus is at a maximum (the half wave-length frequency) and the modulus is again zero reducing to a minimum (negative value) when the modulus crosses the dashed line. This alternating pattern repeats as frequency increases but the swing between maximum and mimimum decreases progressively due to viscous attenuation.

B. The complex input impedance of a section of the same tube compared to that of a second model when a second tube of smaller bore and higher wave velocity (stiffer wall) was connected to the distal end. The modulus and phase of the larger tube, blocked at its distal end, are shown by the solid lines and are essentially the same as in Fig. A (the phase angle here is in the opposite sense, i.e. it is negative towards the top of the diagram). The changes in impedance due to the junction are shown by the dashed line. Whereas the completely blocked tube has a reflection coefficient (R_f) of 1·0 the junction has an $R_f = 0.6$ (calculated from eqns. 12.11 *et seq.*). The fluctuation of both modulus and phase is similar in sequence to those of the blocked tube but are smaller in amplitude (the phase angles are all shifted upwards a little because the phase of the characteristic impedance of the tubes is different). The frequencies at which maxima and minima of the phase occur is also shifted slightly because of the phase angle of the incomplete reflection coefficient. (The inflection of the phase of the dashed line at the lowest frequency is an artifact due to some remaining reflection from the far end of the distal tube.)

speaking it equals the phase of the characteristic impedance; in water-filled models, such as this, the value of α is initially about 10–12 at 2 Hz so that the phase of the characteristic impedance ($\varepsilon_{10}/2$) is initially about 4° and diminishes with increasing frequency so that it is only 1–2° at 14 Hz.) The phase thereafter becomes positive, reaching a maximum value where the modulus is that of the characteristic impedance, and again falls to zero at the frequency of the half wave-length antinode; it then swings to a negative minimum when the relative modulus is again one and is again zero when the three-quarter wave-length node is reached.

This pattern is followed when the incident and reflected pressure waves are in phase at the point of reflection, as in this case with reflection at a completely closed end. Creating a model with a single reflection point with a reflection coefficient less than 1·0 is rather more difficult. This experiment was also done by fusing the tube used in the experiment described above with a long length of a narrower tube with thicker walls. The characteristic wave-velocity of the proximal tube was approximately 14 m/sec while in the distal tube, which was smaller in bore, it was approximately 26 m/sec and so had a higher impedance. The second tube was of such a length that no reflections from its distal end returned to the site of the junction. (In this case the junction was made by sealing one tube inside the other with rubber solution; the use of a short, e.g. 2 cm, section of glass, or other rigid tubing, is, however, permissible because, although the first junction of elastic to rigid tube will cause a positive reflection this is virtually completely cancelled by the distal rigid tube to rubber connection which creates a corresponding negative reflection separated in time only by the transmission time through the short rigid section.)

The comparison of measurements made with the two models is shown in Fig. 13.1B. The variations in the amplitude of the modulus are smaller now that the reflection coefficient is only 0·6, but the nodes and antinodes occur at the same frequencies. The oscillations in phase are also reduced, though to a lesser degree, and again are close to the original pattern. The points of zero phase are, however, shifted slightly, which can be attributed to the fact that at a reflection coefficient of 0·6 the phase angle between incident and reflected wave, although small, will be measurably larger than zero.

RELATIONS OF PRESSURE AND FLOW WAVES IN VARIOUS PARTS OF THE ARTERIAL TREE

McDonald (1960) illustrated the simultaneous change in amplitude and form of the pressure and flow waves at five sites from the ascending aorta to the saphenous artery. At that time, however, it was necessary to draw on data from four different laboratories to provide the illustration. With the advent of multi-channel electromagnetic flowmeters in the last decade it has become possible to eliminate the uncertainties of comparing different experiments and techniques by doing simultaneous measurements at multiple sites on the same animal. Figure 13.2 illustrates five pressure and flow waves recorded in a dog in the ascending aorta, thoracic aorta, proximal and distal abdominal aorta and femoral artery. Flow is recorded as linear flow velocity to eliminate the factor that volume flow is reduced in smaller arteries because of the small cross-sectional area.

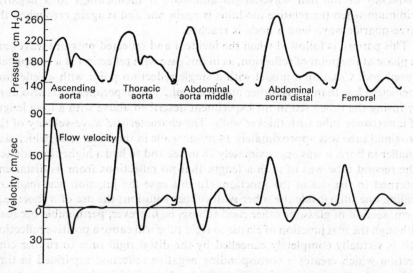

Fig. 13.2. The pressure pulses and the oscillatory flow velocity curves measured simultaneously at four sites in the aorta; the femoral pressure and flow curves are added from a different experiment but matched with corresponding aortic curves. It can be seen that the oscillation in pressure increases with distance from the heart but that the oscillation in flow velocity shows a progressive decrease. This is due to the increase in impedance with increasing distance from the heart as discussed in the text.

Purely by visual inspection it can be seen that while the overall pressure oscillation (discussed in Ch. 12) increases with travel away from the heart, the flow oscillation decreases markedly. There is thus a marked overall increase in impedance progressively towards the periphery. This is found equally in other arteries as shown by Fig. 13.3 where the pressure and flow are recorded simultaneously in the carotid artery, ascending aorta and superior mesenteric and femoral arteries. Figure 13.4 is the original 1960 diagram which shows the further marked drop in flow pulsation between the femoral artery and its saphenous branch (which are recorded simultaneously by the high-speed cinematographic technique). The extrapolations by broken lines in this last figure are based on the assumption that both pressure and flow are not oscillatory in the capillaries. While direct visual observation shows that normally capillary flow is virtually non-pulsatile, it cannot be stated categorically that this is true of the pressure. The extremely narrow bore of

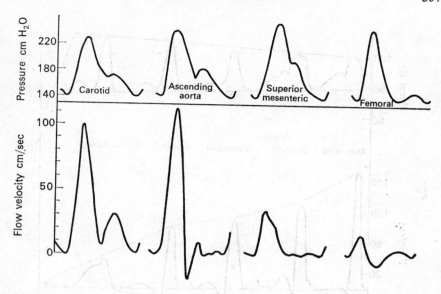

Fig. 13.3. The pressure pulses and oscillatory flow velocity curves measured simultaneously in carotid artery, ascending aorta, superior mesenteric and femoral arteries. As in Fig. 13.2 it can be seen that the pressure pulses increase with increasing distance from the heart while the flow velocity oscillation decreases. This is especially marked in the superior mesenteric and femoral arteries while the change in the carotid artery is quite small.

capillaries has prevented direct measurement of pressure with manometer systems of sufficiently good frequency response to record oscillatory pressures; allowing for the very high impedance of the capillary bed it is conceivable that there remains an appreciable pressure oscillation without a measurable flow oscillation. Considerable pressure oscillations have been measured in arterioles (Rappaport *et al.*, 1959; Wiederhielm *et al.*, 1964) and microscopy shows pulsatile flow in this region. With arteriolar vasodilatation the flow in the systemic capillaries also shows pulsatile variation. Flow and pressure in the lower resistance capillaries of the lung is normally pulsatile; Caro and McDonald (1961) estimated that approximately 25 per cent of the arterial pressure oscillation may be transmitted through the capillaries of the lung.

The moduli of the impedances calculated from the pressure and flow curves illustrated in Fig. 13.2 are shown in Fig. 13.5. The units of the impedance are here (and in Fig. 13.6) shown in terms of linear flow velocity (dyn sec/cm³) to eliminate the effect of taking the volume flow in a single vessel and hence the velocity characterizes the impedance of all vessels of that order of branching. An earlier estimate of the impedance at three different sites calculated from simultaneous pressure measurements and apparent phase velocity is given in Fig. 13.6 and shows similar impedance modulus patterns. (The relation

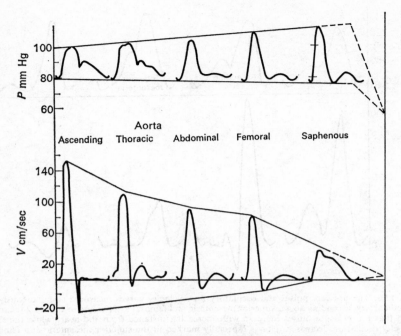

Fig. 13.4. A diagrammatic comparison of the behaviour of the pressure and flow velocity pulses from the ascending aorta until the saphenous artery. As far as that point the oscillatory pressure is greatly increasing, and is about twice the oscillation in the ascending aorta. Thereafter it begins to decrease (see Figs. 12.16 and 12.17) and this is indicated by the broken lines. The flow oscillations diminish with increasing distance from the origin of the aorta; the continuing decrease until steady flow is achieved in the microcirculation is again indicated by broken lines.

As noted before this disparate behaviour of the pressure and flow curves indicates that the impedance, or ratio of pressure/flow oscillation, is increasing.

between the apparent wave velocity and the modulus of impedance is discussed below.)

From these diagrams we see that the variations of the modulus of the impedance with frequency indicate that in peripheral situations such as the femoral and saphenous arteries the effects of reflection are very marked. By contrast, the effects of reflection in more central regions such as the thoracic aorta are greatly reduced due to the attenuation of reflected waves arising from peripheral terminations. Similar conclusions were drawn from the detailed analysis of the travelling pressure wave made in Ch. 12. In the ascending aorta there is very little change in the amplitude of the impedance at frequencies above 2 Hz; while this is in large part due to the effects of attenuation of reflected waves it is also probable from the analysis of the behaviour of pressure waves and of the impedance that an interaction between pressure waves from the fore- and hind-parts of the systemic system make this a special case. This is discussed in detail below as the input impedance of the whole

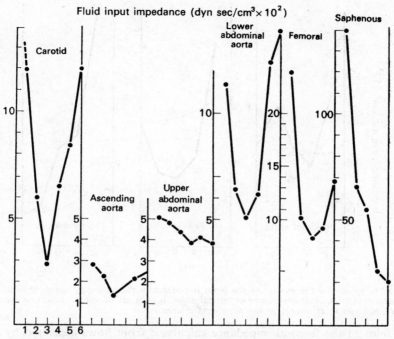

Fig. 13.5. Values for the moduli of the input impedance at the vascular sites of which the flow and pressure pulses are illustrated in Fig. 13.2 (the carotid artery impedance has been calculated from the curves in Fig. 13.3). The first six harmonics are shown for the first four curves and five harmonics for the last two.

It can be seen that in the more peripheral arteries the impedance shows a very marked minimum due to the increased effect of reflections and the general value of the impedance is greatly increased. The ascending and thoracic aorta curves, by contrast, are much lower in value and do not show much influence of reflected waves.

system is of particular importance in considering the pulsatile work load on the heart.

The input impedance of the femoral artery

The impedance of the femoral artery may be taken as typical of peripheral branch arteries because it has been studied in far more detail than any other.

The first published data on the impedance of the femoral artery were those of Randall and Stacy (1956). While this paper is of importance in appreciating the value of the concept of impedance the actual results are dubious because of the nature of the flowmeter. This was a cannulating electromagnetic flowmeter but it was connected to the artery by two 15 cm lengths of polyethylene tubing. This produced great damping of the pulsatile flow and the impedance they measured was, in effect, the impedance of the bed plus a length of plastic tubing. McDonald and Taylor (1959) presented data on the

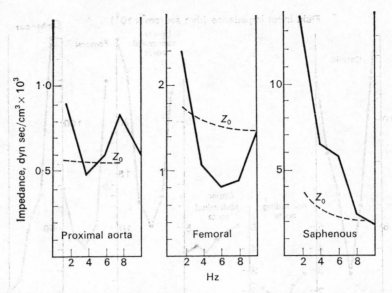

Fig. 13.6. Values for the moduli of the input impedance in the ascending aorta, femoral and saphenous arteries. Note the change in vertical scale in each set of values indicating that the impedance gets much higher in the peripheral arteries.

modulus of the femoral impedance calculated from flows measured by the high-speed cinematograph technique (Fig. 13.7). This showed a well-marked minimum at 13·5 Hz and could be attributed to a 'mean' position of the termination of the bed somewhere between the ankle and the knee. McDonald (1960) also showed data on the changes in impedance with vasoconstriction and vasodilatation. With arteriolar constriction the impedance at the lower frequencies was increased but the fall to the minimum was steeper and the impedance value at the minimum was lower than the 'normal' value. This is the expected behaviour with a marked increase in the reflection coefficient. Conversely, vasodilatation reduced the low frequency values and increased the values around the minimum, thus creating a much flatter curve.

In later (unpublished) data McDonald measured both the modulus and phase of the femoral impedance. The flows here were derived by measuring the pressure-gradient in the proximal femoral artery and using the Womersley equation (6.4). Two runs from this series are illustrated under 'normal' conditions in Fig. 13.8. It can be seen that there is a discrepancy in the modulus in the high harmonics but this is a common finding and is attributable to the measurement errors in these components of small magnitude; in this case, the two phase plots are essentially the same although the phase, being the arctan of the ratio between the small sine and cosine components (Ch. 7), is usually more sensitive to random error of this type.

The modulus shows the same pattern as that seen in Fig. 13.7, being high

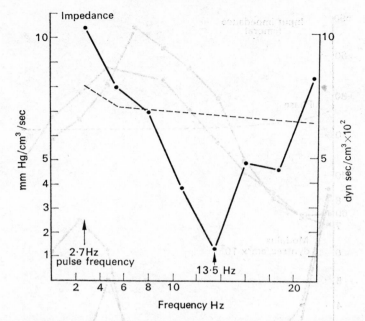

Fig. 13.7. The modulus of the input impedance of the first eight harmonics recorded in the dog femoral artery—full line. The characteristic impedance of the femoral artery is also shown—broken line. The pressure and flow curves from which this curve is calculated is shown as Fig. 6.1.

The pulse frequency in this animal was 2·7 Hz and there is a minimum of impedance at the 5th harmonic—13·5 Hz. One quarter wave-length at this frequency is about 15 cm and, as discussed in the text, the graph indicates that the main site of reflections is at this distance from the point of observation.

Ordinate—input impedance; scale on left in mm Hg sec/cm³; scale on right dyn sec/cm³, i.e. impedance calculated in terms of linear velocity of flow.

at the lowest frequency and falling to a minimum at the fifth harmonic (approximately 12 Hz) and rising to a second maximum representing the half wave-length frequency at the tenth harmonic. The analysis to 12 harmonics is thus able to demonstrate that the rise in amplitude up to the eighth harmonic in Fig. 13.7 is, in fact, approaching an antinodal value. The phase behaves as predicted by Fig. 13.1 and is initially negative and rises to the phase of the characteristic impedance at the frequency where the modulus is at a nodal minimum. It then becomes positive mid-way between the nodal and anti-nodal frequencies and again crosses the characteristic impedance at the tenth harmonic. As this also occurs in the curve where the maximum in the modulus looks dubious the behaviour of the phase confirms that an antinode is in fact occurring at this point.

The input impedance of the femoral bed has also been measured by Gabe (1965*a*) in the human. He also derived flows from the pressure-gradient measured through a double-lumen catheter inserted into the superficial femoral artery but measuring pressures in the external iliac artery. The

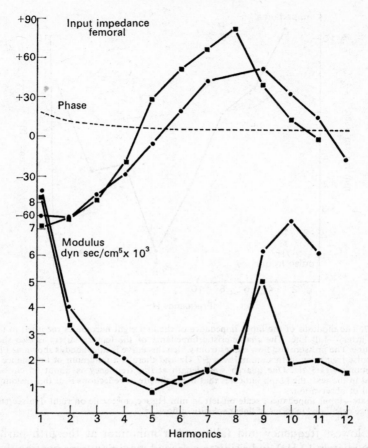

Fig. 13.8. The modulus and phase of the impedance of the dog femoral artery. The two curves in the lower half of the illustration record the modulus measured in two separate cardiac cycles and the two plots in the upper half represent the phase angle of the impedance in the same cycles.

Ordinate: for *phase* degrees—the broken line represents the phase of the characteristic impedance; for modulus the ordinate is dyn sec/cm⁵. Abscissa—order of harmonics; the pulse frequency was 2·4 Hz so that, for example, the fifth harmonic was 12 Hz and the 10th harmonic 24 Hz.

It will be seen that the modulus starts at a high value and then falls to a minimum between the 5th and 7th harmonics and then rises to a new maximum. The impedance phase is initially about −60° and increases rapidly until it crosses the characteristic impedance where the modulus is at a minimum. This, as is seen in Figs. 13.1 and 13.2, confirms that this minimum represents a quarter wave-length frequency. The phase then increases to a maximum and falls again to the line of the characteristic impedance when the modulus in one curve is at a maximum. This indicates that this represents a half wave-length maximum at double the frequency of the quarter wave-length situation.

pattern has a general similarity to that of Fig. 13.8 (see McDonald, 1964), and the differences may be largely attributed to the technical difficulty of measuring a pressure-gradient accurately with a double-lumen catheter and the manometers available in England in the early 1960s.

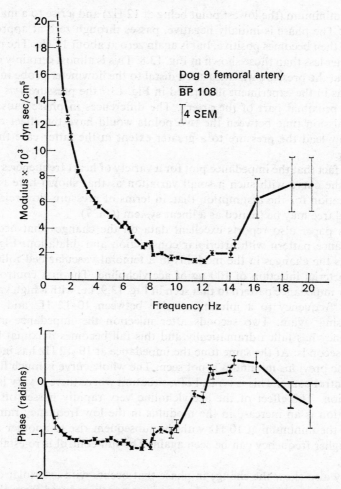

Fig. 13.9. The modulus and phase of the femoral impedance of the dog. This represents the pooled data from 57 cycles in a dog with heart block whose heart was being paced at different frequencies. The pattern to be seen is very similar to that shown in Fig. 13.8. The modulus is very high at the lowest frequency and falls to a minimum between 10 and 14 Hz; at the same frequency the phase, which initially is negative, approximates to zero. This indicates a quarter wave-length frequency range. The modulus then rises while the phase goes to positive maximum and then falls to zero again at about 18 Hz, indicating the half wave-length maximum frequency. (Redrawn from O'Rourke and Taylor, 1966.)

The most detailed study of the input impedance of the femoral bed has been that of O'Rourke and Taylor (1966). They used an electromagnetic flowmeter and the results were analysed by a digital computer. A composite set of values measured in a dog, in which heart-block was induced and a variety of heart-rates imposed by electrical pacing, is shown in Fig. 13.9. This shows again a high value for the modulus of the impedance at the lowest frequencies with a broad minimum (the lowest point being at 12 Hz) and a rise to a maximum at 20 Hz. The phase is initially negative, passes through zero at approximately 12 Hz, then becomes positive, but is again zero at about 18 Hz. The phases are all rather less than those shown in Fig. 13.8. This is almost certainly due to the fact that the pressure was measured distal to the flowmeter probe in this case, whereas in the experiment illustrated in Fig. 13.7 the pressure was measured in the proximal part of the artery. The differences in phase caused by the transmission time between the two points would have the effect of making the flow lead the pressure to a greater extent in the latter case than in the former.

The fact that the impedance plot for a variety of heart frequencies all fall on the same curve with such a small variation as that shown here is a strong justification for the assumption that, in terms of pressure–flow relations, the arterial tree may be treated as a linear system (Ch. 7).

This paper also reports excellent data on the changes that occur in the impedance pattern with arteriolar constriction and dilatation. Figure 13.10 records the changes in the modulus in a femoral vascular bed following the intra-arterial injection of 100 μg of acetylcholine. The first control shows a similar impedance pattern to that seen in Fig. 13.9, i.e. with a high value at the lowest frequency to a minimum value between 10–12 Hz and thereafter increasing again. Two seconds after injection the impedance at the low frequency has fallen dramatically and this fall becomes maximal between 6 and 8 seconds. At the same time the impedance at 10–12 Hz has increased so that the previous minimum is not seen. The whole curve is much flatter than the control curve. This is typical of a situation where there is very little wave-reflection. The effect of the acetylcholine very rapidly passes off; the first indication is an increase in the modulus in the low frequency range but by 30 sec the minimum at 10 Hz with the subsequent rise to another maximum at a higher frequency can be seen again. The full control is re-established by 44 sec.

They also show the change in phase that occurs with arteriolar dilatation. The negative phase in the low frequency is greatly reduced from the normal value of -1.0 radian to about -0.25 radian and the most positive value at (14 Hz) but the crossover through zero phase remains between 8–10 Hz. With vasoconstriction there is an increase in the negative phase at low frequency but again the crossover through zero phase occurs at the same frequency and there is a tendency for the positive phases thereafter to be more positive than the control. The changes in vasoconstriction shown are, however, less than with vasodilatation.

By simulating these results on a computer model of the circulation (Taylor, 1966a) the reflection coefficient under control conditions at the arteriolar termination was estimated to be 0.8. During vasoconstriction this increased to 0.95 and during the extremes of vasodilatation fell apparently to zero. This

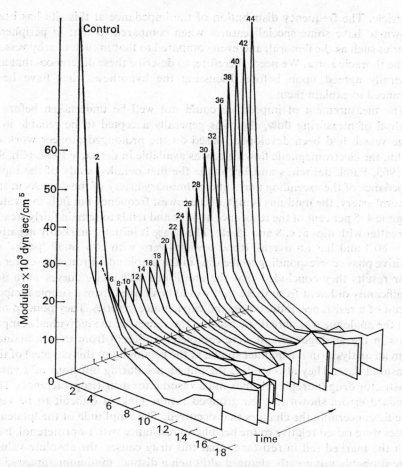

Fig. 13.10. The effect of vasodilatation on the modulus of the vascular impedance. This array of curves shows the time course of the impedance following the intra-arterial injection of 100 μg of acetylcholine. Each curve represents the modulus of one pair of pressure and flow curves and the time, in seconds, following injection is given above each curve. It can be seen that with vasodilatation the curve gets very much flatter largely owing to the dramatic fall in impedance at the lowest frequencies; this effect is maximal at 6–10 sec. As the transient vasodilatation passes off the impedance curve returns to its control form. (From O'Rourke and Taylor, 1966.)

indicates that considerably higher values are possible than had been considered probable in earlier attempts to estimate the reflection coefficient. In view of the quality and detail of this work this is clearly a much better estimate of this parameter than has been made before.

The input impedance in the proximal aorta

It has been noted above that the input impedance measured in the ascending aorta is of especial interest in that it indicates the output load on the left ventricle. The frequency distribution of the impedance at this site has been shown to have some special features when compared to that in peripheral arteries such as the femoral, and even compared to that in such nearby vessels as the thoracic aorta. We need, therefore, to describe these differences that are generally agreed upon before discussing the hypotheses that have been advanced to explain them.

The measurement of impedance could not well be undertaken before a method of measuring flow, that was generally accepted to be reliable in a large vessel, had been developed. Based on the prolonged pioneer work of Kolin, the electromagnetic flowmeter was available in the early 1960s (Ch. 9). In 1963, Patel, deFreitas and Fry made the first detailed study of the input impedance of the ascending aorta and pulmonary artery of the dog. As in the femoral artery, the modulus is high at the lowest frequency but falls to a value of some 4–5 per cent of the resistance at 4 Hz and tends to remain fairly steady thereafter with dips at c. 8 and 18 Hz. The phase is initially markedly negative (c. $-80°$) and has an overall trend towards zero with two small 'peaks' of positive phase corresponding to the dips in the amplitude. From the scatter in their results they concluded that the amplitude and phase curves were not significantly different from those that would be derived from a simple lumped circuit of a resistance, inductance, and capacitance in series. They pointed out that the analogue was unrealistic because the values for the individual components in the analogue circuit were completely different from those obtained from an analysis (in the manner shown at the beginning of this chapter) of the measured data. They also studied the impedance during infusions of a vaso-constrictor drug (norepinephrine) and a vasodilator drug (isoproterenol). The standard errors shown in their grouped results make it difficult to be very specific concerning the changes that occurred. The amplitude of the 'plateau' values were raised relative to the peripheral resistance with isoproterenol, but, with the marked fall in resistance that this drug causes, the absolute values were probably not greatly changed although a distinct minimum appeared at 5 Hz. The phase, throughout the frequency range studied, was negative, but showed little variation. Norepinephrine created a shallow minimum at 4–5 Hz and another one, of lower value, at approximately 12 Hz but the intervening values had a large standard error. The changes with altered peripheral arteriolar activity are neither marked in degree nor clear-cut in definition.

This paper was followed by a study of impedance measurements in man (Patel et al., 1965). The study was conducted in 3 patients undergoing cardiac surgery, so that it was possible to apply a flow probe to the aorta. The distribution of the moduli was essentially the same as those found in the dog. The phases showed more irregularity and several of the points were regarded as unreliable in that they were within the noise level of the recording system.

Another study of the aortic impedance in man was made by Gabe, Karnell, Porjé and Rudewald (1964). Their three patients were not undergoing surgery so that they derived the aortic flow, using the Womersley equation (6.4), from the pressure-gradient measured through a double lumen catheter; this approach had been previously used by Bergel, McDonald and Taylor (1958) in the femoral artery of the dog and has the advantage that it can be used when surgical placement of an electromagnetic flow probe is not possible (at a time when no intravascular devices were available). The subjects were studied before, and during, the infusion of nor-adrenaline. The fundamental cardiac frequency was approximately 1·0 Hz in all cases and, before giving nor-adrenaline, the modulus of the impedance was fairly constant at a value of some 8–10 per cent of the peripheral resistance; the phase was − 60° at the fundamental frequency and increased to some − 10–15° on the third or fourth harmonics and thereafter showed no consistent change. During nor-adrenaline infusion they recorded a marked increase in modulus in the fundamental, falling progressively to the control value between 4–8 Hz and thereafter rising again. This differs from most other reports that have not shown marked changes with vasoactive drugs. The phase of the impedance showed no consistent change during this procedure.

Further studies of impedance in dogs were reported by Attinger et al. (1966, 1967), Noble, Gabe, Trenchard and Guz (1967, in conscious dogs with an implanted probe) and by O'Rourke and Taylor (1967). Later studies were also done in this laboratory by Nichols and McDonald (1973). With regard to the modulus all found a pattern which was essentially similar to that initially reported by Patel et al. (1963). The modulus was relatively high at frequencies below 2 Hz but thereafter tended to remain between 5–10 per cent of the peripheral resistance. Attinger et al. (1967) give a clearer exposition of essentially similar data reported earlier by Attinger et al. (1966). In no cases were there heart rates appreciable below 2 Hz. A typical summary of this type of finding is shown in Fig. 13.11. Noble et al. (1967) compared the impedance in conscious dogs and changed the heart rate by pacing them at four different rates between 158 and 250 beats/min. Neither the modulus nor the phase was significantly altered at any given frequency even though it constitutes a different term in the Fourier series. This again provides evidence that, in terms of pressure and flow relations, the arterial tree behaves as an essentially linear system. Changing the force of contraction of the heart by an intra-coronary injection of calcium gluconate also did not alter the input impedance.

A somewhat larger series of experiments was done by (unpublished) Nichols and McDonald and these are shown in Fig. 13.13. In Fig. 13.12 we find an essentially similar situation to that shown in Fig. 13.11. The heart rate of this group of animals was over a wider range, including some of the effects of vagal stimulation. Again, the fact that there is very little scatter in the points around the line shows that the arterial tree is behaving in a linear manner. In all these cases, we also find that at 2 Hz the phase is markedly negative but

N

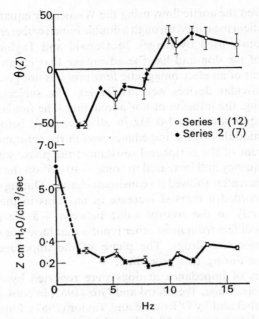

Fig. 13.11. The modulus and phase of the input impedance measured in the ascending aorta. The modulus is shown in the lower part of the figure and the phase is shown, in degrees, in the upper part of the figure. At zero frequency the modulus of the impedance is the peripheral resistance and it falls rapidly to the impedance at 2 Hz. Thereafter, it changes little with increasing frequency. The phase at 2 Hz is about $-50°$ and increases with frequency until it is zero at 7–8 Hz; thereafter, it attains a plateau at about $+25°$. If it were possible to measure pressure and flow at identical points this plateau would be approximately $0°$ (the present discrepancy is largely due to the transmission time between the point of measuring pressure proximal to the flow probe and the centre of the probe itself). (From Attinger *et al.*, 1967.)

increases to zero in the range 4–6 Hz and thereafter increases more slowly. This is similar to the results shown in Fig. 13.11 and in all these three investigations the pressure measurement used was proximal to the flow probe and the transmission time between this point and the middle of the flow probe would give a positive bias to the phase recorded. The magnitude of this effect is discussed below.

The study of aortic impedance by O'Rourke and Taylor (1967) is more detailed in terms of the number of points of the frequency plot. While the previous papers discussed used a standard Fourier analysis of single cardiac cycles, O'Rourke and Taylor used the method of random excitation of the heart to obtain a frequency spectrum from a sequence of pulses over a period of 20–24 sec. This method, described by Taylor (1966*b*, see Ch. 7, p. 166), enabled them to explore the range between 0·25 and 25·0 Hz. They were also concerned with interpreting the pattern in terms of reflections from the arteriolar terminations in the fore- and hind-parts of the body. The typical modulus pattern they describe was high at the lowest frequencies and fell to a mini-

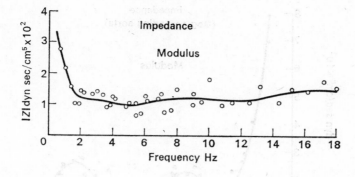

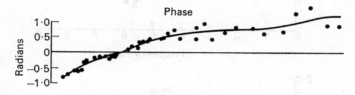

Fig. 13.12. The modulus and phase of the input impedance in the ascending aorta of a set of dogs with differing heart rates, including some slowed by vagal stimulation. As in Fig. 13.11, it can be seen that above 2 Hz (cps) there is very little change in the amplitude of the modulus of the impedance. The phase is initially markedly negative at approximately $-1 \cdot 0$ radian but increases to zero at 4–5 Hz and thereafter the rate of increase is reduced until we get a plateau form at a value of approximately $+1 \cdot 0$ radian. (From Nichols, 1970.)

mum at c. 2 Hz and then rose slightly to a maximum and fell again to a second minimum at 4–5 Hz and thereafter remained relatively constant (Fig. 13.14). Figure 13.15 shows a similar pattern and both are similar to Fig. 13.13. They pointed out that at a region where a single reflecting site dominates the pattern (as in the thoracic aorta, Fig. 13.17), the frequency at which the second minimum is seen would be a maximum (half wave-length impedance). They considered, therefore, that the second minimum represented the quarter wave-length minimum of the reflection effects from the shorter arterial system of the fore-part of the body. A plot of the calculated values of impedance in a model consisting of a T-tube with one limb half the length of the other is shown below (Fig. 13.18) and demonstrates this effect. In other impedance plots (Fig. 13.16) this sequence of two minimums with an intervening maximum is, however, barely seen and the relative constancy of amplitude at frequencies above 2 Hz is similar to that seen in earlier figures. These two slightly differing patterns were also seen in the results of Nichols and McDonald (Figs. 13.12 and 13.13). The phase pattern differs from the ones previously discussed in that it remained negative, or virtually so, throughout the frequency range. The pressure in these experiments was measured on the distal (downstream) side of the flow probe and is probably the main reason

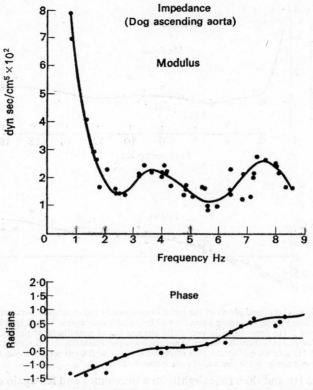

Fig. 13.13. A similar set of ascending aorta impedance plots to those shown in Fig. 13.12. This group has been extracted because they show a distinct modulus minimum at 2 Hz and again at about 6 Hz. For greater detail the frequency scan has been cut short at 9 Hz but the modulus from there out to 20 Hz is flat and shows no further fluctuation with frequency. The presence of the two minima is attributed to the separate reflection effects from the fore-part and hind-part of the arterial tree. This is discussed further in the text. (Nichols and McDonald, unpublished.)

for the discrepancy between the findings reported by the various groups discussed here; there was, however, considerable variation in the phase patterns recorded in different experiments. A rise in mean arterial pressure or the infusion of norepinephrine caused a shift of the curve to the right. Vasodilator drugs decreased the steepness of the curve at low frequencies but produced no significant change in the higher frequency part of the curve. A set of control values in the thoracic aorta is shown in Fig. 13.17, for comparison with those in the ascending aorta. The effects of halothane, phenylephrine and trimetaphan on the aortic input impedance was recently reported by Gersh *et al.* (1972). They found that halothane administration had no consistent effects on the input impedance, phenylephrine markedly increased the mean term, but had little effect on the oscillatory component of the impedance; and trimetaphan markedly decreased the mean term, but

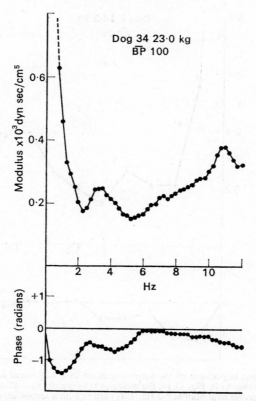

Fig. 13.14. The input impedance of the ascending aorta in the dog analysed by spectral analysis of a long series of waves when the heart was beating irregularly. The peripheral resistance was $7 \cdot 71 \times 10^3$ dyn sec/cm^5 at zero frequency and it can be seen that it falls rapidly to a value of about $0 \cdot 2 \times 10^3$ dyn sec/cm^5 at 2 Hz then rises to a hump and falls to a second minimum at 5 Hz. After this it climbs somewhat to 10 Hz and the remainder of the curve up to 20 Hz (not shown in the graph); it remained flat at about $0 \cdot 34 \times 10^3$ dyn sec/cm^5 which was taken to be the characteristic impedance. The phase angle is about $- 1 \cdot 4$ radians at $1 \cdot 0$ Hz and thereafter increases but never becomes positive; the progression shows an oscillation at the frequencies of the 2 minima.

With this type of pattern it is postulated that the first minimum represents the quarter wave-length frequency of the reflecting sites of the hind-part of the arterial tree while the second minimum, at roughly double the frequency, represents the quarter wave-length frequency of the shorter fore-part of the body. With only one reflecting site the double frequency would represent a half wave-length and there would be a maximum. This pattern is to be compared with that in Fig. 13.13. (Redrawn from Fig. 1 of O'Rourke and Taylor, 1967.)

caused a moderate increase in the oscillatory component of the impedance.

As noted above, the findings of Nichols and McDonald were substantially the same as those of previous workers. Figures 13.12 and 13.13 show two sets of data from Fourier analysis of a series of single cycles selected at varying heart rates in individual dogs; slowing of the heart rate was due to vagal stimulation and increase in rate due to electric pacing. The scatter was more pronounced in the small amplitude, higher frequency components but

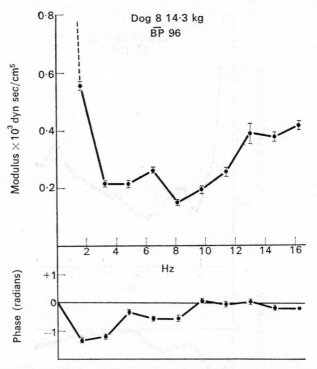

Fig. 13.15. The input impedance of the ascending aorta in a dog based on the analysis of 25 successive pulse waves. As in Fig. 13.14, the modulus falls rapidly to a minimum around 4·0 Hz and then forms a second minimum at 8·0 Hz. This pattern with a second minimum at a frequency about double that of the first one is also seen in Fig. 13.13 and appears to be one of the two standard patterns seen in the ascending aorta.

The phase pattern is similar to that seen in Fig. 13.14 but in this case is very close to zero above 10 Hz. As the impedance is representing the characteristic impedance at those frequencies the phase angle should be virtually zero. In all O'Rourke and Taylor's figures the pressure is measured slightly downstream from the flow so that the transmission time bias will be in the direction of a negative phase angle. (Redrawn from O'Rourke and Taylor, 1967.)

the overall scatter is small. Remarkably, the scatter is less in the phase than in the modulus data. As noted above, the modulus distribution is similar to that found by O'Rourke and Taylor in that in some two distinct minima with an intervening maximum may be seen (Figs. 13.13, 13.14 and 13.15) while a commoner finding is that there is little change in amplitude above 2 Hz (Fig. 13.12). The phase is between −1·0 and −1·15 radians below 1·0 Hz and comes close to zero or crosses it at 4–5 Hz and ultimately reaches a value of +0·5–1·0 Hz.

The component of the phase of the impedance that is due to transmission time between the points at which the flow and the pressure are measured has been estimated and the modified value of the phase is shown in Figs. 13.19 with a broken line. In all experiments two pressure measurements were made

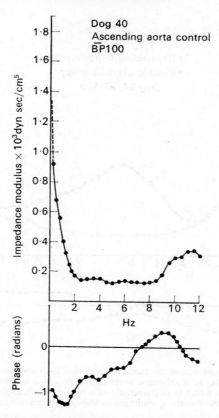

Fig. 13.16. The input impedance of the ascending aorta of a dog derived from a spectral analysis of a period about 20 sec long when the heart was beating irregularly. The modulus plot is different from those in the previous three figures in that it falls from a high value to a low value at 2 Hz and then remains at virtually this value until 9 Hz when it climbs slightly. This flat pattern is the second of the characteristic ways in which the modulus of the aortic impedance behaves and is similar to that seen in Fig. 13.12. (Part of Fig. 6, O'Rourke and Taylor, 1967.)

and the phase-velocity calculated for each harmonic (Nichols and McDonald, 1972). (The phase-velocity was being used in a method for estimating stroke volume, see Ch. 15.) The flow was assumed to be the flow at the mid-point of the flow probe; the distance from the pressure-measuring point and the middle of the flow was usually 15–20 mm and the wave velocity c. 4·0 m/sec. The transmission time would thus appear to be trivial but, in terms of phase angle, it constitutes quite a considerable correction.

INTERPRETATION OF THE AORTIC IMPEDANCE PATTERN

The impedance in the aorta is a measure of the opposition to flow that the ventricle has to overcome in pumping out blood. More properly, as O'Rourke

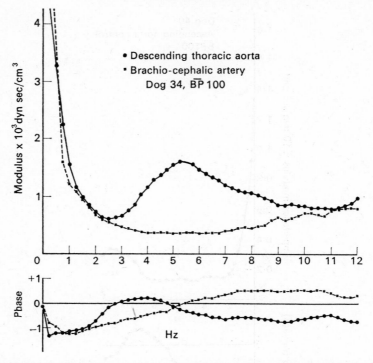

Fig. 13.17. The input impedance of the thoracic aorta (full line) and the brachiocephalic artery (broken line). The modulus of the thoracic aorta falls rapidly to a minimum at 2·5 Hz and rises to a maximum at 5·0 Hz which is characteristic of a pattern in which the reflected waves were arising from one site. This creates a minimum at the quarter wave-length frequency which is double the former.

The impedance of the brachiocephalic artery is similar to that of the thoracic aorta at low frequencies but once it has fallen to a low value at 3 Hz it remains virtually the same without oscillations thereafter. It will be noted that the impedance crosses the zero line for the thoracic aorta at both 2·5 and 5·0 Hz. As seen in Figs. 13.1A and 13.1B the phase should be zero when the modulus is either at a true minimum or a maximum. (Redrawn from Fig. 4, O'Rourke and Taylor, 1967.)

and Taylor have pointed out, the term to consider is that relating the pressure that is in phase with the flow; that is $|Z| \cos \varphi$. It is for this reason that the discussion above, of the true phase distribution with frequency, is of some importance. Calculated in this way O'Rourke and Taylor found that the in-phase impedance above 2 Hz is one-fiftieth, or less, of the peripheral resistance. The constancy of this value for frequencies above this value has the result that an increase in heart-rate will not carry a load penalty as it would if the impedance pattern showed the presence of marked minima and maxima such as that seen in the thoracic aorta (Fig. 13.17).

The contrast in patterns between that typical of the thoracic aorta and the one typical of the ascending aorta has been the subject of some speculation. It has already been seen (Ch. 12) that the influence of reflected waves, in

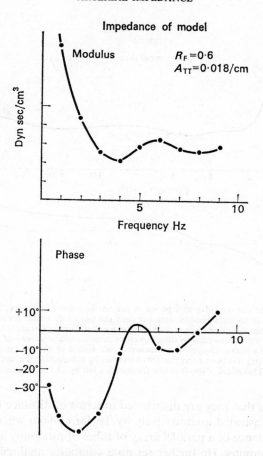

Fig. 13.18. The input impedance of a simple model representing the arterial tree. A short stub (the ascending aorta) connects to an asymmetric T-tube in which one limb is half the length of the other. This represents approximately the lengths of the fore-part and hind-parts of the arterial tree. The reflection coefficient at both ends is assumed to be the same and is taken as being 0·6.

It can be seen that the modulus falls to a minimum at 4·0 Hz, then rises and falls to a second minimum at 8 Hz. This is to be compared to impedance plots in Figs. 13.13, 13.14 and 13.15 when a similar pair of minima are to be seen. Likewise the phase angle is seen to cross the zero line twice as it does in Fig. 13.15. (Unpublished data of U. Gessner.)

terms of the relative amplitudes of the maxima and minima of pressure (Figs. 12.4 and 12.5) or impedance (Fig. 13.1), diminishes with greater distance from the periphery. This is due to the effects of wave-attenuation with travel. Nevertheless the contrast between the effects of reflection seen in the thoracic aorta and the ascending aorta is too marked to be attributed solely to this cause in the lower frequency terms. One factor that operates in smoothing the effects of the reflected waves from individual arteriolar beds (which, as O'Rourke and Taylor, 1966, pointed out, may have a reflection coefficient of

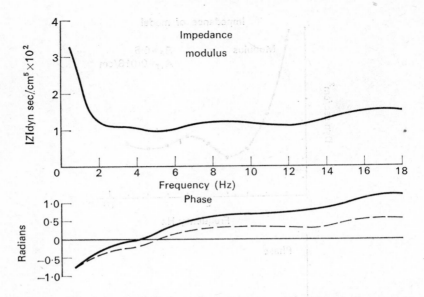

Fig. 13.19. A plot of the modulus and phase of the aortic input impedance. The portion of the impedance phase due to transmission time between the points at which pressure and flow were measured. In this case the pressure was measured at a point 2 cm upstream from the centre of the flow probe and the wave transmission time therefore causes a spurious lead of the pressure phase (positive phase). The wave-velocity was measured and found to be 400 cm/sec. The measured phase (unbroken line) has been corrected (broken line) by subtracting the angle representing the transmission time. This effect is small at low frequencies but by 18 Hz amounts to 0·63 radians.

0·8 or higher) is that they are distributed in terms of distance from the heart. This was demonstrated quantitatively by Taylor (1966*a*) when he calculated the input impedance of a parallel array of tubes of randomly assorted lengths on a digital computer. He further set up a computer analogue of the whole vascular tree as a branching assembly of tubes and showed that the input impedance pattern found in the ascending aorta could be simulated well by such a model. This was extended in a second paper (1966*b*) to include some properties of wave-transmission in peripheral arteries. These papers emphasized the importance of (a) the distributed nature of the terminal beds in minimizing or obliterating the formation of nodes and antinodes of impedance due to reflection and (b) the role of the non-uniform elastic properties of the arteries (Ch. 12) in keeping the input impedance in the aorta very low in comparison to the terminal impedance of the arterioles and capillaries.

Another factor that was not explicitly stated in these papers is created because the ascending aorta is a single tube feeding into two subdivisions of the arterial tree of unequal length; a short system supplying the head and fore-limbs and a longer system supplying the trunk and hind-limbs. McDonald (1965) considered this in very simplistic terms. From the anatomical diagram in Fig. 2.10, we may lump the branches of the two subdivisions of the system together and consider them as an 'eccentric T-tube' with the short arm, representing the ascending aorta, connecting it to an oscillatory pump, the heart. The lengths of the two limbs are such that the long one is approximately twice the length of the short one. This is also implicit in the finding of O'Rourke and Taylor (1967) that the minimum of impedance due to reflections from the fore-part of the body is twice the frequency of the minimum due to reflections from the hind-part of the body. At very low frequencies the input impedance will approach that of the terminal impedance because, in terms of wave-length, it is very close. At a frequency where the long limb is a quarter wave-length the origin will be at a node of impedance; the short limb, however, will only be one-eighth of a wave-length and will still be elevated. In the common trunk the impedance will be a mean of the high and low values. At double this frequency the long limb will be a half wave-length and its input impedance will be at an antinode while the short limb will be a quarter wave-length and its input impedance will be at a node; again the high and low values will cancel out. A plot of the modulus and phase of the impedance of such a simple model, calculated by Gessner, is shown in Fig. 13.18; Gessner extended this model in a series of studies to include the effects of wall-viscosity and elastic non-uniformity but the differences from this simple model is only a matter of degree. If the frequency is doubled again the antagonistic effects will disappear because the short limb is now a half wave-length and the long one a whole wave-length and both input impedances will be at an antinode; at this higher frequency, however, the effects of attenuation will become marked (as can be seen in the behaviour of the moduli of pressure displayed in Figs. 12.4 and 12.10) and the additive effect would be minimized. This concept of the 'competing' effect of reflections from the fore- and hind-parts of the body (McDonald, 1960) was independently conceived and tested by O'Rourke and Taylor (1967) by studying the changes in the input impedance of the aorta due to clamping the anterior branches of the arch of the aorta or the thoracic aorta. As might be expected, the findings in the arterial tree are less clear-cut than would be seen in the simple model but support the validity of the concept.

This account has been based on the considerable experimental evidence in the dog. It has always been assumed that the human circulation would behave in the same way, in the absence of any comparable surveys in man. A recent paper by Mills et al. (1970) has provided some evidence that the analogy that has been assumed is not so exact as has been thought. They used an intravascular electromagnetic flow probe (Mills and Shillingford, 1967) to study pressure and flow in a group of patients (Gabe et al., 1969—see Ch. 15) from which the input impedance has been calculated. This provides a far wider survey of flow patterns and impedances in one man than is available in the dog. A most interesting phenomenon that they observed is a 'hump' on the velocity curve in the innominate artery occurring in the later part of systole which is apparently travelling away from the heart because it arrives later in the right subclavian artery (Fig. 13.20). It can also be related to the inflexion

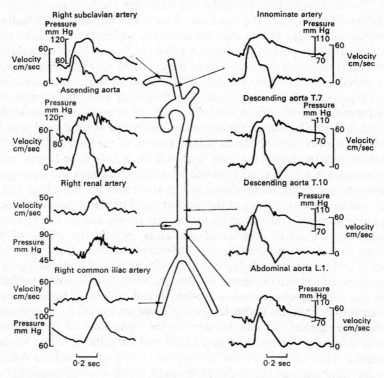

Fig. 13.20. Simultaneous pressures and blood velocity patterns recorded with a catheter-tip electromagnetic flowmeter at numerous points in the human arterial tree. (All were taken from one patient with the exception of the right renal artery and the right common iliac artery. (Redrawn from Mills *et al.*, 1970.)

that is commonly seen in the decelerating limb of the ascending aorta flow curve. The authors interpret this wave as one that has been reflected from the lower part of the body and returned to the arch of the aorta. This is supported by the finding that when the arterial pressure is lowered by a Valsalva manœuvre (in which the intrathoracic pressure is raised by a forcible attempt at expiration with a closed glottis) the arrival of the 'second' innominate wave is delayed into diastole; this is related to the reduction of wave-velocity due to the change in pressure and implies that this wave has travelled over the whole system. It is somewhat puzzling, however, that their velocity records do not show clear evidence of this wave in the distal aorta; in the presence of the marked attenuation that exists in the arterial system it would be much larger there and might be expected to cause more change in the systolic wave form than can be seen (and because we are considering the velocity of flow, the effect of a reflected volume of blood would diminish as it returned into vessels of larger cross-section).

The one important difference that the impedance graphs have, from those in the dog, is in the ascending aorta. After the initial fall to a lower level at 4–5 Hz there is a sharp rise at 7 Hz and then it falls again. The rise at one value in the higher harmonics is occasionally seen in any experimental determination in the dog but can be attributed to the potential errors in the ratio of small components of pressure and flow; in this series, however, it was seen repeatedly and so cannot be dismissed in this manner (although the statistical variation is not given). There is also some rise in the 7–10 Hz frequency range in the ascending aorta impedances calculated by Gabe *et al.* (1964). This peak thus would appear to be an anti-node although there is no clear minimum at 3–4 Hz that should represent the corresponding node. Again, it is puzzling that no sign of such an anti-node in the descending aorta; in the human ten harmonics only extends out to 10–11 Hz but the shift in frequency of such an antinode due to moving closer to the reflection site would not be expected to move it out of this range in the thoracic aorta.

The authors have discussed the evidence for their interpretation very persuasively and their main findings are beyond question. It would appear from this report that reflection from the lower part of the arterial system in the human is much greater relative to that of the upper (or anterior) part of the system than it is in the dog. In view of the fact that the normal posture in man is upright a difference of this kind is not altogether surprising and, as they point out, this modifies interpretations based on considering the effects of the eccentric position of the heart. This important paper also emphasizes the value of a flow-measuring device that can be easily moved into different regions of the arterial system.

As in more peripheral arteries the effects caused by reflected waves diminish with increasing frequency due to wave attenuation. The input impedance thus tends to become constant at the value of the characteristic impedance system. O'Rourke and Taylor (1967) specified this as the input impedance above 15 Hz (as the measurement errors in the small harmonic components tend to introduce scatter into these results a mean of values above 3–4 Hz will give virtually the same value for the modulus). The phase of the characteristic impedance has the value of $+\varepsilon_{10}/2$. At 15 Hz the value of the parameter α will be approximately 25–30 in the dog and the value of $\varepsilon_{10}/2$ will be about $1°$.

Theoretically then, it is to be expected that the phase of the input impedance should be very close to zero at the higher frequencies; the discussion of the published data shows that there is some uncertainty about this. The negative value of the impedance phase at low frequencies fits, with the elevated value of the modulus, the interpretation that the system at these frequencies is less than a quarter wave-length, and that there is a marked interaction with reflected waves. The fairly steady progression of the phase towards zero with increasing frequency accords with the concepts, outlined above, that the formation of nodes and antinodes is smoothed out by the interaction of reflected waves from various regions.

The effect of reflections in the ascending aorta are only seen, to any marked degree, then, at low frequencies and are already small at the normal resting frequency of the heart. Above this frequency there is little change in the amplitude, which is very low in terms of the magnitude of the steady-flow resistance. This low value is due to elastic non-uniformity (or 'taper') of the arterial tree which allows the heart to pump into distensible vessels and decouples it effectively from the peripheral resistance and its fluctuations. This concept was most explicitly set out by Taylor (1964) and is of the greatest value in understanding how the heart is able to adjust its rate of pumping and output without having to alter its work output dramatically. The apparent freedom from reflection effects is due to the distributed nature of the arteriolar terminations and, in particular, to the interaction of reflected waves from the asymmetrical lengths of the arterial tree anterior and posterior to the heart. This eccentric situation of the heart is so universal in land vertebrates (even in the snake the heart is located about 1/4 to 1/3 of the body-length from the head) that it is surprising that its evolutionary significance in giving flexibility to the functioning of the heart has not previously been considered.

The input impedance of the pulmonary artery

Measurement of the pulsatile flow in the pulmonary artery was made (in the cat) as early as 1951 by Baxter and Pierce using a Pitot-tube flowmeter but they did not calculate impedance (although this was done from their data by Caro and McDonald (1961) and the results shown to be consistent with their findings in the rabbit). Engelberg and DuBois (1959) derived values for the impedance of the pulmonary arterial bed of the rabbit from static measurements; the compliance of the whole bed was measured after embolizing the arterioles and the mass of the blood and the normal peripheral resistance were measured. Assuming that the system was so short that it could be treated as a lumped system they set up these values in a simple electrical analogue circuit consisting of an inductance (mass of the blood) and a capacitance (compliance) with the resistance connected in parallel across the capacitance. They derived values of 800 dyn sec/cm^5 at 1·0 Hz falling to a low minimum value of 8 dyn sec/cm^5 at 4·0 Hz and thereafter rising continuously with frequency (at 20 Hz it was c. 1000 dyn sec/cm^5).

The input impedance of the perfused pulmonary bed of the rabbit was studied by Caro and McDonald (1961) using a sinusoidal pump of variable frequency imposed on a steady flow. They found (Fig. 13.21) that there was a

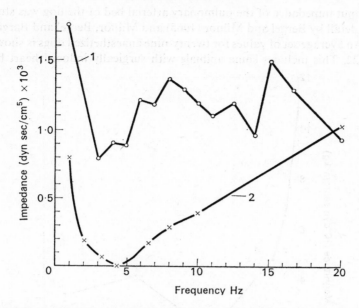

Fig. 13.21. The input impedance of the pulmonary artery of a rabbit. The upper line (with circles) represents the mean values of the modulus of the impedance measured in the perfused lungs using a sinusoidal pump. There is a minimum at 3–4 Hz followed by a rise to a maximum at 7–8 Hz followed by a fall to a second minimum at 14 Hz.

The lower line (with crosses) is a plot of the impedance of the pulmonary tree calculated by Engelberg and DuBois on the assumption that the whole system was so short that it could be taken as a lumped system. It can be seen that this curve shows a minimum also at 4 Hz but that the values are much lower than the actual impedance. Beyond the minimum the curve rises steadily without interruption. (From Caro and McDonald, 1961.)

minimum at 3–4 Hz rising to a maximum at 7–8 Hz and a further, less distinct, minimum around 16–17 Hz. While the first minimum was at approximately the same frequency as that predicted by Engelberg and DuBois its amplitude was much higher (800 as compared to 8 dyn sec/cm⁵). The phase of the impedance showed a lot of scatter and was only reported later (McDonald, 1964) but were fairly consistently negative to varying degrees.

The first adequate studies in the living animal (dog) were reported by Patel, deFreitas and Fry (1963) using a Kolin-type electromagnetic flow-meter. Their results for the modulus were similar to those of Caro and McDonald but the maximum at around 8 Hz was less distinct; their findings have been confirmed by later work. Infusion of norepinephrine made this maximum more distinct while the vasodilator drug, isoproterenol, made the amplitude fairly constant above 3 Hz. Their findings with regard to phase were initially negative (c. −30° at 2 Hz) and became increasingly negative throughout the frequency range; the finding of later work is that the phase pattern (as might be expected) is essentially the same as that in the ascending aorta and it is not easy to explain these earlier results.

The input impedance of the pulmonary arterial bed of the dog was studied
in more detail by Bergel and Milnor (1965) and Milnor, Bergel and Bargainer
(1966). An average set of values for twenty-nine anaesthetized dogs is shown in
Fig. 13.22. This includes some animals with surgically induced heart block

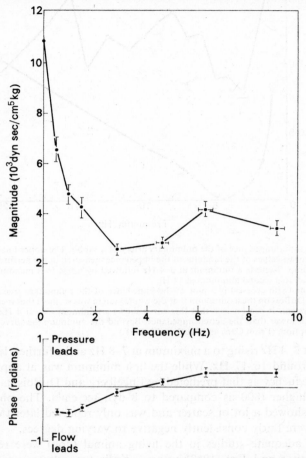

Fig. 13.22. Pulmonary vascular input impedance in anaesthetized, open-chest dogs. The points
represent mean values in 29 animals; the bars represent ±1 standard error of the mean. It can
be seen that the modulus falls to a minimum at 3 Hz and at about the same frequency the phase
crosses the zero-line indicating that this frequency represents the quarter wave-length situation.
At 6 Hz there is a slight maximum representing the half wave-length situation. (Redrawn from
Milnor *et al.*, 1966.)

and a pulse-frequency as low as 0·40 Hz (Milnor *et al.*, 1966). As in the
ascending aorta the impedance modulus tends towards the peripheral resistance at the lowest frequencies and falls to a minimum at 3 Hz but then climbs
to a low maximum around 6 Hz and thereafter falls. The phase is initially
−0·5 radians and increases with frequency, becoming zero between 3 and 4

Hz and levels off at c. $+0.25$ radians above 6 Hz. By pacing hearts with surgical heart block they demonstrated that the value of the impedance at any frequency was independent of the heart rate, i.e. it behaved as a linear system. Infusion of serotonin shifted the curve to the right and this increase of the frequency at the minimum was attributed (Bergel and Milnor, 1965) to the increase in smooth-muscle tone causing an increase in wave velocity (Bargainer, 1967) and so, in essence, shortening of the system in terms of wavelength.

The main difference between this pulmonary impedance pattern and that seen in the asecnding aorta is that it is possible to distinguish, in the former, a minimum followed by a maximum at double the frequency which would thus represent a node and antinode due to some synchronizing of reflected waves. While the absence of such a finding in the ascending aorta was attributed, in the previous section, to the asymmetry in length of the two major subdivisions of the systemic tree, its presence in the pulmonary artery is presumed to be due to the symmetry of the two major subdivisions of the pulmonary vascular beds to the two lungs.

The input impedance of the pulmonary artery in man has been studied by Milnor *et al.* (1969, 1972). They measured the pressure-gradient with a differential manometer connected to a double-lumen catheter passed into the artery through the heart and calculated the flow using the Womersley equation. Ten subjects were studied, of which three had a normal pulmonary artery pressure and the remainder had mitral stenosis and pulmonary hypertension of varying degree. In all cases the pattern of the frequency distribution of the impedance modulus was similar to that seen in the dog and the rabbit. The modulus fell from a relatively high value at low frequencies to a minimum which varied between 2 and 5 Hz and thereafter showed minor oscillations up to 12 Hz. The phase was negative at low frequencies and, with increasing frequency, increased to cross the zero line between 3 and 9 Hz in 7 cases, or remained negative throughout in the other 3 cases. The characteristic impedance was taken as the mean of the values above the minimum; it averaged 23 dyn sec/cm^5 (range 20–29) in the 3 cases with normal pulmonary artery pressure compared to the peripheral resistance which ranged from 59 to 133 dyn sec/ cm^5; in the cases with pulmonary hypertension the mean characteristic impedance was 46 dyn sec/cm^5 (range 25–76) compared to peripheral resistances which ranged from 156 to 680 dyn sec/cm^5. This method of estimating flow from differential pressure appeared to be more reliable in these human studies than in those reported by O'Rourke and Milnor (1971) in the dog, where it was found that theory considerably underestimated the resistive component, an effect thought to be due, possibly, to tapering of the pulmonary artery. The different findings might, therefore, be due to the larger size of the pulmonary trunk in man which enabled a pressure-gradient over a 30 mm interval to be measured without encroaching on the valve, or the region of the bifurcation.

THE INPUT IMPEDANCE AND ITS RELATION TO THE WORK LOAD AND EXTERNAL POWER OUTPUT OF THE HEART

The external work on one ventricle is commonly calculated as the product of the stroke volume (V) and the mean pressure during systole in the artery into which it is ejected. This is a measure of the potential work and to this should be added the kinetic energy due to imparting a velocity (v) to the blood ejected. The kinetic energy (K) is given by

$$K = \frac{1}{2}mv^2 = \frac{1}{2}\rho Vv^2$$

The total work is thus given by

$$W = \bar{P}V + \frac{\rho Vv^2}{2} \qquad\qquad \textbf{13.1}$$

Power $(\dot{W})$ is the rate of doing work (i.e. work per unit time) and at any moment the rate of doing the potential work is given by

$$\dot{W} = PQ \qquad\qquad \textbf{13.2}$$

which can be continuously calculated and plotted with the aid of a computer and is a useful parameter for studying ventricular function. Figure 13.23

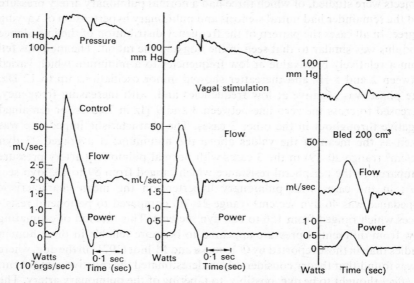

Fig. 13.23. The method of deriving the continuous power output of the ventricle. This is shown for three conditions—control, during vagal stimulation and after a haemorrhage of 200 ml. The pressure and flow curves are shown in each case and the power is obtained by multiplying them together continuously (eqn. 13.2). It can be seen that the power output is more sensitive to changes in haemodynamic conditions than either the pressure or flow considered alone.

shows some examples of plots of the instantaneous power output of the left ventricle under varying conditions. The external stroke work performed is the integral of the potential power over the cycle (as the flow is virtually zero during diastole it is immaterial whether the integration is performed for the period of systole or of the whole cycle, T).

$$W = \int_0^T P . Q dt$$

that is, the area under the curve.

The kinetic power $\dot{K}$ is given by

$$\dot{K} = \frac{\rho}{2} \frac{dV}{dt} v^2 \qquad \textbf{13.3}$$

The velocity, v, is the volume flow ($Q = dV/dt$) divided by the cross-sectional area, A, so that eqn. 13.3 becomes

$$\dot{K} = \frac{\rho}{2} . \frac{Q^3}{A^2} \qquad \textbf{13.4}$$

and again the kinetic work is given by integration. Milnor $et\ al.$ (1966) concerned themselves primarily with the average power. If the flow is sampled J times at intervals of time Δt the average total kinetic power, $\dot{K}_T$ (if the flow of the jth sample is Q_j), is given by

$$\dot{K}_T = \frac{\rho}{2A^2 J} \sum_{j=0}^{J} Q_j^3 \qquad \textbf{13.5}$$

In order to analyse the power output of the right ventricle into mean oscillatory and kinetic terms Milnor $et\ al.$ used the Fourier series to separate the mean pressure and flow power from the oscillatory component of power by utilizing the calculated impedance. The mean power term is the product of the mean pressure and flow.

$$\dot{W}_m = \bar{P}\bar{Q} \qquad \textbf{13.6}$$

As the modulus of the impedance $|Z_n| = |P_n|/|Q_n|$ then $|P_n| = |Z_n| \cdot |Q_n|$ for the nth harmonic, and the oscillatory in-phase (or 'resistive') power is

$$\dot{W}_0 = \frac{1}{2} \sum_{n=1}^{N} |Q_n|^2 |Z_n| \cos \varphi_n \qquad \textbf{13.7}$$

where φ_n is the phase of the impedance of the nth harmonic.

The computation of the kinetic power from the Fourier series is cumbersome because it leads to an unwieldy number of terms so that it is easier to use eqn. 13.5.

The total power is thus given by

$$\dot{W}_T = \dot{W}_M + \dot{W}_0 + \dot{K}_T \qquad \qquad \textbf{13.8}$$

The kinetic power was separated into mean and oscillatory parts by calculating the kinetic power of the mean terms and subtracting it from the total kinetic power to give the oscillating component. The same terms were estimated for the pulmonary veins and the difference between that and the arterial power represented the dissipation of power in the pulmonary vascular bed. The average results found by Milnor *et al.* (1966) are illustrated graphically in Fig. 13.24. The power is expressed in milliwatts; $1 \text{ mW} = 1 \times 10^4 \text{ erg}$

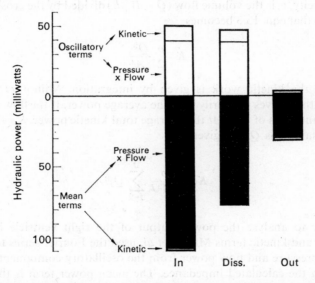

Fig. 13.24. Average hydraulic power at the inlet (pulmonary artery) and the outlet (pulmonary vein near left atrium) of the pulmonary bed of dogs. The difference between the two is power dissipated (Diss.) by flow through the pulmonary vessels. Power associated with mean pressure and flow (mean terms) and that associated with pulsations of pressure and flow (oscillatory terms) are indicated separately as are the pressure-energies and kinetic energies per unit time. (Fig. 3 from Milnor *et al.*, 1966.)

sec^{-1}. In terms of percentages the oscillatory power ($\dot{W}_0$) was c. 37 per cent of the mean power ($\dot{W}_M$) (25 per cent of the total power) and the kinetic power ($\dot{K}_T$) was 7 per cent of the total power ($\dot{W}_T$). (Of the kinetic power some 90 per cent was due to the oscillatory flow.)

The functional effect in terms of power output with changes in heart rate are shown in terms of the power dissipated in Fig. 13.25 assuming

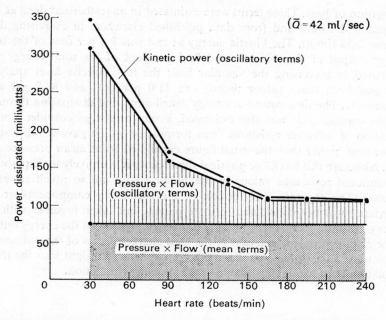

Fig. 13.25. A composite diagram of the relation between heart rate (abscissa) and power dissipated in the pulmonary bed (ordinate—in milliwatts) for a constant mean pulmonary blood flow of 42·0 ml/sec. It is assumed that output power is not changed with heart rate. It can be seen that input power and power dissipated are reduced when the heart rate increases; this amounts to a reduction by one-half when the rate is increased from 60–180 beats/min. (Redrawn from Fig. 5, Milnor et al., 1966.)

that the mean pulmonary blood flow remains constant throughout. It can be seen that, for a mean flow of 42 ml/sec the power dissipated falls from 350 mW at a heart rate of 0·5 Hz to 100 mW at 2·5 Hz and above. This emphasizes the economy for the heart, for it can eject considerably increased volumes of blood per unit time with no increase in external energy dissipation by increasing its rate of pumping.

A corresponding detailed analysis of the energy dissipation in the systemic bed and the power output of the left ventricle has not yet been published. Intuition would indicate that the analysis of the power output of the ventricular muscle gives us more information about its functional capacity than that given solely by measurement of the stroke volume or pulsatile flow. The lead given by Milnor, Bergel and Bargainer's paper should have fruitful clinical applications.

The energy dissipation in the pulmonary vascular bed has also been analysed by Skalak, Wiener, Morkin and Fishman (1966a, b) in two papers of which the first is theoretical and the second experimental. They delineated the distribution of energy delivered to the pulmonary circulation by the right ventricle into strain energy of the vessel walls, kinetic energy of the blood and dissipation of heat. These terms were estimated in anaesthetized dogs at rest (output 1·52 1/min) and from data published elsewhere in exercising dogs (output 2·35 1/min). The kinetic energy at rest was 9·4 per cent of the total energy output of the ventricle and 81·5 per cent of the total energy was dissipated in traversing the vascular bed; the low exercise level analysed increased both these values slightly—to 11·0 per cent and 83·2 per cent respectively. The time course of energy distribution and dissipation throughout the cardiac cycle was also estimated. From the energy considerations a definition of 'effective resistance' was formulated which gave a value some 20 per cent higher than the usual figure calculated from mean pressure and flow. Although this has more physical significance it is unlikely to displace the conventional resistance values in use because they are so much easier to measure. The separate contribution of the oscillatory components or the impedance was not considered in these papers, but taken together with the paper of Milnor et al. (1966) we have a detailed analysis of the energy output of the right ventricle in relation to the load characteristics of the pulmonary circulation. This, in fact, gives a more comprehensive insight into the lesser circulation than the data available in the systemic circulation.

14

Wave-velocity and Attenuation

The velocity of travel of the waves of pressure and flow created by ventricular ejection has been invoked as an important parameter in all the analyses of the behaviour of the arterial tree that have been considered to this point. At first thought this is one of the easiest measurements to make. Nevertheless, there is some uncertainty in the results that have been obtained and it is well to define what it is we wish to measure. Although the value desired can equally well be obtained from the travel of the flow wave as from the pressure pulse it is technically much easier to measure pressure and all studies up to now have only considered the pressure wave. Here the main experimental problem centres around the fact that the pressure changes dramatically in shape as it travels and so raises difficulties in establishing a single value that is definitive for the whole compound.

The shape of the pressure wave

The changes in form of the pulse-wave (Fig. 14.1) have already been noted in Ch. 12 but may be recapitulated briefly here:

A. The amplitude of the pressure wave increases as it travels away from the heart—the so-called 'peaking' of the pulse.
B. The rate of rise of the wave increases and the wave-front becomes steeper (largely due to the increase in amplitude noted in A).
C. The sharp inflection at the incisura becomes rounded and disappears.
D. The slight positive wave in the diastolic portion of curve 1 (ascending aorta) is gradually replaced by a slow but marked dip. In the femoral and saphenous curves we see this dip followed by a second jump (named the dicrotic notch and dicrotic wave respectively).

In his classic monograph on the 'Pressure pulses in the cardiovascular system' Wiggers (1928) attributed these changes to four factors:

1. Damping of waves as they travel.
2. Various components of the wave travelling at different velocities.
3. Annihilation or amplification of the components of the pulse by reflected waves.

389

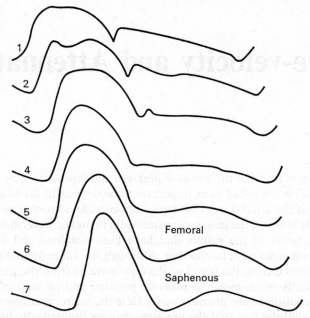

Fig. 14.1. A series of pulse-waves recorded along the arterial tree to show the changes in form that occur as it is propagated. This illustrates one of the problems in defining the velocity of a travelling wave that changes shape progressively.

4. The occurrence of natural vibrations in various parts of the arterial tree.

From the discussion in Ch. 12, we have seen that the evidence is almost entirely against the concept of 'natural vibrations', or resonances as they were later postulated. Otherwise the main modification of the list today would be to add two other factors:

5. The effects of the increasing elastic stiffness of arteries with increasing distance from the heart together with the narrowing of the vessels as they branch. These effects may be summed in terming them as the increase in characteristic impedance as they approach the periphery.
6. The non-linear elastic behaviour of arteries with increasing distension.

Items 1 and 2 are a restatement of the components of the wave-propagation constant (Ch. 11, p. 291)—attenuation and the variation of the velocity of sinusoidal waves with frequency. Attenuation of waves in the arterial system is considered later in this chapter. Its effect on the form of the pressure wave is most distinctly seen in the relatively rapid disappearance of the incisura, which, like any such sharply defined feature, represents the presence of small high-frequency components.

The variation of wave velocity with frequency has been considered theoretically and experimentally in hydraulic models in Ch. 11 where it was seen to be due to the viscosity of the liquid within the tube and to the viscous component of the visco-elastic walls. (There are, of course, large variations in apparent phase velocity in different regions due to reflected waves but these are considered as one of the effects of reflections.) The frequency dependence of velocity causes *dispersion* of the wave. This can be seen clearly in Fig. 12.1 where an initially sharp transient wave becomes rounded and spread out (dispersed) as it travels. In such a case the initial transient has a wide range of frequency components and the illustration shows it after successive 'round-trips' in a rubber tube about 10 m long. The periodic pressure wave has a much more limited array of frequency components and the distance it travels in the arterial tree is very much shorter. As the analysis in Ch. 11 shows, the difference in velocity with frequency is only marked in the fall that occurs when the parameter α is less than 3; in the dog this will begin to be the case for the fundamental frequency of the pulse in arteries of the calibre of the femoral artery and will apply to the first two harmonics in the saphenous artery. In these vessels, however, the proximity of the terminal arterial bed produces marked reflection effects on the measured (apparent) phase velocity, which mask it. The effects of dispersion, therefore, will be small and have proved impossible to detect.

Of the changing characteristics of the pressure pulse the development of the dicrotic wave (item D) is clearly due to the effect of reflected waves. Reflected waves also play a large part in the 'peaking' of the wave (item A) but the analysis presented in Ch. 12 showed that the non-uniform elastic properties of the arteries—the 'elastic' taper—(plus the geometrical taper) contribute an equally large part to this striking feature of the travelling pressure pulse.

The change in slope of the wave-front (item B) is principally due to the increase in amplitude because it is found that the time interval from the beginning of the rise (or 'foot' of the wave) to the point of maximum pressure remains virtually unchanged. However, the arteries are known to have strikingly non-linear elastic properties in that their elastic modulus increases with increasing distension and Barnard et al. (1966) showed that this would cause a slight increase in the slope of the wave-front of a travelling wave.

We thus see that the factors that cause a change in shape of the wave are generally involved with the velocity of the components of the wave. For practical purposes, however, we need a single characteristic value; this is especially true in relating the elastic properties of the wall to the velocity of wave propagation. This has an important clinical application in the study and diagnosis of arterial disease. The changes that occur in the arterial wall in atherosclerosis and in the ageing process cause an increase in elastic modulus and hence an increase in wave velocity. The practical problems of establishing criteria of normality have so far rendered most of the work on this subject inconclusive. Good measurements are also needed to test the numerous theoretical analyses of wave propagation that have appeared in the past decade. Some of these were briefly noted in Ch. 11. The link between this theoretical work and its clinical application is most clearly stressed in Willem Klip's doctoral thesis of 1962 where he states that the work was started in response to the question, three years previously, from a leading cardiologist: 'How can we measure the wave velocity accurately?' The pursuit of this problem has involved his whole research effort since then and involved the writing of an extensive book on cardiovascular biophysics (Klip, 1969). Other important contributions have come from Mirsky (1967a, b; 1968) on propagation in an orthotropically elastic tube; from Atabek and Lew (1966) on propagation in an initially stressed orthotropic tube, and from Anliker and his group in a series of papers dealing with a variety of conceptual models together with extensive experimental tests of their validity (Maxwell and Anliker, 1968; Anliker and Maxwell, 1967). A valuable review of the topic is that by Skalak (1966).

What is the true wave-velocity?

This rhetorical question was put, in the light of the problems recapitulated above, by McDonald and Taylor in their 1959 review. It cannot be said that we can give an answer today that is any more definitive than they could then. For a wave that shows dispersion due to the frequency-dependent velocity of its components the set of waves is regarded as a *group* and the term *group velocity* is used. It is sometimes described as the velocity of the centre of area of the group. In the presence of retrograde waves the concept cannot be applied with any significance. Womersley (1955c) calculated the relative values of the group and phase velocity of an arterial pressure wave assuming that only the dispersion due to the viscous effect of the blood was causing distortion of the wave. He found that in arteries where α was greater than 3 (i.e. in the larger arteries where most measurements are made) the difference between the phase and group velocity would not be more than 2 to $2\frac{1}{2}$ per cent. Müller (1950) also purported to measure the group and phase velocities of a train of sinusoidal waves in a rubber tube variously filled with liquids of different viscosities; however, he used the velocity of the first wave in the train as a measure of group velocity which is not valid. Indeed, because of the discontinuity at this point it will tend to be represented by the higher frequency components; the concept is reinforced by the fact that the two values became virtually identical at 20 Hz.

The velocity of the 'foot' and other points

The method that has been most commonly used in the past has measured the time of travel of the 'foot' of the wave over a known distance. The 'foot' is defined as the point, at the end of diastole, when the steep rise of the wavefront begins. In essence the principle involved is that of determining a point of identity in the travelling wave and to use its velocity as characteristic of the whole wave. In view of the various factors that cause the form of the wave to change, the identity of features of the wave cannot be taken as self-evident.

By analogy with the interaction of a transient wave with reflected waves that it creates (Fig. 12.1) the early part of the wave will be little affected by reflections. Therefore, it is reasonable to treat the early wave-front as a region that maintains its identity in the propagated wave. The 'foot' of the wave-front is, at first sight, the easiest point to recognize; it is, however, clear-cut only when the pressure wave is recorded on a relatively slow time-base. When the sweep speed is increased, as is necessary for recording over short distances, it becomes much more difficult to define with any precision; this can be seen in Fig. 14.1. Various manœuvres have been introduced to avoid this difficulty.

Laszt and Müller (1952a, b, c) defined a point, representing the foot, by extrapolating the wave-front downwards and measuring from the intersection of this line with a straight line extrapolation of the last part of the diastolic curve. Anliker, Histand and Ogden (1968) used a similar technique for the superimposed sine waves that they used. Frank (1905) suggested measuring the velocity of a point at one-fifth of the height of the rising limb. Kapal, Martini and Wetterer (1951) extended this idea by measuring the velocities of four 'corresponding points' on the rising limb and found that they were not appreciably different from each other, nor from the velocity of the foot. They thus confirmed the concept that the rising limb, or wave-front, retains its identity reasonably well.

This concept was utilized by McDonald (1968a) in developing a technique which used a double-beam cathode-ray oscilloscope equipped with an adjustable delay-time between the two beams. Using a double-lumen arterial catheter, with a 5 cm interval between the recording points, introduced through a peripheral artery, he recorded the wave velocity at successive 5 cm intervals along the length of the aorta and at slightly larger intervals in the more peripheral vessels. The sweep of the oscilloscope was triggered from the QRS complex of the electrocardiogram (in peripheral arteries a later trigger is desirable). Initially two pressure waves separated by the transmission time would be seen (Fig. 14.2 top); after carefully monitoring the two waves in terms of amplitude, the proximal pressure recording was then delayed until the wave-fronts were superimposed (Fig. 14.2 lower). The time of delay then represents the time of travel of the wave-front over the known distance. From this the 'wave-front velocity' is easily calculated. The precision of the measurement depends on the rate of sweep and this was used at the highest rate that would allow all the wave-front to be retained on the screen (the illustration in Fig. 14.2 includes all the wave for clarity of explanation). The proportion of the wave-front that can be precisely superimposed is usually at least 75 per cent of the wave amplitude in the thoracic aorta; in the femoral or more distal vessels closer to major reflecting sites the proportion is usually between

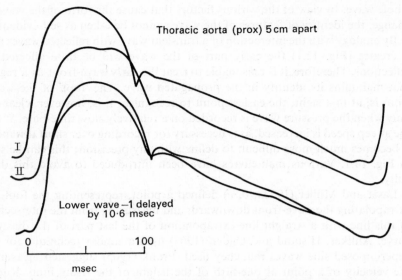

Thoracic aorta (prox) 5 cm apart

I

II

Lower wave −1 delayed
by 10·6 msec

0   100

msec

Fig. 14.2. *Top.* Two pulse-waves recorded (I and II) 5 cm apart in the thoracic aorta of the dog. The levels of the waves have been altered in order to distinguish between them.

Lower. The waves have been set at the same level and the recording of wave I progressively delayed until the two wave-fronts coincided. The delay was then found to be 10·6 msec. It can be seen that about 75 per cent of the rising phase of the pressure wave coincides; this very early part of the wave is not affected by reflection from the periphery and may thus be regarded as the true transmission time as determined by the elastic properties of the wave. It can be seen that the transient notch caused by the closure of the aortic valves also travels at the same velocity because these notches also coincide when the first wave is delayed.

For maximum accuracy the sweep speed of the oscilloscope is increased so that only the rising phase is included. The whole wave is shown here for clarity. (From McDonald, 1968.)

30–50 per cent. The findings of Kapal *et. al* are thus confirmed. Other points of possible identity can also be checked. Where it exists, the incisura can be seen to travel at the same velocity as the wave-front.

The distribution of wave-velocities that were found are illustrated in Fig. 14.3; the velocity over each interval is represented by a point at the middle of the interval. The point representing the ascending aorta is added from a later paper by Nichols and McDonald (1972); they also repeated measurements along the aorta and found them to be in close agreement with those illustrated. The values are also in general agreement with those of Dow and Hamilton (1939) who also measured the wave-velocities (foot-to-foot with intra-arterial catheters over intervals of 5 cm). This paper was, for many years, the only clear evidence of a progressive and marked rise in wave velocity with increasing distance from the heart because the series of measurements were made in the same dog. Laszt and Müller (1952*a*, *b*, *c*) in a series of papers had made careful recordings of the normal pattern of pressure waves throughout the arterial system and measured the wave velocity over intervals of 10–15 cm. A summary of these findings, together with values derived from measure-

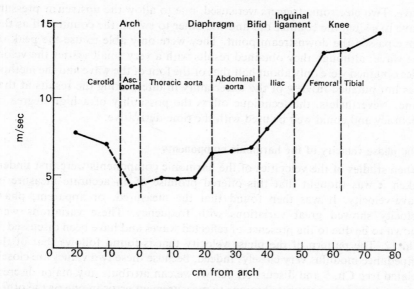

Fig. 14.3. A diagram to show the progressive increase in wave-front velocity of the pulse wave with increasing distance from the heart. The values show the average values from three dogs. The mean pressure was between 130–160 cm H₂O for all readings.

It will be seen that in the ascending aorta the wave-velocity is 4 m/sec, rises slightly to about 4·7 m/sec in the thoracic aorta and finally attains 13–15 m/sec in the femoral and tibial artery. The rise towards the head is also marked but is ultimately less elevated because the distances are shorter. (From Nichols and McDonald, 1972.)

ments of elasticity, is given in Table 14.1. There appear to have been no comparable measurements made in man and all the evidence available is over large intervals such as between the carotid and femoral arteries. Typical values in man are also given in the Table. It is clear that, in the presence of a marked progressive rise, the measurement over a long interval will only give an average value. In attempts to relate this to the elasticity measured in arterial segments such an average value will be of little use.

Another method of measuring the wave velocity which is closely linked to that described above has been used by Fry and his colleagues (Greenfield and Fry, 1962, Patel *et al.*, 1969). In this the time-derivative of the pulse-wave is recorded and the transit time of the peak of the derivative is measured. As this point of maximum rate of rise in pressure is usually about half-way up the wave-front, or somewhat earlier, this falls within the area that can always be matched in the method of McDonald (1968*a*) and is thus essentially the same measure. This technique could be easily adapted to the delay-line method and might well be better than using the actual wave-front as it would provide a steeper slope for matching. It also might usefully be adapted to the technique that was tested by Hale, McDonald, Taylor and Womersley (1955), who used a quartz oscillator counter chronometer to measure the transit time of the wave. Two electronic triggers were used, one to allow the upstream pressure wave to switch the counter on, and the other to switch the counter off as the wave passed the downstream point. They were only able to use the peak of the wave; although they obtained results with a very small scatter the velocities obtained were only about half that of the foot of the wave and the method was not pursued in view of the uncertainty in interpreting the results at that time. Nevertheless, the technique offers the possibility of a high degree of accuracy and could well be used with the time-derivative.

The phase velocity of the harmonic components

When studies of the velocities of the harmonic components were first undertaken it was thought that this offered promise of an accurate measure of wave-velocity. It was then found that the measured, or apparent, phase velocity showed great variations with frequency. These variations were shown to be due to the presence of reflected waves and have been discussed in Ch. 12. The pattern of the phase velocity that is found follows that of the impedance modulus very closely; indeed, because these two values are closely related (see Ch. 6 and discussion below) we can attribute any major discrepancy between the two distributions to measurement error in one or the other. Especially where the apparent phase velocity is high, this error is most likely to be in the phase velocity because the phase shift is small and the phase discrimination using A–D converters and magnetic tape recording is rarely less than $\pm 1°$. In all situations the apparent phase velocity is high for components of the pulse-wave below 2 Hz. In the ascending aorta (following the modulus pattern seen in Ch. 13) it fluctuates little as shown in Fig. 14.4. In a peripheral

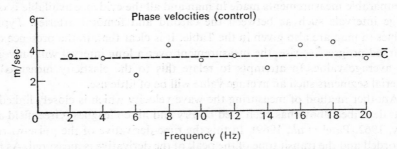

Fig. 14.4. The phase velocity of the first ten harmonics of the pulse wave in the ascending aorta when the heart frequency is 2 Hz. It will be seen that above this frequency there is little change in phase-velocity with frequency. The mean value is shown by the broken line and this is found to be very close to the wave-front velocity. (Nichols and McDonald, unpublished.)

artery such as the femoral the fluctuations (like that of the modulus) are still marked above 2 Hz but, nevertheless, have usually become very small above 8–10 Hz. The disappearance of reflection effects at these higher frequencies is due to two causes: (1) the attenuation of the reflected waves becomes progressively greater with frequency, and the interaction with the centrifugal wave therefore becomes much less; (2) as the phase velocity is measured over a finite interval this produces some averaging of the changes and, as the frequency increases, the measuring interval forms a progressively greater fraction of a wave length and the averaging effect becomes dominant.

Relationship of the apparent phase velocity to the wave-front velocity

The fluctuations of apparent phase velocity were shown by Taylor (1957*a, b*) to be around the velocity which is characterized by the elastic properties of the tube. The relatively steady value of phase velocity that is attained in the higher frequency components is, in fact, found to be in good agreement with wave-velocities measured from the foot of the wave. McDonald (1968*a*) also found that there was good agreement with the wave-front velocity. Further, he found that the mean value of the apparent phase velocity* above 2–2·5 Hz (which were the slowest rates of the fundamental frequency in this series) was very close to the wave-front velocity which was measured in the aorta. The mean taken over this frequency range was not so good because the deviations due to reflections were much greater. Figure 14.5 shows the distribution of

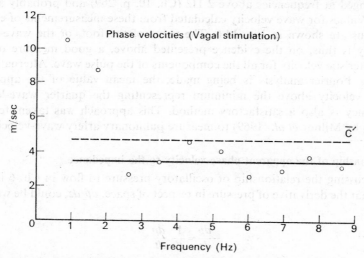

Fig. 14.5. The distribution of phase velocities of the pulse-wave in the ascending aorta when the heart-rate has been slowed to below 1 Hz by vagal stimulation. It can be seen that the velocity is elevated in the lowest two harmonics but that the variation above 2 Hz is quite small. The mean value of all the harmonics is shown by the broken line but is significantly higher than the mean value of the harmonics above (solid line). This latter value coincides with the wave-front velocity. Nichols and McDonald, unpublished.)

* Because the phase velocity is a reciprocal function of the phase difference which is measured, the mean velocity is properly calculated from the mean phase shift rather than taking the mean of the calculated velocities. This was not done by McDonald (1968*a*) but was by Nichols and McDonald (1972) in the ascending aorta. In this latter situation where the fluctuations of velocity above 2 Hz are small the discrepancy between the two calculated values is small but in more peripheral vessels it may be appreciable.

velocities in an experiment where the heart had been slowed by vagal stimulation. The mean of all values is shown by the broken line and is substantially higher than the mean of the values above 2 Hz, shown by the solid line. This latter value was virtually identical with the wave-front velocity; for this situation the matching of the mean value of the phase velocity above 2 Hz is always extremely close to the wave-front velocity.

McDonald and Taylor (1959) concerned themselves with the steady value which the apparent phase velocities attained at the higher frequencies and argued that the similarity of this value to the velocity of the foot was due to the fact that the sharp inflection there would be largely determined by the higher frequency components. They assumed that the visco-elastic properties of the arterial wall would cause a progressive increase in the dynamic elastic modulus (and hence the wave velocity) with frequency as with all classical visco-elastic materials. Thus the foot-to-foot wave velocity would represent the characteristic wave velocity of the higher frequency components but not the velocity of the main low frequency terms. The work of Bergel (1960, 1961b), however, showed that the dynamic elastic modulus remains virtually unchanged at frequencies above 2 Hz (Ch. 10, p. 269) and probably above 1 Hz. Values for wave velocity calculated from these measurements of elastic modulus are shown in Fig. 14.6. The value of the foot, or the wave-front velocity is thus, on the evidence presented above, a good measure of the characteristic velocity for all the components of the pulse wave. Alternatively, when a Fourier analysis is being made, the mean value of the apparent phase velocity above the minimum representing the quarter wave-length frequency is also a satisfactory method. This approach was taken, for example, by Milnor et al. (1969) to measure pulmonary artery wave-velocity.

Relationship of the apparent phase-velocity to the impedance

In discussing the relationship of oscillatory pressure to flow in Ch. 6 it was seen that the derivative of pressure in respect of space, dp/dz, could be written as

$$-\frac{dp}{dz} = \frac{1}{c'} \cdot \frac{dp}{dt}$$ **14.1**

where c' is the apparent phase velocity, i.e.

$$c' = \frac{\omega . \Delta z}{\Delta \varphi}$$ **12.7**

Writing an harmonic of the pressure, P, as $M \cos (\omega t - \varphi)$ we see that

$$\frac{dp}{dz} = -\frac{\omega}{c'} M \sin (\omega t - \varphi)$$ **14.2**

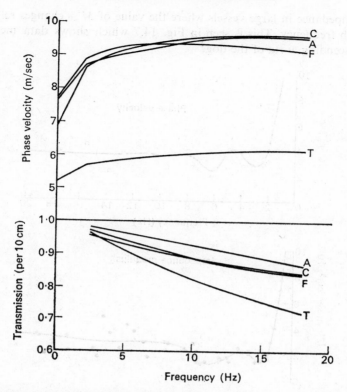

Fig. 14.6. The upper part of this figure shows the change of velocity in various arteries with frequency where only the visco-elastic changes dependent on frequency are considered. The values are calculated from the dynamic elastic modulus measured in an isolated segment of artery. This demonstrates that the high phase-velocity found at low frequencies (Fig. 14.5) is not due to inherent elastic behaviour but is due to wave-reflection.

The arteries used were thoracic aorta—T, abdominal aorta—A, femoral artery—F, and carotid artery—C. (From Bergel, 1960.)

and the equation for flow becomes

$$Q = \frac{\pi R^2}{\rho c'} . M . M'_{10} \sin (\omega t - \varphi - \pi/2 + \varepsilon_{10}) \qquad \textbf{14.3}$$

The modulus of the impedance is then

$$|Z| = \frac{|P|}{|Q|} = \frac{\rho c'}{\pi R^2 . M'_{10}} \qquad \textbf{14.4}$$

For a given artery the ratio $\rho/\pi R^2$ remains the same; while the modulus of the Bessel function, M'_{10}, is dependent on the value of α it does not change greatly in the larger arteries as it is asymptotically approaching its limit. Therefore, the apparent phase velocity will vary fairly closely with the modulus

o

of the impedance in large vessels where the value of M'_{10} changes relatively little with frequency. This is seen in Fig. 14.7 which shows data measured in the ascending aorta of the dog.

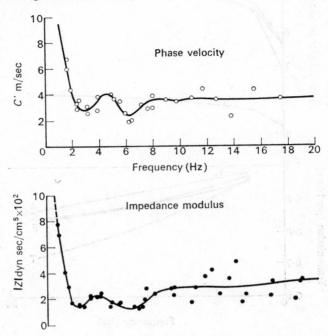

Fig. 14.7. A comparison of the changes in phase-velocity in the ascending aorta of the dog with the changes in impedance modulus. They are seen to be very closely paralleled and may be both attributed to the effects of wave reflection.

The accuracy of the relationship is further illustrated in Fig. 14.8 where the moduli calculated from the apparent phase velocity are compared with those derived from the Fourier analysis of a flow curve recorded at the same time.

The use of transient excitation to measure wave-velocity

All the methods of measuring wave-velocity that have been discussed above have used the pressure-wave created by systolic ejection. The presence of wave reflection has posed a problem in interpreting these results. To avoid this, Landowne (1957b) developed a method in which a transient spike of pressure could be superimposed on the pulse wave by tapping the artery sharply with a solenoid operated mechanism. The transit time of the spike between two points in the arteries of the arm was measured and its velocity of propagation determined. In his experiment the spike was created in the brachial artery (of patients) and the pressure measured at one position in that artery and another

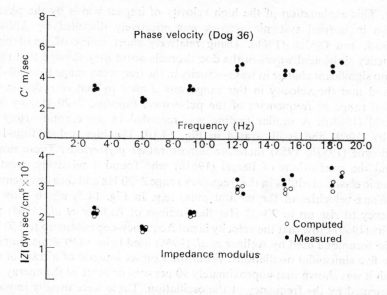

Fig. 14.8. To show that the parallelism of phase velocity and impedance modulus is not fortuitous, the phase velocity is shown in the upper part of this figure. In the lower part, the values of the impedance modulus are calculated from eqn. 14.4 and shown to correspond very closely to the values directly measured from the pressure and flow. (From Nichols, 1970.)

in the radial artery. The transient impulse showed marked attenuation and no reflected waves were seen; even if present they would have been quite distinct from the brief impulse. The velocities that he recorded were, however, much higher than those recorded by the more usual methods. McDonald and Taylor (1959) assumed that this was due to an increase of elastic stiffness at the high frequencies which constituted the brief transient. This explanation has proved to be untenable in the light of the work of Bergel (1961*b*) and others, particularly of Anliker and his group, who have made a detailed study of the propagation velocity of transient waves and trains of waves at a high frequency.

The impact waves produced in Landowne's experiments would have a large non-axisymmetric component and Anliker and Maxwell (1967) and Maxwell and Anliker (1968) showed theoretically that, under certain circumstances, non-axisymmetrical waves could have a velocity which was much higher than the characteristic one. In their own experiments, which repeated the technique as far as possible, they were, however, unable to find the same high values, so that it remains in doubt whether this explanation applied to the earlier results. The suggestion by McDonald and Taylor (1959) that the phase-velocity would rise markedly at high frequencies appeared to be supported by the results of Landowne (1957*a*) who imposed long trains of sinusoidal pressure waves on excised umbilical arteries (which have a very high proportion of muscle in the

wall). This explanation of the high velocity of impact waves by the phenomenon in normal systemic arteries was effectively dispelled by Anliker,
Histand, and Ogden (1968). Using relatively short trains of small high-
frequency sinusoidal waves in the dog thoracic aorta they showed that there
was no significant change in wave-velocity in the frequency range from 40–140
Hz and that the velocity in this range was similar to that recorded in the
normal range of frequencies of the pulse-wave (approx. 2–20 Hz) by Mc-
Donald (1968a). A similar finding was recorded in the carotid artery by
Moritz (1969) and is illustrated in Fig. 14.10. The high values found by
Landowne (1957b, 1958) therefore remain rather mysterious. These results
extend the conclusions of Bergel (1961b) who found a relatively constant
dynamic elastic modulus in the frequency range 2–20 Hz and measurements of
the phase-velocities of the natural pulse (e.g. in Fig. 14.5) which show no
tendency to rise up to 20–25 Hz; the findings of Anliker et al. (1968) and
Moritz (1969) show that the velocity is not frequency-dependent up to 150 Hz.

The technique used by Anliker et al. (1968) used (Fig. 14.9) short trains of
some five sinusoidal oscillations. From the Fourier integral of a train of this
length it was shown that approximately 90 per cent or more of the energy was
represented by the frequency of the oscillation. These were usually imposed
with a mechanical oscillator applied to the wall. The non-axisymmetric
component that this produces was found to be attenuated very rapidly so that
if the proximal pressure measurement was made at some 5–6 cm distant this
wave was found to be virtually axisymmetrical. The advantages of this technique were (a) that the superimposed waves were of small amplitude so that
they could be assumed to be propagated linearly, (b) short trains of high-
frequency oscillations are attenuated to such a degree that no reflected waves
are created, and (c) as the excitation was very brief compared to the length of
the cardiac cycle the propagation velocity could be tested at various parts of
the cycle. This last facility was especially used to test the effect of changes in
distending pressure on the wave-velocity.

The effect of arterial distension on wave-velocity

The fact that an increase in mean arterial pressure increases the pulse-wave
velocity was appreciated by Frank (1905, 1920). It was later studied in detail
by Bramwell and Hill (1922). They used excised arterial segments which they
filled with mercury to slow the wave velocity and so allow more accurate
measurements of the transit time. They concluded that the foot-to-foot wave-
velocity increased proportionately with the diastolic pressure. This concept
was extended in another brief paper (Bramwell and Hill, 1923) to assuming
that each portion of the wave travelled at the characteristic velocity associated
with the pressure at that point. They thus postulated that the portion of the
wave at the systolic peak would ultimately overtake the foot and that 'breakers'
would be created like those of ocean waves on a shelving shore. This analogy

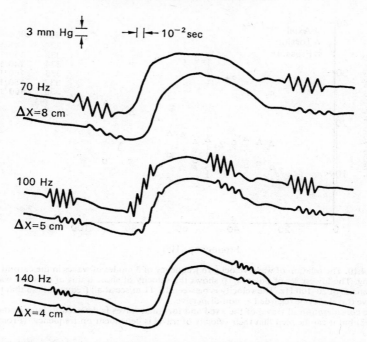

Fig. 14.9. An illustration of the technique used by Anliker and his colleagues to measure the velocity of radial waves. An external vibrator imposed short trains of high frequency waves on the intact vessel and the resultant pressure was recorded at two points a known distance apart. The velocity of travel can thus be calculated from the transmission time. From the downstream recording it can be seen how rapidly these waves are attenuated so that there is no possibility of reflected waves being created and interacting with the centrifugal wave. The frequencies used are far higher than those that can be detected in the natural waves but as it was also shown that the velocity of pressure waves is virtually independent of frequency (see Fig. 14.10), they may be taken as a measure of the velocity of the normal pulse-wave. (From Anliker, Histand and Ogden, 1968.)

was, one feels, more picturesque than realistic. Measurements of the velocity of the peak of the wave have not borne out this prediction. It was noted above that Hale, McDonald, Taylor and Womersley (1955) found that the peak of the wave in the femoral artery actually appeared to travel at a considerably lower velocity than the foot. It is also apparent by inspection of the changing form of the pulse wave (Figs. 12.12, 14.1 and 14.2) that points of equal pressure on the rising and falling phases of the pulse do not necessarily have the same velocity, while the incisura travels at the same velocity as the foot of the wave although at a considerably higher pressure. Taylor (McDonald and Taylor, 1959) found that while the foot-to-foot velocity correlated well with the mean arterial pressure (and with the minimum diastolic pressure) the velocity of the point of maximum pressure correlated very poorly with it. The fallacy inherent in many of these concepts is the assumption that arbitrary points selected on two successive curves have a specific identity.

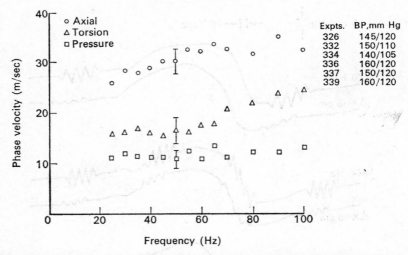

Fig. 14.10. The relation of wave-velocity to frequency of 3 modes of waves in the carotid artery of the dog. The lowest set of points (☐) shows the velocity of short trains of pressure waves from frequencies of 20–100 Hz. The velocity is between 10–11 m/sec at all frequencies so that this mode of wave travel may be regarded as non-dispersive.

The consideration of travel of the axial and torsional waves is deferred to later in the chapter (p. 408) but it can be seen that their velocity of travel is dependent on frequency. (From Moritz, 1969.)

By using brief transient excitation, Anliker *et al.* (1968) were able to study the velocity of a discrete wave at the various pressures of the successive phases of the cardiac cycle. They also varied the mean pressure by vagal slowing or arrest of the heart and by brief periods of aortic occlusion either proximal or distal to the thoracic aorta where all their measurements were made. A typical distribution of the velocity of the transient waves with pressure is shown in Fig. 14.11. This shows a change in velocity from c. 3·7 m/sec at 30 mm Hg to 4·2 m/sec at 80 mm Hg and thereafter a faster rise to approx. 6·0 m/sec at 120 mm Hg. These values are similar to those found for the wave-front velocity in the thoracic aorta (4·4–4·8 m/sec) by McDonald (1968a). This type of behaviour is to be expected from the non-linear elastic properties of arteries which was discussed in Ch. 10, and it is the most detailed study of this important phenomenon. Nevertheless, the relation of the velocity of a transient wave superimposed during systole to the elastic properties of the wall is somewhat complicated by the effect of the blood flow velocity on the transmission of the pressure wave.

Relationship of flow velocity to pressure wave-velocity

By the terms of the simple analysis of the Moens-Korteweg equation (eqn. 10.56) the presence of a steady-flow will increase the wave-velocity by the amount of the stream-velocity. That is if the Moens-Korteweg velocity is c_0,

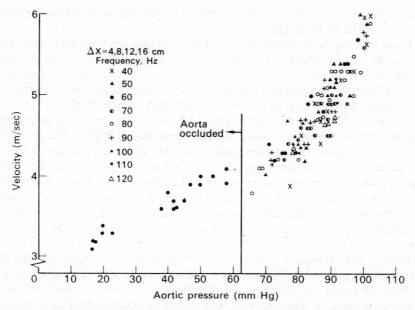

Fig. 14.11. The velocity of small imposed transient waves at different transmural pressures. The lowest pressures are recorded during partial aortic occlusion; to the right of the vertical line the velocities are taken to be those of the pressures during diastole and systole. As the blood flow velocity is high during systole this velocity will be added to the wave-velocity, so that the measured wave velocity is not entirely due to the elastic behaviour of the wall. (From Anliker, Histand and Ogden, 1968.)

and the flow velocity $\overline{V}$, then the pressure wave will travel at a velocity $\overline{c}$ such that

$$\overline{c} = c_0 + \overline{V} \qquad\qquad 14.5$$

in the downstream direction, and

$$\overline{c} = c_0 - \overline{V} \qquad\qquad 14.6$$

in the upstream direction.

Müller (1950) tested this experimentally in hydraulic models and found that the downstream wave-velocity was somewhat less than $c_0 + \overline{V}$ while the upstream velocity was somewhat greater than $c_0 - \overline{V}$. His measurements were made from the front of a long train of sinusoidal waves, and in a long rubber tube would be somewhat in error due to dispersion. However, the discrepancies were about 17 per cent and it is doubtful whether dispersion can account for all of this. His results have not been repeated, nor fully explained. In a theoretical study Morgan and Ferrante (1955) indicated that with a viscous liquid the wave-velocity in the direction of the stream would be slightly in excess of the sum $c_0 + \overline{V}$, while for an inviscid fluid it would be slightly less. The differences predicted, however, were small and would be very difficult to detect over short distances of wave travel. This theoretical problem has been further studied by Wells (1969).

These analyses were based on the assumption that the stream-velocity was (a) steady and (b) small in relation to wave-velocity. When considering the phase-velocity in arteries these conditions are met; as the phase-velocity is derived from the analysis of a complex cardiac cycle it clearly must be related to the mean flow velocity. In the thoracic aorta this is normally from 0·15–0·25 m/sec while the wave-velocity is from 4·5–5·0 m/sec. In more peripheral arteries the flow velocity is lower and the wave-velocity higher. The pulsatile flow velocity, however, reaches peak velocities which are of the order of 1·0 m/sec or more in the aorta of an anaesthetized dog and can be much higher with an increased cardiac output. When the velocity of travel of a very short transient is measured it is modified by the flow velocity at that moment in the cardiac cycle. Thus the increased wave-velocity measured during systole will be due not only to the increase of pressure but also due to the high flow rates that occur in systole. This has been studied in detail by Histand (1969). Extending the technique used by Anliker, Histand, and Ogden (1968), he arranged the position of the mechanical stimulator so that the wave-velocity in both upstream and downstream directions could be measured. While a marked increase in wave-velocity was found in the downstream direction during systole (as shown by the higher pressure points in Fig. 14.11) the velocity in the upstream direction showed virtually no difference during diastole or systole. This last finding was interpreted as meaning that the increase in velocity due to the increase in pressure during systole was cancelled by the fast flow rate due to ventricular contraction. Conversely, the increase in wave-velocity with pressure seen in Fig. 14.11 (all measured in the downstream direction) is partly due to the high rates of flow in systole. Histand tested this hypothesis by differencing the downstream and upstream wave velocities measured at different points in the cardiac cycle and derived a flow curve which fitted quite well with a flow-velocity curve measured with a Pieper catheter-tip flowmeter (Pieper and Paul, 1969).

When the wave-velocity is measured from the mean phase-velocity this value is derived from the whole wave and will only be affected by the mean blood flow velocity which is very low compared to the pressure wave-velocity. Such values are shown at various mean pressures in Fig. 14.12A. These velocities were measured in the ascending aorta of the dog. It can be seen that the velocity remains unchanged at c. 4 m/sec from a pressure of 60–110 mm Hg and then begins to rise but only reaches 5·5 m/sec at 160 mm Hg. This dependence on pressure should be compared to that seen in Fig. 14.11 where the high pressure values were taken in systole where blood-flow velocity is high (c. 1 m/sec). In 14.12B a comparable set of values is shown which were measured during the infusion of norepinephrine. Wave-velocity is virtually unchanged up to a pressure of 100 mm Hg but thereafter there is an appreci-

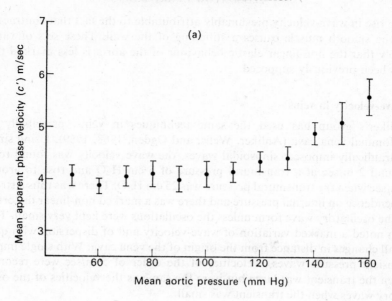

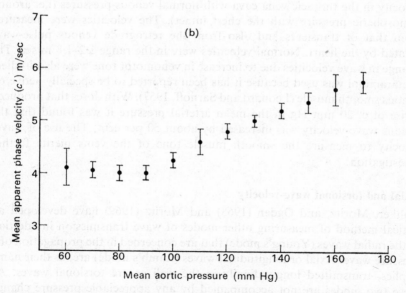

Fig. 14.12A. The mean apparent phase velocity in the ascending aorta of the dog. The arterial pressure was varied by a controlled pressure reservoir (barostat) over the range 50–160 mm Hg.

B. A similar set of values during the infusion of nor-adrenaline. The contraction of the smooth muscle in the wall adds to its elastic stiffness causing an increase in wave velocity at pressures above 100 mm Hg.

These results are discussed in the text. (From Nichols and McDonald, 1972.)

able rise in wave-velocity presumably attributable to the fact that contraction of the smooth muscle causes a stiffening of the wall. These sets of values imply that the non-linear elastic behaviour of the aorta is less marked than has been previously supposed.

Wave-velocity in veins

Anliker's group has used the same techniques in veins, principally the abdominal vena cava (Anliker, Wells, and Ogden, 1968, 1969). Using small, hydraulically imposed, sinusoidal waves, the wave velocity was found to be around 2 m/sec at a transmural pressure of 5 cm H_2O and rose to around 5 m/sec when the transmural pressure was 25 cm H_2O. There was thus a strong dependence on internal pressure and there was a marked non-linear distortion of the oscillatory wave form unless the oscillations were kept very small. They also noted a marked variation of wave-velocity and of dispersion with quite small changes in distance from the origin of the vena cava. With single impact transient pressure waves,, velocities of the order of 5 m/sec were recorded when the transient was large but were the same as the velocities of the oscillatory waves when the transient was small.

In this laboratory, preliminary studies have been made of the wave-velocity in the thoracic vena cava with normal venous pressures (i.e. around atmospheric pressure with the chest intact). The velocities were measured from that of transients and also from the retrograde venous pulse-wave created by the heart. Normal velocities were in the range 1·2–1·8 m/sec. The change in wave velocities due to increase in venomotor tone were also studied. Metaraminol was used because it has been reported to be specially active on venous smooth muscle (Leonard and Sarnoff, 1957). With doses that produced a rise of c. 20 mm Hg in the mean arterial pressure it was found that the venous wave-velocity was increased by about 50 per cent. The use of wave-velocity to measure the smooth muscle tone of the veins merits further investigation.

Axial and torsional wave-velocity

Anliker, Moritz, and Ogden (1968) and Moritz (1969) have developed an optical method of measuring other modes of wave transmission in addition to the radial waves (Young's mode) that are concerned in the propagation of a pressure wave. Axial or longitudinal waves (Lamb's mode) are, as their name implies, transmitted longitudinally in the wall as are torsional waves. As these two modes are not accompanied by any appreciable pressure change their measurement in arteries is difficult; it had not previously been undertaken. The technique used was to fit a collar on the common carotid artery and impose short trains of sinusoidal axial or torsional motions by means of an electromagnetic shaker. Target markers were attached to the artery and their movement observed with two electro-optical tracking devices which recorded the transit time, between 2 markers, of a wave travelling in the wall.

The average results from measurements made in the carotid arteries of 31 dogs are shown in Fig. 14.10. In the range of frequencies from 20 to 100 Hz the pressure wave-velocity was approximately 10·0 m/sec and showed no dispersion. The axial mode, by contrast, was markedly dispersive and increased from 24 m/sec at 20 Hz to 33 m/sec at 100 Hz. The velocity of torsional waves was intermediate in value and also dispersive. They ranged from c. 15 m/sec at 20 Hz to 22 m/sec at 100 Hz.

It was also demonstrated that an axial wave created by the heart beat could be recorded in the proximal carotid artery. Its form was similar to that of the aortic pressure wave; the amplitude of the wave was somewhat less than 0·4 mm but was rapidly attenuated; at a distance of 10 cm it was reduced to about one-third this amplitude. Both axial and torsional waves showed a much greater attenuation (by a factor of about 4) than that of the pressure waves.

Wave attenuation in arteries

When there is no interference by reflected waves the attenuation of a travelling wave is easily measured by recording its amplitude at two points z cm apart. Using the equation

$$|P_z| = |P_0| e^{-az} \qquad \textbf{11.14}$$

the value of the attenuation coefficient a is thus determined.

With the high frequency trains of waves used by Anliker and his group the condition of wave propagation in one direction only is met, and they determined their attenuation coefficients in this manner. To standardize this term the attenuation (or its complement the transmission) it is usually expressed as the attenuation per wave-length (i.e. $e^{-a\lambda}$, eqn. 11.15).

For pressure waves in the thoracic aorta the value of $a\lambda$ (termed K in their papers) fell between 0·7 and 1·0, and showed no significant variation in the frequency range 40–200 Hz. In the carotid artery the value of K fell between 0·8 and 1·5 for pressure waves. By comparison for axial waves the values of K ranged from 4·0–6·5; for torsional waves it was found to be dependent on the amplitude of the wave created but in the range tested the value of K was between 3·5 and 5·0.

As the transmission per wave-length in a typical visco-elastic medium such as a rubber tube (Fig. 11.8) is markedly dependent on frequency it is necessary, before using these values in analysing the propagation characteristics of the natural pulse wave, to measure the attenuation over the frequency range of the significant harmonic components of the pulse. This is more difficult than for the high-frequency range because of the presence of reflected waves. To measure the attenuation *in vivo* under these circumstances requires the measurement of the pressure at three equally spaced points; the principle of the method was outlined in the last section of Ch. 11.

Experimentally, the difficulties of the method are centred around the placement and precise matching of 3 manometer systems. Rarely can one position the manometer so that the proximal and distal ones are precisely equidistant from the centre one; provided the difference between the two interval is small, this can be overcome by using an iterative computing technique as was done by McDonald and Gessner (1968). The relatively small attenuation per cm in the lower frequency terms makes it necessary to use as long an interval as possible and these authors found that a suitably long over-all interval of 15–18 cm without the intervention of major branching could only be achieved in the thoracic aorta and common carotid arteries; even so there was considerable scatter in the results. The method presupposes that the propagation constant is unchanged throughout the length studied, i.e. its elastic properties and internal diameter remain approximately constant. After a few experiments it was decided that the changes in wave-velocity along the thoracic aorta (McDonald, 1968*a*, Fig. 14.3) and the changes in bore (Ch. 2, p. 46) were too great to satisfy this condition and all further experiments were made on the carotid artery. Gabe (personal communication) later made extensive studies on the thoracic aorta and also had difficulties with the problem of homogeneity. These technical limitations clearly restrict the survey of attenuation throughout the arterial tree by this method.

The first predictions of attenuation were made by Bergel (1961*b*) from the measurement of the complex elastic properties of excised vessels. This technique has also been used by Learoyd and Taylor (1966) and extended to the study of arteries *in vivo* by Gow and Taylor (1968). The results from the 3-point method in the thoracic aorta are therefore compared (Fig. 14.14) to those obtained from isolated vessels and also the results obtained by Anliker *et al.* (1968) with a view to establishing norms for future studies on other arteries.

The calculated values for wave velocity and transmission over a 10 cm interval from Bergel (1961*b*) are shown in Fig. 14.6. The values obtained in the excised thoracic aorta (maintained in oxygenated Krebs solution to preserve the viability of the smooth-muscle component) by McDonald and Gessner (1968) are displayed in Fig. 14.13. They are compared to the values obtained by Bergel and also to the attenuation to be expected due to the viscosity of the blood alone when the wall is expected to be purely elastic as in the Womersley formulation discussed in Ch. 11. The curve representing Bergel's results are compatible with those of McDonald and Gessner, although the latter show a higher attenuation, because the wave velocity determined by Bergel was higher (so that 10 cm was a smaller fraction of a wave-length). The value of the attenuation term per wave-length was also compatible with those

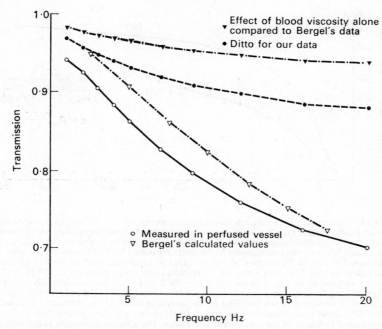

Fig. 14.13. A display of values derived for the attenuation of a pressure wave travelling 10 cm in the thoracic aorta of a dog. The lowest line (–o–) shows the values obtained at frequencies from 1–10 Hz by McDonald and Gessner (1968) in the isolated vessel. They are compared to those calculated by Bergel (1961) for the same vessel and illustrated in Fig. 14.6. (The values calculated by Bergel are indicated by the line -◁–◁–◁)

determined by Anliker *et al.* (1968). This is most simply demonstrated by the calculation of the transmission per wave-length for the thoracic aorta which is displayed graphically against the value of α in Fig. 14.14 (the graph only includes the high frequency values up to 60 Hz as it is known that they remain constant thereafter.) Again, a comparison is made with a graph of the predicted attenuation in a longitudinally restrained elastic tube (an extension of Fig. 11.8). In both Figs. 14.13 and 14.15 the measured attenuation in the artery is much higher (i.e. the transmission is much lower) than that due to the viscosity of the blood alone and the major component is due to the 'viscous' component of the wall.

In the carotid artery the attenuation per wave-length is higher, but, because the wave-velocity is also higher, the attenuation per 10 cm (Fig. 14.15) is comparable to that in the thoracic aorta. Again the larger values in the data of McDonald and Gessner over those of Bergel in the perfused vessel were due, in part, to the fact that in the former case the wave-velocity was about 7 m/sec (Fig. 14.3) while in Bergel's it was somewhat above 9 m/sec (Fig. 14.6). In the *in vivo* carotid the attenuation varied from values close to those in the perfused isolated carotid to values that were considerably higher although

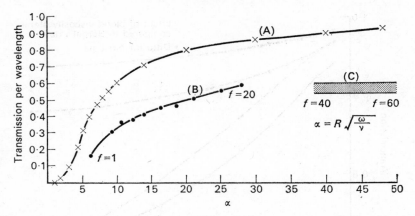

Fig. 14.14. A demonstration of the attenuating properties of the arterial wall over a wide range of values of α. All values are for the dog thoracic aorta. Graph A shows the transmission (which is the complement of the attenuation) of the wave when damping is only due to the viscosity of the blood. Graph B shows the transmission in the aorta measured by McDonald and Gessner (1968) and displayed in Fig. 14.13. Graph C shows the range of values recorded by Anliker, Histand and Ogden (1968) for the frequency range 40–60 Hz (the same range holds up to 120 Hz but is not shown for reasons of space). It is clear that graphs B and C could be reasonably extrapolated together. This again shows that the attenuation due to the viscosity of the blood only contributes one-quarter or one-third of the damping of the travelling wave. In the thoracic aorta the wave-length will be about 10 cm when the frequency is 50 Hz so that a wave-component of the frequency will be damped by about 40 per cent over that distance. The abscissa represents values of α so that the results may be generalized.

the wave-velocity was the same, or somewhat higher. The data on the vessel in the living animal are more limited than in the perfused artery because only the frequency components of the pressure wave could be used and once they became small in the higher harmonics the results were indeterminable. Values for the transmission per wave-length are shown for the carotid artery in Fig. 14.15, which emphasizes how much less the transmission is when compared to Womersley's model. The transmission characteristics are consistent with the values for the carotid artery reported by Moritz (1969). Giving vasoconstrictor drugs tended to increase the attenuation. The findings all tend to support Bergel's conclusion that the viscous element in the wall is largely represented by the smooth-muscle component. In Bergel's experiments the vessel was filled with saline and suspended in air so that the smooth muscle was presumed to be completely relaxed. In McDonald and Gessner's experiments the wall was oxygenated even in the isolated arteries and the somewhat greater attenuation is probably due to the more active state of the smooth muscle.

The data in the dynamic elastic modulus of human arteries recorded by Learoyd and Taylor (1966) is comparable to that of Bergel in dogs and the calculated attenuation is comparable to the values discussed above.

The attenuation in pulmonary vessels has not been measured in any comparable way. The transmission of pressure waves from the main pul-

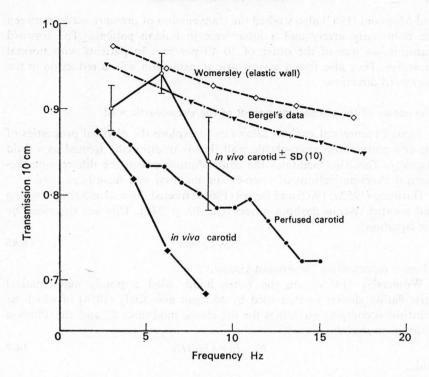

Fig. 14.15. Three sets of values (solid lines) for the transmission over 10 cm in the carotid artery of the dog measured by McDonald and Gessner (1968). The upper two broken lines show respectively the values obtained from the Womersley equations using a perfectly elastic wall and the values calculated by Bergel (1961) in Fig. 14.6. The values obtained by McDonald and Gessner show greater damping and this may be attributed to the fact that the vascular smooth muscle was in a more active state. It is assumed that the smooth muscle contributed a large part of the viscous properties of the arterial wall.

monary artery to a lobar vein was studied by Caro and McDonald (1961) in the perfused rabbit lung. At 3–5 Hz (the frequency of the minimum for the input impedance) the mean pressure oscillation created by the sinusoidal pump was ±0·32 SE; in a lobar vein the amplitude was 0·62 cm H_2O ±0·12 SE. This indicates a transmission of almost 25 per cent. In the experiment with the lowest peripheral resistance the transmission was approx. 45 per cent. Maloney *et al.* (1968) performed somewhat similar experiments in the perfused dog lung but studied lower frequencies and were also concerned with changes in alveolar pressure. They found that oscillatory flow transmission was approx. 75 per cent at 0·03 Hz, approx. 50 per cent at 0·1 Hz and approx. 30 per cent at 1·0 Hz. They also found the same values for transmission from vein to artery although Caro, Bergel, and Seed (1967) had found that transmission was markedly asymmetrical under certain conditions. Caro, Harrison, and Mognoni (1967) also studied the transmission of pressure waves between the pulmonary artery and a lobar vein in human patients. The forward transmission was of the order of 30–40 per cent in patients with normal pressures. They also found asymmetric transmission with a reduction in the backward direction.

The nature of the viscous component of the visco-elastic wall

A further theoretical analysis allows us to explore the physical properties of the component in a visco-elastic wall that is traditionally treated as a fluid viscosity. This also facilitates the comparison between the different mathematical characterizations of visco-elastic material that have been used.

Hardung (1952a, 1962) and Bergel (1961b) treated the wall as a simple spring and parallel viscous dashpot model (Ch. 10, p. 249). This was described by the equation

$$E' = E_{dyn} + i\eta\omega \qquad \textbf{10.45}$$

where η represents a Newtonian viscosity.

Womersley (1955c), on the other hand, used a purely mathematical formulation similar to that used by Morgan and Kiely (1954) in which he substituted complex quantities for the elastic modulus, E, and the Poisson ratio, σ, so that

$$E_c = E(1 + i\omega\Delta E) \qquad \textbf{14.7}$$

and

$$\sigma_c = \sigma(1 + i\omega\Delta\sigma) \qquad \textbf{14.8}$$

The result of this substitution was explored by Taylor (1959b) in his analysis of the visco-elastic properties of a rubber-tube hydraulic model (Ch. 11, p. 303). In place of the Womersley equation for the complex velocity, c, in terms of the Moens–Korteweg velocity, c_0,

$$c_0/c = (X - iY) \qquad \textbf{11.16}$$

we write

$$c_0/c = (X - iY)(1 - i\omega W) \qquad \textbf{11.30}$$

where

$$W = \left(\frac{\Delta E}{2} + \frac{\Delta\sigma}{3} \right) \qquad \textbf{11.31}$$

The phase velocity c_1 is then given by

$$c_1 = \frac{c_0}{X\left(1 - \frac{Y}{X}\omega W\right)} \qquad \textbf{11.32}$$

and, as Taylor showed, the values found for c_1 in the rubber tube approximated closely to those predicted by Womersley for the longitudinally restrained ('tethered') elastic tube (eqn. 11.26).

Similarly, for the transmission per wave-length for the elastic tube, which is

$$\exp - 2\pi \frac{Y}{X} \qquad \textbf{11.18}$$

we write

$$\exp \left[\left(-2\pi\frac{Y}{X} \right) \left(1 + \frac{X}{Y}\omega W \right) \left(1 - \frac{Y}{X}\omega W \right)^{-1} \right] \qquad \textbf{11.33}$$

In terms of the propagation constant

$$\gamma = a + ib \qquad \textbf{11.11}$$

the transmission per wave-length is given by

$$\exp - 2\pi a/b$$

so that from the values of a and b measured by McDonald and Gessner (1968) and the tabulated values of X and Y (Womersley, 1957a) we can calculate the value of ωW from the equation

$$\omega W = \frac{[(a/b)(X/Y)] - 1}{(a/b) + (X/Y)} \qquad \textbf{14.9}$$

The values for ωW calculated for the carotid artery by McDonald and Gessner are shown in Fig. 14.16. It can be seen that they are fairly constant over the whole frequency range; this is true of the comparable values calculated from Bergel's data. The term W is thus strongly frequency dependent as is shown in Fig. 14.17. As W represents the 'viscous' component it can be seen that this behaviour is very different from that of a component with a simple Newtonian viscosity (Ch. 2). To try to account for this in terms of the spring and dashpot model Bergel (personal communication) tested a wide variety of arrays of many spring and dashpot components on a computer in an endeavour to mimic this behaviour but found no satisfactory analogue. Thus, while the term viscous component is used for convenience, it must be realized that it has properties very different from the viscosity normally encountered in liquids.

The relation between the terms incorporated in W and those used in eqn. 10.45 for the single spring and parallel dashpot analogy may be shown in the following way. The elastic modulus of a cylindrical tube maintained at constant length was expressed by Bergel (eqn. 10.38) thus

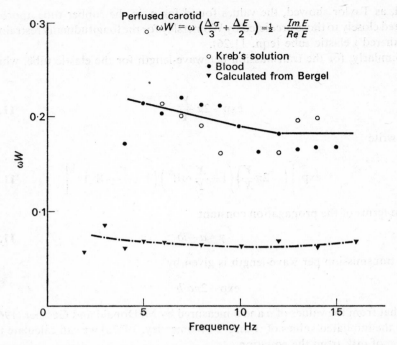

Fig. 14.16. Graphs of the values extracted from the data for transmission in the carotid artery for the function $\omega W = \omega(\varDelta\sigma/3 + \varDelta E/2)$ where $\varDelta\sigma$ and $\varDelta E$ are the imaginary parts of Poisson ratio and the elastic modulus ωW is thus equivalent to the Hardung formulation $\eta\omega$ (p. 251) where η is taken as the viscosity of the arterial wall.

The lines of our data are both almost parallel to the abscissa, so that ωW shows little frequency dependence. (From McDonald and Gessner, 1968.)

$$E = \frac{\varDelta P}{\varDelta R} \cdot \frac{2(1 - \sigma^2)r^2 R}{R^2 - r^2}$$

where R is the external radius and r the internal radius.

If a viscous element is introduced into the wall there will be a phase difference, φ, between $\varDelta P$ and $\varDelta R$. Thus we can write

$$\frac{\varDelta P}{\varDelta R} = \frac{\varDelta P'}{\varDelta R'} \cdot e^{i\phi} = \frac{E_c}{(1 - \sigma_c^2)} \cdot \frac{(R^2 - r^2)}{2r^2 R} \qquad \textbf{14.10}$$

By comparing this with Hardung's complex elastic modulus (eqn. 10.45) we see that

$$E' = E_c = E_{\mathrm{dyn}}(1 + i\eta\omega/E_{\mathrm{dyn}}) = E_{\mathrm{dyn}}(1 + i\omega\varDelta E)$$

and by treating the complex Poisson ratio, σ_c, in a similar way,

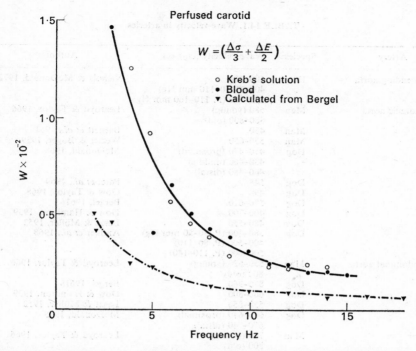

Fig. 14.17. Graphs to show the values of the term W representing the viscous element in the arterial wall at frequencies from 2–20 Hz. These values have been extracted from the data of Fig. 14.16. It can be seen that the value of the viscous term falls markedly with increase of frequency. It is thus very different in behaviour from the viscosity of a liquid and is unlike that of most plastic solids. It is to this property of arterial wall viscosity that we may attribute the unique behaviour of the arterial wall in which wave-velocity and attenuation per wave length do not vary with frequency. (From McDonald and Gessner, 1968.)

$$\frac{\Delta P'}{\Delta R'} \cdot e^{i\varphi} = \frac{(R^2 - r^2)}{2r^2 R} \cdot \frac{E_{\mathrm{dyn}}}{1 - \sigma^2_{\mathrm{dyn}}} [1 + i(\Delta E + \tfrac{2}{3}\Delta\sigma)] \qquad \textbf{14.11}$$

and when $\sigma = 0.5$ we find that

$$\tan \varphi = \frac{\eta\omega}{E_{\mathrm{dyn}}} = \omega(\Delta E + \tfrac{2}{3}\Delta\sigma) = 2\omega W \qquad \textbf{14.12}$$

or,

$$\omega W = \tfrac{1}{2} \tan \varphi \qquad \textbf{14.13}$$

where φ is the phase component of the dynamic elastic modulus measured by Bergel.

While this analysis shows that there now exists a reasonable structure on which to base studies of the visco-elastic properties of arteries it is a field in which a lot more experimental information is required. Data on the wave-

TABLE 14.1. Wave-velocity in arteries

Artery	Species	Wave-velocity (cm/sec)	Authors
Ascending aorta	Dog	400–404	Nichols & McDonald, 1972
		400 (P. 50–110 mm Hg)	
		429–500 (P. 110–160 mm Hg)	
Thoracic aorta	Man	580 (young)	Learoyd & Taylor, 1966
		680–800 (old)	
	Man	480	Barnett et al., 1961
	Man	550–650	Wezler & Böger, 1939
	Dog	410–470 (proximal)	McDonald, 1968
		430–460 (middle)	
		460–480 (distal)	
	Dog	548	Patel et al., 1969
	Dog	490	Gow & Taylor, 1968
	Dog	570–610	Bergel, 1961b
	Dog	400–700	Dow & Hamilton, 1939
	Dog	480–550	Laszt & Müller, 1952
	Dog	380–400 (P. 30–80 mm Hg)	Anliker et al., 1968
		400–500 (P. 80–110)	
		500–600 (P. 110–140)	
Abdominal aorta	Man	550–620 (young)	Learoyd & Taylor, 1966
		800 (old)	
	Dog	870–960	Bergel, 1961b
	Dog	600–800	Dow & Hamilton, 1939
	Dog	550–850	Laszt & Müller, 1952
	Dog	600–640 (proximal)	McDonald, 1968
		670–740 (distal)	
Iliac	Man	700 (young)	Learoyd & Taylor, 1966
		800 (old)	
	Dog	700–800	McDonald, 1968
Femoral	Man	1,800 (young)	Learoyd & Taylor, 1968
		1,300 (old)	
	Man	800	Kapal et al. (1951)
	Dog	800–1,200	Dow & Hamilton, 1939
	Dog	850–1,300	Laszt & Müller, 1952
	Dog	830–1,030	McDonald, 1968
Popliteal	Dog	1,220–1,310	McDonald, 1968
Tibial	Dog	1,040–1,430	McDonald, 1968
Carotid	Man	800–1,200	Bramwell et al., 1923
	Dog	610–740 (proximal)	McDonald, 1968
		700–780 (distal)	
	Dog	860–970	Bergel (1961a)
	Dog	1,000–1,100	Moritz, 1969
Pulmonary	Man	182	Caro & Harrison, 1962
	Man	168	Milnor et al., 1969
	Dog	267–275	Bargainer (1967)
Measurements over long segments			**Data from Bergel, 1960**
Carotid to femoral	Man	450–500	Broemser & Ranke, 1930
Carotid to femoral	Man	500–600	Hallock, 1934
Femoral to dorsalis pedis	Man	900	Bazett & Dryer, 1922
		880	Bazett, et al., 1935
Brachial to radial	Man	850	Bazett & Dryer, 1922
Carotid to radial	Man	500–600	Hickson & McSwiney, 1925
Carotid to radial	Man	600	Hemingway et al., 1928
Carotid to radial	Man	600–700	Hallock, 1934
Carotid to brachial	Man	470	Fulton & McSwiney, 1930
Brachial to radial	Man	870	Fulton & McSwiney, 1930
Carotid to radial	Man	900	Bazett et al., 1935
Carotid to radial	Man	750–900	Wezler & Böger, 1936

velocity of arteries of dogs is still of a piecemeal nature while in the human it can only be described as sketchy. The energy dissipation during wave travel which is expressed as attenuation is probably the most important parameter in arterial haemodynamics which has received very little attention and which can only be examined experimentally. The unusual visco-elastic properties of arteries compared to those of synthetic plastics, for example, make the analysis of theoretical models of the arterial wall virtually useless without more experimental data.

15
Methods of Monitoring Cardiac Output in Man

In terms of the practical clinical application of haemodynamic studies the problems associated with the care of patients suffering from coronary infarction, or during the immediate post-operative period following myocardinal infarction, are pre-eminent.

The introduction of cardiac catheterization in the late 1940s made possible the reliable measurement of cardiac output using the Fick principle, or indicator-dilution methods. Both these techniques, however, average the output over a period of time and cannot follow the ventricular ejection on a beat-to-beat basis. Also, they can only be repeated at intervals.

In the acutely ill patient the desirability of monitoring parameters of ventricular function continuously has long been appreciated. The development of manometers that could measure arterial pressure accurately through catheters that were small enough to introduce intra-arterially and leave in position throughout the acute period of the patient's illness naturally led to a concentration of methods for deriving flow from pressure. The introduction of the electro-magnetic flowmeter as a standard method for measuring arterial flow did not, in effect, change this situation because the conventional flow probe required surgical procedures for both placing it on the artery, and later, removing it. It has, however, been used on occasion during surgical operations. The recent development of catheter-tipped flowmeters (Ch. 9) has raised hopes of a more direct method of monitoring flow than in the methods deriving it from pressure, but their reliability in patients has not, to date, been tested in a systematic fashion.

The aim of any technique used to monitor the heart output on a beat-to-beat basis is, naturally, to obtain as much information as possible about the *functional state of the ventricle*. Methods to be discussed below can be said to fall loosely into two categories in this respect—those that can only measure stroke volume and those that measure the pulsatile flow pattern throughout systole. Where these are derived from aortic pressure records the correspondence between pressures and flows are, of course, available. This means that if stroke volume alone is measured estimates of the peripheral resistance and the external work per stroke may also be made. If the pulsatile flow curve and the pressure pulse curve can be recorded then not only the stroke work and peripheral resistance, but also the continuous power output and the input impedance, can be recorded. Parameters derived from these records, such as the peak acceleration of flow or external power, or peak power output, can be regarded as giving us more information about ventricular performance than that from the stroke volume alone. Noble *et al.* (1966) put forward evidence that the maximum acceleration of flow was the best single parameter indicating the contractile state of the ventricular muscle; from physical principles the peak power output, or the rate of rise of the power output, would be more reliable and has been under investigation in this laboratory (Boone, 1972). While the clinical value of such secondary parameters has not been adequately tested the possibilities for the future need to be born in mind when assessing methods for monitoring patients. It has been clear throughout the survey of haemodynamics in this book that an adequate measure of circulatory conditions requires simultaneous information about both pressure and flow. This has, in part, been one of the limitations in the application of intra-arterial flow probes; in some forms there has been no provision for simultaneous pressure measurement, while in others measurement of pressure is difficult due to the necessity of making the whole assembly so small.

The necessity for making the measurements on ventricular output immediately available have, in the past, placed a heavy premium on simplicity of methods of calculation. The widespread availability of digital computers in special centres such as intensive care units where data measured in acutely ill patients is continuously processed on-line by a computer (e.g. Sheppard *et al.* 1968), has enormously widened the scope of methods that may be used, in terms of complexity of the calculations required, and of the possibility of deriving secondary parameters such as those discussed above. The discussion of such methods can therefore be widened, and made more realistic in terms of possible application than in a previous outline by McDonald (1960).

THE ASSESSMENT OF ACCURACY OF METHODS USED

In assessing any method of measurement it is clearly necessary to know the probable error of the standards against which it is compared. This is especially so in considering the methods of deriving flow from pressure because of the uncertainties in measuring flow by any method. If the two methods to be compared are not used simultaneously, there are additional factors to consider in the minor fluctuations that undoubtedly occur in the cardiac output even when the circulatory system is in a stable steady-state. The variation with the phases of respiration is the best known and defined of these. In addition, there seems little doubt that there is a small random fluctuation in the volume ejected during successive cardiac cycles. Even with dogs in an extremely stable circulatory condition with no detectable respiratory variation personal measurements of the largest harmonic components of the pressure pulse in the aorta have shown that there is rarely a standard error of less than ± 5 per cent; this variation in pressure oscillation almost certainly represents a similar fluctuation in ventricular output. In a method such as the indicator-dilution technique which measures the total flow over a period of time the estimate of stroke volume during this period will necessarily be an average which may differ appreciably from estimates by a pressure method which measures the output during a single beat. As in several methods in current use it will be seen below that an initial indicator-dilution estimate is used to calibrate unknown factors in equations, e.g. the cross-sectional area of the aorta, so that this limit to precision must be borne in mind. Conversely, the presence of small variations in ventricular output puts a limit on the possible or useful accuracy in methods of measuring the volume ejected in individual beats; in other words a decision needs to be made as to how large a change in stroke volume or peak flow is physiologically or clinically significant.

In this laboratory, before initiating an extensive study of various methods by which flow may be derived from pressure, some attempt was made to estimate the inherent error in the methods used for comparison. Using a digital computer programme to analyse the dye curve, the flow measured by indicator-dilution was compared by Kerr and Kouchoukos between pairs of estimates made during the same period. The right atrium was the site of injection and simultaneous curves were recorded of the flow in the central aorta and in the femoral artery. The correlation coefficient (r) was 0·985 and the regression line was $y = 0·937x + 88·0$ ml/min, SE $= \pm 7$ per cent ($N = 60$) (see Kouchoukos, Sheppard and McDonald, 1970). The standard error here is essentially the same as the best that has been recorded in the literature. As the electromagnetic flowmeter was used as the standard in most investigations of the last decade a comparison was then made between our electromagnetic flowmeter (Statham-Medicon) and simultaneous indicator-dilution measurements. The results were $r = 0·98$, $y = 0·922x + 182$ ml/min, SE $= \pm 10$ per cent ($N = 31$).

It is seen that the SE of the flowmeter against the indicator-dilution method is somewhat greater than those inherent in the latter method alone. The calibration of the electromagnetic flowmeter electrically and in hydraulic models has already been discussed in Ch. 9. The result here indicates that some additional variability is created in the living animal with the probe in place on an artery. Speculation as to the causes of this error does not seem likely to be fruitful as it may be due to the short-circuitry effect through the body fluids analysed by Gessner (1961), asymmetry of flow in the ascending aorta, variability of contact with changes of pressure or other causes. What is apparent is that one is unlikely to find a smaller SE than ± 10 per cent with any method which is compared with the electromagnetic flowmeter.

PULSE CONTOUR OR WINDKESSEL MODELS

The formulas for calculating the stroke volume (SV) from the aortic pressure that fall under this heading are very numerous. The theoretical basis cannot be adequately scrutinized without a detailed discussion of the Windkessel theory largely built up during the earlier years of this century by Otto Frank (1899) and his pupils in Germany; later developments in America were made principally by Remington and Hamilton and their co-workers (Remington, 1952). The subject was reviewed at length by Wezler and Böger (1939) and an excellent recent account is given by Wetterer and Kenner (1968) so that only a brief and simple summary of the principles underlying them are given here.

In this approach the pressure pulse is treated as a transient phenomenon with the system completely at rest at the end of diastole. The systolic rise of pressure is regarded as due to the simultaneous distension of a single elastic chamber (or Windkessel) represented by the larger 'elastic' arteries. In later modifications this excitation was assumed to travel back and forth over the Windkessel creating a 'resonance' or 'fundamental vibration' (Grund-schwingung) which gave rise to the phenomenon of the dicrotic wave seen during diastole in the peripheral arteries. The length of the Windkessel was calculated by the period between this wave and the systolic peak, although there was considerable dispute among different investigators as to whether the termination of the chamber should be regarded as creating an open or closed-end reflection (Wezler and Böger, 1939). As this determined whether the resonance was over a quarter or a half wave-length the difference between the two estimates was large. An example of such a formula is one derived by Frank (1930) and later used by Wezler and Böger (1939) which may be written (with a change of symbols to those used in this book)

$$SV = \frac{\Delta P . A . T}{2\rho c} \qquad \textbf{15.1}$$

where ΔP is the pulse pressure, A the cross-sectional area of the aorta, ρ the density of the blood, c the mean wave-velocity between the central aorta and the femoral artery and T the period of the 'fundamental vibration'. Another formula due to Broemser and Ranke (1931) which did not include the concept of the 'fundamental vibration' was

$$SV = K \frac{\Delta P . A . T_S . T_C}{\rho . c . T_D} \qquad \textbf{15.2}$$

where terms common to eqn. 15.1 have the same meaning and T_S, T_D and T_C are, respectively, the duration of systole, diastole, and the entire cycle (i.e. $T_S + T_D$). K is a constant calculated from dimensional criteria. These two formulas were tested by Starr and Schild (1957) by injecting a known volume into the ascending aorta of a cadaver. The correlation coefficient (r) for eqn. 15.1 was 0·64 with a regression line $y = 0·21x + 25$ ml $\pm 11·0$ ml SD; this standard deviation was ± 24 per cent. A similar scatter was found with eqn. 15.2. Starr and Schild (1957) found that the correlation coefficient was actually increased to 0·74 (regression line $y = 0·34x + 8$ ml ± 8 ml SD) by reducing the RHS of eqn. 15.1 to only $\Delta P/c$.

The Georgia group (Remington and Hamilton, 1945, 1947; Remington, Hamilton and Dow, 1945; Hamilton and Remington, 1947; Remington et al., 1948, and Remington, 1952) studied the problem in detail, especially in terms of the non-uniform elasticity of the arterial tree. By this means they quantitated the time course of the distension of the elastic chamber. This led to the concept (Remington, 1952) of 'serial' Windkessels. They also tested the relation of the pulse pressure alone to the stroke volume. Hamilton (1953, 1962) regarded this as good a measure of stroke volume and stated that the pulse pressure (in mm Hg) was approximately equal to the stroke index (ml/m^2 of body surface). Remington (1954) also published a table by which the cardiac index could be predicted from the pulse pressure. Brotmacher (1957) compared the cardiac output in patients measured by the Fick principle with that calculated by the formula of Starr et al. (1953), that of Remington et al. (1948) and the pulse-pressure relation of Hamilton (1953). He also reviewed comparisons made by previous workers. The results were not subjected to statistical analysis but the results using the method of Remington et al. (1948) were somewhat better than the others. Of 107 patients at rest, the discrepancy was less than 1·0 l/min in 47 and greater than 2·1 l/min in 36 (the corresponding figures for the Starr method was 38 and 44, and for the Hamilton method 41 and 38 respectively).

Simpler approaches than that of the full mathematical derivations of the Windkessel theory have also been used. These are based on the concept that the rise in pressure is a linear measure of the increased volume injected while the rate of drainage through the capillary bed is given by the rate of fall in pressure during diastole. One such method introduced by Warner et al. (1953) has, in a somewhat modified form, been used to monitor cardiac patients (Warner, Gardner, and Toronto, 1968). In this method the increment of pressure over the whole arterial bed is defined as the 'end-systolic mean distending pressure' (Pmd) so that the systolic uptake is

$$\text{Uptake} = \text{Pmd} \times K \qquad 15.3$$

where K is a constant of proportionality.

To average the pressure over the whole bed the transmission time was measured between the central aorta and the femoral artery. In the later paper, it was standardized at 80 msec. The difference between the mean pressure during the last 80 msec of systole and the last 80 msec of diastole in the central aortic pulse defined the term Pmd. The drainage from the bed during systole (Sd) was defined by the ratios of the areas under the pressure curve during systole (Sa) and diastole (Da) respectively (again treating the systolic drainage as beginning 80 msec before the initial systolic rise in pressure and diastolic drainage starting 80 msec before the closure of the aortic valves). The areas were calculated from a level of 20 mm Hg above zero; this is based on the statement by Remington, Hamilton, and Dow (1945) that flow out of the arterial bed ceases at a mean arterial pressure of 20 mm Hg (Guyton, on the other hand, e.g. Guyton, 1966, gives 7 mm Hg as the equilibrium pressure).

The systolic drainage is thus given by

$$Sd = \frac{Sa}{Da}. Uptake \qquad \textbf{15.4}$$

and this needs to be added to the uptake represented by eqn. 15.3. Then, substituting the term for uptake from 15.3, the equation for stroke volume becomes

$$SV = K \times Pmd + \frac{Sa}{Da}. K. Pmd = K. Pmd \left(1 + \frac{Sa}{Da}\right) \qquad \textbf{15.5}$$

The 1953 paper tested this in thirteen patients (forty-four determinations) by comparing the results with cardiac outputs measured by the Fick or indicator-dilution methods. Comparisons were made at rest, during moderate exercise, and during a 70° body tilt. The comparison showed that the method predicted the direction of change in output correctly in all cases and this was the declared purpose of the method. In terms of quantitative comparison the standard deviation was ± 10 per cent.

The important idea introduced by this paper was that the constant K could be determined experimentally for each subject by comparing the pressure estimate with the first measurement by the standard method. Previous pressure methods had predicted any constant of this sort either from theoretical considerations (e.g. the period of the 'fundamental vibration', eqn. 15.1) or from generalized values for arterial distensibility as in the various Remington methods. By determining K empirically for each patient individual variations between subjects could be accounted for. This modification has been used in most subsequent methods.

In the later survey by Warner *et al.* (1968) eqn. 15.4 had been modified by using the square root of the distending pressure in place of the actual value, so that the equation became

$$SV = K_1 \sqrt{(Pmd)}. (1 + Sa/Da) \qquad \textbf{15.6}$$

No reason was given for the substitution.

The authors reported that, in humans, 'measurements by the two methods agreed as well as repeated determinations by the dye method', over a range of heart rates from 55–120 beats/min and during rest and exercise. In dogs under a variety of circulatory changes the correlation coefficient ranged from 0·90–0·98 in individual experiments.

Warner et al. (1953) also compared the results from using eqn. 15.4 with other simpler formulations including the pulse-pressure alone. They obtained the best results with their own method.

USE OF THE 'WATER-HAMMER' FORMULA

The so-called 'water-hammer' equation of hydrodynamics appears to have been first derived by Allievi (1909); it has already been introduced in Ch. 10. In its simplest form for a thin-walled elastic tube, filled with an inviscid liquid of density ρ, the pressure of a transient pulse is given by

$$P = \rho . \bar{V} . c \qquad \text{11.1}$$

where c is the velocity of wave propagation and $\bar{V}$ is the average velocity across the tube of the rate of flow created. As $\bar{V}$ is $Q/\pi R^2$ this substitution may be made and, by rearrangement, we have

$$Q = \frac{P . \pi R^2}{\rho c} \qquad \text{15.7}$$

The analogy with eqn. 15.1 is clear; eqn. 15.7 gives the rate of volume flow and, in the Frank formula (15.1), the stroke volume is calculated by multiplying by $T/2$ (half the period of the 'fundamental vibration').

Equation 15.7 may be generalized to include the effects of viscosity in the liquid and the Poisson's ratio of the wall from the equation for the characteristic impedance (Chs. 6 and 13):

$$\frac{P}{Q} = Z_0 = \frac{\rho c_0}{\pi R^2 (1 - \sigma^2)^{\frac{1}{2}} (M'_{10})^{\frac{1}{2}}} e^{j\epsilon_{10}/2} \qquad \text{6.26}$$

or

$$Q = \frac{P . \pi R^2 (1 - \sigma^2)^{\frac{1}{2}} . (M'_{10})^{\frac{1}{2}}}{\rho c_0} e^{j\epsilon_{10}/2} \qquad \text{15.8}$$

The value of $(M'_{10})^{1/2}$ tends to 1·0 in the limit as the parameter α becomes large, i.e. as viscosity tends to zero.

The water-hammer formula was discussed in a brief paper by Evans (1958) who found a reasonable prediction of the results of Warner et al. (1953). It was also emphasized by McDonald and Taylor (1959) and McDonald (1960). The latter pointed out that it provides the rationale for using the pulse-pressure as a measure of stroke volume. Provided the rise in pressure in systole is not modified by reflection, eqn. 15.7 shows its relation to the peak flow velocity during systolic ejection. If the assumption is made that the peak velocity varies directly as the stroke volume then it will also provide a prediction of the latter. Experimental evidence appears to show that the ejection flow wave form is approximately triangular, and does not greatly vary from this. Therefore, provided that the length of systole does not vary, there is some basis for this assumption. On the other hand, if the pulse-pressure represented only the pressure generated by the peak flow during ejection the peaks on the two curves would coincide. Figure 12.2 has shown that they do not.

A survey of possible methods for deriving the ventricular outflow from pressure measurements were initiated in this laboratory in 1967. For clinical use any method that uses a single pressure channel has advantages and, to start with, a pressure-contour method was chosen. The method chosen for the first test in dogs was one of those tested by Warner *et al.* (1953). It was

$$SV = K.Psa\,(1 + T_S/T_D) \qquad\qquad \textbf{15.9}$$

where K is an arbitrary constant derived by an initial comparison with a standard method (as introduced by Warner *et al.*, 1953). Psa is the 'systolic area of pressure'; this is the area above the diastolic pressure and below the systolic part of the aortic pressure curve and limited by a vertical line through the incisura marking the closure of the aortic valves (Fig. 15.1).

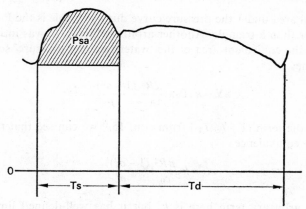

Fig. 15.1. A diagram to show the measurements of the Pressure-systolic area—Psa—used to calculate stroke volume. The area is under the systolic portion of the pressure pulse that is above the minimal diastolic pressure and limited by a vertical line drawn through the incisura which marks the closure of the aortic valves. (From Kouchoukos *et al.*, 1970.)

T_S and T_D are the respective lengths of systole and diastole. The results of this investigation have been reported by Kouchoukos, Sheppard, and McDonald (1970) and are discussed below. While the approach had initially been that of an empirical test the results were sufficiently encouraging to attempt to analyse the equation further with a view to determine the components incorporated in the term K, in order to give an insight into the conditions that made some of the results unreliable.

The term $(1 + T_S/T_D)$ derives from a formulation by Remington (1952) and is designed to allow for the fact that there is drainage out of the aorta during systole (see Fig. 12.2). In other words, the 'water-hammer' is conceived as imposed on a tube in which the pressure is falling. It cannot be deduced from eqn. 15.8; it was retained because, although testing showed that the omission of the term did not greatly change the statistical correlation, it was, in most cases, better when this term was used.

The derivation made started with eqn. 15.8 with the further approximation that M'_{10} was given the value of 1.0. Again, making the approximation (for simplicity) that the form of the flow curve is triangular (see Fig. 12.2) the stroke volume is given by

$$SV = \tfrac{1}{2}.T_S.\hat{Q} \qquad\qquad\qquad \textbf{15.10}$$

where $\hat{Q}$ is the peak flow.

If the pressure were solely determined by the rate of ventricular ejection, the equivalent area under the pressure could be written in the same form and we would write (from eqn. 15.8)

$$SV = (\tfrac{1}{2}T_S.)\dot{P}\pi \, \frac{R^2}{c_0}.\frac{(1-\sigma^2)^{\frac{1}{2}}}{\rho} \qquad\qquad \textbf{15.11}$$

The actual area under the pressure curve during systole is the Psa which is clearly larger than a triangle. Another arbitrary factor, k, was introduced to reduce it to the equivalent area of the 'water-hammer pressure' so that eqn. 15.11 becomes

$$SV = k.\text{Psa}.\frac{\pi R^2}{c_0}.\frac{(1-\sigma^2)^{\frac{1}{2}}}{\rho} \qquad\qquad \textbf{15.12}$$

Omitting the term $(1 + T_S/T_D)$ from eqn. 15.9 we can see that the term K now has the equivalence

$$K = k.\frac{\pi R^2}{c_0}.\frac{(1-\sigma^2)^{\frac{1}{2}}}{\rho} \qquad\qquad \textbf{15.13}$$

The only arbitrary term here is k, but it has well-defined limits. If the pressure curve is rectangular and the flow curve triangular then it will have the value 0·5; if both are the same geometrical shape then it will be 1·0. In a series of pressure and flow curves that were measured its value ranged from 0·58 to 0·74 so that its variation is limited. It increases under conditions of peripheral vasoconstriction when the distributed reflection contribution to the central pressure wave is greater (Ch. 12).

Of the other terms in eqn. 15.12 it was seen (Ch. 10) that the value of the Poisson ratio, σ, is very close to 0·5; the value of the density of blood was taken as 1·05. The values to be taken for the cross-section area, πR^2, and the wave-velocity, c_0, need further consideration. As the derivation hinges on the value of the peak flow, $\hat{Q}$, the arteries to be considered are those traversed by the pressure wave from the beginning of flow ejection to the time of peak flow, which is of the order of 60 msec. From values for wave-velocity given in Ch. 14, it is found that the distance travelled in that time in the aorta is approximately that from the heart to the diaphragm. Thus the ascending and thoracic aorta will be involved plus equivalent lengths of the arteries to the head and fore-limbs. From measurements of the cross-sectional area of the ascending aorta and the relative sizes of the other vessels, given in Ch. 2, a weighted mean value for the area πR^2 was calculated; a similar mean value for c_0 was also approximated. The values of K thus predicted from eqn. 15.12 (after conversion from CGS to those in which K was empirically calibrated) were from 0·92–3·68; the measured values ranged from $K = 0·89$–3·37. In view of the approximations necessarily made, the agreement is good enough to support the general validity of the derivation. In a subsequent study on patients by Kouchoukos, Sheppard, McDonald and Kirklin (1969) it was found that the K values were larger in proportion to the larger size of the aorta in humans.

As the method using pulse pressure as the measure of stroke volume is, as noted, also related to the water-hammer formula it was also tested in dogs by Kouchoukos *et al.* (1970). As anticipated from the restrictive assumptions on which it is based, the correlation remained reasonably good while the pulse-frequency and peripheral resistance remained fairly constant. As the summary below shows, the circulatory conditions and stroke volume were deliberately varied over as wide a range as possible and, under these circumstances, the correlation of pulse pressure was consistently worse than that determined by the area method.

Kouchoukos *et al.* (1970) studied twelve dogs in which the heart rate ranged from 35 (vagal stimulation) to 207 beats/min (pacing of sinoatrial node). The mean arterial pressure was varied from 24 (haemorrhage or occlusion of the inferior cava) to 166 mm Hg (nor-adrenaline or dextran infusion). The total range of the measured stroke volume was from 2·4–28·1 ml. For a total of 541 cardiac cycles studied the correlation coefficient was 0·93; the regression line was SV (Psa) = 1·04 SV (emf) + 0·21 ml ± SEE 1·75 ml (± 17·4 per cent of mean); the mean SV (emf) was 9·46 ml compared to the mean SV (Psa) of 10·06 ml. This line, with the 95 per cent confidence limits of the mean value, is illustrated in Fig. 15.2.

The regression line was eminently satisfactory but the SEE indicated that there was a larger scatter than is desirable in a method on which to base clinical judgments. On analysis of the results of the individual interventions used it was found that while in those that solely modified cardiac output the correlation was good, the use of drugs that acted on vascular smooth muscle caused very poor correlation between the derived and measured stroke volumes. Thus with dextran infusion, $r = 0·97$, with vagal stimulation, $r = 0·99$,

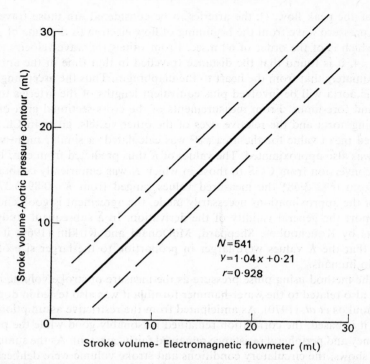

Fig. 15.2. The regression line and Standard Error of Estimate of the means (parallel broken lines) for all the points measured by Kouchoukos *et al.* (1970).

with atrial pacing, $r = 0.98$, with occlusion of the inferior vena cava, $r = 0.97$; on the other hand, infusion of norepinephrine gave $r = 0.77$ (slope 0.72, intercept $+2.38$ ml); isoproterenol gave $r = 0.70$ (slope 0.51, intercept $+6.30$ ml) and metaraminol (Aramine) $r = 0.77$ (slope 0.85, intercept $+2.10$ ml). Figure 15.3 illustrates the results with venous occlusion and with isoproterenol.

These drugs caused considerable changes in the peripheral resistance. In assessing the components of the factor K (eqn. 15.13) this would create an increased reflected component in the Psa area and alter the arbitrary constant, k. However, this did not alter sufficiently to account for a very large proportion of the discrepancy. Of the other terms the factor $\pi R^2/c_0$ is the only one that can change. With an increase of mean arterial pressure the area πR^2 will increase. Owing to the non-linear elastic properties of the arterial wall (Chs. 10 and 14) it becomes stiffer with increasing distension. Thus with an increase of πR^2 the value of c_0 also increases so that the ratio of the two changes much less than they both do individually. Using the data of Anliker *et al.* (1968) it was calculated that over a pressure change from 100–150 mm Hg there would be a negligible change in the value of $\pi R^2/c_0$. In discussing

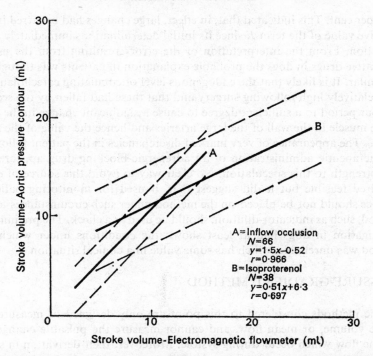

Fig. 15.3. The regression lines and variability for two of the interventions in the series illustrated in Fig. 15.2. The data for occlusion of venous inflow shows that if the cardiac output alone is altered the prediction of stroke volume by the Psa method remains accurate. The data for the intervention with isoproterenol shows that a drug which alters the condition of the peripheral circulation causes prediction of stroke volume to become very poor. This is attributed to the change in arteriolar diameter which alters the reflected wave component and also changes in the elastic behaviour of the large arteries due to changes in vascular smooth muscle tone. (From Kouchoukos *et al.*, 1970.)

the effects of the smooth muscle in the arterial wall (Ch. 10) it was shown that contraction of this muscle component could increase the effective elastic modulus of the wall without changing the radius. Kouchoukos *et al.* (1970) thus postulated that this was the cause of failure of the method when vaso-active drugs were used.

Following the successful tests in the dog the method was used for the study of patients in the immediate post-operative period following cardiac surgery. All were in an Intensive Care Unit where the measurements made were fed on-line to an IBM 1800 digital computer. Parallel paired indicator-dilution (cardiogreen) estimations were made at intervals. During the first 24 hours after operation 95 determinations by both methods were made in 31 patients. The statistical analysis was $r = 0.95$, $y = 1.07x - 1.8$ ml with SEE ± 16 per cent (range of stroke volumes 15–98 ml). This compared very favourably with the results in dogs. In the second 24 hours after operation 24 determinations were made in 12 patients and here $r = 0.70$, $y = 0.70x + 6.8$ ml and the SEE

P

± 31 per cent. This indicated that, in effect, large changes had occurred in the effective value of the term K since its initial determinations immediately after operation. From the interpretation of the errors resulting from the use of vasocative drugs in dogs the probable explanation in patients was thought to be similar. It is likely that the endogenous level of circulating catecholamines was relatively high following surgery and that these had fallen by the second 24-hour period to a sufficient degree to cause a significant change in the tone of the muscle in the wall of the large arteries and hence the value of the term $\pi R^2/c_0$. The appearance of very marked discrepancies in the patient following the therapeutic administration of an adrenergic-blocking drug appeared to lend strength to this speculation. No clear way to avoid this source of error appeared feasible but it did suggest that, if used for monitoring patients, reliance should not be placed on the method under such circumstances and a method, such as indicator-dilution, should be used as a check. The preliminary investigation in dogs had at least shown the conditions under which the method was unreliable, which has some value in a clinical situation.

PRESSURE-GRADIENT METHOD

All the methods considered to this point are only designed to measure the stroke volume, or mean flow, and cannot measure the pulsatile changes in volume flow which occur during systole. Moreover, their derivation in some cases assumes a certain form for the flow curve and so cannot be used to predict it. The fact that the stroke volume is an integral of the oscillatory flow curve makes it less susceptible to errors introduced by the use of broad assumptions. As pointed out at the beginning of this chapter much more additional information about ventricular function is available if both the pulsatile pressure and flow wave forms are known. While the physiological significance of such features as the fluctuations of power output have only been casually explored, it seems to be an important field to study. It may not prove to be as informative as studies of intra-ventricular parameters but the risk to patients from instruments introduced into already diseased hearts is very much higher than that from catheters only introduced as far as the ascending aorta.

The only parameter of pressure which can be used to predict the time course of arterial flow reliably is the pressure-gradient. This relation is based on sound hydrodynamic principles with a minimum of primary assumptions (Ch. 6). This requires the measurement of two pressures separated by a small, known, interval. In the past this was a considerable limitation because, although double-lumen catheters were available, they were rather large and apt to cause arterial damage at the site of introduction. However, for some years now double-lumen catheters have been available which are no bigger than many single lumen ones commonly introduced intra-arterially (e.g. the

Fox-Fry catheter, USCI, Glen Falls, N.Y.). Their use requires more care in ensuring a good frequency response, but we have been using it routinely in our laboratory without difficulty. Catheters fitted with two microtransducers are now available for this purpose (e.g. Millar Instruments Co., Houston, Texas). Because the amplitude of the pressure-gradient is very small in comparison to the total pressure the calibration and matching of the two manometers must be accurate. To increase the amplitude the interval between pressure measurements is made as large as possible but is restricted by the distance between major branches. This creates especial difficulty in the ascending aorta of the dog where the available distance between the aortic valve and the origin of the brachiocephalic artery is commonly only 3 cm, and rarely more than 4 cm. In man, however, the longer ascending aorta does not create so severe a problem and a 5 cm interval can easily be used (Barnett, Greenfield and Fox, 1961). Although, for precision in testing methods, Fry and his colleagues have often used somewhat larger intervals they have recorded good results with 4 cm intervals (e.g. Greenfield and Fry, 1965a).

However, many workers have preferred to derive the pressure-gradient from the time-derivative of the pressure and much of the discussion below will be concerned with the additional approximations that this involves.

The use of the true pressure-gradient to measure outflow from the ventricle has largely stemmed from Fry's laboratory, using the equation (6.11) introduced by Fry, Mallos, and Casper (1956). It was first used in humans by Barnett, Greenfield and Fox (1961). Until 1962 when they had established the reliability and accuracy of the Kolin-type electromagnetic flowmeter (Greenfield et al., 1962) they had no way to check the accuracy of their predicted results. The first tests against a flowmeter were by Greenfield, Patel, Barnett, and Fox (1962) and by Jones and Griffin (1962); in both these papers the time derivative of the pressure was used. The sources of possible error in their gradient method were discussed by Greenfield and Fry (1962), and later Greenfield and Fry (1965a) made a careful comparison of the flows derived by the Fry and the Womersley equations with those measured, in the thoracic aorta of the dog, by an electromagnetic flowmeter. The comparison was expressed in terms of the means of the amplitude and phase difference of each of the first 5 harmonics in each of the six dogs that they studied. The agreement between all three sets of results was good, although that between the two calculated flows was somewhat better than either of them with the recorded flow. This appears to be the only direct comparison between the Fry and Womersley equations applied to the pressure-gradient in the aorta. The pulsatile flow in the ascending aorta was derived by the Womersley equation in man for the purpose of calculating the input impedance by Gabe, Karnell, Porjé and Rurewald (1964)—see Ch. 13, p. 366. This showed its feasibility in man although it was not tested against any other method. To simplify the calculations required Gabe (1965*a*, *b*) has developed a method where they can be rapidly solved on an analogue computer.

The first reported measurement of pressure-gradient was by Porjé and Rudewald in 1957. They developed their own equation for computing flow which was, in essence, an integration of the pressure-gradient in respect to time; this was initially done numerically and, later, by electrical integration (Rudewald, 1962). Tests were done on hydraulic models (Porjé and Rudewald, 1960, 1961) and these papers also report numerous uses of it in man for the study of cardiac patients, especially those with aortic valvular lesions. The emphasis was more on diagnosis than on determining output, but these studies have aroused too little attention in England and America.

Because of some of the technical difficulties in measuring an accurate gradient many have used a 'derived' gradient from the time-derivative of the pressure wave and the wave-velocity (eqn. 6.7). A failing of this approach, which was pointed out when it was first used by McDonald (1955), was that the mean value of the time-derivative would be zero and so there was no way to calculate the mean flow. While, theoretically, this is correct, it has little experimental validity because the mean value of the actual gradient is so small. For example, calculation from the Poiseuille equation (2.3) shows that, in a human ascending aorta, with a flow of 5 l/min and a diameter of 2·5 çm the pressure drop over an interval of 5 cm will be only 0·014 mm Hg. This is far too small to measure so that indirect means of deriving it have to be used. The usual one, in the ascending aorta, is to adjust the synthesized flow so that the flow in late diastole is zero. This was introduced by Fry *et al.* (1956) and was also used by Porjé and Rudewald (1957) and has been adapted for use on a digital computer by McDonald and Nichols (1973). The other criticisms centre around the value to be taken for wave-velocity and are discussed below.

The introduction of the *time-derivative method* for estimating the pressure-gradient as a feasible means of measuring stroke volume is due to Jones, Hefner, Bancroft and Klip (1959). They took the original Fry equation (6.11) and made the substitution

$$\frac{dp}{dz} = -\frac{1}{c} \cdot \frac{dp}{dt} \qquad\qquad 6.7$$

so that it became

$$\frac{1}{c} \cdot \frac{dp}{dt} = \frac{dw}{dt} + aw(t) \qquad\qquad 15.14$$

and solved it with the same analogue device as used by Fry.

The 'resistance' term a was found by adjustment until the diastolic flow velocity was zero. The integral of the flow wave was then matched against the stroke volume measured by the dye-dilution method. This produced a calibration factor K which was thereafter used to convert the analogue results to ml of stroke volume. The wave velocity in this treatment is assumed to be independent of frequency for the underlying assumption in using eqn. 6.7 is that the wave is distorted as it travels and, among other factors, is not influenced by wave reflection. The wave-velocity was not measured so that the term $1/c$ is a component of the factor K. As the Fry equation measures flow velocity this has to be multiplied by the cross-sectional area, πR^2, to convert to volume flow. The term $\pi R^2/c$ thus becomes the variable component of K as in the pressure-contour methods, used by Warner *et al.* (1953, 1968) and Kouchoukos *et al.* (1970) which were discussed above. As we saw there, this ratio will not vary very much with passive changes of mean pressure but will be likely to change under the influence of vasoactive drugs.

The results that they obtained for their whole series of experiments were good. The correlation coefficient was 0·97, and the regression line $y = 1·1x - 45$ ml/min ($N = 66$). The SEE was not given. In the series of eight dogs the stroke volume was altered over a considerable range by altering the pressure in the left atrium with an adjustable reservoir. In six of the dogs the authors said that infusions of epinephrine and methoxamine were also given, but there was no statement as to how many of the total 66 cycles analysed these conditions applied, nor what doses were used. As we saw with the results of Kouchoukos *et al.* (1970), vasoactive drugs caused a poor correlation while changes in output due to purely cardiac effects had a very good correlation. The circumstances of the experimental procedures may be the reason why the later papers by Jones and his colleagues never reported such good results. Jones and Griffin (1962) compared the flow by the time-derivative method with an electromagnetic flowmeter in dogs. The correlation coefficient was 0·93 (regression line $y = 0·90x + 9·2$ ml ± 13·4 per cent SD). Stroke output was altered by withdrawal, and later retransfusion, of blood and also by the administration of nitroglycerine and amyl nitrite. Comparisons of peak flows were made, with a rather poorer correlation coefficient of 0·85 (regression line $y = 0·97x + 0·2 ± 17·5$ per cent).

The method was subsequently used in man by Jones, Russell and Dalton (1966) and Jones and Reeves (1968); the subjects were patients with cardiac disease of widely different degrees who were being given exercise tests. The statistical data for the earlier paper was $r = 0·90$, ($N = 73$) $y = 1·23x - 1·09$ l/min ± 1·85 l/min SD; for the later paper it was $r = 0·93$, $y = 0·87x + 0·77$ l/min/m². The comparison was made with either the Fick or the indicator-dilution method.

The computer analysis of the Fry method was modified by Boyett, Stowe and Becker (1966) by using a servo-mechanism to adjust the potentiometer representing the friction factor a in the equation. In five dogs subjected to progressive haemorrhages the statistical summary was $r = 0·92$, $y = 1·03x - 0·06$ l/min. This suggests that no apparent improvement was made by the increased sophistication of the analogue computer analysis.

The method has also been compared with the electromagnetic flowmeter in dogs, in terms of the peak flow in systole, by Greenfield, Patel, Barnett, and Fox (1962) and Greenfield and Fry (1965b). Greenfield *et al.* recorded a range of correlation coefficients from 0·91–0·98 in each of ten dogs, with regression lines ranging in slope from $y = 1·64x - 17·6$ ml/sec to $y = 0·84x + 9·62$ ml/sec with SEE ranging from 2·4–8·9 per cent. Greenfield and Fry recorded similar results in six dogs with $r = 0·91–0·98$, and $y = 1·53x - 9·6$ ml/sec to $y = 0·80x + 11·6$ ml/sec and SEE $\pm 6·2$ per cent – 17·0 per cent. In this paper they were especially concerned with the analytic basis of the method and found that with the standard values for inductance and resistance that they had determined for calculating flow from the pressure-gradient and the increased value for the wave-front velocity the resultant curve was very similar in form to the pressure curve (see Ch. 6, p. 136) and the results were, consequently, much in error. Only by adjusting the analogue to arbitrary values that produced a flow curve similar to that of the flowmeter could they produce the results given above. They pointed out that the variables, in effect, determine the impedance but did not elaborate the point. As is seen below in relation to the discussion on the results of McDonald and Nichols, the error in the form of the curve is, in large part, due to a failure to incorporate the phase of the input impedance. The other source of error is due to the fact that, due to wave reflection, the value of c varies with frequency (Figs. 12.6, 14.5); this, however, will only be important at pulse frequencies below 2·0 Hz in most dogs. The paper by Mills *et al.* (1970) indicates that this critical frequency also applies to humans, so that the pulse rate will be below this frequency.

To eliminate this error McDonald and Nichols (1973) used two pressure recordings 3–5 cm apart in the ascending aorta; both curves were subjected to Fourier analysis and the apparent phase-velocity, c', calculated for each of the ten harmonics used. This value of c', and the time-derivative of the proximal pressure, were then incorporated in the Womersley equation (6.4). With two pressure measurements the pressure-gradient could have been used; the reasons for adopting this modified method, first suggested by McDonald (1960), were (1) in a method designed for clinical use it obviated the necessity for the very precise calibration matching of two manometer systems while, with modern high-frequency manometers, the phase shift could be held both small and constant over a long period, (2) it was hoped to analyse further, as had Greenfield and Fry, the potential errors of the time-derivative method using a constant value for c introduced by Jones *et al.* (1959). The steps leading to the equation that is used for calculating the flow by the method using the apparent phase velocity are as follows:

It was seen that a pressure-gradient of simple harmonic form, with modulus M_g and phase φ_g, may be written

$$\frac{dp}{dz} = M_g \cos (\omega t - \varphi_g) \qquad \textbf{15.15}$$

and also

$$\frac{dp}{dz} = -\frac{1}{c'} \frac{dp}{dt}$$ **15.16**

and the volume flow produced by this gradient is

$$Q = \frac{\pi R^2 M_g M'_{10}}{\omega \rho} \sin (\omega t - \varphi_g + \varepsilon_{10})$$ **15.17**

An harmonic component of the pressure is similarly written

$$p(t) = M_p \cos (\omega t - \varphi_p)$$ **15.18**

so that the time-derivative is

$$\frac{dp}{dt} = -\omega M_p \sin (\omega t - \varphi_p)$$ **15.19**

or, as $-\sin (\theta) = +\cos (\theta + \pi/2)$,

$$\frac{dp}{dt} = \omega M_p \cos (\omega t - \varphi_p + \pi/2)$$ **15.20**

and eqn. 6.7 or 15.16 becomes

$$\frac{dp}{dz} = \frac{\omega M_p}{c'} \cos (\omega t - \varphi_p + \pi/2)$$ **15.21**

from which we obtain

$$Q = \frac{\pi R^2 . M_p . M'_{10}}{\rho c'} \sin (\omega t - \varphi_p + \varepsilon_{10} + \pi/2)$$ **15.22**

As two pressures P_1 and P_2 were recorded at a distance Δz apart we have any given harmonic component represented by

$$P_1 = M_1 \cos (\omega t - \varphi_1)$$

and

$$P_2 = M_2 \cos (\omega t - \varphi_2)$$

and the phase shift is

$$\Delta \varphi = (\varphi_1 - \varphi_2)$$

and the velocity that this component travels, i.e. the apparent phase velocity (Chs. 12 and 14) is given by

$$c' = \frac{\omega . \Delta z}{\Delta \varphi}$$ **12.7**

Thus, in terms of what is actually measured directly, eqn. 15.22 becomes

$$Q = \frac{\pi R^2}{\omega} \cdot \frac{\Delta \varphi M_p . M'_{10}}{\Delta z} \cdot \sin \left(\omega t - \varphi_p + \varepsilon_{10} + \pi/2 \right) \qquad \textbf{15.23}$$

where the values of M_p and φ_p taken were those of the pressure, P_1, closest to the aortic valve. (For computing purposes the factor π was cancelled out by writing $\pi R^2/\omega = R^2/2f$.)

The computing procedure may be summarized briefly. The pressure pulses were sampled at 10 msec intervals, starting at the R wave of the ECG and stopping at the next R wave. Ten harmonic components were computed in the modulus and phase form and also the phase shift $\Delta \varphi$ for each harmonic. (In early experiments comparisons were made with a sampling interval of 5 msec and using 20 harmonics but the gain in precision—as witness the variance data discussed in Ch. 7—was so trivial as not to justify the considerable increase in computing time needed.) The values of the parameter α were then calculated from the pulse frequency derived from the cycle length and using standard values of $\rho = 1.05$ and $\mu = 0.04P$; the radius was estimated by measuring the external circumference of the ascending aorta and assuming a ratio of wall-thickness to external radius, h/R (Ch. 10) of 0.16. The modulus and phase of the Bessel function (M'_{10} and ε_{10}) were calculated for each harmonic from three terms of the series expansion

$$M'_{10} = 1 - \frac{\sqrt{2}}{\alpha} + \frac{1}{\alpha^2} \qquad \textbf{15.24}$$

$$\varepsilon_{10} \text{ (radians)} = \frac{\sqrt{2}}{\alpha} + \frac{1}{\alpha^2} + \frac{19}{24 \cdot \sqrt{2} . \alpha^3} \qquad \textbf{15.25}$$

The lowest α recorded was approximately 8.0 and for this and higher values this expansion gives values always accurate to 3 significant figures.

The computation of the flow for each harmonic (eqn. 15.23) then only required the addition of the measured values for Δz and πR^2 together with the appropriate value of $\Delta \varphi$ and f for each harmonic (and a factor for converting pressure from mm Hg to CGS units). These were then summed at 10 msec intervals to give the ordinates of the synthesized flow curve. However, the mean value of a sine wave over a cycle is zero and so the synthesized flow curve, the sum of a set of sine waves, will also have a mean value of zero. This results in all the ordinates for the diastolic portion of the curve being negative; in experimentally measured curves we know that the diastolic flow is very close to zero. The average negative value of the synthesized curve is, therefore, the value of the mean flow and needs to be added throughout the cycle to represent the real situation. Where the Fry electrical analogue was used this adjustment was made manually; in the present procedure the computer was programmed to calculate a mean of all the negative values of the synthesized flow and this was printed out as the value for mean flow and added to all the ordinates of the curve for plotting.

The overall results for 720 determinations (35 of these were compared against dye-dilution; the remainder against a flowmeter) in 30 dogs and 1 pig are illustrated in Fig. 15.4 for mean flow over a range from 4·5–64·6 ml/sec;

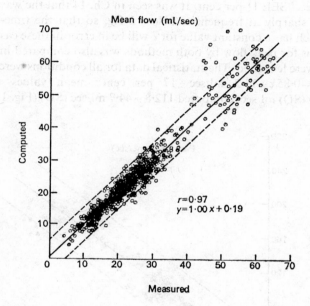

Fig. 15.4. A diagram to the individual points and the regression line for the prediction of stroke volume in the method used by McDonald and Nichols (1973). This method uses the time-derivative of the pressure and the apparent phase velocity to calculate the pressure gradient. The broken lines are drawn through the 95 per cent confidence limit of the Standard Error of the Estimate (SSE).

These values with a slope of unity, a correlation coefficient of 0·97 and an SEE of ±12 per cent show that stroke volume is predicted very well by this method.

the regression line and 95 per cent confidence limits are also shown. The numerical statistical data were: $r = 0·97$, $y = 1·000x + 0·19$ ml/sec, SEE ±12 per cent. Comparison of the mean values obtained showed that, for measured flow, it was 25·32 ± 12·16 (SD) ml/sec and for computed flow 25·49 ± 12·57 (SD) ml/sec, and perhaps gives a clearer idea of the precision of the flow prediction. Ten different interventions were used to alter cardiac output and mean arterial pressure; these were essentially the same as those used by Kouchoukos *et al.* (1970). The number of determinations with vasoactive drugs comprised 336 of the total number and the results with adrenaline, nor-adrenaline, isoproterenol, and metaraminol were not appreciably different from the overall totals. (These results are set out in detail by Nichols, 1970, and McDonald and Nichols, 1973.)

Isoproterenol, for example, which gave particularly poor results with the contour method (Fig. 15.3) had the following statistical analysis: $r = 0.94$, $y = 1.10x - 1.21$ ml/sec $\pm$ SEE 10 per cent. For slow pulse-frequencies (< 1.5 Hz) with vagal stimulation the statistical data were: $r = 0.96$, $y = 0.96x + 0.76$ ml/sec $\pm$ SEE 11 per cent. It was seen in Ch. 14 that the wave-velocity values rose sharply at frequencies below 2 Hz, so that the time-derivative method which has a constant value for c will be in error in these cases.

The values for peak flow by both methods was also compared but in these the results were less good. The statistical data for all conditions were: $N = 573$, $r = 0.91$, $y = 0.85x + 13.2$ ml/sec ± 17 per cent; mean values measured, 128.1 ± 52.9 (SD) ml/sec, computed 112.8 ± 44.7 ml/sec (SD) (Fig. 15.5). Thus

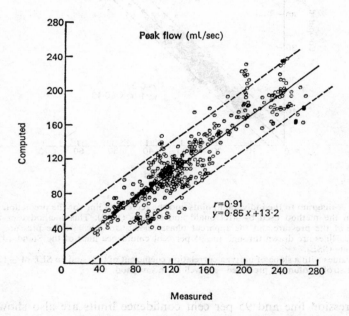

Fig. 15.5. The scatter of points and regression lines of the prediction of *peak* flow by the method of McDonald and Nichols (1973). Comparison with values in Fig. 15.4 show that peak flow is not predicted so accurately by this method as is stroke volume. The reasons for this discrepancy are discussed in the text and are also illustrated in Fig. 15.6.

it can be seen that the computed values all tend to be low and this is particularly marked where the heart rates were slowed by vagal stimulation where the slope of the regression line was only 0.55. By comparison, a control group where all the pulse-frequencies were > 2 Hz the data were: $N = 122$, $r = 0.97$, $y = 0.91x + 5.4$ ml/sec $\pm$ SEE 9 per cent. The probable reason for the discrepancy for peak flow is to be found in a consideration of the initial assumptions made in this method.

These assumptions made here include, as do all the others, those underlying the Womersley and Fry equations which were discussed in Ch. 6. In addition the pressure-gradient method primarily predicts the linear velocity of flow, averaged across the artery, and to predict volume flow the assumptions must be made that, not only is the cross-sectional area of the ascending aorta known, but it remains constant with variations of mean arterial pressure. (This also applies to the use of an intra-arterial flowmeter.) This assumption is clearly subject to a fair amount of error and it is surprising that the observed discrepancies are not greater; comparison with the flow measured by an electromagnetic flowmeter may artificially improve the comparison because the presence of a circumarterial probe will limit expansion over an appreciable proportion of the interval over which the gradient is measured. The assumptions made in using the time-derivative of the pressure (eqn. 6.7) have been discussed above. In using the apparent phase velocity as the appropriate value for the wave velocity the hope was to remove the restriction made by assuming that there were no reflections. In comparing the flow as a function of the pulsatile arterial pressure with the flow as a function of the pressure-gradient we are, in effect, comparing the input impedance with the longitudinal impedance. The close relation of the apparent phase velocity with the input impedance was originally explored by Taylor (1959c) and has been discussed in a section of Ch. 14. The modulus of the input impedance is given by

$$|Z| = \frac{\rho c'}{\pi R^2 M'_{10}} \qquad \textbf{14.4}$$

The close fit for the measured against the calculated values of the input impedance modulus is illustrated in Fig. 14.8.

The apparent phase velocity, however, has no phase component, so that the input impedance phase given by use of eqn. 15.23 will be the same as that of the longitudinal impedance, i.e. ε_{10}. This will always have a small positive value varying from about $10°$ at the lowest frequencies used to 1–$2°$ in the highest harmonics. In addition, when using eqn. 15.23, there will be an additional component due to transmission between the points of measuring P_1 and the flow; this is already present in the measured impedance phase (see p. 372). By contrast the phase of the input impedance (Fig. 13.19) is markedly negative at the low frequencies and becomes positive above 4–5 Hz. As a result the synthesized curve will be distorted by errors in the phases of the components relative to each other. This can be seen in some examples of computed curves (Fig. 15.6). The 'spreading' of the synthesized curve that results from the error in the relative phases of the components causes a reduction in

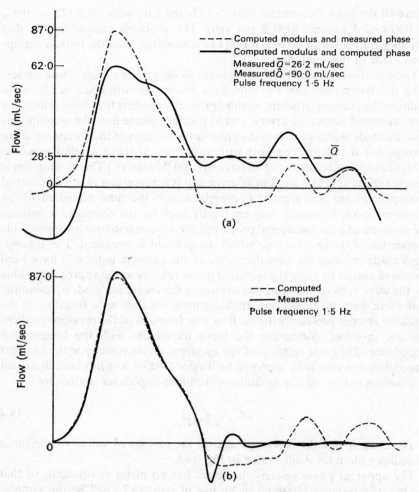

Fig. 15.6. The method of using apparent phase velocity and the time-derivate of the pressure wave predicts the modulus of the harmonic components very accurately, as was seen in Ch. 14. The method, however, does not calculate the phase difference between the pressure and the flow but only predicts the phase of the characteristic impedance. As a result, the resynthesis of the flow shows major deviations from the true flow curve due to the phase shift in the low-frequency components (which are also the largest in amplitude).

(a) This drawing illustrates this error. The computed resynthesis is shown by the solid line which shows the flow pattern computed without phase correction. The broken line shows the resynthesis using the measured phase differences between flow and pressure. The horizontal broken line shows the mean flow value. The flow curves show marked differences in shape, and discrepancies in peak flow can be seen. Because the moduli are calculated accurately, the integral of the flow curve, which determines mean flow, is accurate.

(b) The corrected flow curve in (a) is here compared to actual measured flow curve and it can be seen that there is a close match during the period of systolic ejection. There are minor discrepancies during the period of zero diastolic flow but this is due to the fact that more harmonic terms are needed to resynthesize a straight, or nearly straight, line. (From McDonald and Nichols, 1973.)

the height of the peak; this accounts for the statistical findings that the predicted peak flow is too low.

To test the hypothesis that has been advanced as the cause of this discrepancy a number of computed flow curves were calculated a second time using the measured phase of the input impedance (derived from the measured flow). The change in form resulting from this is illustrated in one example in Fig. 15.6(a) and Fig. 15.6(b), where it is seen that the new fit of the systolic flow curve is very good. As, in our measurements, the phase of the impedance is reasonably linear with frequency, it suggests that an arbitrary correction for phase (as a function of frequency) might be added to the computation to improve the prediction of peak flow and the form of the flow curve. This has not, however, been tested yet.

In spite of this distortion the mean flow is well predicted. This is because stroke volume (a function of mean flow) is an integral of the flow curve and will not be altered by small rearrangements of relative phase of the harmonic components; this is also shown in Fig. 15.6(a). It was seen above that other methods (e.g. Jones and Griffin, 1962) found that the prediction of peak flow was not as good as that of the stroke volume and this can be attributed to the same cause even though they did not actually perform a Fourier analysis.

As in the case of the Fry pressure-gradient method the method of McDonald and Nichols had not yet been tested as a monitoring technique in patients. From the results in dogs they merit testing in a clinical situation. Neither are susceptible to the unpredictable changes in wall-elasticity and, hence, of wave-velocity, due to the catecholamines. This is probably especially important in the study of patients with acute myocardial infarction, who are likely to have marked fluctuations of endogenous catecholamines (in addition to their therapeutic use).

The recent development of catheter-tip flowmeters holds out great promise for the continuous monitoring of ventricular outflow in patients. Warbasse *et al.* (1969) used the catheter-tip model described by Bond and Barefoot (1967) to compare the flow it measured with that measured by a conventional flow probe in twelve experiments in dogs. Flows were recorded in the ascending aorta, thoracic aorta and abdominal aorta (four experiments at each site); comparisons were made of peak flow and also of the complete cycle as sampled at 10-msec intervals. The measurement of peak flow and complete cycles showed correlation coefficients between 0·97 and 0·99 (with one exception of 0·94 for all points in complete cycles in the ascending aorta). The slopes were all reasonably close to 1·0; the highest value was 1·18 in the peak flow series and 1·24 in the other, the lowest was 0·84 in both series. The conversion from velocity to volume flow appears to have been achieved by comparison with the flow cuff probe but, although this obviates a calibration problem that would occur in patients, the small scatter of the results is excellent. It suggests that the potentialities of this type of instrument are great. Pressures were not recorded but the facility to do so was built into the instrument they used. As there is no blood entering the transducer it was not found necessary to use anticoagulant drugs. In another study, Nolan *et al.* (1969) used the Biotronex catheter-tip meter in five normal dogs and in four dogs with chronic aortic valve insufficiency. In the normal series a comparison of the electrical deflection of the two meters showed a correlation coefficient of 0·96 for the mean deflection and 0·95 for the peak deflection; the corresponding regression lines were $y = 1·05x + 0·09 \pm 12·7$ per cent and $y = 1·06x + 1·56 \pm 12·4$ per cent. In the four animals with aortic regurgitation the stroke volumes ejected show the statistical analysis $r = 0·95$, $y = 0·89x + 2·53$ ml ($\pm 1·71$ ml SE) while for the regurgitant flow (mean value 3·43 ml compared to 12·8 ml stroke volume) $r = 0·92$, $y = 0·99x + 0·71 \pm 0·91$ ml SE. The conversion to volume flow was made by comparison with indicator-dilution measurement of flow. Because, in this instrument, the blood flows through an open cylinder at the top it was found essential to give heparin (3 mg/kg) to prevent coagulation. The design, however, permitted the establishment of a zero velocity flow level by advancing the catheter until it was in contact with a valve cusp. Again pressures were not recorded and it does not appear to be possible with this instrument.

As pointed out early in the chapter, much more haemodynamic information can be achieved by simultaneous measurement of pressure and flow than by measurement of flow alone. Such a study has been carried out in patients by Gabe *et al.* (1969) using the Mills intravascular probe (Mills and Shillingford, 1967). Twenty-three patients with a considerable range of cardiac disease were studied; pressure and flow were measured in the pulmonary artery, the ascending, the thoracic, and the abdominal aorta and their branches, right subclavian, innominate, renal and iliac arteries. The impedances calculated from these and other studies in terms of flow velocity (Mills *et al.*, 1970) have been discussed in Ch. 13. In order to derive volume flow the aortic diameter was measured radiologically in nine patients by contrast angiography. The stroke volume measured with the flowmeter was compared with that derived from the indicator-dilution technique. Only thirteen determinations were made and the correlation coefficient was 0·73. No anticoagulants were used.

This investigation shows the feasibility of the use of this type of flowmeter in human beings. One of the problems has been size; both the Mills probe and the one used by Warbasse *et al.* (1969) were the diameter of a no. 8 (French) catheter. This might be regarded as a little large for a probe left in position for a prolonged period. The present commercial version of the Mills probe (1970) has been reduced to that of a no. 7 catheter. The illustration of the Biotronex probe used by Nolan *et al.* (1969) appears to show a tip of almost 4 mm in diameter which would be prohibitively large for routine insertion; also these authors report that a considerable dose of anticoagulant needed to be given.

Other factors also need to be considered: the possible leakage of current from the tip and the heating effect in the blood. The Mills probe has been cleared by British safety standards in both these respects.

Thus, while the intravascular flow probe is not yet a standard method it has the great advantage of a direct measurement of flow and is likely, in the future, to become the method of choice.

The Theoretical Analysis of Manometer Behaviour

Simple harmonic motion is defined in the following way: If a body moves so that its acceleration is always proportional, and opposite in sign to its displacement from an equilibrium position, it is said to execute simple harmonic motion.

If we take as an example a mass (M) hanging on the end of a spring of elastance, S, then if the mass is displaced a distance x from the equilibrium position, the force exerted by the spring will be Sx, which must balance the acceleration; thus

$$M \cdot \frac{d^2x}{dt^2} = -Sx \qquad\qquad 1$$

If we test for a solution in the form $x = Be^{pt}$, we find

$$p^2 = -S/M$$
$$\therefore \; p = \pm i\sqrt{(S/M)} \qquad\qquad 2$$

so that the solution is

$$x = C_1 e^{i\sqrt{(S/M)} \cdot t} + C_2 e^{-i\sqrt{(S/M)} \cdot t} \qquad\qquad 3$$

where C_1 and C_2 are constants which may be determined from the initial conditions. If, when $t=0$, the body is at the limit of its oscillation then its velocity, $dx/dt = 0$ and we set $x = A$.

Then from eqn. 3 we have

$$\left(\frac{dx}{dt}\right)_{t=0} = i\sqrt{(S/M)} \cdot C_1 - i\sqrt{(S/M)} \cdot C_2 = 0$$

so that $C_1 = C_2$
but $x = C_1 + C_2 = A$
$\therefore \; C_1 = C_2 = A/2$
so that eqn. 3 becomes

446

$$x = A \frac{(e^{t\sqrt{(S/M)}t} + e^{-t\sqrt{(S/M)}t})}{2}$$

$$= A \cos \left[\sqrt{\left(\frac{S}{M}\right)} t \right] \qquad \qquad 4$$

which is the familiar form of simple harmonic motion described by a cosine wave where the circular frequency (ω_0) is given by

$$\omega_0 = \sqrt{\frac{S}{M}} \qquad \qquad 5$$

Damped simple harmonic motion is the condition where there is a resistance to the motion that is proportional to the velocity (viscous damping). If we call this reistance factor R the equation of motion corresponding to eqn. 1 is

$$\frac{M d^2 x}{dt^2} = -Sx - R \frac{dx}{dt}$$

or

$$M . \frac{d^2 x}{dt^2} + R \frac{dx}{dt} + Sx = 0 \qquad \qquad 6$$

again putting x in the form Be^{pt} we obtain

$$Mp^2 + Rp + S = 0 \qquad \qquad 7$$

$$\therefore \ p = -\frac{R}{2M} \pm \sqrt{\left(\frac{R^2}{4M^2} - \frac{S^2}{M^2}\right)} \qquad \qquad 8$$

for convenience we can write

$$\beta_0 = \frac{R}{2M} \qquad \qquad 9$$

and as in eqn. 5

$$S/M = \omega_0^2$$

so that

$$x = e^{-\beta_0 t}[C_1 e^{\sqrt{(\beta_0^2 - \omega_0^2)}t} + C_2 e^{-\sqrt{(\beta_0^2 - \omega_0^2)}t}] \qquad \qquad 10$$

The behaviour of x in eqn. 10 is determined by the relative values of β_0 and ω_0 and falls into one of three categories (i) $\beta_0 > \omega_0$ (ii) $\beta_0 < \omega_0$ and (iii) $\beta_0 = \omega_0$.

In (i) $\beta_0^2 - \omega_0^2$ is positive, the exponents in eqn. 10 are real and the terms in the square brackets become a hyperbolic function. In terms of the mass-spring analogue we have used, there is now a dashpot in parallel, and the mass, when displaced and released, never oscillates but slowly returns to the equilibrium position. This is often called 'dead-beat' motion and the system is spoken of as 'over-damped'.

(ii) $\beta_0 < \omega_0$, $\beta_0^2 - \omega_0^2$ is negative and its square root is imaginary. Taking the same initial conditions as for eqn. 3 we obtain the solution

$$x = \frac{A\omega_0^2}{\omega_0^2 - \beta_0^2} \, e^{-\beta_0 t} \, \cos\left[(\omega_0^2 - \beta_0^2)^{\frac{1}{2}} t - \tan^{-1}\frac{\beta_0}{(\omega_0^2 - \beta_0^2)^{\frac{1}{2}}}\right] \qquad \textbf{11}$$

which represents a sinusoidal oscillation that diminishes exponentially. We note that the 'damped natural frequency' is given by $\sqrt{(\omega_0^2 - \beta_0^2)}$ which is plainly less than ω_0, the natural frequency of the undamped system with the same mass and spring-stiffness.

(iii) In the special case where $\beta_0 = \omega_0$ the solution of eqn. 10 becomes

$$x = Ae^{-\beta_0 t}(1 + \beta_0 t) \qquad \textbf{12}$$

This resembles dead-beat motion and is the limiting aperiodic case which is called *critical damping*. Damping coefficients are usually expressed as a ratio of this value, i.e. $\beta = \beta_0/\omega_0$. It is important to note that it is defined in terms of free vibrations and that the effect of damping where there are forced vibrations is somewhat different.

When a system that would oscillate naturally in simple harmonic motion is driven by a force that also varies harmonically it is said to be in a state of forced vibration. If there is no damping the resultant motion of the system is compounded of oscillations at both the natural and the driving frequencies. As in any real situation there is some damping the oscillation at the natural frequency dies away and the system only responds to the driving frequency. This is the 'steady-state' condition that has been discussed in Ch. 7, i.e. the state after disturbances due to 'starting-up' have died away.

If the driving oscillation is $K \sin \omega t$ while the natural frequency of the system is ω_0 as before, then the equation of motion is now (cp. eqn. 6)

$$M\frac{dx^2}{dt^2} + R\frac{dx}{dt} + Sx = SK \sin \omega t \qquad \textbf{13}$$

and its steady-state solution is, using ω_0 (eqn. 5) and β_0 (eqn. 9),

$$x = \frac{\omega_0^2 K}{\sqrt{[(\omega_0^2 - \omega^2)^2 + 4\beta_0^2\omega^2]}} \, \sin\left[\omega t - \tan^{-1}\frac{2\beta_0\omega}{\omega_0^2 - \omega^2}\right] \qquad \textbf{14}$$

If K and ω_0 are put $= 1 \cdot 0$ and ω is expressed as a fraction, γ, of ω_0 this is identical to eqn. 8.10.

If the damping is so small that β_0^2 can be neglected, it can be seen that the amplitude of the response, A, is given approximately by

$$A = \frac{\omega_0^2 K}{(\omega_0^2 - \omega^2)} \qquad \textbf{15}$$

and will become very large when ω approaches ω_0—the condition of resonance.

Under the same conditions the phase lag is zero for all values except $\omega = \omega_0$ when it becomes indeterminate; in effect the phase lag changes rapidly from 0° to 180°. As the damping increases the phase lag changes progressively with frequency but when $\omega = \omega_0$ it is always 90°. The changes in phase and in amplitude have already been illustrated in Figs. 8.1 and 8.2.

In applying these equations more precisely to the hydraulic system of the manometer it is necessary to establish the equivalent terms of the generalized oscillatory system that we have considered up to this point. When there is a change in pressure there is movement of a volume of fluid, V, into or out of the system. Under dynamic conditions the effect of such fluid movement can be regarded as determined by its kinetic energy (as Noble, 1953, does) or more rigorously by the analysis of the physical behaviour of oscillations set up by a generator in a fluid-filled system of varying cross-section (as by Hansen, 1950). The velocity of flow with a given change of volume is inversely proportional to the cross-sectional area of the channel. The effective 'mass' and the effective 'resistance' are thus almost wholly dominated by the dimensions of the narrowest channels—the approximation is of the order of the ratio of the squares of the cross-sectional area of the manometer chamber and that of the needle or cannula. As the ratio of these areas is at least 20:1 it can be seen that the error is about 1/400. The second approximation that is made by Hansen (1950) is that the pressure-flow relationship under oscillatory conditions is that of Poiseuille's equation (2.3). As a result he has rewritten the equation of motion (6) for free vibrations in the following form:

$$\rho \, \frac{L}{\pi r^2} \cdot \frac{d^2 V}{dt^2} + \frac{8 \mu L}{\pi r^4} \cdot \frac{dV}{dt} + EV = 0 \qquad\qquad 16$$

(where V is the volume flow).

In Frank's (1903) original equation the second term (on LHS) was replaced by

$$\frac{k}{\pi r^2} \cdot \frac{dV}{dt}$$

where k was a constant to be determined experimentally. E is the pressure-volume modulus (i.e. $\Delta P / \Delta V$ and not the Young's modulus as in Ch. 8).

Rewriting eqn. 16 so that it is more easily comparable with eqn. 12 (i.e. dividing by $\rho l / \pi r^2$, and putting the density $\rho = 1\cdot 0$) we obtain

$$\frac{d^2 V}{dt^2} + \frac{8 \mu}{r^2} \cdot \frac{dV}{dt} + \frac{E \pi r^2 V}{L} = 0 \qquad\qquad 17$$

whence we write (equation 8.4).

$$\omega_0 = \sqrt{\frac{\pi r^2 E}{L}}$$

The damping term β_0 (i.e. $R/2M$) is similarly

$$\beta_0 = \frac{4\mu}{r^2} \qquad\qquad \mathbf{18}$$

As the ratio of the damping to critical damping ($\beta_0 = \omega_0$) is normally used we write

$$\beta = \frac{4\mu}{r^3} \sqrt{\frac{L}{\pi E}}$$

It is in this term, and in all the other manometer characteristics that involve the damping, e.g. the resonant frequency, that errors due to using the Poiseuille resistance will be apparent. Lambossy (1952b) investigated in detail the changes in predicted manometer characteristics that result from using the pressure-flow relationship of oscillatory flow in place of the approximation used by Hansen. It will be easier here to use the terms derived from Womersley's equations. In Ch. 8 the fluid resistance for oscillatory flow was given (eqn. 8.9) and is illustrated in Fig. 6.13. The new expression for β_0, in place of eqn. 18, becomes

$$\beta_0 = \frac{\mu}{2r^2\rho} \cdot \frac{\alpha^2}{M'_{10}} \sin \varepsilon_{10} \qquad\qquad \mathbf{19}$$

The values of M_{10}'/α^2 and ε_{10} are tabulated in Table A and are determined by the term α.

The effect of using the oscillatory fluid resistance in eqn. 19, in place of the Poiseuille resistance (eqn. 18) will be to increase the damping constant as the frequency increases. As α is a function of the radius of the cannula as well as the frequency this effect will vary in degree with the size of tube used and is best illustrated by taking some numerical cases.

In one of Hansen's (1949) examples (that Lambossy, 1952b, also analysed) the characteristics of the manometer were predicted from the dimensions of the apparatus. The calculated value for the damping was 0·22. Now the radius of the needle was 0·0158 cm so that, water-filled, at 6 c/sec the value of $\alpha \doteqdot 0.95$ and the damping calculated from eqn. 19 will be less than 1 per cent greater than that calculated from Hansen's own equation. At the resonant frequency (predicted to be 115 c/sec) the value of $\alpha \doteqdot 4.25$ and the damping will be 20 per cent higher than calculated by the Hansen eqn., i.e. 0·26 in place of 0·22.

Lambossy (1952b) reached similar conclusions and calculated some of the ancillary effects, e.g. a slightly lower resonant frequency. It is also of interest to note that the frequency-amplitude curve for 'optimal' damping, which is that for $\beta = 0.707$ (Fig. 8.1) with the simple theory, occurs with $\beta = 0.8$ with the modified equation in this example.

This effect must be regarded as being of minor significance. The only situation in which this error might be worth correcting for is that of a manometer calibrated by the free vibration method (Ch. 8). This method, in effect, calculates the damping at the resonant frequency and so, in the working range, it will tend to be too high. Let us take an example from one of our own manometers—with a needle of radius 0.02 cm the resonant frequency was found to be 198 c/sec ($\alpha = 7.1$) and the damping at this frequency was 0.1. Applying the correction, this damping is reduced to 0.063 at 30 c/sec ($\alpha = 2.75$) and 0.06 at 2 c/sec ($\alpha = 0.7$) which is appreciably smaller. The phase error, however, is only c. $1.5°$ at 30 c/sec with damping of 0.1 and would be actually c. $1.0°$ if the corrected value were used. The corresponding change in amplitude distortion is to reduce it from 2 per cent to 1.9 per cent. Thus if we use manometers of high natural frequency and low damping so that we can neglect the errors in the low frequency range then we find that the actual errors are in fact smaller than predicted. If the damping is higher through using very fine needles the discrepancy will also be small because the change in fluid resistance is very small when α is small; for example the increase is less than 1.4 per cent for α 0.0–2.0.

Direct calibration with a generator over the frequency range that it is desired to measure experimentally does not, of course, require any adjustment. It is, in any case, difficult to build a calibration apparatus of sufficient accuracy to detect these deviations from the simple theory of Hansen. The more precise form of the solution, with an estimate of the changes it produces, has been given here in an easily computable form to enable more precise calculation to be made when it is desirable.

TABLE A. M'_{10}/α^2 and ε_{10} tabulated for values of α from 0 to 10

α	M'_{10}/α^2	ε_{10}	α	M'_{10}/α^2	ε_{10}	α	M'_{10}/α^2	ε_{10}	α	M'_{10}/α^2	ε_{1}
0·00	0·1250	90·00	2·50	0·0855	44·93	5·00	0·0302	18·65	7·50	0·0147	11·87
0·05	0·1250	89·98	2·55	0·0837	43·88	5·05	0·0297	18·43	7·55	0·0146	11·78
0·10	0·1250	89·90	2·60	0·0819	42·86	5·10	0·0292	18·23	7·60	0·0144	11·70
0·15	0·1250	89·79	2·65	0·0802	41·86	5·15	0·0287	18·02	7·65	0·0142	11·61
0·20	0·1250	89·62	2·70	0·0784	40·90	5·20	0·0282	17·83	7·70	0·0140	11·53
0·25	0·1250	89·40	2·75	0·0767	39·96	5·25	0·0278	17·63	7·75	0·0139	11·45
0·30	0·1250	89·14	2·80	0·0750	39·05	5·30	0·0273	17·44	7·80	0·0137	11·37
0·35	0·1250	88·83	2·85	0·0734	38·17	5·35	0·0269	17·26	8·85	0·0136	11·29
0·40	0·1250	88·47	2·90	0·0717	37·32	5·40	0·0264	17·08	7·90	0·0134	11·21
0·45	0·1249	88·07	2·95	0·0701	36·50	5·45	0·0260	16·90	7·95	0·0133	11·14
0·50	0·1249	87·61	3·00	0·0685	35·70	5·50	0·0256	16·73	8·00	0·0131	11·06
0·55	0·1248	87·11	3·05	0·0670	34·93	5·55	0·0252	16·56	8·05	0·0130	10·98
0·60	0·1248	86·57	3·10	0·0655	34·18	5·60	0·0248	16·39	8·10	0·0128	10·91
0·65	0·1247	85·97	3·15	0·0640	33·46	5·65	0·0244	16·23	8·15	0·0127	10·84
0·70	0·1246	85·33	3·20	0·0626	32·77	5·70	0·0240	16·07	8·20	0·0125	10·77
0·75	0·1244	84·65	3·25	0·0612	32·09	5·75	0·0237	15·91	8·25	0·0124	10·70
0·80	0·1243	83·91	3·30	0·0598	31·45	5·80	0·0233	15·76	8·30	0·0122	10·63
0·85	0·1240	83·14	3·35	0·0585	30·82	5·85	0·0230	15·61	8·35	0·0121	10·56
0·90	0·1238	83·32	3·40	0·0572	30·22	5·90	0·0226	15·46	8·40	0·0120	10·49
0·95	0·1235	81·45	3·45	0·0559	29·64	5·95	0·0223	15·32	8·45	0·0119	10·42
1·00	0·1232	80·55	3·50	0·0547	29·08	6·00	0·0220	15·18	8·50	0·0117	10·36
1·05	0·1228	79·60	3·55	0·0535	28·53	6·05	0·0216	15·04	8·55	0·0116	10·29
1·10	0·1224	78·61	3·60	0·0523	28·01	6·10	0·0213	14·90	8·60	0·0115	10·22
1·15	0·1219	77·59	3·65	0·0512	27·51	6·15	0·0210	14·77	8·65	0·0114	10·16
1·20	0·1213	76·53	3·70	0·0501	27·02	6·20	0·0207	14·63	8·70	0·0112	10·10
1·25	0·1207	75·44	3·75	0·0490	26·55	6·25	0·0204	14·50	8·75	0·0111	10·04
1·30	0·1200	74·31	3·80	0·0480	26·10	6·30	0·0201	14·38	8·80	0·0110	9·97
1·35	0·1193	73·16	3·85	0·0470	25·66	6·35	0·0199	14·25	8·85	0·0109	9·91
1·40	0·1185	71·98	3·90	0·0460	25·24	6·40	0·0196	14·13	8·90	0·0108	9·85
1·45	0·1176	70·77	3·95	0·0451	24·83	6·45	0·0193	14·01	8·95	0·0107	9·79
1·50	0·1166	69·54	4·00	0·0441	24·43	6·50	0·0191	13·89	9·00	0·0106	9·73
1·55	0·1156	68·30	4·05	0·0432	24·05	6·55	0·0188	13·77	9·05	0·0104	9·68
1·60	0·1144	67·03	4·10	0·0424	23·68	6·60	0·0185	13·66	9·10	0·0103	9·62
1·65	0·1133	65·76	4·15	0·0415	23·32	6·65	0·0183	13·54	9·15	0·0102	9·56
1·70	0·1120	64·47	4·20	0·0407	22·98	6·70	0·0181	13·43	9·20	0·0101	9·51
1·75	0·1107	63·18	4·25	0·0399	22·64	6·75	0·0178	13·32	9·25	0·0100	9·45
1·80	0·1093	61·89	4·30	0·0391	22·32	6·80	0·0176	13·21	9·30	0·0099	9·40
1·85	0·1078	60·59	4·35	0·0384	22·00	6·85	0·0173	13·11	9·35	0·0098	9·34
1·90	0·1063	59·30	4·40	0·0376	21·70	6·90	0·0171	13·00	9·40	0·0097	9·29
1·95	0·1047	58·02	4·45	0·0369	21·40	6·95	0·0169	12·90	9·45	0·0096	9·24
2·00	0·1031	56·74	4·50	0·0362	21·11	7·00	0·0167	12·80	9·50	0·0096	9·18
2·05	0·1015	55·47	4·55	0·0355	20·84	7·05	0·0165	12·70	9·55	0·0095	9·13
2·10	0·0998	54·22	4·60	0·0349	20·56	7·10	0·0163	12·60	9·60	0·0094	9·08
2·15	0·0980	52·98	4·65	0·0342	20·30	7·15	0·0161	12·50	9·65	0·0093	9·03
2·20	0·0963	51·77	4·70	0·0336	20·05	7·20	0·0159	12·41	9·70	0·0092	8·98
2·25	0·0945	50·57	4·75	0·0330	19·80	7·25	0·0157	12·31	9·75	0·0091	8·93
2·30	0·0927	49·39	4·80	0·0324	19·55	7·30	0·0155	12·22	9·80	0·0090	8·88
2·35	0·0909	48·24	4·85	0·0319	19·32	7·35	0·0153	12·13	9·85	0·0089	8·84
2·40	0·0891	47·11	4·90	0·0313	19·09	7·40	0·0151	12·04	9·90	0·0088	8·79
2·45	0·0873	46·01	4·95	0·0308	18·86	7·45	0·0149	11·95	9·95	0·0088	8·74
2·50	0·0855	44·93	5·00	0·0302	18·65	7·50	0·0147	11·87	10·00	0·0087	8·69

TABLE B. The function $(1 - F_{10})$ for values of α from $0(0 \cdot 1)10$. The function is defined in eqns. 6.2 and 6.3 (Reprinted from Womersley (1958a) by kind permission of the U.S. Air Force.)

α	$1 - F_{10}(\alpha)$ Real	Imaginary	α	$1 - F_{10}(\alpha)$ Real	Imaginary	α	$1 - F_{10}(\alpha)$ Real	Imaginary	α	$1 - F_{10}(\alpha)$ Real	Imaginary
0·0	0·0000	0·0000	2·5	0·3784	0·3774	5·0	0·7159	0·2416	7·5	0·8109	0·1704
0·1	0·0000	0·0012	2·6	0·4061	0·3768	5·1	0·7215	0·2376	7·6	0·8134	0·1684
0·2	0·0000	0·0050	2·7	0·4322	0·3744	5·2	0·7269	0·2337	7·7	0·8159	0·1664
0·3	0·0002	0·0112	2·8	0·4568	0·3706	5·3	0·7320	0·2300	7·8	0·8182	0·1645
0·4	0·0005	0·0200	2·9	0·4797	0·3657	5·4	0·7369	0·2264	7·9	0·8206	0·1627
0·5	0·0013	0·0312	3·0	0·5010	0·3600	5·5	0·7417	0·2229	8·0	0·8228	0·1608
0·6	0·0027	0·0448	3·1	0·5207	0·3536	5·6	0·7463	0·2195	8·1	0·8250	0·1590
0·7	0·0050	0·0608	3·2	0·5389	0·3468	5·7	0·7508	0·2163	8·2	0·8272	0·1573
0·8	0·0084	0·0791	3·3	0·5557	0·3398	5·8	0·7551	0·2131	8·3	0·8292	0·1556
0·9	0·0134	0·0994	3·4	0·5712	0·3327	5·9	0·7593	0·2100	8·4	0·8313	0·1539
1·0	0·0202	0·1215	3·5	0·5856	0·3256	6·0	0·7633	0·2070	8·5	0·8333	0·1523
1·1	0·0292	0·1452	3·6	0·5988	0·3185	6·1	0·7672	0·2041	8·6	0·8352	0·1507
1·2	0·0407	0·1699	3·7	0·6111	0·3116	6·2	0·7710	0·2013	8·7	0·8371	0·1491
1·3	0·0549	0·1953	3·8	0·6225	0·3049	6·3	0·7746	0·1985	8·8	0·8390	0·1475
1·4	0·0718	0·2208	3·9	0·6331	0·2984	6·4	0·7782	0·1959	8·9	0·8408	0·1460
1·5	0·0917	0·2458	4·0	0·6430	0·2921	6·5	0·7816	0·1932	9·0	0·8426	0·1446
1·6	0·1143	0·2698	4·1	0·6522	0·2860	6·6	0·7849	0·1907	9·1	0·8443	0·1431
1·7	0·1395	0·2921	4·2	0·6609	0·2802	6·7	0·7882	0·1882	9·2	0·8460	0·1417
1·8	0·1668	0·3123	4·3	0·6691	0·2747	6·8	0·7913	0·1858	9·3	0·8477	0·1403
1·9	0·1959	0·3300	4·4	0·6769	0·2693	6·9	0·7943	0·1834	9·4	0·8493	0·1389
2·0	0·2262	0·3449	4·5	0·6842	0·2642	7·0	0·7973	0·1811	9·5	0·8509	0·1376
2·1	0·2572	0·3569	4·6	0·6911	0·2593	7·1	0·8002	0·1789	9·6	0·8525	0·1363
2·2	0·2884	0·3660	4·7	0·6978	0·2546	7·2	0·8030	0·1767	9·7	0·8540	0·1350
2·3	0·3192	0·3723	4·8	0·7041	0·2501	7·3	0·8057	0·1745	9·8	0·8555	0·1337
2·4	0·3494	0·3761	4·9	0·7101	0·2458	7·4	0·8083	0·1724	9·9	0·8569	0·1325
2·5	0·3784	0·3774	5·0	0·7159	0·2416	7·5	0·8109	0·1704	10·0	0·8584	0·1312

The High-speed Cinematograph Technique for Measuring Blood Flow Velocity

This technique was developed by McDonald in the 1950s for the direct measurement of pulsatile blood-flow velocity in medium-sized arteries at a time when no reliable blood-flow meters were available. By the early 1960s the electromagnetic flowmeter had been greatly improved and thoroughly evaluated. As it has been commercially available for the past decade, together with ultrasonic flowmeters, the high-speed cinematograph method may be regarded as obsolete for its original purpose, and an account of it has been omitted from Ch. 9. However, I still receive queries as to the possible use of the technique of flow-velocity measurement in small vascular beds such as in the mesentery or the retina, and so the technical account of how it can be used for flow measurement is reprinted here from McDonald (1960).

High-speed cinematography

The velocity of blood flow can be estimated by filming the movement of some visible discontinuity that moves with the blood. This has the advantage that it may be used on an intact vessel with no more interference than is required by surgical exposure and the cannulation of a side-branch for injection of a marker substance. Furthermore it is a direct observational method. The rate of filming required to record arterial flow velocities is, however, of the order of 1,000 frames/sec so that a special camera has to be used and observations must be limited to very short periods. It is not, therefore, a method strictly comparable with the use of a meter.

The essentials of the method have been described by McDonald (1952a) where bubbles of air were used as the 'marker'. Oxygen was later substituted for air to diminish the risk of gas embolism. Bubbles of gas can be fairly easily photographed through the wall of arteries up to about 4 mm in external diameter. Larger vessels, in my experience, have walls that are too thick to be sufficiently translucent.

The need to form a clear photographic image determines the choice of marker. Bubbles are by far the best that we have found. Ideally one single spherical bubble filling the lumen of the vessel should be injected in each cardiac cycle. In practice, oxygen is injected at the rate of about 0·1 ml/sec with a tuberculin syringe to form a train of bubbles. A bubble just filling the

454

vessel travels at a velocity very close to the average flow velocity (Womersley, unpublished).

Injections of dyes, although they might seem preferable, are of little value in measuring flow velocity. With a dye that mixes with the blood the only movement that can be analysed is the 'front', or profile, of the dye. Thus for each injection of dye only one observation is possible. Secondly, the profile is seen as a shadow diminishing in density towards the axis and so is impossible to delimit precisely—the optical opacity of the blood renders this especially difficult. Essentially the same problem occurs in cineradiography with radiopaque material and may introduce an error that possibly accounts for some of the extraordinarily high velocities reported by Reynolds *et al.* (1952). Thirdly, there is no simple relation between axial velocity and mean velocity in pulsating flow as there is in a Poiseuille-type flow as we discussed above (Ch. 5). The use of dye is, however, valuable in studying the flow pattern; it is also preferable, possibly, in very small vessels, such as those in the rabbit ear studied by Widmer (1957).

The camera rate at which the flow must be filmed is determined by three factors: (1) the actual length of exposure on the individual frames of film, (2) the degree of optical magnification, and (3) the peak velocity of flow. Of these the exposure on the frame is the most important and is obviously linked with the repetition rate of the camera. With the usual type of high-speed camera a repetition rate of at least 1,000 frames/sec is necessary to avoid visible movement on each frame. This corresponds to an effective frame exposure of about 200 μsec. With the use of synchronized electronic flashes a short frame exposure could be made independent of camera speed but it would still be necessary to film at up to 3–400/sec to follow systolic flow. The power unit for a discharge tube working at that rate would have to be very large. Such a unit would, however, simplify many of the lighting problems. Factors 2 and 3 above are linked together as, although the peak velocities in the smaller vessels are lower, one must magnify them optically to see sufficient detail and the apparent velocity on the film (which determines camera speed) remains much the same. It is desirable for analysis to have the optical field large enough to encompass the movement of a bubble throughout one cardiac cycle. In the dog femoral artery this is of the order of 5 cm but is less in the rabbit aorta.

The camera used in my experiments was the Eastman high-speed camera. This works on the principle of traversing the film continuously behind a revolving block of glass so that the image follows the film. Several different makes of camera are now available on this principle. Some have repetition rates of up to 10,000 frames/sec and more but the lowest effective speed for the purpose should always be used as the length of the event that can be photographed is inversely proportional to the camera running speed. While the camera is accelerating to its steady speed the film cannot be used for analysis and this wastage increases with the speed used. When the effective film run becomes less than 1 sec the problems of synchronizing the injection become very difficult (16 mm film has 40 frames per foot length so that a 100 ft reel has 4,000 frames).

When the exposure of the individual frames is about 1/5,000 sec a high intensity of incident light is required. I have used continuous lighting with a Mazda MEC/U compact source mercury/cadmium high pressure arc in a quartz bulb. On continuous running this is rated at 1 kW but it can be over-run at 3, 5 or 10 kW for short pulses coincidentally with the running of the camera. It is rarely necessary to use more than 5 kW. With this setting the lens aperture was usually f.8. The film used has been Kodak positive reversal Super XX or, preferably, Super X for its finer grain. Faster films with accept-able grain size are becoming available.

Blood-pressure is recorded simultaneously through a second cannula in a side-branch with a capacitance manometer and synchronized with the film by a flashing light in the picture area whose pulses are recorded on the second beam of a double-beam cathode-ray oscilloscope.

To analyse the results precisely the film is projected on to a motor-driven drum rotating at 90° to the line of the artery. The movement of the bubble is then traced manually on to the moving paper (McDonald, 1955b). The result-ant curve (Fig. A.1) has time as the abscissa and the distance travelled by the bubble (which is what the film record shows) as ordinate. This curve, in fact, represents the distance the blood has flowed throughout the cycle, and for many purposes, such as the study of hyperaemia, is the most valuable form of the flow curve. However, the conventional representation of phasic flow is in terms of a velocity curve and, to derive this, the total flow curve must be differentiated. Graphic differentiation has usually been used. If the slope at any point is y/x then

$$\text{Velocity} = \frac{y}{x} \times \frac{\text{camera speed (f.p.s.)}}{\text{projector speed (f.p.s.)}} \times \frac{\text{drum paper rate (cm/sec)}}{\text{magnification of projected image}}$$

The mean velocity throughout the cycle is easily determined from the slope of the line joining the beginning of two successive systoles. The differentiation of the curve may be performed by a Fourier series if the ordinates are measured from the sloping abscissa representing the mean flow.

The errors inherent in the method are small. They may be due (1) to the introduction of bubbles of gas into the circulation or (2) to the discrepancies between the rate of travel of the bubble and the rate of flow of the liquid. The main factor under the heading (1) is gas embolism. Under the heading (2) are (a) the possibilities of the bubble being carried in the axial streams, (b) the flow characteristics of large bubbles and (c) surface tensions effects causing 'sticking' of the bubble.

(1) Gas embolism of any significant amount can be avoided by injecting

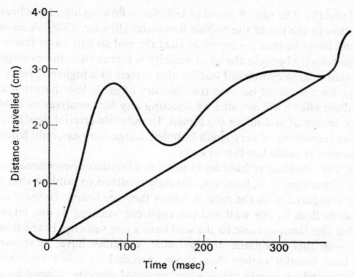

Fig. A.1. An example of the method of analysing a high-speed ciné film of oxygen bubbles in an artery. The film is projected so that the axis of the artery lies vertically on a rotating paper-covered drum (see McDonald, 1955b). The movement of the bubble is then traced and the resultant curve represents distance travelled (vertically) in respect to time (horizontal movement of the drum). The slope is, therefore, a measure of the velocity of the bubble and, hence, of the blood carrying it. Reversal of slope indicates backflow. The slope of the straight line represents the mean velocity; it can be seen that the total travel of the bubble in one cycle is about 3 cm.

The record shown here is from a dog femoral artery while there was an occluding cuff at 40 mm Hg obstructing the venous return. The backflow phase is very marked.

only very small volumes of gas. Ideally one bubble is needed in each cardiac cycle. If the femoral artery has an internal diameter of 3 mm then a spherical bubble filling it has a volume of 0·014 ml. It can be seen that the amount of gas injected, even if 4 or 5 bubbles are injected per cycle, is rarely more than about 0·2–0·25 ml in the course of a film run which lasts about 1 sec. Furthermore, only a small fraction of this will reach the minute vessels, where embolism occurs, within the short time of the film run. If this caused a significant difference then there would be a change in shape of the flow curve in successive cardiac cycles, and this has not been observed. The danger of embolism lies in the accumulation of gas in the capillary bed due to successive injections. When air was used (McDonald, 1952a) it was found that after several runs there was an alteration in flow pattern which was attributed to embolism. Since then oxygen has been substituted for air and no such effect has been observed. As film runs are rarely made at intervals of time shorter than 20 min it appears that the oxygen is totally absorbed. In large arteries the use of oxygen, in small injections at considerable intervals of time, does not cause any modification of flow pattern due to obstruction of the vascular bed. In much smaller vessels the possibility of gas embolism causing an alteration in flow would be greater.

2(a) and (b). The rate of travel of bubbles in flowing liquid has been studied in relation to the use of the bubble flowmeter (Bruner, 1948). A small bubble will tend to move into the centre of the tube and so will travel faster than the average velocity because the axial velocity is higher than the average. Bruner states that a large cylindrical bubble also travels at a higher velocity than the average for the blood because the viscosity of air is less than that of blood. Both these effects are avoided by rejecting any film analyses of bubbles that are not spherical and filling the lumen. In pulsatile arterial flow I have never seen the formation of very small bubbles. Large ones are only formed when an injection is made too fast in error.

2(c). The 'sticking' of bubbles in tubes is a familiar phenomenon in physiological apparatus. It is, however, virtually confined to bubbles that are small in size compared with the tube in which they are found. In these cases they commonly float to one wall and the apparent 'sticking' is due largely to the fact that the laminae close to the wall have a low velocity. In the flow records made with this technique the pulsatile velocities have, as shown in Fig. 11.2, been usually higher than those recorded by other methods so that this factor, which would cause a low recorded velocity, cannot be the cause of the discrepancy.

The errors that arise in practice are due to the technical problem of obtaining a good photographic image. Extraneous highlights on the artery and changes in the translucency of the artery may make analysis of some films very difficult, and inaccuracies may be introduced which are hard to eliminate. This often necessitates the rejection of a proportion of the records. The method of analysis by tracing the movement of the bubble also implies an observational error which can only be minimized by repeated analyses by more than one observer. The character of the image makes it impossible to use a photographic method of recording the rate of travel of the bubble as seen in the projected film. These factors constitute practical limitations to the usefulness of the method as a technique for the experimental recording of blood flow. McDonald (1955a) showed that the velocities of flow recorded by this method were in good agreement with those calculated from the pressure-gradient, or the time-derivative of the pressure curve. This gives us confidence in the method as no other has been simultaneously checked in this fashion and few different meters have shown much agreement one with the other. It should be remembered, however, that the direct measurement is of *velocity* of flow and that where *volume* flows have been reported they are derived secondarily. Some volume flow curves previously reported (McDonald, 1955a) have undoubtedly been too high due to over-estimation of the internal radius of the artery.

As regards the cinematographic method of recording flow velocity, the peak values may be rather high—possibly as much as 25 per cent in some cases. This doubt is based on current estimations of arterial impedance (Ch. 13) and may prove to be unjustified.

References

ABBOTT, B. C. and LOWY, J. (1958). Contraction in molluscan smooth muscle, *J. Physiol.*, **141**: 385–97.

ALBRITTON, E. C. (1952). *Standard values in blood*. Philadelphia: Saunders.

ALEXANDER, R. S. (1953). The genesis of the aortic standing wave. *Circulat. Res.* **1**: 145–51.

ALEXANDER, R. S. (1954). The influence of constrictor drugs on the distensibility of the splanchnic venous system, analysed on the basis of an aortic model. *Circulat. Res.*, **2**: 140–47.

ALFONSO, S. (1966). A thermodilution flowmeter. *J. appl. Physiol.*, **21**: 1883–86.

ALLIEVI, L. (1909). *Allgemeine Theorie über die verändliche Bewegung des Wassers in– Leitungen.* Berlin: Springer. Cited by Karreman, G. (1952).

ANDRES, R., ZIERLER, K. L., ANDERSON, H. M., STAINSBY, W. N., CADER, G., GHAYYIB, A. S. and LILIENTHAL, J. L. JR. (1954). Measurement of blood flow and volume in the forearm of man; with notes on the theory of indicator-dilution and on the production of turbulence, hemolysis, and vaso-dilation by intravascular injection. *J. clin. Invest.*, **33**: 482–504.

ANLIKER, M. and MAXWELL, J. A. (1967). The dispersion of waves in blood vessels. Biomech. Symp., ASME, New York, pp. 47–67.

ANLIKER, M. and RAMAN, K. R. (1966). Korotkoff sounds at diastole—a phenomenon of dynamic instability of fluid-filled shells. *Int. J. Solids Struct.* **2**: 467–91.

ANLIKER, M., HISTAND, M. B. and OGDEN, E. (1968). Dispersion and attenuation of small artificial pressure waves in the canine aorta. *Circulat. Res.*, **23**: 539–51.

ANLIKER, M., MORITZ, W. E. and OGDEN, E. (1968). Transmission characteristics of axial waves in blood vessels. *J. Biomech.*, **1**: 235–46.

ANLIKER, M., WELLS, M. K. and OGDEN, E. (1969). The transmission characteristics of large and small pressure waves in the abdominal vena cava. *IEEE Trans. Biomed. Eng.*, BME-16: 262–73.

APÉRIA, A. (1940). Haemodynamical Studies. *Skand. Arch. Physiol.*, **83**: Suppl. 1–230.

APTER, J. T. (1966). Correlation of visco-elastic properties of large arteries with microscopic structure. I. Methods used and their justification. III. Circumferential viscous and elastic constants measured in vitro. *Circulat. Res.*, **19**: 104–21.

APTER, J. T. (1967). Correlation of visco-elastic properties of large arteries with microscopic structure. IV. Thermal responses of collagen, elastin, smooth muscle, and intact arteries. *Circulat. Res.*, **21**: 901–18.

APTER, J. T. and MARQUEZ., E. (1968). Correlation of visco-elastic properties of large arteries with microscopic structure. *Circulat. Res.*, **22**: 393–404.

APTER, J. T., RABINOWITZ, M. and CUMMINGS, D. H. (1966). Correlation of visco-elastic properties of large arteries with microscopic structure. II. Collagen,

459

elastin and muscle determined chemically, histologically, and physiologically. *Circulat. Res.*, **19**: 104–21.

ARNDT, J. O. (1969). Uber die Mechanik der intaken A. Carotis communis des Menschen unter verschiedenen Kreislaufbedingungen. *Arch. Kreisl.-Forsch.*, **59**: 153–97.

ARNDT, J. O., KLAUSKE, J. and MERSCH, F. (1968). The diameter of the intact carotid artery in man and its change with pulse pressure. *Pflügers Arch. ges. Physiol.*, **301**: 230–40.

ARNDT, J. O., STEGALL, H. F. and WICKE, H. J. (1971). Mechanics of the aorta in vivo. *Circulat. Res.*, **28**: 693–704.

ASCHOFF, J. and WEVER, R. (1956). Die Funktionsweise der Diathermie Thermostromuhr. *Pflügers Arch. ges. Physiol.*, **262**: 133–51.

ATABEK, H. B. and LEW, H. S. (1966). Wave propagation through a viscous incompressible fluid contained in an initially elastic tube. *Biophys. J.*, **6**: 481–503.

ATABEK, H. B., CHANG, C. C. and FINGERSON, L. M. (1964). Measurement of laminar oscillatory flow in the inlet length of a circular tube. *Phys. in Med. Biol.*, **9**: 219–27.

ATTINGER, E. O. (1964). Elements of theoretical hydrodynamics. In *Pulsatile Blood Flow*, ed. O. E. Attinger., pp. 15–76. New York: McGraw-Hill.

ATTINGER, E. O., ANNE, A. and MCDONALD, D. A. (1966). Use of fourier series for the analysis of biological systems. *Biophys. J.*, **6**: 291–304.

ATTINGER, E. O., SUGAWARA, H., NAVARRO, A. and ANNE, A. (1966). Pulsatile flow patterns in distensible tubes. *Circulat. Res.*, **18**: 447–56.

ATTINGER, E. O., SUGAWARA, H., NAVARRO, A., MIKAMI, T. and MARTIN, R. (1967). Flowpatterns in the peripheral circulation of the anesthetized dog. *Angiologica*, **4**: 1–27.

ATTINGER, E. O., SUGAWARA, H., NAVARRO, A., RICETTO, A. and MARTIN, R. (1966). Pressure-flow relations in dog arteries. *Circulat. Res.*, **19**: 230–46.

ATTINGER, F. M. L. (1968). Two-dimensional in-vitro studies of femoral arterial walls of the dog. *Circulat. Res.*, **22**: 829–40.

BAEZ, S., LAMPORT, H. and BAEZ, A. (1960). Pressure effects in living microscopic vessels. In *Flow Properties of Blood*, ed. Copley, A. L. and Stainsby, G. London: Pergamon Press.

BAKER, D. W. (1965). The Doppler shift principle applied to flow and displacement measurement. *Engineering in Medicine and Biology*, Proceedings 18th Annual Conference, p. 172.

BAKER, D. W. (1966). Pulsed ultrasonic flowmeter. *Meth. med. Res.*, **11**: 107–17. Chicago: Year Book Medical Publishers.

BAKER, D. W., STEGALL, F. and SCHLEGEL, W. A. (1964). A sonic transcutaneous blood flowmeter. *Engineering in Medicine and Biology*, Proceedings 17th Annual Conference, p. 76.

BALDES, E. J. and HERRICK, J. F. (1937). Thermostromuhr with D.C. heater. *Proc. Soc. exp. Biol. Med.*, **37**: 432.

BALL, G. and GABE, I. T. (1963). Sinusoidal pressure generator for testing differential manometers. *Med. Electron. Biol. Engng*, **1**: 237–41.

BARCLAY, A. E., FRANKLIN, K. J. and PRICHARD, M. M. L. (1944). *The foetal circulation and cardiovascular system, and the changes that they undergo at birth.* Oxford: Blackwell.

BARGAINER, J. D. (1967). Pulse wave velocity in the pulmonary artery of the dog. *Circulat. Res.*, **20**: 630–37.

BARNARD, A. C. L., HUNT, W. A., TIMLAKE, W. P. and VARLEY, E. (1966a). A theory of fluid flow in compliant tubes. *Biophys. J.*, **6**: 717–24.

BARNARD, A. C. L., HUNT, W. A., TIMLAKE, W. P. and VARLEY, E. (1966b). Peaking of the pressure pulse in fluid-filled tubes of spatially varying compliance. *Biophys. J.*, **6**: 735–46.

BARNETT, C. H. and COCHRANE, W. (1956). Flow of viscous liquids in branched tubes. *Nature (Lond.)*, **177**: 740–42.

BARNETT, G. O., GREENFIELD, J. C. JR. and FOX, S. M. (1961). The technique of estimating the instantaneous aortic blood velocity in man from the pressure gradient. *Amer. Heart J.*, **62**: 359–66.

BARNETT, G. O., MALLOS, A. J. and SHAPIRO, A. (1961). Relationship of aortic pressure and diameter in the dog. *J. appl. Physiol.*, **16**: 545–48.

BARR, G. (1931). *A monograph of viscometry.* Oxford: University Press.

BAXTER, I. G. and PEARCE, J. W. (1951). Simultaneous measurement of pulmonary arterial flow and pressure using condenser manometers. *J. Physiol.*, **115**: 410–29.

BAXTER, I. G., CUNNINGHAM, D. J. C. and PEARCE, J. W. (1952). Comparison of cardiac output determinations in the cat by direct Fick and flowmeter methods. *J. Physiol.*, **118**: 299–308.

BAYLISS, L. E. (1952). Rheology of blood and lymph. In *Deformation and flow in biological systems*, ed. Frey-Wissling, A., pp. 354–418. Amsterdam: North-Holland Publishing.

BAYLISS, L. E. (1959). The axial drift of the red cells when blood flows in a narrow tube. *J. Physiol.*, **149**: 593–613.

BAYLISS, L. E. (1960). The anomalous viscosity of blood. In *Flow properties of blood*, ed. Copley, A. L. and Stainsby, G. pp. 29–62. Oxford: Pergamon Press.

BAYLISS, L. E. (1962). The rheology of blood. In *Handbook of Physiology*, Sec. 2 (Circulation), Vol. 1, ch. 8. Washington: American Physiological Society.

BAYLISS, L. E. (1965). Flow of suspensions of red blood cells in capillary tubes. Changes in the 'cell-free' marginal sheath with changes in the shearing stress. *J. Physiol.*, **179**: 1–25.

BAYLISS, W. M. (1902). On the local reactions of the arterial wall to changes in internal pressure. *J. Physiol.*, **28**: 220.

BAZETT, H. C. (1941). In *Macleod's physiology in modern medicine*, ch. 23, p. 408. London: Kimpton.

BEALES, J. S. M. and STEINER, R. E. (1972). Radiological assessment of arterial branching coefficients. *Cardiovasc. Res.*, **6**: 181–86.

BELL, E. T. (1965). *Men of mathematics*, New York: Simon & Schuster.

BELLHOUSE, B. J. (1972). Fluid mechanics of a model mitral valve and left ventricle. *Cardiovasc. Res.*, **6**: 199–210.

BELLHOUSE, B. J. and BELLHOUSE, F. H. (1968). Mechanism of closure of the aortic valve. *Nature (Lond.)*, **217**: 86–87.

BELLHOUSE, B. J. and BELLHOUSE, F. H. (1969). Fluid mechanics of model normal and stenosed aortic valves. *Circulat. Res.*, **25**: 693–704.

BELLHOUSE, B. J. and REID, K. G. (1968). A bio-engineering study of the geometry and fluid dynamics of the aortic root. *Report*, Dept. of Engineering, Univ. of Oxford.

BELLHOUSE, B. J., BELLHOUSE, F. H. and REID, K. G. (1968). Fluid mechanics of the aortic root with application to coronary flow. *Nature (Lond.)*, **219**: 1059–61.

BENCHIMOL, A., STEGALL, H. F., MAROKO, P. R., GARTLAN, J. L. and BRENER, L. (1969). Aortic flow velocity in man during cardiac arrhythmias measured with the Doppler catheter-flowmeter system. *Amer. Heart J.*, **78**: 649–59.

BENNINGHOF, A. (1930). Blutgefässe und Herz. In *Handbuch der Mikroscopischen Anatomie des Menschen.* Berlin: Springer.

BERGEL, D. H. (1960). *The visco-elastic properties of the arterial wall.* Ph.D. thesis, University of London.

BERGEL, D. H. (1961*a*). The static elastic properties of the arterial wall. *J. Physiol.*, **156**: 445–57.

BERGEL, D. H. (1961*b*). The dynamic elastic properties of the arterial wall. *J. Physiol.*, **156**: 458–69.

BERGEL, D. H. and GESSNER, U. (1966). The electro-magnetic flowmeter. *Meth. med. Res.*, **11**: 70–82. Chicago: Year Book Medical Publishers.

BERGEL, D. H. and MILNOR, W. R. (1965). Pulmonary vascular impedance in the dog. *Circulat. Res.*, **16**: 401–15.

BERGEL, D. H. and SCHULZ, D. L. (1971). Arterial elasticity and fluid dynamics. *Progr. Biophys. molec. Biol.*, **22**: 1–36. Oxford and New York: Pergamon Press.

BERGEL, D. H., MCDONALD, D. A. and TAYLOR, M. G. (1958). A method for measuring arterial impedance using a differential manometer. *J. Physiol.*, **141**: 17–18P.

BERGMANN, C. (1937–38). Die 'Stromborste,' ein electrischer Geschwindigkeitsmesser für Flüssigkeiten. II. Stromkanüle und electrische Messanordnung. *Z. Biol.*, **98**: 536–43.

BETTICHER, A., MAILLARD, J. and MÜLLER, A. (1954). Un manomètre differential à transmission électrique entièrement alimenté sur le réseau alternatif, pour mesurer la vitesse d'écoulement dans des tuyaux et des vaisseaux sanguins. *Helv. physiol. Acta.*, **12**: 112–22.

BEVERIDGE, W. I. B. (1957). *The art of scientific investigation.* New York: Modern Library, Random House.

BINGHAM and JACKSON (1918). *Bur. Stand. J. Res., Wash.*, **14**: 75; p. 1993 in *Handbook of chemistry and physics*, 35th edn. ed. Hodgman, C. D., Weast, R. C. and Wallace, C. W., Cleveland, Ohio: Chemical Rubber Publishing.

BIRCHER, M. E. (1921). Clinical diagnosis by the aid of viscosimetry of the blood with special reference to the viscosimeter of W. R. Hess. *J. Lab. clin. Med.*, **7**: 134–47.

BIRKHOFF, G. (1960). *Hydrodynamics.* Princeton: University Press.

BLACKMAN, R. B. and TURKEY, J. W. (1958). *The measurement of power spectra from the point of view of communications engineering.* New York: Dover Publications.

BLUM, E. (1919). Die Querschnittbezeihungen zwischen Stamm und Asten in Arteriensystem. *Pflügers Arch. ges. Physiol.*, **175**: 1–19.

BOND, R. F. and BAREFOOT, C. A. (1967). Evaluation of an electro-magnetic catheter tip velocity-sensitive blood flow probe. *J. appl. Physiol.*, **23**: 403–9.

BOONE, M. N. (1972). Peak power as an index of myocardial contractility. Ph.D. Dissertation, University of Alabama in Birmingham.

BORGNIS, F. E. and FRUTIGER, P. (1969). An improved ultrasonic flowmeter. *Cardiologia*, **54**: 193–204.

BOYETT, J. D., STOWE, D. E. and BECKER, L. H. (1966). Evaluation of aortic blood velocity computed from the pressure pulse. U.S. Air Force School of Aerospace Medicine, SAM-TT-66-75, 1–6.

BRAMWELL, J. C. and HILL, A. V. (1922). The velocity of the pulse wave in man. *Proc. roy. Soc. B.*, **93**: 298–306.

BRAMWELL, J. C. and HILL, A. V. (1923). The formation of 'breakers' in the transmission of the pulsewave. *J. Physiol.*, **57**: lxxiii–lxxiv.

BRANDT, A. and BUGLIARELLO, G. (1966). Concentration redistribution phenomena in the shear flow of monolayers of suspended particles. *Trans. Soc. Rheol.*, **10:1**, 229–51.

BRECHER, G. A. (1954). Cardiac variations in venous return studied with a new bristle flowmeter. *Amer. J. Physiol.*, **176**: 423–40.

BRECHER, G. A. (1956). *Venous return*. New York: Grune & Stratton.

BRECHER, G. A. (1960). Bristle flowmeter. *Meth. med. Res.*, **8**: 307–21. Chicago: Year Book Medical Publishers.

BRECHER, G. A. and HUBAY, C. A. (1954). A new method for direct recording of the cardiac output. *Proc. Soc. exp. Biol.* (*N. Y.*), **86**: 464–67.

BROEMSER, P. (1928–29). Der Differentialsphygmograph. Eine methode zur Registrierung der Kurve des Ablaufes der Strömungsgeschwindigkeit des Blutes in uneröffneten Arterien. *Z. Biol.*, **88**: 264–76.

BROEMSER, P. (1930). Anwendung mathematischer Methoden auf dem Gebiet der physiologischen Mechanik. In *Abderhalden's Handbuch der biologischen Arbeitsmethoden*, Abt. V, Teil 1, p. 81.

BROEMSER, P. and RANKE, O. F. (1931). Uber die Messung des Schlagvolumen des Herzens auf unblutigen Weg. *Z. Biol.*, **90**: 467–507.

BROTMACHER, L. (1957). Evaluation of derivation of cardiac output from blood pressure measurements. *Circulat. Res.*, **5**: 589–93.

BRUNS, D. L. (1959). A general theory of the causes of murmurs in the cardiovascular system. *Amer. J. Med.*, **27**: 360–74.

BUCHANAN, J. W. JR. and SHABETAI, R. (1972). True power dissipation of catheter tip velocity probes. *Cardiovasc. Res.*, **6**: 211–13.

BUGLIARELLO, G. (1964). Phase separation in suspensions flowing through bifurcations: a simplified hemodynamic model. *Science*, **143**: 469–71.

BUGLIARELLO, G. and HAYDEN, J. W. (1962). High-speed microcinematographic studies of blood in vitro. *Science*, **138**: 981–83.

BUGLIARELLO, G. and HSIAO, G. C. (1965). The mechanism of phase separation at bifurcations: an introduction to the problem in the microcirculatory system. *Bibl. anat.*, **7**: 363–67.

BUGLIARELLO, G. and HSIAO, G. C. (1970). A mathematical model of the flow in the axial plasmatic gaps of the smaller blood vessels. *Biorheology*, **7**: 5–36.

BUGLIARELLO, G. and SEVILLA, J. (1970). Velocity distribution and other characteristics of steady and pulsatile blood flow in fine glass tubes. *Biorheology*, **7**: 85–107.

BUGLIARELLO, G., KAPUR, C. and HSIAO, G. C. (1965). The profile viscosity and other characteristics of blood flow in a non-uniform shear field. In *Proc. 4th int. Congr. Rheol.* Part 4, ed. Copley, A. L. pp. 351–70. New York: Interscience.

BUGLIARELLO, G., DAY, H. J., BRANDT, A., EGGENBERGER, A. J. and HSIAO, G. C. (1968). Model studies of the hydrodynamic characteristics of an erythrocyte. I. Method, apparatus and preliminary results. In Copley, A. L. (1968), *Hemorheology*. pp. 305–24. London: Pergamon Press.

BURTON, A. C. (1954). Relation of structure to function of the tissues of the walls of blood vessels. *Physiol. Rev.*, **34**: 619–42.

BURTON, A. C. (1965). *Physiology and Biophysics of the Circulation*. Chicago: Year Book Medical Publishers.

CAPPELEN, C. (ED.) (1968). *New findings in blood flowmetry*. Oslo: Universitetsforlaget.

CAREW, T. E., VAISHNAV, R. N. and PATEL, D. J. (1968). Compressibility of the arterial wall. *Circulat. Res.*, **23**: 61–68.

CARLETON, R. A., BOWYER, A. F. and GRAETTINGER, J. S. (1966). Overestimation of left ventricular volume by the indicator-dilution technique. *Circulat. Res.* **18**: 248–55.

CARO, C. G. (1966). The dispersion of indicator flowing through simplified models of the circulation and its relevance to velocity profile in blood vessels. *J. Physiol.*, **185**: 501–19.

Q

CARO, C. G. and MCDONALD, D. A. (1961). The relation of pulsatile pressure and flow in the pulmonary vascular bed. *J. Physiol.*, **157**: 426–53.

CARO, C. G., BERGEL, D. H. and SEED, W. A. (1967). Forward and backward transmission of pressure waves in the pulmonary vascular bed of the dog. *Circulat. Res.*, **20**: 185–93.

CARO, C. G., FITZ-GERALD, J. M. and SCHROTER, R. C. (1971). Atheroma and arterial wall shear. Observation, correlation and proposal of a shear dependent mass transfer mechanism for arterogenesis. *Proc. roy. Soc. Lond. B.*, **177**: 109–59.

CARO, C. G., HARRISON, G. K. and MOGNONI, P. (1967). Pressure wave transmission in the human pulmonary circulation. *Cardiovasc. Res.*, **1**: 91–100.

CASSON, N. (1959). A flow equation for pigment-oil suspensions of the printing-ink type. In *Rheology of disperse system*, ed. Mill, C. C. pp. 84–102. London: Pergamon Press.

CHANG, C. C. and ATABEK, H. B. (1961). The inlet length for oscillatory flow and its effects on the determination of the rate of flow in arteries. *Phys. in Med. Biol.*, **6**: 303–17.

CHAUVEAU, A., BERTOLUS, G. and LAROYENNE, L. (1860). Vitesse de la circulation dans les artères du cheval. *J. de la Physiol. de l'homme et des animaux.*

CHICHE, P., KALMANSON, D., VEYRAT, C. and TOUTAIN, G. (1968a). Enregistrement transcutané du flux artériel par fluxmètre directionnel à effet Doppler. *Bull. Med. Soc. Med. Hôp. de Paris*, **119**: 87–95.

CHICHE, P., KALMANSON, D. and VEYRAT, C. (1968b). Etude des courbes de flux artériel obtenues par enregistrement transcutané chez le subjet normal. *Presse méd.*, **76**: 1943–46.

CLARK, R. W. (1971). *Einstein: the life and times.* New York and Cleveland: World Publishing Co.

CLARK-KENNEDY, A. E. (1965). *Stephen Hales.* Ridgewood, New Jersey: Gregg Press. (Originally published 1929, London: Cambridge University Press.)

CLEARY, E. G. (1963). *A correlative and comparative study of the non-uniform arterial wall.* M.D. thesis, University of Sydney, Australia.

COKELET, G. R., MERRILL, E. W., GILLILAND, E. R., SHIN, H., BRITTEN, A. and WELLS, R. E. (1963). The rheology of human blood—measurement near and at zero shear rate. *Trans. Soc. Rheol.*, **7**: 303–17.

COON, G. W. and SANDLER, H. (1967). Ultra-miniature manometer tipped cardiac catheter, *Proc. 20th ACEMB*, **9**: 22.2.

COPENHAVER, W. M. (ED.) (1964). *Baily's textbook of histology.* 15th edn. Baltimore: Williams and Wilkins.

COPHER, G. H. and DICK, B. M. (1928). 'Stream line' phenomena in the portal vein and the selective distribution of portal blood in the liver. *Arch. Surg., Chicago*, **17**: 408–19.

COPLEY, A. L. (ED.) (1965). *Symposium on Biorheology.* New York: Interscience.

COPLEY, A. L. (ED.) (1968). *Hermorheology*, Proceedings First International Conference. Oxford: Pergamon Press.

COPLEY, A. L. and HARTERT, H. H. (EDS.) (1971). *Theoretical and Clinical Hemorheology*, Proceedings Second International Conference. New York: Springer-Verlag.

COTTON, K. L. (1960). *The instantaneous measurement of blood flow and of vascular impedance.* Ph.D. Thesis, University of London.

COULOMB (1798). Cited Hatschek, E. (1928). *The viscosity of liquids.* London: Bell.

COULTER, N. A. JR. and PAPPENHEIMER, J. R. (1949). Development of turbulence in flowing blood. *Amer. J. Physiol.*, **159**: 401–8.

COURNAND, A. F. (1948). Comment on 'right heart catheterization'. *Meth. in Med. Res.*, **1**: 231. Chicago: Year Book Medical Publishers.

COX, R. H. (1968). Wave propagation through a Newtonian fluid contained within a thick-walled, viscoelastic tube. *Biophys. J.*, **8**: 691–709.

COX, R. H. (1969). Comparison of linearized wave propagation models for arterial blood flow analysis. *J. Biomech.*, **2**: 251–65.

COX, R. H. (1970*a*). Blood flow and pressure propagation in the canine femoral artery. *J. Biomech.*, **3**: 131–49.

COX, R. H. (1970*b*). Wave propagation through a Newtonian fluid contained within a thick-walled viscoelastic tube: the influence of wall compressibility. *J. Biomech.*, **3**: 317–35.

DAWES, G. S., MOTT, J. C. and WIDDICOMBE, J. G. (1955). The cardiac murmur from the patent ductus arteriosus in newborn lambs. *J. Physiol.*, **128**: 344–60.

DAWES, G. S., MOTT, J. C., WIDDICOMBE, J. G. and WYATT, D. G. (1953). Changes in the lungs of the new-born lamb. *J. Physiol.*, **121**: 141–62.

DENISON, A. B., SPENCER, M. P. and GREEN, H. D. (1955). A square-wave electromagnetic flowmeter for application to intact blood vessels. *Circulat. Res.*, **3**: 39–46.

DENNIS, J. and WYATT, D. G. (1969). Effect of haematocrit value upon flowmeter sensitivity. *Circulat. Res.*, **24**: 875–85.

DICK, D. E., KENDRICK, J. E., MATSON, G. L. and RIDEOUT, V. C. (1968). Measurement of nonlinearity in the arterial system of the dog by a new method. *Circulat. Res.*, **22**: 101–11.

DIX, F. J. and SCOTT BLAIR, G. W. (1940). On flow of suspensions through narrow tubes. *J. appl. Phys.*, **11**: 574.

DOBRIN, P. B. and DOYLE, J. M. (1970). Vascular smooth muscle and the anisotropy of dog carotid artery. *Circulat. Res.*, **27**: 105–19.

DOBRIN, P. B. and ROVICK, A. A. (1969). Influence of vascular smooth muscle on contractile mechanics and elasticity of arteries. *Amer. J. Physiol.*, **217**: 1644–51.

DODGE, H. T., HAY, R. E. and SANDLER, H. (1962). An angiocardiographic method for directly determining left ventricular stroke volume in man. *Circulat. Res.*, **11**: 739–45.

DODGE, H. T., SANDLER, H., BALLEW, D. W. and LORD, J. D. (1960). The use of biplane angiocardiography for the measurement of left ventricular volume in man. *Amer. Heart J.*, **60**: 762–76.

DOW, P. (1956). Estimations of cardiac output and central blood volume by dye dilution. *Physiol. Rev.*, **36**: 77–102.

DOW, P. and HAMILTON, W. F. (1939). An experimental study of the velocity of the pulse wave propagated through the aorta. *Amer. J. Physiol.*, **125**: 60–65.

DREYER, B. (1954). Streamlining in the portal vein. *Quart. J. exp. Physiol.*, **39**: 305–7.

DUGUID, J. B. and ROBERTSON, W. B. (1957). Mechanical factors in atherosclerosis. *Lancet*, 1957/i, 1205–9.

DWIGHT, H. B. (1961). *Mathematical tables*, 3rd edn. New York: Dover Publications.

EINSTEIN, A. (1906). Eine neue Bestimmung der Moleküldimensionen. *Ann. Physik.*, **19**: 289–306.

ELLIS, E. J., GAUER, O. H. and WOOD, E. H. (1951). An intracardiac manometer: its evaluation and application. *Circulation*, **3**: 390–98.

ENGLEBERG, J. and DUBOIS, A. B. (1959). Mechanics of pulmonary circulation in isolated rabbit lungs. *Amer. J. Physiol.*, **196**: 401–14.

EVANS, R. L. (1955). On the mechanism of turbulent flow in a liquid. Proceedings Fourth Midwestern Conference on Fluid Mechanics. *Res. Bull. Purdue Exp. Stn*, **128**: 235–43.

*Q

EVANS, R. L. (1956). Elasticity of vessel walls. *Amer. J. Physiol.* **187**: 597.

EVANS, R. L. (1958). Cardiac output and central pressure data. *Nature (Lond.)*, **181**: 1471–72.

EVANS, R. L. (1962). Pulsatile flow in vessels whose distensibility and size vary with site. *Phys. in Med. Biol.*, **7**: 105–16.

FABRE, P. (1932). Utilisation des forces électromotrices d'induction pour l'enregistrement des variations de vitesse des liquides conducteurs: un nouvel hémodromographe sans palette dans le sang. *C. R. Acad. Sci. (Paris)*, **194**: 1097.

FEDER, W. and BAY, E. B. (1959). The d.c. electromagnetic flowmeter and its application to blood flow measurement in unopened vessels. *IRE Trans. med. Electron.*, M.E.–6: 240.

FENN, W. O. (1957). Changes in length of blood vessels on inflation. In *Tissue elasticity*, ed. Remington, J., pp. 154–67. Washington: American Physiological Society.

FICH, S., WELKOWITZ, W. and HILTON, R. (1966). Pulsatile blood flow in the aorta. *Biomedical Fluid Mechanics Symposium*. New York: ASME.

FISCHER, G. M. and LLAURADO, J. G. (1966). Collagen and elastin content in canine arteries selected from functionally different vascular beds. *Circulat. Res.*, **19**: 394–99.

FOLKOW, B. (1964). Description of myogenic hypothesis. *Circulat. Res.*, **14–15**: Suppl. 1, 279–87.

FOLKOW, B. and LÖFVING, B. (1956). The distensibility of the systemic resistance blood vessels. *Acta physiol. scand.*, **38**: 37–52.

FRANK, O. (1899). Die Grundform des arteriellen Pulses. Erste Abhandlung. Mathematische Analyse. *Z. Biol.*, **37**: 483–526.

FRANK, O. (1903). Kritik der elastischen Manometer. *Z. Biol.*, **44**: 445–613.

FRANK, O. (1905). Der Puls in den Arterien. *Z. Biol.*, **46**: 441–553.

FRANK, O. (1906). Die Analyse endlicher Dehnungen und die Elastizität des Kautschuks. *Ann. Physik*, **21**: 602–8.

FRANK, O. (1920). Die Elastizität der Blutegefässe. *Z. Biol.*, **71**: 255–72.

FRANK, O. (1925). Die Moensschen Schliessungs- und Offnungsschwingungen als gekoppelte Schwingungen. *Z. Biol.*, **83**: 1–7.

FRANK, O. (1926a). Die Theorie der Pulswellen. *Z. Biol.*, **85**: 91–130.

FRANK, O. (1926b). Der arterielle Puls. *S.-B. Ges Morph. U. Physiol.*, *München*, **37**: 33–54.

FRANK, O. (1926c). Das Altern der Arterien. *S.-B. Ges. Morph. U. Physiol.*, *München*, **37**: 23–32.

FRANK, O. (1927). Die Theorie der Pulswellen. *Z. Biol.*, **85**: 91–130.

FRANK, O. (1927–28). Der Ablauf der Geschwindigkeit in der Aorta. *S.-B. Ges. Morph. U. Physiol.*, *München*, **38**: 1–7.

FRANK, O. (1928a). Das Aufblähen von Schläuchen und kugelförmigen Blasen. *Z. Biol.*, **88**: 93–104.

FRANK, O. (1928b). Die Elastizität der Blutgefässe, II. Mitt. *Z. Biol.*, **88**: 105–18.

FRANK, O. (1926c). Modell fur die Strömung im Aortenbogen. *Z. Biol.*, **88**: 245–48.

FRANK, O. (1928d). Der Ablauf der Strömungsgeschwindigkeit in den Gefässen. *Z. Biol.*, **88**: 250–63.

FRANK, O. (1929). Kurze Bemerkungen über die Bestimmungen der Blutgeschwindigkeit. *S.-B. Ges. Morph. U. Physiol.*, *München*, **39**: 19–22.

FRANK, O. (1930). Schätzung des Schlagvolumens des menschlichen Herzens auf Grund der Wellen- und Windkesseltheorie. *Z. Biol.*, **90**: 405–9.

FRANKE, E. O. (1966). Physiologic pressure transducers. *Meth. med. Res.*. **11**: 137–61 Chicago: Year Book Medical Publishers.

FRANKLIN, D. L., BAKER, D. W. and RUSHMER, R. F. (1962). Ultrasonic transit-time flowmeter. *IRE Trans. biomed. Engng*, ME–9: 44–49.

FRANKLIN, D. L., ELLIS, R. M. and RUSHMER, R. F. (1959). Aortic blood flow in dogs during treadmill exercise. *J. appl. Physiol.*, **14**: 809–12.

FRANKLIN, D. L., SCHLEGEL, W. and RUSHMER, R. F. (1961). Blood flow measured by Doppler frequency shift back-scattered sound. *Science*, **134**: 564–65.

FRANKLIN, K. J. (1937). *A monograph on veins*. Springfield, Illinois: Thomas.

FRANKLIN, K. J. (1961), *William Harvey: Englishman, 1578–1657*. London: Mac-Gibbon & Kee.

FRANKLIN, P. (1958). *An introduction to Fourier methods and the Laplace transformation*. New York: Dover Publications.

FRASHER, W. G., WAYLAND, H. and MEISELMAN, H. J. (1968). Viscometry of circulating blood in dogs. I. Heparin injection. II. Platelet removal. *J. appl. Physiol.*, **25**: 751–60.

FREIS, E. D. and HEATH, W. C. (1964). Hydrodynamics of aortic blood flow. *Circulat. Res.*, **14**: 105–16.

FRONEK, A. (1972). Analysis of recent developments in blood flow measurement. In *Biomechanics: Its Foundations and Objectives*, eds. Fung, Y. C., Perrone, N. and Anliker, M. Englewood Cliffs, New Jersey: Prentice-Hall.

FRONEK, A. and GANZ, V. (1960). Measurement of flow in single blood vessels including cardiac output by local thermodilution. *Circulat. Res.*, **8**: 175–82.

FRY, D. L. (1959a). Certain aspects of hydrodynamics as applied to the living cardiovascular system, *IRE Trans. med. Electron.*, ME–6: 252–58.

FRY, D. L. (1959b). Measurement of pulsatile blood flow by the computed pressure gradient technique, *IRE Trans. med. Electron.*, ME–6: 259–64.

FRY, D. L. (1966). General considerations in selecting a flow detection technique. *Meth. med. Res.*, **11**: 44–69. Chicago: Year Book Medical Publishers.

FRY, D. L. (1968). Acute vascular endothelial changes associated with increased blood velocity gradients. *Circulat. Res.*, **22**: 165–97.

FRY, D. L. (1969a). Certain histological and chemical responses of the vascular interface to acutely induced mechanical stress in the aorta of the dog. *Circulat. Res.*, **24**: 93–108.

FRY, D. L. (1969b). Certain chemorheologic considerations regarding the blood vascular interface with particular reference to coronary artery disease. *Circulation*. **39–40**: Suppl. 4, 38–57.

FRY, D. L. and GREENFIELD, J. C. JR. (1964). The mathematical approach to hemodynamics, with particular reference to Womersley's theory. In *Pulsatile Blood Flow*, ed. Attinger, E. O., pp. 85–99. New York: McGraw-Hill.

FRY, D. L., GRIGGS, D. M. JR. and GREENFIELD, J. C. JR. (1964). Myocardial mechanics: tension-velocity-length relationships of heart muscle. *Circulat. Res.*, **14**: 73–85.

FRY, D. L., MALLOS, A. J. and CASPER, A. G. T. (1956). A catheter tip method for measurement of the instantaneous aortic blood velocity. *Circulat. Res.*, **4**: 627–32.

FRY, D. L., NOBLE, F. W. and MALLOS, A. J. (1957). An evaluation of modern pressure recording systems. *Circulat. Res.*, **5**: 40–46.

FUCHS, R. F. (1900). Zur Physiologie und Wachstummsmechanik des Blutgefässystems. *Arch. ges. Physiol.*, **28**: 7.

FULTON, J. F. (1966). *Selected readings in the history of physiology*, Springfield, Illinois: Thomas.

FUNG, Y. C., ZWEIFACH, B. W. and INTAGLIETTA, M. (1966). Elastic environment of capillary bed. *Circulat. Res.*, **19**: 441–61.

GABE, I. T. (1965a). Arterial blood flow by analogue solution of the Navier–Stokes equation. *Phys. in Med. Biol.*, **10**: 271–80.

GABE, I. T. (1965b). An analogue computer deriving oscillatory arterial blood flow from the pressure gradient. *Phys. in Med. Biol.*, **10**: 407–15.

GABE, I. T. (1972). Pressure Measurement in Experimental Physiology. In *Cardiovascular Fluid Dynamics*, Vol. 1, ed. Bergel, D. H. London and New York: Academic Press.

GABE, I. T., KARNELL, J., PORJÉ, I. G. and RUDEWALD, B. (1964). The measurement of input impedance and apparent phase velocity in the human aorta. *Acta physiol. scand.*, **61**: 73–84.

GABE, I. T., GAULT, J. H., ROSS, J. JR., MASON, D. T., MILLS, C. J., SHILLINGFORD, J. P. and BRAUNWALD, E. (1969). Measurement of instantaneous blood flow velocity and pressure in conscious man with a catheter-tip velocity probe. *Circulation*, **40**: 603–14.

GALLE, K. R. (1966). Thermal flowmeters. *Meth. med. Res.*, **11**: 94–106. Chicago: Year Book Medical Publishers.

GANZ, V., HLAVOVA, A., FRONEK, A., LINHART, J. and PREROVSKY, J. (1964). Measurement of blood flow in the femoral artery in man at rest and during exercise by local thermodilution. *Circulation*, **30**: 86–89.

GAUER, O. H. and GIENAPP, E. (1950). Miniature pressure recording device. *Science*, **112**: 404.

GEROVA, M. and GERO, J. (1967). Effector mechanisms induced by baroreceptor stimulation. In *Baroreceptors and Hypertension*. pp. 225–33. Oxford: Pergamon Press.

GERSH, B. J., PRYS-ROBERTS, C., REUBEN, S. R., and SCHULTZ, D. L. (1972). The effects of halothane on the interactions between myocardial contractility, aortic impedance and left ventricular performance. II. Aortic input impedance, and the distribution of energy during ventricular ejection. *Brit. J. Anaesth.*, **44**: 767–75.

GESSNER, U. (1961). Effects of the vessel wall on electromagnetic flow measurement. *Biophys. J.*, **1**: 627–37.

GESSNER, U. (1972). Vascular Input Impedance. In *Cardiovascular Fluid Dynamics*, Vol. I, ed. Bergel, D. H. London and New York: Academic Press.

GESSNER, U. and BERGEL, D. H. (1964). Frequency response of electro-magnetic flowmeters. *J. appl. Physiol.*, **19**: 1209.

GILINSON, P. J. JR., DAUWALTER, C. R. and MERRILL, E. W. (1963). A rotational viscometer using an a.c. torque to balance loop and air bearing. *Trans. Soc. Rheol.*, **7**: 319–31.

GIRARD (1813). Cited Hatschek, E., *The viscosity of liquids*. London: Bell, 1928.

GOLDMAN, S. C., MARPLE, N. B. and SCOLNICK, W. L. (1963). Effects of flow profile on electromagnetic flowmeter accuracy. *J. appl. Physiol.*, **18**: 652.

GOLDSMITH, H. L. and MASON, S. G. (1961). Axial migration of particles in Poiseuille flow. *Nature (Lond.)*, **190**: 1095–96.

GOLDSMITH, H. L. and MASON S. G. (1964). Some model experiments in haemodynamics. 2nd Europ. Conf. on Microcirc., Pavia, 1962, *Bibl. anat.*, **4**: 462–78.

GOLDSMITH, H. L. and MASON, S. G. (1966). Further comments on the radial migration of spheres in Poiseuille flow. *Biorheology*, **3**: 33–36.

GOLDSTEIN, S. (1938). *Modern developments in fluid dynamics*. 2 vols. Oxford: Clarendon Press.

GORLIN, R. (1958). Normal variations in venous oxygen content. *Meth. med. Res.*, **7**: 69. Chicago: Year Book Medical Publishers.

GOW, B. S. (1966). An electrical caliper for measurement of pulsatile arterial diameter changes in vivo. *J. appl. Physiol.*, **20**: 1122–26.

GOW, B. S. and TAYLOR, M. G. (1968). Measurement of viscoelastic properties of arteries in the living dog. *Circulat. Res.*, **23**: 111–22.

GRAHN, A. R., PAUL, M. H. and WESSEL, H. U. (1969). A new direction-sensitive probe for catheter-tip thermal velocity measurements. *J. appl. Physiol.*, **27**: 407–12.

GREEN, A. E. and ADKINS, J. E. (1960). *Large elastic deformations and non-linear continuum mechanics.* Oxford: Clarendon Press.

GREEN, A. E. and ZERNA, W. (1960). *Theoretical elasticity.* Oxford: Clarendon Press.

GREEN, H. D. (1944). Circulation: physical principles. In *Medical physics*, ed. Glasser, O. New York: Yearbook Publishers.

GREEN, H. D. (1948). Pulsatile flow meters. *Meth. med. Res.*, **1**: 101–8. Chicago: Year Book Medical Publishers.

GREEN, H. D. (1950). Circulatory system: physical principles. In *Medical physics*, Vol. II, ed. Glasser, O. Chicago: Year Book Publishers.

GREEN, J. H. (1954). A manometer. *J. Physiol.*, **125**: 4–6P.

GREENFIELD, J. C. JR. and FRY, D. L. (1962). Measurement errors in estimating aortic blood velocity by pressure gradient. *J. appl. Physiol.*, **17**: 1013–19.

GREENFIELD, J. C. JR. and FRY, D. L. (1965a). Relationship between instantaneous aortic flow and the pressure gradient. *Circulat. Res.*, **17**: 340–48.

GREENFIELD, J. C. JR. and FRY, D. L. (1965b). A critique: relationship of the time derivative of pressure to blood flow. *J. appl. Physiol.*, **20**: 1141–47.

GREENFIELD, J. C. JR. and PATEL, D. J. (1962). Relation between pressure and diameter in the ascending aorta of man. *Circulat. Res.*, **10**: 778–81.

GREENFIELD, J. C. JR., PATEL, D. J., BARNETT, G. O. and FOX, S. M. (1962). Evaluation of the pressure time derivative method for estimating peak blood flow. *Amer. Heart J.*, **64**: 101–5.

GREENFIELD, J. C. JR., PATEL, D. J., MALLOS, A. J. and FRY, D. L. (1962). Evaluation of Kolin type electromagnetic flowmeter and the pressure gradient technique. *J. appl. Physiol.*, **17**: 372–74.

GREENFIELD, J. C. JR., TINDALL, G. T., DILLON, M. L. and MAHALEY, M. S. (1964). Mechanics of human carotid artery in vivo. *Circulat. Res.*, **15**: 240–46.

GREGG, D. E. and GREEN, H. D. (1939). Phasic blood flow in coronary arteries obtained by a new differential manometric method. *Proc. Soc. exper. Biol. Med.*, **41**: 597–98.

GREGG, D. E., PRITCHARD, W. H. and SHIPLEY, R. E. (1948). Changes in arterial inflow in the dog's leg following venous occlusion: evaluation of results obtained with different types of flow recorders. *Amer. J. Physiol.*, **153**: 153–58.

GRODINS, F. S. (1962). Basic concepts in the determination of vascular volumes by indicator-dilution methods. *Circulat. Res.*, **10**: 429–46.

GROOM, A. C., MORRIS, W. B. and ROWLANDS, S. (1957). The difference in circulation times of plasma and corpuscles in the cat. *J. Physiol.*, **136**: 218–25.

GUTH, E. (1947). Muscular contraction and rubber-like elasticity. *Ann. N.Y. Acad. Sci.*, **47**: 715–66.

GUYTON, A. C. (1963). *Circulatory physiology: cardiac output and its regulation.* Philadelphia: Saunders.

GUYTON, A. C. (1966). *Textbook of medical physiology*, 3rd edn. Philadelphia: Saunders.

HALE, J. F., MCDONALD, D. A. and WOMERSLEY, J. R. (1955). Velocity profiles of oscillating arterial flow, with some calculations of viscous drag and the Reynolds number. *J. Physiol.*, **128**: 629–40.

HALE, J. F., MCDONALD, D. A., TAYLOR, M. G. and WOMERSLEY, J. R. (1955). The counter chronometer method for recording pulse-wave velocity. *J. Physiol.*, **129**: 27P.

HALES, S. (1727). *Vegetable staticks*. Republished 1961. London: Scientific Book Guild.

HALES, S. (1733). *Statical essays: containing haemastaticks*, reprinted 1964, No. 22, History of Medicine series, Library of New York Academy of Medicine. New York: Hafner Publishing.

HAMILTON, W. F. (1953). The physiology of the cardiac output. *Circulation*, **8**: 527–43.

HAMILTON, W. F. (1962). Measurement of the cardiac output. In *Handbook of physiology*, Section 2: Circulation, I: 551–84. Washington: American Physiological Society.

HAMILTON, W. F. and DOW, P. (1939). An experimental study of the standing waves in the pulse propagated through the aorta. *Amer. J. Physiol.*, **125**: 48–59.

HAMILTON, W. F. and REMINGTON, J. W. (1947). Measurement of stroke volume from the pressure pulse. *Amer. J. Physiol.*, **148**: 14.

HAMILTON, W. F., BREWER, G. and BROTMAN, I. (1934). Pressure pulse contours in the living animal. I. Analytical description of a new high-frequency hypodermic manometer with illustrative curves of simultaneous arterial and intracardiac pressure. *Amer. J. Physiol.*, **107**: 427–35.

HANSEN, A. T. (1949). Pressure measurement in the human organism. *Acta physiol. scand.*, **19**: Suppl. 68.

HANSEN, A. T. and WARBURG, E. (1950). A theory for eastic liquid-containing membrane manometers. General part. *Acta physiol. scand.*, **19**: 306–32.

HARDUNG, V. (1952). Uber eine Methode zur Messung der dynamischen Elastizität und Viskosität kautschukähnlicher Körper, insbesondere von Blutgefässen und anderen elastischen Gewebteilen. *Helv. physiol. Acta.*, **10**: 482–98.

HARDUNG, V. (1953). Vergleichende Messungen der dynamischen Elastizität und Viskosität von Blutgefässen, Kautschuk und synthetischen Elastomeren. *Helv. physiol. Acta*, **11**: 194–211.

HARDUNG, V. (1957). Zum Gebrauch des Pitot-Rohres bei nichtstationärer Stromung. *Arch. Kreisl.-Forsch.*, **26**: 337–48.

HARDUNG, V. (1958). Wellenwiderstand und Impedanzen der geraden Schlauchleigung. *Arch. Kreisl.-Forsch.*, **29**: 77–88.

HARDUNG, V. (1962). Propagation of pulse waves in viscoelastic tubing. In *Handbook of physiology: Circulation*: Vol. I, ed. Hamilton, W. F. and Dow, P. p. 107. Washington: American Physiological Society.

HARDUNG, V. (1964a). Die Bedeutung der Anistropie und Inhomogenität bei der Bestimmung der Elastizität der Blutgefässe, I. Mitteilung. *Angiologica* (Basel), **1**: 141–55.

HARDUNG, V. (1964b). Die Bedeutung der Anistropie und Inhomogenität bei der Bestimmung der Elastizität der Blutgefässe, II. Mitteilung. *Angiologica* (Basel), **1**: 185–96.

HARKNESS, M. L. R., HARKNESS, R. D. and MCDONALD, D. A. (1957). The collagen and elastin content of the arterial wall in the dog. *Proc. roy. Soc. B.*, **146**: 541–51.

HARVEY, W. (1628). *De Motu Cordis*, Frankfurt: William Fitzer. Translated as *Movement of the heart and blood in animals* by Franklin, K. J. (1957). Oxford: Blackwell Scientific Publications.

HATSCHEK, E. (1928). *The viscosity of liquids*. London: Bell.

HAUGEN, M. G., FARRELL, W. R., HERRICK, J. F. and BALDES, E. J. (1955). An ultrasonic flowmeter. *Proc. nat. Electron. Conf.*, **11**: 1–11.

HAYNES, R. H. (1961). The rheology of blood. *Trans. Soc. Rheol.*, **5**: 85–101.

HAYNES, R. H. and BURTON, A. C. (1959). Axial accumulation of cells and the rheology of blood. *Proceedings First National Biophysics Conference*. pp. 452–59. Yale: University Press.

HELPS, E. P. W. and MCDONALD, D. A. (1954). Observations on laminar flow in veins. *J. Physiol.*, **124**: 631–39.

HERRICK, J. F. (1942). Poiseuille's observations on blood flow lead to a law in hydrodynamics. *Amer. J. Phys.*, **10**: 33–39.

HESS, W. R. (1908). Die Viskosität des Blutes bei Gesunden. *Dtsch. Arch. klin. Med.*, **94**: 404–8.

HESS, W. R. (1911). Blutviskosität und Blutkörperchen. *Pflügers Arch. ges. Physiol.*, **140**: 354.

HESS, W. R. (1917). Uber die periphere Regulierung der Blutzirkulation. *Pflügers Arch. ges. Physiol.*, **168**: 439–90.

HESS, W. R. (1927). Die Verteilung von Querschnitt, Widerstand, Druckgefälle und Strömungsgeschwindigkeit im Blutkreislauf. *Handb. d. normale u. path. Physiol.* (*Bethe*), Bd. VII, Teil 2, pp. 904–33. Berlin: Springer.

HESSE, M. (1926). Uber die Pathologischen Veranderungen der Arterien der oberen Extremität. *Virchows Arch. path. Anat. Physiol.*, **261**: 225–52.

HILL, L. (1900). The mechanism of the circulation of blood. In *Textbook of physiology*, ed. Schäfer, E. A. Vol. II. Edinburgh: Pentland.

HISTAND, M. B. (1969). An experimental study of the transmission characteristics of pressure waves in the aorta. *Stanford Univ. Report* No. SUDAAR–369.

HOLT, J. P. (1956). Estimation of the residual volume of the ventricle of the dog's heart by two indicator dilution techniques. *Circulat. Res.*, **4**: 187–95.

HOLT, J. P. (1966). Symposium on measurement of left ventricular volume. II. Indicator dilution methods: indicators, injection, sampling and mixing problems in measurement of ventricular volume. *Amer. J. Cardiol.*, **18**: 208–25.

HOSIE, K. F. (1957). *Studies on the mechanics of the aorta in vitro*. Ph.D. dissertation, University of Minnesota.

HÜRTHLE, K. (1920). Uber die Bezeihung zwischen Durchmesser und Wandstärke der Arterien nebst Schätzung des Anteils der einzelnen Gewebe am Aufbau der Wand. *Pflügers Arch. ges. Physiol.*, **183**: 253–70.

IBERALL, A. S. (1950). Attenuation of oscillatory pressures in instrument lines. U.S. Dept. of Commerce, Res. Paper RP2115, *J. Res. Nat. Bur. Stands.*, **45**: 85–108.

IBERALL, A. S. (1967). Anatomy and steady flow characteristics of the arterial system with an introduction to its pulsatile characteristics. *Math. Biosci.*, **1**: 375–95.

INOUYE, A. and KOSAKA, H. (1959). A study of flow patterns in carotid and femoral arteries of rabbits and dogs with the electromagnetic flowmeter. *J. Physiol.*, **147**: 209–20.

INOUYE, A., KUGA, H. and USUI, G. (1955). A new method for recording pressure flow diagrams applicable to peripheral blood vessels of animals and its application. *Jap. J. Physiol.*, **5**: 236–49.

JAGER, G. N., WESTERHOF, N. and NOORDERGRAAF, A. (1965). Oscillatory flow impedance in electrical analog of arterial system: representation of sleeve effect and non-Newtonian properties of blood. *Circulat. Res.*, **16**: 121–33.

JAHNKE, E. and EMDE, F. (1945). *Tables of functions*. New York: Dover Publications.

JANICKI, J. S. and PATEL, D. J. (1968). A force gauge for measurement of longitudinal stresses in a blood vessel in situ. *J. Biomech.*, **1**: 19–21.

JANSSEN, S., ASCHOFF, J., BAUMGARTNER, G., GRUPP, G., HIERHOLZER, K., HILLE, H., OBERDORF, A., RUMMEL, W. and WEVER, R. (1957). Vergleich und Kritik verschiedener Durchblutungs-Messmethoden. *Pflügers Arch. ges. Physiol.*, **264**: 198–216.

JOCHIM, K. E. (1948). Electromagnetic flow meter. *Meth. med. Res.*, 1: 108–15. Chicago: Year Book Medical Publishers.

JOHANSEN, K. and MARTIN, A. W. (1965). Comparative aspects of cardiovascular function in vertebrates. *Handbook of physiology*, Section 2, Circulation, Vol. III: 2583–2614.

JOHNS, R. J. (1968). Is biomedical engineering fulfilling its destiny? The Samuel Armstrong Talbot Memorial Lecture, 9th IBM Medical Symposium, Burlington, Vermont: 13–21.

JOHNSON, P. C. (1969). Hemodynamics. *Ann. Rev. Physiol.*, 31: 331–52.

JOLY, M. (1968). Notice biographique sur J. M. L. Poiseuille, in *Hemorheology*, ed. Copley, A. L. pp. 29–31. New York: Pergamon Press.

JONES, M. A. S. and WYATT, D. G. (1970). The surface temperature of electromagnetic velocity probes. *Cardiovasc. Res.*, 4: 388–97.

JONES, W. B. and GRIFFIN, J. B. (1962). Comparison of computed aortic blood velocity with that of electromagnetic flowmeter. *J. appl. Physiol.*, 17: 482.

JONES, W. B. and REEVES, T. J. (1968). Total cardiac output response during four minutes of exercise. *Amer. Heart J.*, 76: 209–16.

JONES, W. B., RUSSELL, R. O. JR. and DALTON, D. H. JR. (1966). An evaluation of computed stroke volume in man. *Amer. Heart J.*, 71: 746–50.

JONES, W. B., HEFNER, L. L., BANCROFT, J. R. and KLIP, W. (1959). Velocity of blood flow and stroke volume obtained from pressure pulse. *J. clin. Invest.*, 38: 2087–90.

KALMANSON, D., TOUTAIN, G., NOVOKOFF, N., and DERAI, C. (1972). Retrograde catheterization of left heart cavities in dogs by means of an orientable directional Doppler catheter-tip flowmeter: A preliminary report. *Cardiovascular Research*, 6: 309–18.

KALMANSON, D., VEYRAT, C. and CHICHE, P. (1968). Aspects morphologiques de l'onde de flux artériel enregistrée par voie transcutanée chez le sujet normal. *Bull. Mém. Soc. Méd. Hôp. de Paris*, 119: 743–52.

KALMANSON, D., VEYRAT, C. and CHICHE, P. (1969a). Etude des variations physiologiques du retour veineux droit enregistré par voie transcutanée au niveau de la veine jugulaire interne. I. Variations respiratoires. *Arch. Malad. Coeur Vaisseaux*, 62: 1293–1310.

KALMANSON, D., VEYRAT, C. and CHICHE, P. (1969b). Variations physiologiques du retour veineux enregistré par voie transcutanée au niveau de la veine jugulaire interne. II. Variations extra-respiratoires. *Arch. Malad. Coeur Vaisseaux*, 62: 1386–1403.

KALMANSON, D., VEYRAT, C. and CHICHE, C. (1970). Venous return disturbances produced by arrhythmias. *Cardiovasc. Res.*, 4: 279–90.

KAPAL, E., MARTINI, F. and WETTERER, E. (1951). Uber die Zuverlässigkeit der bisherigen Bestimmungsart der Pulswellengeschwindigkeit. *Z. Biol.*, 104: 75–86.

KARREMAN, G. (1952). Some contributions to the mathematical biology of blood circulation. Reflections of pressure waves in the arterial system. *Bull. math. Biophys.*, 14: 327–50.

KAUFMANN, W. (1963). *Fluid mechanics*. Translated by E. G. Chilton. New York: McGraw-Hill.

KENNER, T. and WETTERER, E. (1963). Studie über die verschiedenen Definitionen des Elastizitätsmoduls in der Haemodynamik. *Z. Biol.*, 114: 11–24.

KHOURI, E. M. and GREGG, D. E. (1963). Miniature electromagnetic flowmeter applicable to coronary arteries. *J. appl. Physiol.*, 18: 224–27.

KHOURI, E. M., GREGG, D. E. and LOWENSOHN, H. S. (1968). Flow in the major branches of the left coronary artery during experimental coronary insufficiency in the unanesthetized dog. *Circulat. Res.*, **23**: 99–109

KING, A. L. (1947). Waves in elastic tubes: velocity of the pulse wave in large arteries. *J. appl. Physics*, **18**: 595–600.

KING, A. L. (1950). Circulatory system: arterial pulse; wave velocity. In *Medical physics*, Vol. 2, ed. Glasser, O. Chicago: Year Book Medical Publishers.

KING, A. L. and LAWTON, R. W. (1950). Elasticity of body tissues. In *Medical physics*, Vol. 2, ed. Glasser, O. Chicago: Year Book Medical Publishers.

KINNEN, E. (1966). Thermistor tipped catheter instrumentation for measuring pulsatile blood flow. *Proc. ann. Conf. Engng Med. Biol.*, **8**: 110.

KLIP, W. (1961). Anomalous viscosity of blood and the 'summation phenomenon'. *Circulat. Res.*, **9**: 1380–83.

KLIP, W. (1969). *Theoretical Foundations of Medical Physics*. 2 Vols. Alabama: University of Alabama Press.

KLIP, W. and KLIP, D. A. B. (1964). Phase velocity and damping of torsional waves in thin-walled tubes of infinite length. In *Pulsatile blood flow*, ed. Attinger, E. O. pp. 323–30. New York: McGraw-Hill.

KLIP, W., VAN LOON, P. and KLIP, D. A. B. (1967). Formulas for phase velocity and damping of longitudinal waves in thick-walled viscoelastic tubes. *J. appl. Phys.*, **38**: 37–45.

KOBER, G. and ARNDT, J. O. (1970). Die Druck-Durchmesser-Beziehung der A. carotis communis des wachen Menschen. *Pflügers Arch. ges. Physiol.*, **214**: 27–39.

KOLIN, A. (1936). An electromagnetic flowmeter. Principle of the method and its application to blood flow measurements. *Proc. Soc. exp. Biol. Med.*, **35**: 53–56.

KOLIN, A. (1937). An electromagnetic recording flowmeter. *Amer. J. Physiol.*, **119**: 355.

KOLIN, A. (1944). Electromagnetic velometry. I. A method for the determination of fluid velocity distribution in space and time. *J. appl. Phys.*, **15**: 150–64.

KOLIN, A. (1945). An alternating field induction flowmeter of high sensitivity. *Rev. Scient. Instrum.*, **16**: 109–16.

KOLIN, A. (1960). Blood flow determination by electromagnetic method. In *Medical physics*, Vol. 3, ed. Glasser, O. pp. 141–55. Chicago: Year Book Medical Publishers.

KOLIN, A. (1969a). A radial field electromagnetic intravascular flow sensor. *IEEE Trans. Biomed. Engng*, BME 16: 220–21.

KOLIN, A. (1969b). A new principle for electromagnetic catheter flowmeters. *Proc. Nat. Acad. Sci.*, **63**: 357–63.

KOLIN, A. (1970). A new approach to electromagnetic blood flow determination by means of catheter in an external magnetic field. *Proc. Nat. Acad. Sci.*, **65**: 521–27.

KOLIN, A. and WISSHAUPT, R. (1963). Single-coil coreless electromagnetic blood flowmeters. *IEEE Trans. Biomed. Electron.* BME–10: 60–67.

KOLIN, A., ARCHER, J. and ROSS, G. (1967), An electromagnetic catheter-flowmeter. *Circulat. Res.*, **21**: 889–99.

KORTEWEG, D. J. (1878). Cited Lambossy, P. (1950).

KOUCHOUKOS, N. T., SHEPPARD, L. C. and MCDONALD, D. A. (1970). Estimation of stroke volume in the dog by a pulse contour method. *Circulat. Res*, **26**: 611–23.

KOUCHOUKOS, N. T., SHEPPARD, L. C., MCDONALD, D. A. and KIRKLIN, J. W. (1969). Estimation of the stroke volume from the central arterial pressure contour in post-operative patients. *Surg. Forum*, **20**: 180–82.

KRAFKA, J. JR. (1939). Comparative study of the histophysics of the aorta. *Amer. J. Physiol.*, **125**: 1–14.

KRAMER, K., LOCHNER, W. and WETTERER, E. (1963). Methods of measuring blood flow. *Handbook of Physiology*, Section 2: Circulation, Vol. II: 1277–1324. Washington: American Physiological Society.

KROVETZ, L. J. (1965a). On the experimental determination of laminar-turbulent transitions in liquid flow. *Phys. in Med. Biol.*, **10**: 261–70

KROVETZ, L. J. (1965b). The effect of vessel branching on haemodynamic stability. *Phys. in Med. Biol.*, **10**: 417–70.

KROVETZ, L. J. and CROWE, W. J. (1967). Studies of arterial branching in models using flow birefringence. *Digest, 7th int. Conf. med. biol. Engng, Stockholm:* 158.

KEUTHER, F. W., HIGGS, R. W. and RICHARDS, A. M. (1966). A point sensor of pulsatile blood flow velocity for use in the human body. *Proc. ann. Conf. Engng, Med. Biol.*, **8**: 112.

KÜMIN, K. (1949). *Bestimmung des Zähigkeitskoeffizienten für Rinderblut bei Newtons' schen Strömungen in Verschieden weiten Röhren und Kapillaren bei physiologischer Temperatur*, Inaug. Diss. Freiburg: Schweiz.

KUNZ, A. L. and COULTER, N. A. JR. (1967). Non-Newtonian behavior of blood in oscillatory flow. *Biophys. J.*, **7**: 25–36.

LAMB, H. (1898). On the velocity of sound in a tube as effected by the elasticity of the walls. *Manchester Mem.*, **43**: 1.

LAMB, H. (1932). *Hydrodynamics*, 5th edn (reprinted 1953). Cambridge: University Press.

LAMBOSSY, P. (1950), Aperçu historique et critique sur le problème de la propagation des ondes dans un liquide compressible enfermé dans un tube elastique. *Helv. physiol. Acta*, **8**: 209–27.

LAMBOSSY, P. (1952a). Oscillations forcées d'un liquide incompressible et viscueux dans un tube rigide et horizontal. Calcul de la force de frottement. *Helv. phys. Acta*, **25**: 371–86.

LAMBOSSY, P. (1952b). Manomètres a l'observation des variations de la pressure sanguine. *Helv. physiol. Acta*, **10**: 138–60.

LAMPORT, H. (1955). Hemodynamics. In *Fulton's textbook of physiology*, 17th edn, pp. 589–611. Philadelphia: Saunders.

LANDES, G. (1949). Die Berechnung des Schlagvolumens mit Berücksichtigung der Reflexionen, verteilter Elastizität, Masse und Reibung. *Arch. Kreisl.-Forsch.*, **15**: 1.

LANDOWNE, M. (1957a). Pulse wave velocity as an index of arterial elastic characteristics. In *Tissue elasticity*, ed. Remington, J. W. pp. 168–76. Washington: American Physiological Society.

LANDOWNE, M. (1957b). A method using induced waves to study pressure propagation in human arteries. *Circulat. Res.*, **5**: 594–601.

LANDOWNE, M. (1958). Characteristics of impact and pulse wave propagation in brachial and radial arteries. *J. appl. Physiol.*, **12**: 91–97.

LASZT, L. and MÜLLER, A. (1951a). Uber den Druckverlauf im linken Ventrikel und Vorhof und in den Aorta ascendens. *Helv. physiol. Acta*, **9**: 55–73.

LASZT, L. and MÜLLER, A. (1951b). Gleichzeitige Druckregistrierung in beiden Herzkammern, in der Aorta und der Pulmonalis. *Helv. physiol. Acta*, **9**: 326–37.

LASZT, L. and MÜLLER, A. (1951c). Uber die Druckverhältnisse im bereiche des Aortenbogens. *Helv. physiol. Acta*, **9**: 442–53.

LASZT, L. and MÜLLER, A. (1952a). Uber den Druckverlauf im Bereiche der Aorta. *Helv. physiol. Acta*, **10**: 1–19

LASZT, L. and MÜLLER, A. (1952b). Gleichzeitige Druckmessung in der Aorta abdominalis und ihren Hauptästen. *Helv. physiol. Acta*, **10**: 259–72.

LASZT, L. and MÜLLER, A. (1952c). Vergleich der Druckverhältnisse in den Gefässen des Halses und der oberen Extremitäten mit dem Drucke in der Aorta ascendens. *Helv. physiol. Acta*, **10**: 469–81.

LASZT, L. and MÜLLER, A. (1957). Uber Druck- und Geschwindigkeitsverhältnisse im Coronar Kreislauf des Hundes. *Helv. physiol. Acta*, **18**: 38–54.

LAURENS, P., BOUCHARD, F., BRIAL, E., CORNU, C., BACULARD, P. and SOULIE, P. (1959). Intra-cardiac sound and pressure recording by means of a micromanometer. *Archiv. Malad. Coeur Vaisseaux*, February.

LAWTON, R. W. (1954). The thermoelastic behavior of isolated aortic strips in the dog. *Circulat. Res.*, **2**: 344–53.

LAWTON, R. W. (1955). Measurements on the elasticity and damping of isolated aortic strips in the dog. *Circulat. Res.*, **3**: 403–8.

LAWTON, R. W. and GREENE, L. C. (1956). A method for the in situ study of aortic elasticity in the dog. Report No. NADC–MA–5603, AMAL, U.S. Nav. Air Dev. Cent.

LAWTON, R. W. and KING, A. L. (1950). The elasticity of soft body tissues. *Scient. Mon.*, **71**: 258–60.

LEAROYD, B. M. and TAYLOR, M. G. (1966). Alterations with age in the visco-elastic properties of human arterial walls. *Circulat. Res.*, **18**: 278–92.

LEE, Y. W. (1960). *Statistical theory of communication*. New York: Wiley.

LEITZ, K. H. and ARNDT, J. O. (1968). Die Durchmesser-Druck-Beziehung des intakten Gefässgebietes der A. carotis communis von Katzen. *Pflügers Archiv. ges. Physiol.*, **301**: 50–69.

LEONARD, E. and SARNOFF, S. J. (1957). Effect of aramine-induced smooth muscle contraction on length-tension diagrams of venous strips. *Circulat. Res.*, **5**: 169–74.

LEUSEN, I., DEMEESTER, G. and BOUCKAERT, J. J. (1954). Influence des reflexes sino-carotidiens due le débit cardiaque et la résistance peripherique après hémorragie. *Arch. int. Physiol.*, **62**: 535–39.

LEVY, M. N. (1958). Relative influence of variations in arterial and venous pressures on resistance to flow. *Amer. J. Physiol.*, **192**: 164–70.

LEVY, M. N. and SHARE, L. (1953). The influence of erythrocyte concentration upon the pressure-flow relationships in the dog's hind limb. *Circulat. Res.*, **1**: 247–55.

LEVY, M. N., BRIND, S. H., BRANLIN, F. R. and PHILLIPS, F. A. (1954). The relationship between pressure and flow in the systemic circulation of the dog. *Circulat. Res.*, **2**: 372–80.

LEWIS, D. H., DEITZ, G. W., WALLACE, A. D. and BROWN, J. R. JR. (1959). Intracardiac phonocardiography. *Prog. cardiovasc. Dis.*, **2**: 85–96.

LIGHTHILL, M. J. (1956). Physics of gas flow at very high speeds. *Nature (Lond.)*, **178**: 343–45.

LIGHTHILL, M. J. (1969). Motion in narrow capillaries from the standpoint of lubrication theory. In *Circulatory and Respiratory mass transport*, ed. Wolstenholme, G. E. W. and Knight, J. pp. 85–104. Boston: Little, Brown.

LILLY, J. C. (1942). Electrical capacitance diaphragm manometer. *Rev. scient. Instrum.*, **13**: 34.

LINDEN, R. J. (1958). A hydraulic pressure wave generator. *J. Physiol.*, **142**: 44–46.

LINFORD, R. G. and RYAN, N. W. (1965). Pulsatile flow in rigid tubes. *J. appl. Physiol.*, **20**: 1078–82.

LING, S. C. and ATABEK, H. B. (1966). Measurement of aortic blood flow in dogs by the hot-film technique. *Proc. 19th ann. Conf. Engng Med. Biol.*, **8**: 113.

LING, S. C., ATABEK, H. B., FRY, D. L., PATEL, D. J. and JANICKI, J. S. (1968). Application of heated-film velocity and shear probes to hemodynamic studies. *Circulat. Res.*, **23**: 789–801.

LLOYD, R. A. (1971). *An evaluation of the thermodilution method for measuring ventricular volumes.* Ph.D. Thesis, University of Alabama in Birmingham.

LLOYD, R. A. and MCDONALD, D. A. (1971). Thermal indicator mixing in the heart (in vitro). *Fed. Proc.*, **30**: 703.

LOVE, A. E. H. (1944). *A treaties on the mathematical theory of elasticity.* 4th edn. New York: Dover Publications.

LUCHSINGER, P. C., SACHS, M. and PATEL, D. J. (1962). Pressure-radius relationship in large blood vessels of man. *Circulat. Res.*, **11**: 885–88.

LUCHSINGER, P. C., SNELL, R. E., PATEL, D. J. and FRY, D. L. (1964). Instantaneous pressure distribution along the human aorta. *Circulat. Res.*, **15**: 503–10.

LUNDHOLM, L. and MOHME-LUNDHOLM, E. (1966). Length at inactivated contractile elements, length-tension diagram, active state and tone of vascular smooth muscle. *Acta physiol. scand.*, **68**: 347–59.

LYNCH, P. R. and BOVE, A. A. (1968). Patterns of blood flow through the intact heart and its valves. In *Prosthetic heart valves*, ed. Brewer, L. A. Springfield, Illinois: Thomas.

LYNCH, P. R. and BOVE, A. A. (1969). Geometry of the left ventricle as studied by a high speed cineradiographic technique. *Fed. Proc.*, **28**: 1330–33.

MACHELLA, T. E. (1936). The velocity of blood flow in arteries in animals. *Amer. J. Physiol.*, **115**: 632–44.

MALL, F. (1888). *König. Sächs. Ges. Wiss. Abhandl. Math. Cl.*, **14**: 151 (cited by Iberall, 1967).

MALL, F. (1905). Cited by Iberall, 1967.

MALLOS, A. J. (1962). An electrical caliper for continuous measurement of relative displacement. *J. appl. Physiol.*, **17**: 131–34.

MALONEY, J. E., BERGEL, D. H., GLAZIER, J. B., HUGHES, J. M. B. and WEST, J. B. (1968). Transmission of pulsatile blood pressure and flow through the isolated lung. *Circulat. Res.*, **23**: 11–24.

MAREY, E. S. (1881). *Le circulation du sang à l'état physiologique et dans des maladies.* Paris: Masson.

MARSHALL, R. J. and SHEPARD, J. T. (1959). Effect of injections of hypertonic solutions on blood flow through the femoral artery of the dog. *Amer. J. Physiol.*, **197**: 951–54.

MASON, D. T., GABE, I. T., MILLS, C. J., GAULT, H. J., ROSS, J. JR., BRAUNWALD, E. and SHILLINGFORD, J. P. (1970). Application of the catheter-tip electromagnetic velocity probe in the study of the central circulation in man. *Amer. J. Med.*, **49**: 465–71.

MAXWELL, J. A. and ANLIKER, M. (1968). The dissipation and dispersion of small waves in arteries and veins with viscoelastic wall properties. *Biophys. J.*, **8**: 920–50.

MCCUTCHEON, E. P. and RUSHMER, R. F. (1967). Korotkoff sounds. An experimental critique. *Circulat. Res.*, **20**: 147–61.

MCDONALD, D. A. (1952). The occurrence of turbulent flow in the rabbit aorta. *J. Physiol.*, **118**: 340–47.

MCDONALD, D. A. (1953). Lateral pulsatile expansion of arteries. *J. Physiol.*, **119**: 28P.

MCDONALD, D. A. (1955). The relation of pulsatile pressure to flow in arteries. *J. Physiol.*, **127**: 533–52.

MCDONALD, D. A. (1960). *Blood flow in arteries*. Monog. Physiol. Soc. London: Edward Arnold; Baltimore: Williams & Wilkins.

MCDONALD, D. A. (1964). Frequency dependence of vascular impedance. In *Pulsatile blood flow*, ed. Attinger, E. O. pp. 115–33. New York: McGraw-Hill.

MCDONALD, D. A. (1965a). Wave propagation in the arterial tree. *Proc. ann. Conf. Engng Med. Biol.*, **7**: 1.

MCDONALD, D. A. (1965b). The flow properties of blood as a factor in the stability of pulsatile flow. *Symp. on Biorheology*. pp. 205–13. New York Interscience.

MCDONALD, D. A. (1968a). Regional pulse-wave velocity in the arterial tree. *J. appl. Physiol.*, **24**: 73–78.

MCDONALD, D. A. (1968b). Hemodynamics. *Ann. Rev. Physiol.*, **30**: 525–56.

MCDONALD, D. A. and GESSNER, U. (1968). Wave attenuation in visco-elastic arteries. In *Hemorheology*, ed. Copley, A. L. pp. 113–25. Oxford: Pergamon Press.

MCDONALD, D. A. and HELPS, E. P. W. (1954). *Streamline flow in veins* (film), description in Copley and Stainsby (eds), *Flow properties of blood*. 1960, p. 395. Oxford: Pergamon Press. Film available from Wellcome Foundation, London, or American Heart Association, New York.

MCDONALD, D. A. and NICHOLS, W. W. (1973). Cardiac output derived from the time derivative and phase velocities of the aortic pressure wave. *Med. biol. Engng* (in press).

MCDONALD, D. A. and POTTER, J. M. (1951). The distribution of blood to the brain. *J. Physiol.*, **114**: 356–71.

MCDONALD, D. A. and TAYLOR, M. G. (1956). An investigation of the arterial system using a hydraulic oscillator. *J. Physiol.*, **133**: 74P.

MCDONALD, D. A. and TAYLOR, M. G. (1959). The hydrodynamics of the arterial circulation. In *Progr. Biophys.* **9**: 107–73. London: Pergamon Press.

MCKUSICK, V. A. (1957). Cardiovascular sound: a clinical survey. *Circulation*, **16**: 424–27.

MCKUSICK, V. A. (1958). *Cardiovascular sound in health and disease*. Baltimore: Williams and Wilkins.

MCLACHLEN, N. W. (1941). *Bessel functions for engineers*. Oxford: University Press.

MCLEOD, F. D. JR. (1967). A directional Doppler flowmeter. *Digest 7th int. Conf. med. biol. Engng*: 213.

MCLEOD, F. D. JR. (1970). Calibration of CW and pulse Doppler flowmeters. *Proc. 23rd ann. Conf. Engng Med. Biol.*, **12**: 271.

MCMILLAN, I. K. R. (1955). Aortic stenosis. A post-mortem cinephotographic study of valve action. *Brit. Heart.*, **17**: 56–62.

MCMILLAN, I. K. R., DALEY, R. and MATHEWS, M. B. (1952). The movement of aortic and pulmonary valves studied post-mortem by colour cinematography. *Brit. Heart J.*, **14**: 42–46.

MEIER, P. and ZIERLER, K. L. (1954). On the theory of the indicator-dilution method for the measurement of blood flow and volume. *J. appl. Physiol.*, **6**: 731–44.

MEISNER, J. E. and REMINGTON, J. W. (1962). Pulse contour changes in carotid and foreleg arterial systems. *Amer. J. Physiol.*, **202**: 527–35.

MEISNER, J. E. and RUSHMER, R. F. (1963a). Eddy formation and turbulence in flowing liquids. *Circulat. Res.*, **12**: 455–63.

MEISNER, J. E. and RUSHMER, R. F. (1963b). Production of sounds in distensible tubes. *Circulat. Res.*, **12**: 651–58.

MELLANDER, S. and RUSHMER, R. F. (1960). Venous blood flow recorded with an isothermal flowmeter. *Acta physiol. scand.*, **48**: 13.

MERRILL, E. W. (1969). Rheology of blood. *Physiol. Rev.*, **49**: 863–88.

MERRILL, E. W., GILLILAND, E. R., LEE, T. S. and SALZMAN, E. W. (1966). Blood rheology: effect of fibrinogen deduced by addition. *Circulat. Res.*, **18**: 437–66.

MERRILL, E. W., BENIS, A. M., GILLILAND, E. R., SHERWOOD, T. K. and SALZMAN, E. W. (1965). Pressure-flow relations of human blood in hollow fibers at low flow rates. *J. appl. Physiol.*, **20**: 954–67.

MERRILL, E. W., MARGETTS, W. G., COKELET, G. R. and GILLILAND, E. R. (1965). The Casson equation and rheology of the blood near shear zero. In *Proceedings Fourth International Congress on Rheology*, Part 4, ed. Copley, A. L. pp. 135–43. New York: Interscience.

MERRILL, E. W., MARGETTS, W. G., COKELET, G. R., BRITTEN, A., SALZMAN, E. W., PENNELL, R. B. and MELIN, M. (1965). Influence of plasma proteins on the rheology of human blood. In *Proceedings Fourth International Congress on Rheology*, Part 4, ed. Copley, A. L. pp. 601–11. New York: Interscience.

MERRILL, E. W., GILLILAND, E. R., COKELET, G. R., BRITTAIN, A., SHIN, H. and WELLS, R. E. (1963a). Rheology of blood flow in the microcirculation. *J. appl. Physiol.*, **18**: 255–60.

MERRILL, E. W., GILLILAND, E. R., COKELET, G. R., BRITTAIN, A., SHIN, H. and WELLS, R. E. (1963b). Rheology of human blood near and at zero flow: effects of temperature and hematocrit levels. *Biophys. J.*, **3**: 199–213.

MILLS, C. J. (1966). A catheter-tip electromagnetic velocity probe. *Phys. in Med. Biol.*, **11**: 323–24.

MILLS, C. J. (1972). Measurement of Pulsatile Flow and flow velocity. In *Cardiovascular Fluid Dynamics*, Vol. 1, ed. Bergel, D. H. London and New York: Academic Press.

MILLS, C. J. and SHILLINGFORD, J. P. (1967). A catheter-tip electromagnetic velocity probe and its evaluation. *Cardiovasc. Res.*, **1**: 263–73.

MILLS, C. J., GABE, I. T., GAULT, J. H., MASON, D. T., ROSS, J., BRAUNWALD, E. and SHILLINGFORD, J. P. (1970). Pressure-flow relationships and vascular impedance in man. *Cardiovasc. Res.*, **4**: 405–17.

MILNOR, W. R. (1968). Chapter 3 in *Medical physiology*, ed. Mountcastle, V. B. p. 26. St. Louis: C. V. Mosby.

MILNOR, W. R. (1972). Pulmonary hemodynamics. In *Cardiovascular Fluid Dynamics*, Vol. 2, ed. Bergel, D. H. London and New York: Academic Press.

MILNOR, W. R., BERGEL, D. H. and BARGAINER, J. D. (1966). Hydraulic power associated with pulmonary blood flow and its relation to heart rate. *Circulat. Res.*, **19**: 467–80.

MILNOR, W. R., CONTI, C. R., LEWIS, K. B. and O'ROURKE, M. F. (1969). Pulmonary arterial pulse wave velocity and impedance in man. *Circulat. Res.*, **25**: 637–49.

MIRSKY, I. (1967a). Wave propagation in a viscous fluid contained in an orthotropic elastic tube. *Biophys. J.*, **7**: 165–86.

MIRSKY, I. (1967b). Pulse velocities in an orthotropic elastic tube. *Bull. math. Biophys.*, **29**: 311–18.

MIRSKY, I. (1968). Pulse velocities in initially stressed cylindrical rubber tubes. *Bull. math. Biophys.*, **30**: 299–308.

MITCHELL, J. R. A. and SCHWARTZ, C. J. (1965). *Arterial disease*. Philadelphia: Davis.

MOENS, A. I. (1878). *Die Pulskurve*, Leiden.

MORGAN, G. W. and FERRANTE, W. R. (1955). Wave propagation in elastic tubes filled with streaming liquid. *J. acoust. Soc. Amer.*, **27**: 715–25.

MORGAN, G. W. and KIELY, J. P. (1954). Wave propagation in a viscous liquid contained in a flexible tube. *J. acoust. Soc. Amer.*, **26**: 323–28.

MORITZ, W. E. (1969). Transmission characteristics of distension, torsion and axial waves in arteries, Stanford Univ. Rep. No. SUDAAR-373.

MÜLLER, A. (1950). Uber die Fortpflanzungsgeschwindigkeit von Druckwellen in dehnbaren Röhren bei ruhender und strömender Flüssigkeit. *Helv. physiol. Acta*, **8**: 228–41.

MÜLLER, A. (1951). Uber die Abhängigkeit der Fortpflanzungsgeschwindigkeit und der Dämpfung der Druckwellen in dehnbaren Röhren von deren Wellenlange. *Helv. physiol. Acta*, **9**: 162–76.

MÜLLER, A. (1954a). Uber die Verwendung des Pitot-Rohres zur Geschwindigkeitsmessung. *Helv. physiol. Acta*, **12**: 98–111.

MÜLLER, A. (1954b). Uber die Verwendung des Castelli-Prinzips zur Geschwindigkeitsmessung. *Helv. physiol. Acta*, **12**: 300–15.

MÜLLER, O. and SHILLINGFORD, J. P. (1955). A manometer for differential and single pressure measurements. *J. Physiol.*, **127**: 2P.

NAVIER (1827). Cited Prandtl and Tietjens, *Fundamentals of Hydro- and Aeromechanics*. New York: Dover Publications (1934).

NEUMASTER, T. and KROVETZ, L. J. (1964). A method for producing transparent models of blood vessels. *J. appl. Physiol.*, **19**: 1184–86.

NEWMAN, F. H. and SEARLE, V. H. L. (1957). *The General Properties of Matter*. 5th edn. London: Edward Arnold.

NICHOLS, W. W. (1970). *Cardiac output derived from the aortic pressure*. Ph.D. dissertation, University of Alabama in Birmingham.

NICHOLS, W. W. and MCDONALD, D. A. (1972). Wave-velocity in the proximal aorta. *Med. biol. Engng*, **10**: 327–35.

NOBLE, M. I. M. (1968). The contribution of blood momentum to left ventricular ejection in the dog. *Circulat. Res.* **23**: 663–70.

NOBLE, M. I. M., GABE, I. T. and GUZ, A. (1967). Blood pressure and flow in the ascending aorta of conscious dogs. *Cardiovasc. Res.*, **1**: 9–20.

NOBLE, M. I. M., TRENCHARD, D. and GUZ, A. (1966a). Left ventricular ejection in conscious dogs. *Circulat. Res.*, **19**: 139–52.

NOBLE, M. I. M., TRENCHARD, D. and GUZ, A. (1966b). Effect of changing heart rate on cardiovascular function in the conscious dog. *Circulat. Res.*, **19**: 206–13.

NOLAN, S. P., FISHER, R. D., DIXON, S. H. and MORROW, A. G. (1969). Quantification of aortic regurgitation with catheter-tip velocitometer. *Surgery*, **65**: 876–83.

NOORDERGRAAF, A. (1970). Chapter on Hemodynamics in *BioEngineering*, ed. Schwann, H. New York: McGraw-Hill.

NOORDERGRAAF, A., JAGER, G. N. and WESTERHOF, N. (EDS.) (1963). *Circulatory analog computers*, Proc. of Symposium on Development of Analog Computers in the Study of Mammalian Circulatory Systems. Amsterdam: North-Holland Publishing.

NOORDERGRAAF, A., VERDOUW, P. D., VAN BRUMMELEN, A. G. W. and WIEGEL, F. W. (1964). Analog of the arterial bed. In *Pulsatile blood flow*, ed. Attinger, E. O. New York: McGraw-Hill.

NYGAARD, K. K., WILDER, M. and BERKSON, J. (1935). The relation between the viscosity of the blood and the relative volume of erythrocytes (hematocrit value). *Amer. J. Physiol.*, **114**: 128–31.

OHLSSON, N.-M. (1962). Left heart and aortic blood flow in the dog. *Acta radiol.*, Suppl. 213.

OPATOWSKI, I. (1967). Elastic deformations of arteries. *J. appl. Physiol.*, **23**: 772–78.

O'ROURKE, M. F. (1965a). *Pressure and flow in arteries*. M.D. Thesis, University of Sydney, Australia.

O'ROURKE, M. F. (1965b). Dynamic accuracy of the electromagnetic flowmeter. *J. appl. Physiol.*, **20**: 142–47.

O'ROURKE, M. F. (1967a). Steady and pulsatile energy losses in the systemic circulation under normal conditions and in simulated arterial disease. *Cardiovasc. Res.*, **1**: 313–26.

O'ROURKE, M. F. (1967*b*). Pressure and flow waves in systemic arteries and the anatomical design of the arterial system. *J. appl. Physiol.*, **23**: 139–49.

O'ROURKE, M. F. and MILNOR, W. R. (1967). Pulsatile pulmonary arterial flow computed from differential pressures. *Fed. Proc.*, **26**: 269.

O'ROURKE, M. F. and MILNOR, W. R. (1971). Relation between differential pressure and flow in the pulmonary artery of the dog. *Cardiovasc. Res.*, **5**: 558–65.

O'ROURKE, M. F. and TAYLOR, M. G. (1966). Vascular impedance of the femoral bed. *Circulat. Res.*, **18**: 126–39.

O'ROURKE, M. F. and TAYLOR, M. G. (1967). Input impedance of the systemic circulation. *Circulat. Res.*, **20**: 365–80.

O'ROURKE, M. F., BLAZEK, J. V., MORREELS, C. L. JR. and KROVETZ, L. J. (1968). Pressure wave transmission along the human aorta. *Circulat. Res.*, **23**: 567–79.

PAPPENHEIMER, J. R. (1954). Differential conductance manometer. *Rev. scient. Instrum.*, **25**: 912–17.

PARDUE, D. R., HEDRICH, A. L., ROSE, J. C. and KOT, P. A. (1967). Ultrasonic catheter-tip probe for measuring blood flow velocity. *Circulation*, **35-36**: Suppl. 2, 204.

PATEL, D. J. (1969). Mechanical properties of large blood vessels. In *The pulmonary circulation and interstitial space*, ed. Fishman, A. P. and Hecht, H. H. Chicago: University of Chicago Press.

PATEL, D. J. and FRY, D. L. (1964). In situ pressure-radius-length measurements in ascending aorta of anesthetized dogs. *J. appl. Physiol.*, **19**: 413–16.

PATEL, D. J. and FRY, D. L. (1966). Longitudinal tethering of arteries in dogs. *Circulat. Res.*, **19**: 1011–21.

PATEL, D. J. and FRY, D. L. (1969). The elastic symmetry of arterial segments in dogs. *Circulat. Res.*, **24**: 1–8.

PATEL, D. J., DEFREITAS, F. M. and FRY, D. L. (1963). Hydraulic input impedance to aorta and pulmonary artery in dogs. *J. appl. Physiol.*, **18**: 134–40.

PATEL, D. J., GREENFIELD, J. C. JR. and FRY, D. L. (1964). In vivo pressure-length-radius relationship of certain blood vessels in man and dog. In *Pulsatile blood flow*, ed. Attinger, E. O. pp. 293–302. New York: McGraw-Hill.

PATEL, D. J., JANICKI, J. S. and CAREW, T. E. (1969). Static anisotropic elastic properties of the aorta in living dogs. *Circulat. Res.* **25**: 765–79.

PATEL, D. J., MALLOS, A. J. and FRY, D. L. (1961). Aortic mechanics in the living dog. *J. appl. Physiol.*, **16**: 293–99.

PATEL, D. J., DEFREITAS, F., GREENFIELD, J. C. JR. and FRY, D. L. (1963). Relationship of radius to pressure along the aorta in living dogs. *J. appl. Physiol.*, **18**: 1111–17.

PATEL, D. J., GREENFIELD, J. C. JR., AUSTEN, W. G., MORROW, A. G. and FRY, D. L. (1965). Pressure-flow relationships in the ascending aorta and femoral artery of man. *J. appl. Physiol.*, **20**: 459–63.

PERONNEAU, P. A. and LEGER, F. (1969). Doppler ultrasonic pulsed blood flowmeter. *Proc. 18th int. Congr. med. biol. Engng, Chicago*, 10–11.

PERONNEAU, P. A., HINGLAIS, J., PELLET, M. and LEGER, F. (1970*a*). Vélocimètre sanguin par effet Doppler à émission ultra-sonore pulsée. A. Description de l'appareil——Résultats. *L'onde Electrique*, **50**: 3–18.

PERONNEAU, P. A., HINGLAIS, J. R. and PELLET, M. M. (1970*b*). Doppler ultrasonic pulsed flowmeter: velocity profiles studied in blood vessels. *Proc. 23rd ann. Conf. Engng Med. Biol.*, **12**: 273.

PETERSON, L. H. (1954). The dynamics of pulsatile blood flow. *Circulat. Res.*, **2**: 127–39.

PETERSON, L. H. and SHEPARD, R. B. (1955). Symposium on applied physiology in modern surgery; some relationships of blood pressure to cardiovascular system. *S. Clin. N. Amer.*, **35**: 1613–28.

PETERSON, L. H., JENSEN, R. E. and PARNELL, J. (1960). Mechanical properties of arteries in vivo. *Circulat. Res.*, **8**: 622–39.

PHILLIPS, F. A., BRIND, S. H. and LEVY, M. N. (1955). The immediate influence of increased venous pressure upon resistance to flow in the dog's hind leg. *Circulat. Res.*, **3**: 357–62.

PIEMME, T. (1963). Pressure measurement: electrical transducers. *Progr. cardiovasc. Dis.*, **5**: 574–94.

PIEPER, H. P. (1958). Registration of phasic changes of blood flow by means of a catheter-type flowmeter. *Rev. scient. Instrum.*, **29**: 965–67.

PIEPER, H. P. (1963). Catheter-tip flowmeter for measurement of pulmonary arterial blood flow in closed-chest dogs. *Rev. scient. Instrum.*, **34**: 908–10.

PIEPER, H. P. (1964). Catheter-tip flowmeter for coronary arterial flow in closed. chest dogs. *J. appl. Physiol.*, **19**: 1199–1201.

PIEPER, H. P. (1966). Catheter-tip instrument for measuring left ventricular diameter in closed-chest dogs. *J. appl. Physiol.*, **21**: 1412–16.

PIEPER, H. P. and PAUL, L. T. (1968). Catheter-tip gauge for measuring blood flow velocity and vessel diameter in dogs. *J. appl. Physiol.*, **24**: 259–61.

PIEPER, H. P. and PAUL, L. T. (1969). Response of aortic smooth muscle in intact dogs. *Amer. J. Physiol.*, **217**: 154–60.

PIEPER, H. P. and WETTERER, E. (1953a). Elektrische Registrierung der Blutströmungsgeschwindigkeit mit neuartigen Strompendeln. *Verh. dtsch. Ges. Kreisl.-Forsch.*, 19 Tagung: 264–69.

PIEPER, H. P. and WETTERER, E. (1953b). Strompendel für elektrische Registrierung der Blutströmungsgeschwindigkeit. *Z. Biol.*, **105**: 214–23.

PIPES, L. A. (1958). *Applied mathematics for engineers and physicists*, 2nd edn. New York: McGraw-Hill.

PLASS, K. G. (1964). A new ultrasonic flowmeter for intravascular application. *IEEE Trans. biomed. Engng*, BME–11: 154–56.

PLATT, J. R. (1964). Strong inference. *Science*, **146**: 347–53.

POISSON (1831). Cited Prandtl and Tietjens. *Fundamentals of hydro- and aeromechanics*. New York: Dover Publications, 1934.

POOLE, J. C. F. (1964). Regeneration of aortic tissues in fabric grafts of the aorta. *Sym. Zool. Soc. Lond.*, **11**: 131–40.

POOLE, J. C. F., SANDERS, A. G. and FLOREY, H. W. (1958). The regeneration of aortic endothelium. *J. path. Bact.*, **75**: 133–43.

POOLE, J. C. F., SANDERS, A. G. and FLOREY, H. W. (1959). Further observations on the regeneration of aortic endothelium in the rabbit. *J. Path. Bact.*, **77**: 637.

PORJÉ, I. G. (1946). Studies of the arterial pulse wave, particularly in the aorta. *Acta physiol. scand.*, **13**: Suppl. 42: 1–68.

PORJÉ, I. G. and RUDEWALD, B. (1957). Studies on a new theory of determination of some fundamental haemodynamic data in a circulation model, in normal persons and in aortic valvular disease. *Opusc. med.* (*Stockholm*), **2**: 180–293.

PORJÉ, I. G. and RUDEWALD, B. (1960). Further haemodynamic studies with differential pressure technique. *Opusc. med.* (*Stockholm*), **6**: 1–11.

PORJÉ, I. G. and RUDEWALD, B. (1961). Haemodynamic studies with differential pressure techniques. *Acta physiol. scand.*, **51**: 116–35.

PRANDTL, L. (1952). *Essentials of fluid dynamics*. London: Blackie.

PRANDTL, L. and TIETJENS, O. G. (1934). *Fundamentals of hydro- and aeromechanics*. New York: Dover Publications.

PREC, O., KATZ, L. N., SENNETT, L., ROSEMAN, R. H., FISHMAN, A. P. and HWANG, W.

(1949). Determination of kinetic energy of the heart in man. *Amer. J. Physiol.*, **159**: 483–91.

PRITCHARD, W. H., GREGG, D. E., SHIPLEY, R. F. and WEISBERGER, A. S. (1943). A study of flow and pattern responses in peripheral arteries to the injection of vasomotor drugs. *Amer. J. Physiol.*, **138**: 731–40.

PROTHERO, L. and BURTON, A. C. (1961). The physics of capillary flow. I. The nature of the motion. *Biophys. J.*, **1**: 566–79.

RALSTON, H. J. and TAYLOR, A. N. (1945). Streamline flow in the arteries of the dog and cat. *Amer. J. Physiol.*, **144**: 706–10.

RALSTON, H. J., TAYLOR, A. N. and ELLIOT, H. W. (1947). Further studies on streamline blood flow in the arteries of the cat. *Amer. J. Physiol.*, **150**: 52–57.

RANDALL, J. E. (1958). Statistical properties of pulsatile pressure and flow in the femoral artery of the dog. *Circulat. Res.*, **6**: 689–98.

RANDALL, J. E. and STACY, R. W. (1956). Mechanical impedance of the dog's hind leg to pulsatile blood flow. *Amer. J. Physiol.*, **187**: 94–98.

RAPPAPORT, M. B., BLOCK, E. H. and IRWIN, J. W. (1959). A manometer for measuring dynamic pressures in the microvascular system. *J. appl. Physiol.*, **14**: 651–55.

READ, R. C., KUIDA, H. and JOHNSON, J. A. (1958). Venous pressure and total peripheral resistance in the dog. *Amer. J. Physiol.*, **192**: 609–12.

REIN, H. (1928). Die Thermo-Stromuhr. *Z. Biol.*, **87**: 394.

REMINGTON, J. W. (1952). Volume quantitation of the aortic pressure pulse. *Fed. Proc.*, **11**: 750–61.

REMINGTON, J. W. (1954). The relation between stroke volume and the pulse pressure. *Minn. Med.*, **37**: 75–80.

REMINGTON, J. W. (1955). Hysteresis loop behavior of the aorta and other extensible tissues. *Amer. J. Physiol.*, **180**: 83–95.

REMINGTON, J. W. (1957). *Tissue elasticity*. Washington: American Physiological Society.

REMINGTON, J. W. (1962). Pressure-diameter relations of the in vivo aorta. *Amer. J. Physiol.*, **203**: 440–48.

REMINGTON, J. W. (1965). Quantitative synthesis of head and foreleg arterial pulses in the dog. *Amer. J. Physiol.*, **208**: 968–83.

REMINGTON, J. W. (1967). Propagation of transient aortic pulses. *Amer. J. Physiol.*, **212**: 612–18.

REMINGTON, J. W. and HAMILTON, W. F. (1945). The construction of a theoretical cardiac ejection curve from the contour of the aortic pressure pulse. *Amer. J. Physiol.*, **144**: 546–56.

REMINGTON, J. W. and HAMILTON, W. F. (1947). Quantitative calculation of the time course of cardiac ejection from the pressure pulse. *Amer. J. Physiol.*, **148**: 25–34.

REMINGTON, J. W., HAMILTON, W. F. and DOW, P. (1945). Some difficulties involved in the prediction of the stroke volume from the pulse-wave velocity. *Amer. J. Physiol.*, **144**: 536–45.

REMINGTON, J. W., NOBACK, C. R., HAMILTON, W. F. and GOLD, J. J. (1948). Volume elasticity characteristics of the human aorta and prediction of the stroke volume from the pressure pulse. *Amer. J. Physiol.*, **153**: 25.

RÉSAL, H. (1876). Cited Lambossy, P. (1950).

REYNOLDS, S. R. M., LIGHT, F. W., ARDRAN, G. M. and PRICHARD, M. M. L. (1952). The qualitative nature of pulsatile flow in the umbilical vessels, with observations on flow in the aorta. *Johns Hopk. Hosp. Bull.*, **91**: 83–104.

RICHARDS, T. G. and WILLIAMS, T. D. (1953). Velocity changes in the carotid and femoral arteries of dogs during the cardiac cycle. *J. Physiol.*, **120**: 257–66.

RICHARDSON, A. W., DENISON, A. B. JR. and GREEN, H. D. (1952). A newly modified electromagnetic blood flowmeter capable of high fidelity flow registration. *Circulation*, **5**: 430–36.

RICHARDSON, E. G. and TYLER, W. (1929). Cited by Womersley, J. R. (1957*a*).

ROACH, M. R. and BURTON, A. C. (1957). The reason for the shape of the distensibility curves of arteries. *Can. J. Biochem. Physiol.*, **35**: 181–90.

ROBINSON, D. A. (1965). Quantitative analysis of the control of cardiac output in the isolated left ventricle. *Circulat. Res.*, **17**: 207–21.

RONNINGER, R. (1954). Uber eine Methode zur übersichtlichen Darstellung haemo-dynamischer Zusammenhänge. *Arch. Kreisl.-Forsch.*, **21**: 127.

ROSSI, H. H., POWERS, S. H. and DWORK, B. (1953). Measurement of flow in straight tubes by means of the dilution technique. *Amer. J. Physiol.*, **173**: 103–8.

ROWLANDS, S., GROOM, A. C. and THOMAS, H. W. (1965). The difference in circulation times between erythrocytes and plasma in vivo. In *Proceedings Fourth International Congress on Rheology*, Part 4, ed. Copley, A. L. pp. 371–79. New York: Interscience.

RUDEWALD, B. (1962). Haemodynamics of the human ascending aorta as studied by means of a differential pressure technique. *Acta physiol. scand.*, **54**: Suppl. 187.

RUSHMER, R. F. (1955). Pressure-circumference relations in the aorta. *Amer. J. Physiol.*, **183**: 545–49.

RUSHMER, R. F. (1970). *Cardiovascular dynamics*, 3rd edn. Philadelphia: Saunders.

RUSHMER, R. F., BAKER, D. W., JOHNSON, W. L. and STRANDNESS, D. E. (1967). Clinical applications of a transcutaneous ultrasonic flow detector. *JAMA*, **199**: 326–28.

RYMER, T. B. and BUTLER, C. C. (1944). An electrical circuit for harmonic analysis and other calculations. *Phil. Mag.*, **35**: 606–16.

SAFFMAN, P. G. (1956). On the motion of small spheroidal particles in a viscous liquid. *J. Fluid Mech.*, **1**: 540–53.

SCHER, A. M., WEIGERT, T. H. and YOUNG, A. C. (1953). Compact flowmeters for use in the unanesthetized animal, an electronic version of Chauveau's hemo-drometer. *Science*, **118**: 82–84.

SCHLEIER, J. (1918). Der Energieverbrauch in der Blutbahn. *Pflügers Arch. ges. Physiol.*, **173**: 172–204.

SCHULTZ, D. L., TUNSTALL-PEDOE, D. S., LEE, G. DE J., GUNNING, A. J. and BELLHOUSE, B. J. (1969). Velocity distribution and transition in the arterial system. In *Ciba Foundation Symposium on Circulatory and Respiratory Mass Transport*, pp. 172–99. London: Churchill.

SEED, W. A. and WOOD, N. B. (1971). Velocity patterns in the aorta. *Cardiovasc. Res.*, **5**: 319–30.

SEGRÉ, G. (1965). Necklace-like formations in the Poiseuille flow of a suspension of spheres. In *Proceedings Fourth International Congress on Rheology*, Part 4, ed. Copley, A. L. pp. 103–18. New York: Interscience.

SEGRÉ, G. and SILBERBERG, A. (1961). Radial particle displacements in Poiseuille flow of suspensions. *Nature (Lond.)*, **189**: 209–10.

SEGRÉ, G. and SILBERBERG, A. (1962). Behavior of macroscopic rigid spheres in Poiseuille flow. *J. Fluid Mech,*, **14**: 115–35, 136–57.

SEXL, H. (1930). Cited by Womersley, J. R. (1957*a*).

SHEPPARD, L. C., KOUCHOUKOS, N. T., KURTTS, M. A. and KIRKLIN, J. W. (1968). Automated treatment of critically ill patients following operation. *Ann. Surg.*, **168**: 596–604.

SHERCLIFF, J. A. (1962). *The theory of electromagnetic measurement*. Cambridge: University Press.

SHIPLEY, R. E., GREGG, D. E. and SCHROEDER, E. F. (1943). An experimental study of flow patterns in various peripheral arteries. *Amer. J. Physiol.*, **138**: 718–30.

SILBERBERG, A. (1965). Hydrodynamic interaction between particles in suspension. In *Proceedings Fourth International Congress on Rheology*, Part 4, ed. Copley, A. L. pp. 119–24. New York: Interscience.

SIMONS, J. R. and MICHAELIS, A. R. (1953). A cinematographic technique, using ultra-violet illumination for amphibian blood circulation. *Nature (Lond.)*, **71**: 801.

SKALAK, R. (1966). Wave transmission in the arterial tree. In *Biomech.*, ed. Fung, Y. C. New York: ASME.

SKALAK, R., WIENER, F., MORKIN, E. and FISHMAN, A. P. (1966a). The energy distribution in the pulmonary circulation. I. Theory. *Phys. in Med. Biol.*, **11**: 287–94.

SKALAK, R., WIENER, F., MORKIN, E. and FISHMAN, A. P. (1966b). The energy distribution in the pulmonary circulation, II. Experiments. *Phys. in Med. Biol.*, **11**: 437–49.

SOMLYO, A. P. and SOMLYO, A. V. (1968). Vascular smooth muscle Part I. *Pharmacol. Rev.*, **20**: 197–292.

SOMLYO, A. V. and SOMLYO, A. P. (1964). Vasomotor function of smooth muscle in the main pulmonary artery. *Amer. J. Physiol.*, **206**: 1196–1200.

SOUTHWELL, R. V. (1941). *An introduction to the theory of elasticity*. 2nd edn. Oxford: University Press.

SPENCER, M. P. and DENISON, A. B. (1956). The aortic flow pulse as related to differential pressure. *Circulat. Res.*, **4**: 476–84.

SPENCER, M. P. and GREISS, F. C. (1962). Dynamics of ventricular ejection. *Circulat. Res.*, **10**: 274.

SPENCER, M. P., INTAGLIETTA, M. and JOHNSON, D. L. (1964). Transmural gauge for determining the pressure in blood vessels. *Physiologist*, **7**: 261 (abstract).

STACY, R. W. (ED.). (1966). Force, tension, pressure, Section III. *Meth. med. Res.*, **11**: 119–79. Chicago: Year Book Medical Publishers.

STACY, R. W., WILLIAMS, D. T., WORDEN, R. E. and MCMORRIS, R. O. (1955). *Essentials of biological and medical physics*. New York: McGraw-Hill.

STARR, I. (1957). Studies made by simulating systole at necropsy. X. State of peripheral circulation in cadavers. *J. appl. Physiol.*, **11**: 174–80.

STARR, I. and SCHILD, A. (1957). Studies made by simulating systole at necropsy. IX. A test of the aortic compression chamber hypothesis and of two stroke volume methods based upon it. *J. appl. Physiol.*, **11**: 169–73.

STARR, I., SCHNABEL, T. G. and MAYCOCK, R. L. (1953). Studies made by simulating systole at necropsy. II. Experiments on the relation of cardiac and peripheral factors to the genesis of the pulse wave and the ballistocardiogram. *Circulation*, **8**: 44–61.

STAUFFER, H. M., OPPENHEIMER, M. J., STEWART, G. H. and LYNCH, P. R. (1955). Cine-fluorography by image amplifier techniques. *J. appl. Physiol.*, **8**: 343–46.

STEGALL, H. F., RUSHMER, R. F. and BAKER, D. W. (1966). A transcutaneous ultrasonic blood-velocity meter. *J. appl. Physiol.*, **21**: 707–11.

STEGALL, H. F., STONE, H. L., BISHOP, V. S. and LAENGER, C. (1967). A catheter-tip pressure and velocity sensor. *Proc. ann. Conf. Engng Med. Biol.*, **9**: 27.4.

STEHBENS, W. E. (1959). Turbulence of blood flow. *Quart. J. exp. Physiol.*, **44**: 110–17.

STEIN, P. D. and SCHUETTE, W. H. (1969). New catheter-tip flowmeter with velocity flow and volume flow capabilities. *J. appl. Physiol.*, **26**: 851–56.

STOKES (1845). Cited by Prandtl and Tietjens (1934).

SUWA, N., NIWA, T. and FUKASUWA, H. (1963). *Tohoku J. exp. Med.*, **79**: 168–98 (cited by Iberall, 1967).

SAWN, H. J. C. and BECK, W. (1960). Ventricular non-mixing as a source of error in the estimation of ventricular volume by the indicator-dilution technique. *Circulat. Res.*, **8**: 989.

TAYLOR, M. G. (1955). The flow of blood in narrow tubes. II. The axial stream and its formation, as determined by changes in optical density. *Aust. J. exp. Biol. med. Sci.*, **33**: 1–16.

TAYLOR, M. G. (1957a). An approach to the analysis of the arterial pulse wave. I. Oscillations in an attenuating line. *Phys. in Med. Biol.*, **1**: 258–69.

TAYLOR, M. G. (1957b). An approach to the analysis of the arterial pulse wave. II. Fluid oscillations in an elastic tube. *Phys. in Med. Biol.*, **1**: 321–9.

TAYLOR, M. G. (1958a). A simple electrical computer for Fourier analysis and synthesis. *J. Physiol.*, **141**: 23–25P.

TAYLOR, M. G. (1958b). The discrepancy between steady- and oscillatory-flow calibration of flowmeters of the 'Bristle' and 'Pendulum' types: a theoretical study. *Phys. in Med. Biol.*, **2**: 324–37.

TAYLOR, M. G. (1959a). The influence of the anomalous viscosity of blood upon its oscillatory flow. *Phys. in Med. Biol.*, **3**: 273–90.

TAYLOR, M. G. (1959b). An experimental determination of the propagation of fluid oscillations in a tube with a visco-elastic wall; together with an analysis of the characteristics required in an electrical analogue., *Phys. in Med. Biol.*, **4**: 63–82.

TAYLOR, M. G. (1959c). *Wave travel in arteries*. Ph.D. Thesis, University of London.

TAYLOR, M. G. (1964). Wave travel in arteries and the design of the cardiovascular system. In *Pulsatile blood flow*, ed. Attinger, E. O. pp. 343–67. New York: McGraw-Hill.

TAYLOR, M. G. (1965). Wave travel in a non-uniform transmission line, in relation to pulses in arteries. *Phys. in Med. Biol.*, **10**: 539–50.

TAYLOR, M. G. (1966a). The input impedance of an assembly of randomly branching elastic tubes. *Biophys. J.*, **6**: 29–51.

TAYLOR, M. G. (1966b). Wave transmission through an assembly of randomly branching elastic tubes. *Biophys. J.*, **6**: 697–716.

TAYLOR, M. G. (1966c). Use of random excitation and spectral analysis in the study of frequency-dependent parameters of the cardiovascular system. *Circulat. Res.*, **18**: 585–95.

TAYLOR, M. G. (1973). Hemodynamics. *Ann. Rev. Physiol.*, **35**: 87–116.

THOMAS, H. W. (1961). Determination of the concentration changes of fine particulate suspensions flowing through narrow capillary tubes. *Lab. Pract.*, **10**: 771–73.

THOMAS, H. W. (1962). The wall effect in capillary instruments: an improved analysis suitable for application to blood and other particulate suspensions. *Biorheology*, **1**: 41–56.

THOMAS, H. W., FRENCH, R. J., GROOM, A. C. and ROWLANDS, S. (1965). The flow of red cell suspensions through narrow tubes: The (Extracorporeal) determination of the difference in mean velocities of red cells and their suspending phase. In *Proceedings Fourth International Congress on Rheology*, Part 4, ed. Copley, A. L. pp. 381–91. New York: Interscience.

TICKNER, E. G. and SACKS, A. H. (1967). A theory for the static elastic behavior of blood vessels. *Biorheology*, **4**: 151–68.

TIMM, C. (1942). Der Strömungsverlauf in einem Modell der menschlichen Aorta. *Z. Biol.*, **101**: 79–99.

TRELOAR, L. R. G. (1958). *The physics of rubber elasticity*, 2nd edn. Oxford: University Press.

TUNSTALL-PEDOE, D. (1972). Blood velocity measurements in the diagnosis of aortic incompetence. In *Blood Flow Measurement*, ed. Roberts, C. London: Spectre Press.

VON DESCHWANDEN, P., MÜLLER, A. and LASZT, L. (1956). Beitraege zur haemodynamik. *Abstr. Comm. XX Int'l Physiol. Congr., Bruxelles*, 930–31.

VIERHOUT, R. R. and VENDRICK, A. J. H. (1961). Hydraulic pressure generator for testing the dynamic characteristics of catheters and manometers. *J. Lab. clin. Med.*, **58**: 330–33.

WALLACE, J. D., BROWN, J. R. JR., DIETZ, G. W. and ERTUGRUL, A. (1959). Intracardiac acoustics. *J. acoust. Soc. Amer.*, **31**: 712–23.

WALLACE, J. D., BROWN, J. R. JR., LEWIS, D. H. and DIETZ, G. W. (1957). Phonocatheters: their design and application, Part I, *IRE Trans. med. Electron.*, PGME-9: 25–30.

WARBASSE, J. R., HELLMAN, B. H., GILLILAN, R. E., HAWLEY, R. R. and BABITT, H. I. (1969). Physiologic evaluation of a catheter-tip electromagnetic velocity probe. *Amer. J. Cardiol.*, **23**: 424–33.

WARNER, H. R., GARDNER, R. M. and TORONTO, A. F. (1968). Computer-based monitoring of cardiovascular functions in post-operative patients. *Circulation*, **37–38**: Suppl. 2, 68–74.

WARNER, H. R., SWAN, H. J. C., CONNOLLY, D. C., TOMPKINS, R. G. and WOOD, E. H. (1953). Quantitation of beat-to-beat changes in stroke volume from the aortic pulse contour in man. *J. appl. Physiol.*, **5**: 495.

WARNICK, A. and DRAKE, E. H. (1958). IRE National Convention Record, Part 9.

WARREN, J. V. (1948). Determination of cardiac output in man by right heart catheterization. *Meth. med. Res.*, **1**: 224–32. Chicago: Year Book Medical Publishers.

WAYLAND, H. (1967). Rheology and the microcirculation. *Gastroenterology*, **52**: 342–55.

WEALE, F. E. (1967). *An introduction to surgical haemodynamics*, Illinois: Year Book Medical Publishers.

WEBER, E. H. (1850). *Ber. der Sächs. ges. der Wiss.*, 166 (cited Lambossy, P., 1950).

WEBER, E. H. (1851). Uber die Anwendung der Wellenlehre vom Kreislaufe des Blutes und inbesondere auf die Pulslehre. *Müller's Arch. für Anat., Physiol. und Wiss. Med.*, 497–546.

WEBER, E. H. and WEBER, W. E. (1825). *Wellenlehre*. Leipzig: Fleischer.

WEHN, P. S. (1957). Pulsatory activity of peripheral arteries. *Suppl. Scand. J. clin. Lab. Invest.*, **9**: 106 pp. Thesis: Oslo.

WELLS, M. K. (1969). On the determination of the elastic properties of blood vessels from their wave transmission characteristics, Stanford Univ. Rep. No. SUDAAR-368.

WESTERHOF, N. and NOORDERGRAAF, A. (1970). Arterial viscoelasticity: A generalized model. Effect on input impedance and wave travel in the systematic tree. *J. Biomechanics*, **3**: 357–79.

WESTERHOF, N., SIPKEMA, P., VAN DEN BOS, G. C. and ELZINGA, G. (1972). Forward and backward waves in the arterial system. *Cardiovascular Research*, **6**: 648–56.

WETTERER, E. (1937). Eine neue Methode zur Registrierung der Blutströmungsgeschwindigkeit am uneröffneten Gefäss. *Z. Biol.*, **98**: 26.

WETTERER, E. (1944). Eine neue manometrische Sonde mit elektrischer Transmission. *Z. Biol.*, **101**: 332–50.

WETTERER, E. (1956). Die Wirkung der Herztätigkeit auf die Dynamik der Arteriensystems. *Verh. dtsch. ges. Kreisl.-Forsch.*, 22 Tagung: 26–60.

WETTERER, E. (1963). Flowmeters: their theory, construction and operation. In

Handbook of physiology, Circulation II, 1294–1324. Washington: American Physiological Society.

WETTERER, E. and DEPPE, B. (1940). *Z. Biol.*, **100**: 205; also *ibid.*, **99**: 320 (cited by Wetterer, 1954).

WETTERER, E. and KENNER, T. (1968). *Die Dynamik des Arterien-pulses*. New York and Berlin: Springer-Verlag.

WETTERER, E. and PIEPER, H. (1952). Eine neue manometrische Sonde mit elektrischer Transmission. *Z. Biol.*, **105**: 49–65.

WEVER, R. and ASCHOFF, J. (1956). Durchflussmessung mit der Diathermie-Thermostromuhr bei pulsierenden Stromung. *Pflügers Arch. ges. Physiol.*, **262**: 152–68.

WEXLER, L., BERGEL, D. H., GABE, I. T., MAKIN, G. S. and MILLS, C. J. (1968). Velocity of blood flow in normal human venae cavae. *Circulat. Res.*, **23**: 349–59.

WEZLER, K. and BÖGER, A. (1939). Die Dynamik des arteriellen Systems. Der arterielle Blutdruck und seine Komponenten. *Ergebn. Physiol.*, **41**: 292–606.

WEZLER, K. and SINN, W. (1953). *Das Strömungsgesetz des Kreislaufes*. Aulendorf i. Wurtt.: Editio Cantor.

WHITBY, L. E. H. and BRITTON, C. J. C. (1950). *Disorders of the blood*. London: Churchill.

WHITMORE, R. L. (1967). Slip of blood at a wall. *Biorheology*, **4**: 121–22.

WHITMORE, R. L. (1968). *Rheology of the circulation*. Oxford: Pergamon Press.

WHITTAKER, S. R. F. and WINTON, F. R. (1933). The apparent viscosity of blood flowing in the isolated hindlimb of the dog and its variation with corpuscular concentration. *J. Physiol.*, **78**: 339–69.

WIEDERHIELM, C. A. (1966). Transcapillary and interstitial transport phenomena in the mesentery. *Fed. Proc.*, **25**: 1789–98.

WIEDERHIELM, C. A. and BILLIG, L. (1968). Effects of erythrocyte orientation and concentration on light transmission through blood flowing through microscopic blood vessels. In *Hemorheology*, ed. Copley, A. L., pp. 681–94. Oxford: Pergamon Press.

WIEDERHIELM, C. A., BRUCE, R. A. and JOHN, G. G. (1957). Continuous recording of oxygen saturation during cardiac catheterization. *Amer. J. med. sci.*, **233**: 542–45.

WIEDERHIELM, C. A., WOODBURY, J. W., KIRK, S. and RUSHMER, R. F. (1964). Pulsatile pressures in the microcirculation of frog's mesentery. *Amer. J. Physiol.*, **207**: 173–76.

WIGGERS, C. J. (1928). *The pressure pulses in the cardiovascular system*. London: Longmans.

WIGGERS, C. J. and WÉGRIA, R. (1938). Active changes in size and distensibility of the aorta during acute hypertension. *Amer. J. Physiol.*, **124**: 603.

WILLIAMS, T. I. (ED.) (1969). *A biographical dictionary of scientists*. New York: Wiley-Interscience.

WILSON, E. M., RANIERI, A. J. JR., UPDIKE, O. L. and DAMMANN, J. F. JR. (1972). An evaluation of thermal dilution for obtaining serial measurements of cardiac output. *Med. & Biol. Engng.*, **10**: 179–91.

WINTROBE, M. M. (1967). *Clinical haematology*. 6th edn. Philadelphia: Lea & Febiger.

WINTON, F. R. (1926). The influence of length on the responses of unstriated muscle to electrical and chemical stimulation, and stretching. *J. Physiol.*, **61**: 368-82.

WITZIG, K. (1914). Uber erzwungene Wellenbewegungen zäher, inkompressibler Flüssigkeiten in elastischen Röhren. *Inaug. Diss. Bern.* Bern: Wyss.

WOLINSKY, H. and GLAGOV, S. (1964). Structural basis for the static mechanical properties of the aortic media. *Circulat. Res.*, **14**: 400–13.

WOLSTENHOLME, G. E. W. and KNIGHT, J. (EDS.). (1969). *Circulatory and respiratory mass transport*. Boston: Little, Brown.

WOMERSLEY, J. R. (1955*a*). Oscillatory flow in arteries: effect of radial variation in viscosity on rate of flow. *J. Physiol.*, **127**: 38–39P.

WOMERSLEY, J. R. (1955*b*). Method for the calculation of velocity, rate of flow and viscous drag in arteries when the pressure gradient is known. *J. Physiol.*, **127**: 553–63.

WOMERSLEY, J. R. (1955*c*). Oscillatory motion of a viscous liquid in a thin-walled elastic tube. I. The linear approximation for long waves. *Phil. Mag.*, **46**: 199–221.

WOMERSLEY, J. R. (1957*a*). The mathematical analysis of the arterial circulation in a state of oscillatory motion. Wright Air Development Center, Technical Report WADC-TR56-614.

WOMERSLEY, J. R. (1957*b*). Oscillatory flow in arteries: the constrained elastic tube as a model of arterial flow and pulse transmission. *Phys. in Med. Biol.*, **2**: 178–87.

WOMERSLEY, J. R. (1958). Oscillatory flow in arteries: the reflection of the pulse wave at junctions and rigid inserts in the arterial system. *Phys. in Med. Biol.*, **2**: 313–23.

WOOD, G. C. (1954). Some tensile properties of elastic tissue. *Biochim. biophys. Acta*, **15**: 311–31.

WYATT, D. J. (1961). Problems in the measurement of blood flow by magnetic induction. *Phys. in Med. Biol.*, **5**: 289–320, 369–99.

YANOF, H. M. (1961). A trapezoidal-wave electromagnetic blood flowmeter. *J. appl. Physiol.*, **16**: 566–70.

YANOF, H. M. (1965). *Biomedical electronics*. Philadelphia. Davis.

YANOF, H. M., ROSEN, A. L., MCDONALD, N. M. and MCDONALD, D. A. (1963). A critical study of the response of manometers to forced oscillations. *Phys. in Med. Biol.*, **8**: 407–22.

YELLIN, E. L. (1966). Laminar-turbulent transition process in pulsatile flow. *Circulat. Res.*, **19**: 791–804.

YOUNG, T. (1808). Hydraulic investigations, subservient to an intended Croonian lecture on the motion of the blood. *Phil. Trans. roy. Soc.*, **98**: 164–86.

YOUNG, T. (1809). On the functions of the heart and arteries. The Croonian lecture. *Phil. Trans. roy. Soc.*, **99**: 1–31.

ZIERLER, K. L. (1962*a*). Circulation times and the theory of indicator-dilution methods for determining blood flow and volume. *Handbook of physiology*, Section 2: Circulation, Vol. I, pp. 585–615. Washington: American Physiological Society.

ZIERLER, K. L. (1962*b*). Theoretical basis of indicator-dilution methods for measuring flow and volume. *Circulat. Res.*, **10**: 393–407.

Index